CURRENT
Diagnosis & Treatment in Pulmonary Medicine

Edited by

Michael E. Hanley, MD
Associate Professor
Department of Pulmonary Sciences and Critical Care
  Medicine
University of Colorado School of Medicine
  and Denver Health Medical Center

Carolyn H. Welsh, MD
Denver Veterans Affairs Medical Center
Professor
Department of Pulmonary Sciences and Critical Care
  Medicine
University of Colorado Health Sciences Center

Lange Medical Books/McGraw-Hill
Medical Publishing Division

New York   Chicago   San Francisco   Lisbon   London   Madrid   Mexico City
Milan   New Delhi   San Juan   Seoul   Singapore   Sydney   Toronto

Current Diagnosis & Treatment in Pulmonary Medicine

ISBN: 0-07-140259-4 (Domestic)

1 2 3 4 5 6 7 8 9 0 DOC/DOC 0 9 8 7 6 5 4 3

Notice

Medicine is an ever-changing science. As new research and clinical experience broaden our knowledge, changes in treatment and drug therapy are required. The authors and the publisher of this work have checked with sources believed to be reliable in their efforts to provide information that is complete and generally in accord with the standards accepted at the time of publication. However, in view of the possibility of human error or changes in medical sciences, neither the authors nor the publisher nor any other party who has been involved in the preparation or publication of this work warrants that the information contained herein is in every respect accurate or complete, and they disclaim all responsibility for any errors or omissions or for the results obtained from use of the information contained in this work. Readers are encouraged to confirm the information contained herein with other sources. For example and in particular, readers are advised to check the product information sheet included in the package of each drug they plan to administer to be certain that the information contained in this work is accurate and that changes have not been made in the recommended dose or in the contraindications for administration. This recommendation is of particular importance in connection with new or infrequently used drugs.

This book was set in Adobe Garamond by Pine Tree Composition, Inc.
The editors were Isabel Nogueira, Janene Matragrano Oransky, and Regina Y. Brown.
The production supervisor was Sherri Souffrance.
The index was prepared by Barbara Littlewood.
R. R. Donnelley was printer and binder.

ISSN: 1544-631X

This book is printed on acid-free paper.

INTERNATIONAL EDITION ISBN: 0-07-121971-4

To our children, our next generation of students:
Peter Ferguson and Michael and Stephen Hanley.

Contents

SECTION I. EVALUATION OF THE PATIENT WITH PULMONARY DISEASE

SECTION II. DISEASES OF THE AIRWAYS

Authors

Ron Balkissoon, MD, FRCP(C)
Associate Professor, Department of Pulmonary Sciences
and Critical Care Medicine, National Jewish Med-
ical and Research Center, University of Colorado
School of Medicine, Denver
Obstruction of Large Airways

Delos D. Carrier, MD, MSPH
Occupational and Environmental Medicine Resident,
University of Colorado Health Sciences Center,
Denver
pilotmd1@juno.com
Pneumoconiosis

Edward D. Chan, MD
Associate Professor of Medicine, National Jewish Medical
and Research Center; Staff Member, University of
Colorado Health Sciences Center and Denver Veterans Affairs Medical Center, Denver
chane@njc.org
Laboratory Evaluation; Viral & Atypical Pneumonia

Harold R. Collard, MD
Fellow, Department of Pulmonary Sciences and Critical
Care Medicine, University of Colorado Health Sci-
ences Center, Denver
hal.collard@uchsc.edu
Idiopathic Interstitial Pneumonia

Gregory P. Cosgrove, MD
Instructor, Interstitial Lung Disease Program, Pul-
monary Division, Department of Medicine,
NJMRC; Instructor, Division of Pulmonary Sci-
ences and Critical Care Medicine, University of
Colorado Health Sciences Center, National Jewish
Medical and Research Center, Denver
cosgroveg@njc.org
Pulmonary Manifestations of Collagen Vascular Diseases;
Vasculitis & the Diffuse Alveolar Hemorrhage Syndromes

Robert S. Crausman, MD, MMS
Associate Professor of Medicine, Brown Medical
School; Chief, Division of Geriatrics; Director, In-
ternal Medicine Residency Program, Memorial
Hospital of Rhode Island, Pawtucket
robert_crausman@brown.edu
Diseases of the Mediastinum

Joseph T. Crossno, Jr., MD, PhD
Instructor in Pulmonary Medicine, Department of Pulmonary Sciences and Critical Care Medicine, University of Colorado Health Sciences Center, Denver
joseph.crossno@uchsc.edu
Procedures in Pulmonary Medicine

Vera A. DePalo, MD, FCCP
Associate Professor of Medicine, Brown University;
Director, Intensive Care, Memorial Hospital of
Rhode Island, Pawtucket
vera_depalo@brown.edu
Pulmonary Anatomy & Physiology; Diseases of the Medi-
astinum

James H. Ellis, Jr., MD
Clinical Professor of Medicine and Pulmonary Sciences, National Jewish Medical and Research Center, Denver
ellisj@njc.org
Pulmonary Alveolar Proteinosis

Karen A. Fagan, MD
Assistant Professor of Medicine, Department of Pulmonary Sciences and Critical Care Medicine, University of Colorado Health Sciences Center, Denver
karen.fagan@uchsc.edu
Pulmonary Arterial Hypertension

Enrique Fernandez, MD
Professor of Medicine, University of Colorado School
of Medicine; Senior Clinician, Department of Pulmonary Sciences and Critical Care Medicine, National Jewish Medical and Research Center, Denver
fernandeze@njc.org
Chronic Ventilatory Failure

Michael B. Fessler, MD
Instructor, Division of Pulmonary Sciences and Criti-
cal Care Medicine, National Jewish Medical and
Research Center and University of Colorado Health
Sciences Center, Denver
michael.fessler@uchsc.edu
Mechanical Ventilation: Invasive and Noninvasive

Linda M. Fielding, MD
Visiting Associate Professor of Radiology, Department of General Radiology, Denver Health Medical Center
linda.fielding@dhha.org
Diagnostic Imaging

Andrew P. Fontenot, MD
Assistant Professor of Medicine, Division of Pulmonary Sciences and Critical Care Medicine, University of Colorado Health Sciences Center, Denver
andrew.fontenot@uchsc.edu
Sarcoidosis

Stephen K. Frankel, MD
Assistant Professor, Interstitial Lung Disease Program, Division of Pulmonary Medicine, Department of Medicine, National Jewish Medical and Research Center, Denver
frankels@njc.org
Drug-Induced Lung Disease

Mark W. Geraci, MD
Associate Professor of Medicine and Pharmacology; Assistant Chief of Medicine; Director, Gene Expression Facility, Division of Pulmonary Sciences and Critical Care Medicine, Human Medical Genetics Program, University of Colorado Health Sciences Center, Denver
mark.geraci@uchsc.edu
Laboratory Evaluation

Craig S. Glazer, MD, MSPH
Assistant Professor of Medicine, Pulmonary and Critical Care Medicine, University of Texas Southwestern Medical Center at Dallas
craig.glazer@utsouthwestern.edu
Acute Inhalational Injury

Michael P. Gruber, MD
Fellow, Department of Pulmonary Sciences and Critical Care Medicine, University of Colorado Health Sciences Center, Denver
michael.gruber@uchsc.edu
Pneumothorax/Hemothorax

Michael E. Hanley, MD
Associate Professor, Department of Pulmonary Sciences and Critical Care Medicine, University of Colorado School of Medicine and Denver Health Medical Center
mhanley@dhha.org
The History & Physical Examination in Pulmonary Medicine; Pneumothorax/Hemothorax

John E. Heffner, MD
Professor of Medicine, Executive Medical Director, Medical University of South Carolina, Charleston
heffnerj@musc.edu
Empyema

Michael D. Iseman, MD
Professor of Medicine, University of Colorado School of Medicine; Chief, Mycobacterial Disease Division, National Jewish Medical and Research Center, Denver
isemanm@njc.org
Mycobacterial Diseases of the Lungs

David A. Kaminsky, MD
Associate Professor of Medicine, University of Vermont College of Medicine; Attending Physician, Fletcher Allen Health Care, Burlington
dkaminsk@zoo.uvm.edu
Asthma

Robert L. Keith, MD, FCCP
Assistant Professor of Medicine, Department of Pulmonary Sciences and Critical Care Medicine, Denver Veterans Affairs Medical Center/University of Colorado Health Sciences Center
robert.keith@uchsc.edu
Bronchogenic Carcinoma & Solitary Pulmonary Nodules

Karen Kelly, MD
Associate Professor, Division of Medical Oncology, University of Colorado Health Sciences Center, Denver
karen.kelly@uchsc.edu
Pleural Malignancies & Benign Neoplasms of the Lung

Talmadge E. King, Jr., MD
Chief, Medical Services, San Francisco General Hospital; The Constance B. Wofsy Distinguished Professor and Vice-Chairman, Department of Medicine, University of California, San Francisco
tking@medsfgh.ucsf.edu
Idiopathic Interstitial Pneumonia

Kathryn A. Lee, MD
Fellow in Infectious Diseases, University of Colorado Health Sciences Center, Denver
kathryn.lee@uchsc.edu
Viral & Atypical Pneumonia

Kenneth V. Leeper, Jr., MD
Associate Professor of Medicine, Division of Pulmonary, Allergy and Critical Care Medicine, Emory University School of Medicine, Atlanta
kenneth.leeper2@med.va.gov
Bacterial Pneumonia

James P. Maloney, MD
Assistant Professor, Department of Pulmonary and Critical Care Medicine, Medical College of Wisconsin, Milwaukee
jmaloney@mcw.edu
Acute Ventilatory Failure

F. Dennis McCool, MD, FCCP
Professor of Medicine, Brown University; Chief, Pulmonary Critical Care Medicine, Memorial Hospital of Rhode Island, Pawtucket
f_mccool@brown.edu
Pulmonary Anatomy & Physiology

Sarah McKinley, MD
Fellow, Department of Pulmonary Sciences and Critical Care Medicine, University of Colorado Health Sciences Center, Denver
sarah.mckinley@uchsc.edu
Laboratory Evaluation

Marc Moss, MD
Associate Professor of Medicine, Emory University School of Medicine; Director, Medical and Cardiac Intensive Care Units, Grady Memorial Hospital, Atlanta
marc_moss@emoryhealthcare.org
Bacterial Pneumonia

Patrick Nana-Sinkam, MD
Fellow, Division of Pulmonary Sciences and Critical Care Medicine, University of Colorado Health Sciences Center, Denver
patrick.nana-sinkam@uchsc.edu
Pulmonary Thromboembolism

Lee S. Newman, MD, MA
Professor of Medicine and Preventive Medicine/Biometrics, University of Colorado Health Sciences Center; Head, Division of Environmental and Occupational Health Sciences, National Jewish Medical and Research Center, Denver
newmanl@njc.org
Pneumoconiosis

Jerry A. Nick, MD
Associate Professor, Department of Pulmonary Sciences and Critical Care Medicine, National Jewish Medical and Research Center, Denver
nickj@njc.org
Chronic Bronchiectasis & Cystic Fibrosis

Mark R. Nicolls, MD
Assistant Professor of Medicine and Immunology, and Associate Director, Transplantation Immunology, Department of Pulmonary Sciences and Critical Care Medicine, University of Colorado Health Sciences Center, Denver
mark.nicolls@uchsc.edu
Lung Transplantation

James M. O'Brien, Jr., MD
Fellow, Department of Pulmonary Sciences and Critical Care Medicine, University of Colorado Health Sciences Center, Denver
james.obrien@uchsc.edu
Pulmonary Langerhans'-Cell Histiocytosis, Lymphangioleiomyomatosis, & Bronchiolitis Obliterans with Organizing Pneumonia

Polly E. Parsons, MD
Professor of Medicine, University of Vermont College of Medicine; Director, Pulmonary and Critical Care Medicine Unit, Chief of Critical Care Services, Fletcher Allen Health Care, Burlington
polly.parsons@vtmednet.org
Acute Respiratory Distress Syndrome

Thomas L. Petty, MD
Professor of Medicine, University of Colorado Health
  Sciences Center, Denver; Professor of Medicine, Rush-
  Presbyterian-St. Luke's Medical Center, Chicago
tlpdoc@aol.com
Chronic Obstructive Pulmonary Disease

Laurie A. Proia, MD
Assistant Professor of Medicine, Rush Medical College;
  Attending Physician, Infectious Diseases, Rush-
  Presbyterian-St. Luke's Hospital, Chicago
lproia@rush.edu
Fungal Pneumonias

Charles E. Ray, Jr., MD
Associate Professor of Radiology, University of Col-
  orado Health Sciences Center; Chief, Interventional
  Radiology, Denver Health Medical Center
cray@dhha.org
Diagnostic Imaging

Cecile Rose, MD, MPH
Associate Professor of Medicine, University of Colorado Health Sciences Center; Director, Occupational Medicine Clinic, National Jewish Medical
  and Research Center, Denver
rosec@njc.org
Hypersensitivity Pneumonitis

John R. Ruddy, MD
Assistant Professor of Medicine (Clinical), Department of
  Medicine, New York University School of Medicine
john.ruddy@med.nyu.edu
Sleep Apnea & the Upper Airway Resistance Syndrome

Milene T. Saavedra, MD
Instructor, Department of Pulmonary Sciences and
  Critical Care Medicine, University of Colorado
  Health Sciences Center, Denver
milene.saavedra@uchsc.edu
Chronic Bronchiectasis & Cystic Fibrosis

Marvin I. Schwarz, MD
Director, Professor, and Division Head, Division of Pulmonary Sciences and Critical Care Medicine, University of Colorado Health Sciences Center, Denver
marvin.schwarz@uchsc.edu
Vasculitis & the Diffuse Alveolar Hemorrhage Syndromes

John Segreti, MD
Professor, Department of Internal Medicine, Rush
  Medical College; Attending Physician, Rush-
  Presbyterian-St. Luke's Medical Center, Chicago
john_segreti@rush.edu
Pulmonary Complications of HIV Disease

Randy L. Sid, MD
Clinical Assistant Instructor of Medicine, Brown
  Medical School; Chief Resident, Memorial Hospital
  of Rhode Island, Pawtucket
rsid@mail.com
Diseases of the Mediastinum

Benjamin T. Suratt, MD
Assistant Professor of Medicine, Division of Pul-
  monary and Critical Care Medicine, University of
  Vermont College of Medicine and Fletcher Allen
  Health Care, Burlington
benjamin.suratt@uvm.edu
Pleural Effusions, Excluding Hemothorax

E. Rand Sutherland, MD, MPH
Assistant Professor of Medicine, National Jewish
  Medical and Research Center and University of
  Colorado Health Sciences Center, Denver
sutherlande@njc.org
Occupational Asthma

Jason S. Vourlekis, MD, FCCP
Medical Officer, Lung and Upper Aerodigestive
  Cancer Research Group, Division of Cancer Pre-
  vention, National Cancer Institute, National Insti-
  tutes of Health, Department of Health and Human
  Services, Bethesda, MD
vourlekj@mail.nih.gov
Eosinophilic Pneumonias

Yasmine S. Wasfi, MD
Pulmonary Fellow, Division of Pulmonary Sciences
  and Critical Care Medicine, University of Colorado
  Health Sciences Center, Denver
yasmine.wasfi@uchsc.edu
Sarcoidosis

Carolyn H. Welsh, MD
Staff Physician, Medicine and Research Services, Denver Veterans Affairs Medical Center, and Professor, Department of Medicine, Division of Pulmonary Sciences and Critical Care Medicine, University of Colorado Health Sciences Center
carolyn.welsh@med.va.gov
Mechanical Ventilation: Invasive and Noninvasive; Evaluation of Sleepiness & Sleep Disorders Other Than Sleep Apnea: Narcolepsy, Restless Leg Syndrome, & Periodic Limb Movements; Medical Conditions That Often Cause Daytime Sleepiness

Howard West, MD
Medical Oncologist, Swedish Cancer Institute, Seattle
howard.west@swedish.org
Pleural Malignancies & Benign Neoplasms of the Lung

Robert A. Winn, MD
Assistant Professor, Department of Pulmonary Sciences and Critical Care Medicine, University of Colorado Health Sciences Center and Denver Veterans Affairs Medical Center, Denver
robert.winn@uchsc.edu
Laboratory Evaluation

Martin R. Zamora, MD
Associate Professor of Medicine, Department of Pulmonary Sciences and Critical Care Medicine, and Medical Director, Lung Transplant Program, University of Colorado Health Sciences Center, Denver
marty.zamora@uchsc.edu
Lung Transplantation

Preface

This is the first edition of *Current Diagnosis & Treatment in Pulmonary Medicine* in this respected and well-read series of books dedicated to important topics in the practice of clinical medicine.

The book is designed as a resource for practicing clinicians and those in training. It includes in-depth but concise discussions of topics an internist or family medicine physician might independently manage, as well as conditions that require referral to a pulmonary subspecialist. It is intended to be a quick reference to provide the busy clinician and clinician-in-training with clinically relevant information. It is not intended to be an exhaustive review of all aspects of pulmonary science and medicine, but includes references to direct the stimulated reader to more detailed information.

It has been a privilege working with our contributing authors, many of whom are our mentors at the University of Colorado. Our contributor pool draws deeply from the talented physicians, teachers, and investigators who have trained in the University of Colorado pulmonary training program over the years. The quality of this book mirrors the outstanding character of these people; it is a pleasure highlighting their knowledge and extensive clinical experience with this publication.

Michael E. Hanley, MD
Carolyn H. Welsh, MD

Denver, Colorado
September 2003

SECTION I

Evaluation of the Patient with Pulmonary Disease

Vera A. DePalo, MD, FCCP, & F. Dennis McCool, MD, FCCP

Ventilation of the lungs allows exchange of gas between blood and atmospheric air. This chapter will describe the anatomy of the lungs and airways and explain the mechanical properties of the lungs and chest wall that affect the amount of air that is exchanged between the atmosphere and alveoli, how this air is distributed within the lungs, diffusion of alveolar gas into the pulmonary circulation, and control of this process. Mechanical properties of the lungs will be described in the context of the elastic and resistive forces that need to be overcome during inspiration to ventilate the lungs, expiratory flow limitation, and the work and energetics of breathing.

ANATOMY OF THE RESPIRATORY SYSTEM

Major elements of the respiratory system include the chest wall, airways, alveolar–capillary units, pulmonary and bronchial circulations, nerves, and lymphatics. To complete the structure, the pleura is a mesenchymal lining that consists of a visceral layer adhered intimately to the lungs and a parietal layer lining the mediastinum and chest wall.

Chest Wall

The chest wall is composed of the diaphragm and rib cage. The rib cage is composed of the spine posteriorly, the sternum anteriorly, and the ribs and their cartilaginous attachments to the sternum. The rib cage serves as a framework for attachment of respiratory muscles and their ligaments. Respiratory muscles are classified as inspiratory or expiratory although some of them contribute to both actions (Figure 1–1). Inspiratory muscles include the diaphragm, external intercostals, parasternal internal intercostals, scalenes, and sternocleidomastoids. Expiratory muscles include the abdominal wall muscles and the interosseus internal intercostals.

The diaphragm is the major muscle of inspiration and separates the thoracic and abdominal cavities (Figure 1–2). It is composed of a fibrous central tendon and a muscular layer that inserts into the lower rib cage and spine. The component of the diaphragm that inserts anteriorly and laterally into the rib cage is referred to as the costal diaphragm, whereas the portion that inserts posteriorly is the crural diaphragm. The zone of apposition is that part of the diaphragm that is closely apposed to the inner surface of the lower rib cage; it is sandwiched between the internal surfaces of the rib cage and the abdominal cavity. The zone of apposition represents an area in which the lower rib cage is exposed to abdominal pressure. The diaphragm is innervated by the phrenic nerve that originates from the third, fourth, and fifth cervical nerve roots.

Contraction of inspiratory muscles increases the anteroposterior and transverse diameters of the rib cage and expands the anterior abdominal wall. Rib cage and abdominal expansion during inspiration results from coordinated activity of the diaphragm and inspiratory muscles of the rib cage. Diaphragm contraction alone results in outward movement of the lower rib cage and anterior abdominal wall, but produces paradoxical inward motion of the upper rib cage. The outward motion of the upper rib cage that normally occurs during inspiration is due to actions of the inspiratory muscles of the rib cage, the sternocleidomastoid and scalene muscles.

Contraction of inspiratory muscles enlarges the chest wall and underlying lung. The lungs tend to pull

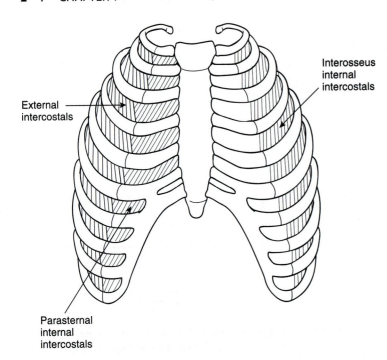

Figure 1–1. Schematic of the rib cage and the intercostal muscles. The parasternal intercostal and external intercostal muscles are important in inspiration. The interosseus internal intercostal muscles are expiratory.

away from the chest wall as the thorax is expanding. This creates subatmospheric or negative intrapleural pressure. Alveolar pressure falls and air enters the airways and lung. The change in intrapleural pressure during inspiration is usually 4–5 cm H_2O subatmospheric. Intrapleural pressure can be measured directly by passing a needle between two ribs and injecting air or fluid to separate the two pleura. Alternatively, pressure can be measured by using a 10-cm-long, thin-walled balloon that is introduced into the esophagus. Intraesophageal pressure reflects intrapleural pressure because the esophagus lies between the lungs and chest wall and is a thin tube with little tone that offers little resistance to transmission of intrathoracic pressure changes.

Usually expiration is a passive event requiring little or no expiratory muscle activity. However, expiration is an active phenomenon when demand for ventilation increases. When abdominal expiratory muscles contract, the abdomen is displaced inward and its anteroposterior diameter is reduced. This increases intraabdominal pressure and displaces the passive diaphragm cephalad into the thoracic cavity. Increased intraabdominal pressure is transmitted into the thoracic cavity, raising alveolar pressure and promoting expiratory airflow. The internal intercostal muscles assist the expiratory muscles of the abdominal wall by constricting the rib cage (Figure 1–3). The diaphragm can also function as an expiratory muscle. With hyperinflation, the diaphragm becomes flattened. In this configuration, diaphragmatic contraction pulls the lower rib cage inward and produces expiratory action.

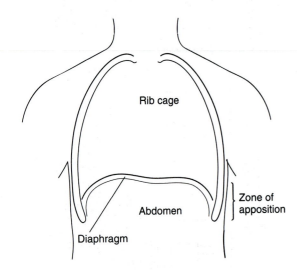

Figure 1–2. Drawing of the chest and abdomen depicting the position of the diaphragm and the zone of apposition.

Airways

The tracheobronchial tree is a series of branching tubes that get narrower and more numerous as they penetrate into the lungs. They consist of the trachea, mainstem

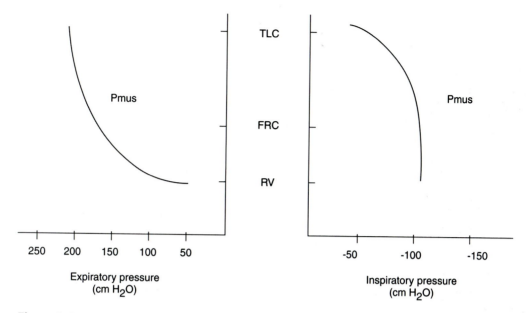

Figure 1–3. Pressure–volume relationships for the inspiratory and expiratory muscles. Inspiratory muscles are strongest at low lung volumes, whereas expiratory muscles are strongest at high volumes.

bronchi, lobar bronchi, segmental and subsegmental bronchi, bronchioles, and terminal bronchioles. The first 16 generations of airways, the conducting airways, lead air to the gas-exchanging lung units but do not directly participate in gas exchange. These airways constitute anatomic dead space (Figure 1–4).

The airway wall is composed of mucosal, submucosal, and fibrocartilaginous layers. The mucosal layer is the most superficial and is in direct contact with inhaled gases and particles. This layer consists of a lining of pseudostratified columnar epithelial cells with hair-like projections, cilia, on their luminal surfaces. Cilia contain longitudinal microtubules with contractile function. The cross-sectional structure of cilia in the lungs is similar to that in other parts of the body and consists of nine peripheral pairs of microtubules surrounding a single central doublet. Sidearms and dynein arms project from each peripheral pair of microtubules and are important for normal ciliary function. Rhythmic beating of cilia transports mucus, cellular debris, and liquid out of distal airways into larger airways and the pharynx where it is expectorated or swallowed. The superficial layer also contains goblet cells that produce mucus. Basal reserve cells are capable of differentiating into either goblet or columnar cells.

The submucosal layer is composed of bronchial mucous glands, smooth muscles, and lymphocytes. Mucous glands produce the majority of the mucus found in airways. As airways penetrate deeper into the lung,

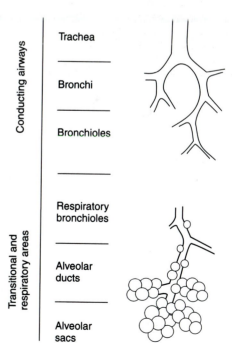

Figure 1–4. Diagram of the branching airways from the trachea down to the respiratory bronchioles and alveolar sacs.

there is less smooth muscle. Changes in smooth muscle tone alter airway diameter. An increase in tone leads to airway constriction. Smooth muscle tone is determined by the autonomic nervous system and mediators released by mast cells and other inflammatory cells. Bronchial-associated lymphoid tissue (BALT) consists of aggregates of lymphocytes located in the submucosa. These lymphocytes participate in lung defense by reacting to airborne pathogens and debris.

The fibrocartilaginous layer provides structural support of airways from the trachea to distal bronchioles. The trachea is a fibromuscular tube supported by C-shaped cartilage anteriorly and laterally and with a posterior smooth muscle wall. Semicircular cartilaginous rings are present in large bronchi, but are replaced by irregularly shaped cartilaginous plates as the bronchi enter the lungs. The outer layer of bronchiolar walls contains no cartilage and is surrounded by connective tissue with elastic fibers.

Alveolar–Capillary Units

Airways may branch up to 23 times before terminating in acini, the gas-exchange units of the lungs (Figure 1–4). Acini are composed of respiratory bronchioles, alveolar ducts, and alveoli. The walls of alveoli are very thin and are composed of two major cell types, type I and type II pneumocytes. Type I pneumocytes are flattened cells with long cytoplasmic extensions that comprise 95% of the alveolar surface. Their major function is gas exchange, which is achieved by passive diffusion. Type I pneumocytes are metabolically inactive. Type II pneumocytes are more numerous and cuboidal in shape. They have greater intracellular metabolic activity and produce surfactant, a complex lipid and protein mixture. Surfactant reduces alveolar surface tension, prevents atelectasis, and removes excess water and material from the alveolar space. Type II pneumocytes are capable of differentiating into type I cells to facilitate lung repair. Alveolar spaces contain large numbers of macrophages that act as an important defense mechanism, scavenging inhaled pathogens and other materials.

Frerking I et al: Pulmonary surfactant: functions, abnormalities and therapeutic options. Intensive Care Med 2001;27:1699. [PMID: 11810113]. (Description of the basic biophysics, physiology, and biochemistry of surfactant, including pathophysiological mechanisms that interfere with surfactant function in some diseases.)

Misuri G et al: Respiratory muscles in internal medicine. Monaldi Arch Chest Dis 1999;54:520. [PMID: 10695324]. (Review of respiratory muscle abnormalities that are associated with various medical illnesses.)

MECHANICAL PROPERTIES OF THE RESPIRATORY SYSTEM

Lung Recoil

Elasticity is the property of matter that causes it to return to its resting shape after deformation by an external force. Elastic properties of the respiratory system can be subdivided into those of the lungs and chest wall. Tissues of the lungs and chest wall are elastic in that external forces stretch them. When the external force is removed, the tissues recoil to their resting position. The pressure generated as lung tissue returns to its resting position is referred to as recoil pressure. The greater the external force applied, the more the lungs are stretched and the greater the volume change and recoil pressure. The degree of stretch is proportional to the change in lung volume. Lung recoil occurs in part because the lungs are composed of airspaces surrounded by a network of collagen and elastin. Because of the structure of these tissues the lungs always have a tendency to recoil inward away from the chest wall; the resting position of the lungs would be an airless state if external forces did not act on them.

Surface forces also contribute to recoil of the lungs. There is a very thin film of liquid that lines alveoli, creating an air–liquid interface. Surface tension in an air–liquid interface results from attracting forces between atoms or molecules within the liquid. Water molecules on the surface of the interface have more of a tendency to be pulled down by the molecules beneath the surface than up to the air over it. This imbalance of molecular forces produces surface tension and results in the surface shrinking to the smallest possible area. The surface tensions from air–liquid interfaces in millions of alveoli contribute to the tendency of the lungs to collapse. Taken in total, the recoil pressure created by surface tension in all the alveoli provides as much lung recoil as do the elastic fibers.

Surfactant, the fluid lining the surface of alveoli, lowers surface tension when the lungs are at lower volumes. Surfactant is secreted by type II pneumocytes. Its main constituent is the phospholipid dipalmitoyl phosphatidylcholine. It is a complex mixture of lipids and proteins, containing 80% phospholipids, 8% other lipids, cholesterol, triacylglycerol, and free fatty acids, and 12% protein. A lower surface tension requires less air pressure to maintain a given radius or volume. Low surface tension reduces the muscular effort necessary to ventilate the lungs and keep them aerated. If surfactant were not present, surface tension would not decrease as alveoli became smaller and the alveoli would collapse completely.

The influence of surface tension is best illustrated by comparing pressure–volume (P–V) curves for lungs inflated with air and those inflated with saline. Filling the lungs with saline eliminates surface active forces; the pressure required to inflate saline-filled lungs is less than half that required to inflate air-filled lungs. Surfactant deficiency has been noted in infants who die of respiratory distress syndrome. Surfactant replacement improves the status of infants suffering from this syndrome.

Recoil pressure of the lungs is measured under static conditions (conditions of no airflow). It is the difference between alveolar (Palv) and pleural (Ppl) pressure and is called transpulmonary pressure (Ptp; Ptp = Palv − Ppl) (Figure 1–5). Transpulmonary recoil pressure can be measured at different lung volumes, thereby defining a number of points on a volume–pressure curve of the lungs. The slope of the volume–pressure curve is the static compliance or stiffness of the lungs. Static compliance is defined as the volume change per unit of pressure change and is described as liters/centimeter H_2O. Normal lung compliance is 0.2 L/cm H_2O. If static compliance is decreased, lung tissue is more rigid and less distensible. This occurs in diseases such as interstitial fibrosis, atelectasis, pulmonary edema, or pneumonia. An increase in compliance occurs in emphysema, a disease that destroys lung elastic fibers.

Compliance can also be measured under dynamic conditions, that is, under conditions of airflow during the respiratory cycle. To measure dynamic compliance, transpulmonary pressures are measured at end inspiration and end expiration. The slope of the line connecting these points on a volume–pressure plot is dynamic compliance. Dynamic compliance is equal to static compliance in normal subjects, even at respiratory rates approaching 90/min. In patients with increased airway resistance, dynamic compliance decreases at higher respiratory rates. Lung units with long time constants may not fill or empty completely before the next inspiration, thus causing an apparent decrease in compliance.

Chest Wall Recoil

The elastic forces of the thoracic cage, if not acted on by an external force such as the pull of the lungs, enlarge the thorax from its resting volume to about 600 mL above it. Expansion of the thorax above its resting volume can be noted when air is introduced into the pleural space. In this instance, the lung becomes smaller and the thorax becomes larger.

At the end of a quiet, tidal volume breath the respiratory system is at its resting position. This is the relaxation volume or functional residual capacity (FRC). At FRC, the recoil of the chest wall is in an inspiratory direction; that is, it causes the thorax to expand. The recoil pressure of the chest wall in this regard is negative at FRC in the sense that it results in expansion of the thorax. It is prevented from expanding by the recoil of the lungs, which causes the lungs to shrink. Chest wall recoil is equal and opposite to lung recoil at FRC (Figure 1–6). During inspiration to modest volumes above FRC, the passive recoil of the chest wall assists inspiration and inspiratory muscles act only against the recoil of the lungs. With inspiration to volumes greater than approximately 600 mL above FRC the passive recoil of the chest wall becomes expiratory (the thorax will shrink if no external force is applied) and inspiratory muscles work to expand both the chest wall and lungs.

Recoil pressure of the chest wall measured under static conditions is the difference between pleural and atmospheric (Patm) pressure and is called trans chest wall pressure (Pcw; Pcw = Ppl − Patm) (Figure 1–5). Transchest wall pressure can be measured at different lung volumes, thereby defining a number of points on a volume–pressure curve of the respiratory system. The slope of this volume–pressure curve is the compliance of the passive chest wall (relaxed respiratory muscles). Normal chest wall compliance is 0.2 L/cm H_2O. Chest wall compliance can also be calculated as the difference between respiratory system and lung compliance. Respiratory system compliance (Crs) is the difference between airway opening pressure and atmosphere at different volumes during relaxation. If data are obtained simultaneously for the lungs (Cl) and the total respira-

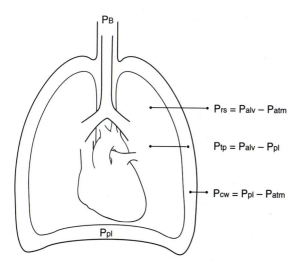

Figure 1–5. Diagram depicting relevant respiratory system pressures. Patm is atmospheric pressure, Palv is alveolar pressure, Ppl is pleural pressure, Ptp is the transpulmonary pressure, Prs is the respiratory system pressure, and Pcw is chest wall pressure.

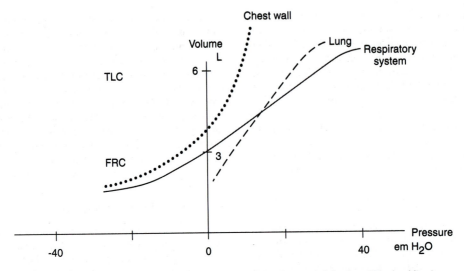

Figure 1–6. The graph demonstrates the elastic contribution of the lung (dashed line) and the relaxed chest wall (dotted line). The solid line represents the sum of the elastic properties of the lung and chest wall, which is the transrespiratory system pressure.

tory system, compliance of the chest wall (Ccw) can be calculated as

$$1/Ccw = 1/Crs - 1/Cl$$

Normal values for healthy individuals are approximately 0.1 L/cm H_2O for total respiratory system compliance. Chest wall compliance may be decreased in kyphoscoliosis, neuromuscular disease, and obesity. The chest wall also progressively stiffens with age.

Airway Resistance

The physical factors determining airway resistance are similar to those governing resistance of fluid flowing in tubes. The magnitude of pressure required to drive fluid through a straight rigid tube depends on the radius and length of the tube and whether the flow is laminar or turbulent. If the dimensions of the tube are constant, the driving pressure (P) required to produce a certain flow ($\dot{V}$) is directly proportional to the viscosity of the fluid:

$$P = K_1\dot{V}$$

where K_1 is a constant that includes the influence of viscosity. When the length and radius of the tube are changed, the pressure needed to produce a given flow varies directly with the length of the tube and inversely with the fourth power of its radius. Combining these factors, resistance (R) is proportional to the length of

the tube (L) and the coefficient of viscosity (μ), and is inversely proportional to the radius (r) as follows:

$$R = P/\dot{V} = 8\mu L/\pi r^4 \text{ (Poiseuille's law)}$$

These relationships are valid when flow is laminar, organized flow with molecules within the stream moving in parallel. However, application of Poiseuille's law for laminar flow in the lungs is limited in several ways. First, the bronchial tree is not composed of smooth cylindrical rigid tubes. Second, the upper airway starts with two irregular tubes in parallel (the nares) followed by tubes in series (the nasopharynx, larynx, and trachea), followed by a complex system of branching and rebranching distensible tubes in parallel (20 to 22 divisions of bronchi, bronchioles, and terminal bronchioles). Finally, when flow becomes turbulent the driving pressure required for a given flow increases.

Disorganized movement of air molecules within the air stream characterizes turbulent flow. Molecules may be moving in different directions, with different velocities, and are often colliding with each other. The density of gas becomes important and viscosity less so with turbulent flow. The pressure needed to produce a given flow is greater when airflow is turbulent and varies with the square of the flow as follows:

$$P = K_2\dot{V}_2$$

where K_2 is a constant that includes the influence of density.

Flow changes from laminar to turbulent when Reynold's number exceeds 2000. Reynold's number is a dimensionless number equal to the product of the density, velocity, and diameter divided by viscosity. Turbulent flow may occur at very high velocities or in tubes with large diameters such as the mainstem bronchi or trachea. Turbulence at low flow rates can occur when there are irregularities in tubes caused by mucus, tumors, foreign bodies, or partial closure of the glottis. It is likely that normal airflow is a combination of both laminar and turbulent flow; the pressure required to produce flow in this setting is described by

$$P = K_1\dot{V} + K_2\dot{V}^2$$

Airway resistance can be calculated by measuring the driving pressure for flow (the difference between alveolar pressure and pressure at the airway opening) and flow through the airways. This can be accomplished with body plethysmography to rapidly measure alveolar pressure and airflow during a panting maneuver. This maneuver is usually performed with the subject panting at a lung volume slightly greater than normal FRC. Airway resistance (Raw) is calculated as alveolar pressure minus airway opening pressure (Pao) divided by flow:

$$Raw = (Palv - Pao)/\dot{V}$$

Airway resistance is approximately 1–1.5 cm H_2O/L/s in adults. It decreases in a hyperbolic fashion as lung volume is increased because airways are wider at higher lung volumes. About half the resistance during quiet breathing is due to resistance of the nasal passages. Airway resistance is often referenced to the lung volume at which it is measured. The reciprocal of resistance is airway conductance.

Several factors influence airway resistance. Smooth muscle constriction results in luminal narrowing and increases airway resistance. An increase in parasympathetic tone constricts airway smooth muscle, whereas an increase in sympathetic tone relaxes airway smooth muscle. In normal subjects, however, there is little or no resting parasympathetic or sympathetic tone. Inhaled irritants, such as smoke, dust, cold air, and chemical irritants, can cause reflex bronchoconstriction. Circulatory factors such as arterial hypoxemia, hypocapnia, and emboli lodging in certain parts of the pulmonary circulation also cause bronchoconstriction. Hypercapnia does not affect airways conductance. Reductions in gas density (such as from breathing mixtures of gases with a high helium concentration) decrease the driving pressure needed for flow and thereby decrease resistance. Conversely, airway resistance is increased during a deep underwater dive because the increased pressure raises gas density.

Airway resistance in patients with asthma is increased because of smooth muscle constriction, bronchial edema, and airway obstruction from mucus. Airway resistance in patients with chronic bronchitis is increased because of airway inflammation, edema, and mucous hypersecretion. There is also hyperplasia of bronchial mucous glands. Airway resistance in patients with emphysema is increased because of loss of elastic tissue that normally supports and keeps open smaller nonrigid airways. During quiet inspiration and expiration there is probably little change in airway resistance because the airways become longer as well as wider.

Expiratory Flow Limitation

Generally, increases in effort at a given lung volume increase pleural pressure and therefore expiratory flow. However, flow eventually becomes limited in that further increases in effort do not cause higher flow. This phenomenon, referred to as expiratory flow limitation, is most apparent at lung volumes less than 80% of total lung capacity (TLC). This region of the expiratory flow volume loop is sometimes referred to as the effort-independent zone.

One explanation of expiratory flow limitation is based on the equal pressure point (EPP) concept. Forced expiration greatly increases both alveolar and pleural pressure; alveolar pressure is greater than pleural pressure in this scenario. The difference between these two pressures is the elastic recoil of the lung and is small relative to the increase in both pressures from the expiratory effort. Pressure in the airways drops down the length of the airways from the alveolus to the mouth (downstream). This pressure drop is related both to frictional heat gain and acceleration of gas (Bernoulli effect). The pressure in the airways at some point equals pleural pressure. This point is referred to as the equal pressure point and normally resides either in the trachea or more proximal airways. Pleural pressure exceeds airway pressure downstream of the EPP. Airways become compressed when pressure outside the airways exceeds pressure within them. As lung volume falls, the effect of the change in recoil pressure is significant, the flow-limiting site moves more peripherally, and flow decreases. The EPP hypothesis is a good but approximate description of flow limitation at high lung volumes.

A second theory is based on principles of fluid dynamics. These principles assert that maximum flow through compliant tubes such as airways is the flow at that point in the system at which fluid velocity equals wave-speed ("wave-speed mechanism"). Wave-speed is the speed at which a small disturbance travels in a compliant tube filled with fluid. The wave-speed depends on the cross-sectional area of the tube and density of the fluid. The location at which the flow-limiting mechanism operates is called a "choke point." When this principle is applied to airways, flow limitation at the choke point results from a complex interaction between transmural pressure (the difference between pressure in the airstream and pressure in the peribronchial space), the area of the airway, and its compliance. These factors vary with lung volume. At high lung volumes, both transmural pressure and the total cross-sectional area in peripheral airways are large, so velocity of flow is low. However, in central airways the total cross-sectional area is low and flow velocity increases. Thus, by the Bernoulli effect, velocity of the airstream increases, thereby decreasing transmural pressure. This reduces the cross-sectional area of the airway further and contributes to flow limitation. At this point, lowering the downstream pressure further does not move more air through the airways. Conditions at the choke point set the upper limits of flow during forced expiration. The choke point normally resides near the tracheal carina at high lung volumes and progresses out to more peripheral airways (the second- and third-generation airways) as lung volume decreases and airways are narrowed.

The segment of airway between the choke point and the airway opening is referred to as the downstream segment. Flow in the downstream segment must equal flow in the upstream segment. However, linear velocities are considerably higher in the downstream segment as the total cross-sectional area of these airways is reduced in comparison to the upstream segments. This occurs for two reasons. First, the lungs are designed in such a manner that the total cross-sectional area of the airways decreases as one moves from the alveoli to the mouth. Second, downstream segments are dynamically compressed because intrapleural pressure is greater than intraairway pressure. The intrapleural pressure may be raised to such an extent that tracheal cross-sectional area is reduced up to 80%. Dynamic compression of the downstream segment is effort dependent, starts at the thoracic inlet, and follows choke points upstream as lung volume diminishes. In contrast, the extrathoracic downstream segment is not exposed to pleural pressure and therefore is not compressed during expiration. Accordingly, the extrathoracic cross-sectional area is greater and the linear velocity of exhaled gas is lower in the extrathoracic trachea.

Abnormally severe expiratory flow limitation, such as seen with chronic obstructive pulmonary disease (COPD), adversely affects pulmonary function by increasing FRC and residual volume (RV). The chest becomes progressively hyperinflated if flow limitation is severe and there is not enough time for complete expiration. Hyperinflation lowers airway resistance; however, progressive increases in FRC limit inspiratory capacity and the ability to increase ventilation. The elastic force at end inspiration also increases as FRC increases. Although this increases the pressure available for expiration it also increases respiratory efforts and leads to tiring of respiratory muscles. An increase in FRC is also disadvantageous because the chest wall is larger than normal resulting in inspiratory muscle inefficiency.

Tissue Resistance

Displacement of the tissues of the lungs, rib cage, diaphragm, and abdominal contents is associated with frictional resistance. Tissue resistance occurs only during motion and is dependent on the velocity of motion. It occurs during inspiration and expiration. Mechanical limitation of movement of the muscles or joints of the thorax provides resistance to inflating the lungs. As more elastic force is dissipated overcoming frictional tissue resistance during expiration, less elastic force is available to overcome airway resistance. Consequently, expiratory flow becomes diminished.

Tissue resistance is the difference between airway resistance and total pulmonary resistance. Airway resistance is measured with body plethysmography as previously described. Pulmonary resistance can also be measured with body plethysmography, but pleural pressure is measured rather than measuring alveolar pressure. Tissue resistance in healthy young men is about 20% of total pulmonary resistance. Diseases such as pulmonary fibrosis, asthma, and kyphoscoliosis can increase tissue resistance. Chest wall resistance may be particularly high in patients with diseases of the chest wall such as kyphoscoliosis.

Work & Oxygen Cost of Breathing

Work is defined as the product of force applied over distance. Work in a fluid system is performed when pressure produces volume change in the system. The cumulative product of pressure and the volume of air moved at each instant is equal to work ($W = PdV$). Work performed on the respiratory system can be done overcoming resistive loads (airway resistance) and elastic loads (recoil of the lungs and chest wall), and in decompressing intrathoracic gas.

During quiet breathing, most of the work of breathing is done to overcome the recoil of the lungs and chest wall. However, when ventilation is increased or the airways are narrowed, much of the work is done to overcome the frictional resistance to airflow. The elastic work is related to the force necessary to overcome the elastic recoil of the lungs and chest wall and to overcome surface tension of alveoli. Resistive work overcomes tissue and airway resistance.

The work performed by inspiratory muscles on the lungs and airways can be calculated from measurements of transpulmonary pressure and volume during breathing ($Wl = Ptp \times dV$). The work performed on the respiratory system and airways can be calculated from measurements of transrespiratory system pressure and volume during passive mechanical ventilation. During passive ventilation, the ventilator performs work displacing the lungs and chest wall as well as flow-resistive work required to generate flow through airways. This work is the area under the P–V curve of the respiratory system ($Wrs = Prs \times dV$). The work performed on the chest wall alone can also be determined during passive mechanical ventilation by measuring trans chest wall pressure rather than trans thoracic pressure. The work performed on the chest wall is calculated as $Wcw = Pcw \times dV$.

The work rate, or power, of breathing is the amount of work performed over time. Respiratory muscle power increases in a curvilinear manner with increasing ventilation. The work of breathing increases disproportionately as minute volume increases. Maximum power output of the respiratory muscles is measured by a maximum voluntary ventilation maneuver. The maximum power that can be sustained is approximately 80% of the maximum voluntary ventilation in normal subjects.

The oxygen consumed by respiratory muscles is normally a small fraction of total body metabolism. Respiratory muscle oxygen consumption during normal, quiet breathing is less than 5% of total body oxygen uptake. The oxygen cost of breathing is greater in patients with emphysema, obese patients, and individuals with chest wall disease. High oxygen cost of breathing is associated with development of inspiratory muscle fatigue.

Oxygen cost of breathing is measured as the change in oxygen consumption from baseline during a respiratory maneuver such as hyperpnea or inspiratory resistive loading. The difference in oxygen consumption between baseline and either hyperpnea or inspiratory resistive loaded breathing is attributed to the respiratory muscles, although nonrespiratory muscles (postural muscles of the back) are likely also involved during these maneuvers.

Efficiency of breathing is calculated as the ratio of work rate over the oxygen cost of breathing. It ranges between 2 and 8% and varies directly with work rate and minute ventilation. The efficiency of breathing is reduced in individuals with tetraplegia or Parkinson's disease.

Distribution of Ventilation

Lower regions of the lungs receive more ventilation per unit volume in the upright position than do upper regions of the lungs. Preferential ventilation to the bases is due to a gradient of intrapleural pressure that is gravity dependent and related to the weight of the lungs as well as the shape of the static pressure–volume curve of the lungs. Intrapleural pressure in the upright position is less negative at the bottom of the lung than at the top. The pressure gradient from top to bottom is about 0.25 cm H_2O per centimeter lung height. The transpulmonary pressure is greatest at the top of the lungs because intrapleural pressure is more negative in this region. Accordingly, alveoli at the top of the lungs are inflated to a greater degree at FRC than are alveoli at the bottom of the lungs (Figure 1–7). Alveoli at the bottom of the lungs are about 40% of their TLC size and will have a large increase in volume for a given change in pleural pressure during inspiration. Alveoli at the top of the lungs are inflated to 70% of TLC size. This causes them to be less compliant than alveoli at the bottom of the lungs and results in smaller increments in volume for the same change in pleural pressure during inspiration. Thus, a greater proportion of inspired gas goes to lower alveoli when inhaling from FRC.

The first part of inspiration from RV is to alveoli at the top of the lungs. When exhaling to RV, alveoli at the top of the lungs may be partially inflated or on the steep portion of their P–V relationship, whereas alveoli in lower lung zones are on the horizontal part of their P–V relationship. Indeed, smaller airways in lower lung zones may be closed and not open until the adjacent pleural pressure becomes less than airway pressure. Thus the first part of inspiration goes almost exclusively to the top of the lung when the breath is initiated from RV. The distribution of ventilation also is altered by supine positioning. In this instance, gravity acts along the anteroposterior axis leading to greater ventilation in more posterior alveolar units.

Factors other than gravity also affect the distribution of ventilation. The concept that the degree of filling of a lung unit depends on the time available for filling is referred to as the time constant of that lung unit. Time constants depend on both lung compliance and airway resistance. Normally airway resistance is sufficiently low that all lung units empty synchronously. Units with long time constants due to disease fill slowly and at high breathing frequencies are relatively poorly ventilated. Areas with short time constants empty first during expiration and areas with long time constants empty later. In disease states in which there are regional differences in compliance and resistance, ventilation will be unevenly distributed. There is also interdependence of lung units. Contiguous units may not move independently of each other. Interdependence promotes a more uniform distribution of ventilation. In addition, collateral channels of ventilation between ad-

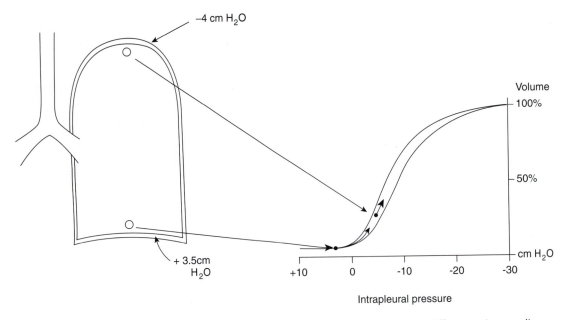

−4 cm H$_2$O

Volume
100%

50%

cm H$_2$O

+ 3.5cm
H$_2$O

+10   0   −10   −20   −30

Intrapleural pressure

Figure 1–7. Intrapleural pressure and its effect on alveolar volume result in regional differences in compliance and ventilation.

jacent alveoli, such as pores of Kohn, contribute to more evenly distributed ventilation.

Celli B: The diaphragm and respiratory muscles. Chest Surg Clin North Am 1998;8:207. [PMID: 9619302]. (Discussion of the anatomy of the muscles that leads to generation of ventilatory pressures and the physiological principles that guide their function.)

Gibson GJ: Lung volumes and elasticity. Clin Chest Med 2001;22: 623. [PMID: 11787655]. (Review of the elastic properties of the respiratory system. Includes the measurements and determinants of lung volumes and their patterns of abnormality in disease.)

VASCULAR SYSTEMS

Vascular systems within the lungs include the pulmonary, bronchial, and lymphatic systems. The pulmonary circulation consists of the pulmonary arterial trunk, right and left pulmonary arteries, lobar arteries, arterioles, capillaries, and pulmonary venules and veins. The right ventricle pumps blood through these structures and blood drains into the left atrium. Its primary function is to deliver blood to alveoli for participation in gas exchange. Barriers to gas exchange include the alveolar epithelium, the capillary endothelium, and the interstitial space between them. This space is normally about 0.2–0.5 μm thick. The pulmonary circulation also acts as a filter and participates in some metabolic functions.

The pulmonary circulation is a low-resistance system and therefore requires less driving pressure than the systemic circulation. Pulmonary vascular resistance is low for the following reasons. First, the amount of smooth muscle surrounding the vessels is small in comparison to the systemic circulation. Second, previously closed vessels can be readily recruited to accommodate increases in blood flow through the lungs. Finally, the thin walled nature of the pulmonary arterioles allows them to distend as intravascular pressure rises. For these reasons, pulmonary vascular resistance remains low when cardiac output is acutely increased.

As with ventilation, distribution of pulmonary blood flow in the upright lung is affected by gravity. Perfusion of a given region of lung is a function of arterial, alveolar and venous pressures (Figure 1–8). Gravity has a greater effect on vessels at the lung bases. Therefore, pulmonary arterial (Pa) and venous (Pv) pressures are greater at the lung bases than at the apex. Both pressures also are greater than alveolar pressure (Pa > Pv > Palv) at the bases. The driving pressure for blood flow in this region of the lungs is the difference between pulmonary arterial and venous pressure. This region is referred to as zone III of the lung. Both pulmonary arterial and venous pressure are reduced toward the apex of the lungs. Alveolar pressure, however, remains constant. Alveolar pressure becomes greater than pulmonary venous pressure at some distance above the lung bases. The driving pressure for blood flow in this

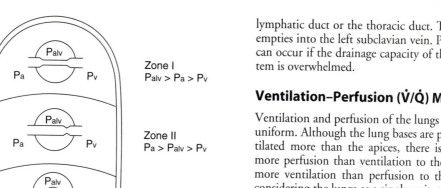

Zone I
$P_{alv} > P_a > P_v$

Zone II
$P_a > P_{alv} > P_v$

Zone III
$P_a > P_v > P_{alv}$

Figure 1–8. Schematic representation of the regional differences in blood flow related to alveolar pressure. P_{alv} is alveolar pressure, P_a is arterial blood pressure, and P_v is venous blood pressure.

region is the difference between pulmonary arterial and alveolar pressure ($P_a > P_{alv} > P_v$). This region is referred to as zone II of the lung. Arterial and venous pressures are even lower at the lung apex. In theory, they may be lowered to the extent that alveolar pressure is now greater than both vascular pressures ($P_{alv} > P_a > P_v$). There is no blood flow in this region under normal conditions. This is referred to as zone I of the lung.

Regional factors also influence the distribution of perfusion. When an area of lung is not well ventilated alveolar hypoxia causes vasoconstriction of the pulmonary circulation. Hypoxemic vasoconstriction reduces blood flow to areas with low ventilation, thereby better matching ventilation and perfusion. This regulation of blood flow is thought to occur at the precapillary arterial vessels.

The bronchial circulation provides a second supply of blood for the lungs. It is part of the systemic circulation; bronchial arterial branches originate from the aorta and drain directly into pulmonary veins. The bronchial circulation carries 1–2% of the cardiac output and supplies nutrients to most intrapulmonary structures, including airways, nerves, lymph nodes, and the visceral pleura (but not the parenchyma). There are anastomoses between the bronchial and pulmonary circulations that provide some perfusion to alveolar tissue in the event of pulmonary artery obstruction.

Lymphatic vessels also occupy the interstitial space of alveolar units. Extraalveolar interstitial fluid enters distal lymphatics and drains into hilar and mediastinal lymph nodes, the cisternae chyli, and either the right

lymphatic duct or the thoracic duct. The thoracic duct empties into the left subclavian vein. Pulmonary edema can occur if the drainage capacity of the lymphatic system is overwhelmed.

Ventilation–Perfusion ($\dot{V}/\dot{Q}$) Mismatch

Ventilation and perfusion of the lungs are not normally uniform. Although the lung bases are perfused and ventilated more than the apices, there is proportionately more perfusion than ventilation to the lung bases and more ventilation than perfusion to the apices. When considering the lungs as a single unit, the ratio of ventilation to perfusion ($\dot{V}/\dot{Q}$) is about 0.8. This average reflects a composite of lung units with $\dot{V}/\dot{Q}$ ratios that range from near "zero" (virtually unventilated) to infinity (virtually unperfused). Ventilation–perfusion mismatch occurs in disease states such as chronic bronchitis, asthma, emphysema, interstitial lung disease, and pulmonary vascular disease.

Control of Breathing

Ventilation is finely adjusted to accommodate wide fluctuations in oxygen consumption and carbon dioxide production. Control of this process is so precise that partial pressures of oxygen (PaO_2) and carbon dioxide ($PaCO_2$) in arterial blood are maintained within a narrow range. This is accomplished by integrated activity of a complex system including central respiratory centers in the brain stem and peripheral receptors in the lungs, airways, chest wall, and blood vessels. Respiratory centers in the brain process information transmitted from peripheral receptors and activate motor neurons innervating the respiratory muscles in a rhythmic fashion.

Carbon dioxide is the most important stimulus in regulating breathing. Changes in carbon dioxide tension are sensed by central and peripheral chemoreceptors. Central chemoreceptors are located in the medulla of the brain and respond to alterations in the concentration of hydrogen ion ($[H^+]$) in the extracellular fluid of the intracerebral interstitial space. Elevation of $PaCO_2$ increases carbon dioxide diffusion across the blood–brain barrier and increases $[H^+]$. Elevation in $[H^+]$ increases minute ventilation.

Peripheral chemoreceptors are located in the carotid vessels and left atrium. The most important peripheral chemoreceptors are the carotid bodies, which are located at the bifurcation of the common carotid arteries. Peripheral chemoreceptors respond to changes in $PaCO_2$ and arterial pH by signaling the respiratory center to alter ventilation. This signal is sent to the brain stem via vagal afferents. In contrast to central chemoreceptors, the carotid bodies also sense changes in arterial oxygen tension. The carotid bodies are therefore entirely responsible for increases in ventilation that accompany hypoxemia.

The respiratory system is richly endowed with sensory fibers that allow adaptation to a variety of chemical and mechanical changes. Mechanoreceptors in the chest wall include muscle spindles and tendon organs. These receptors modulate respiratory drive by sensing misalignment of muscle fibers and inhibit motor activity when the force of contraction reaches potentially injurious levels. Muscle spindles in intercostal muscles and the diaphragm help maintain tidal volume when chest wall movement is impeded. Slowly adapting stretch receptors located within smooth muscle of conducting airways respond to lung inflation to terminate inspiration. Rapidly adapting irritant receptors are located in the epithelium of extrapulmonary airways. A variety of inhaled irritants stimulate these receptors resulting in bronchoconstriction, cough, and mucus secretion. Pulmonary C-fiber receptors located in alveolar walls are stimulated by changes in the interstitial space such as accumulation of fluid or fibrotic tissue. Their stimulation results in rapid shallow breathing and increased respiratory drive. Bronchial C-fiber receptors located in airways and blood vessels respond to chemical stimuli in the bronchial arterial circulation to produce rapid shallow breathing, increased respiratory drive, and mucus secretion.

Gas Exchange

Only the volume of air that ventilates alveoli participates in gas exchange. This volume is the difference between the volume of inhaled air (V_T, tidal volume) and the volume of air that does not participate in gas exchange (V_D, deadspace volume) and is termed alveolar volume or alveolar ventilation. V_A can be calculated from the tidal volume, partial pressure of alveolar carbon dioxide (P_{ACO_2}), and partial pressure of carbon dioxide in mixed expired air (P_{ECO_2}) by the following equation:

$$V_D / V_T = (P_{ACO_2} - P_{ECO_2}) / P_{ACO_2}$$

The partial pressure of carbon dioxide in arterial blood and alveoli at end expiration is essentially identical in healthy individuals. This simplifies the equation to

$$V_D / V_T = (P_{ACO_2} - P_{ECO_2}) / P_{ACO_2}$$

V_D/V_T is normally 0.2–0.35 during quiet breathing. The average tidal volume in an average sized adult is about 500 mL and therefore alveolar volume is about 350 mL.

Alveolar ventilation and the fraction of inspired oxygen (F_{IO_2}) determine the quantity of oxygen delivered

to alveoli. The partial pressure of oxygen in the alveolus is related to the barometric pressure and the partial pressures of other gases in the alveolus by the following equation:

$$P_{AO_2} + P_{AN_2} + P_{ACO_2} + P_{AH_2O} = P_B$$

where P_{AO_2}, P_{AN_2}, P_{ACO_2}, and P_{AH_2O} are the partial pressures of oxygen, carbon dioxide, nitrogen, and water and P_B is barometric pressure.

When breathing ambient air, the pressure of inspired oxygen is the product of the ambient total gas pressure and the fraction of inspired oxygen. That is,

$$P_{IO_2} = (F_{IO_2}) (P_B)$$

Ambient air is humidified after it is inhaled. The addition of water vapor to inspired air reduces P_{IO_2} as it enters alveoli. Finally, carbon dioxide released from pulmonary capillaries into alveoli further reduces the partial pressure of oxygen in the alveolus. The alveolar gas equation describes these relationships as follows:

$$P_{AO_2} = (P_B - P_{H_2O}) (F_{IO_2}) - (P_{ACO_2} / R)$$

where P_{H_2O} is water vapor pressure (47 mm Hg at 37°C) and R is the respiratory exchange ratio ($\dot{V}_{CO_2}/\dot{V}_{O_2}$). In practice, the equation is simplified by substituting P_{ACO_2} for P_{ACO_2}. R is assumed to be 0.8 under most conditions.

Alveolar oxygen must diffuse into the capillaries to complete gas exchange. Effectiveness of this process is assessed by calculating the difference between the alveolar and arterial oxygen concentrations. This is the A–a O_2 gradient or $P_{(A-a)}O_2$:

$$P_{(A-\alpha)O_2} = P_{AO_2} - P_{aO_2}$$

The A–a O_2 gradient is normally less than 10–15 mm Hg but increases with age. The gradient exists even in healthy lungs because of ventilation–perfusion mismatching and the presence of a small right-to-left shunt. Of venous blood 1–3% normally flows into the systemic circulation. This shunt is the result of blood passing through the bronchial and left thebesian vessels (coronary venous blood).

GAS TRANSPORT

Oxygen Transport

Oxygen that has diffused from alveoli into capillaries dissolves in blood and binds to hemoglobin. Binding of oxygen to hemoglobin accounts for the vast majority of oxygen delivered by blood. The hemoglobin molecule is a complex protein composed of four polypeptide chains (2α and 2β), each of which contains a heme moiety that is able to bind oxygen. The hemoglobin sites are not fully saturated with oxygen under normal conditions. Percent saturation (SO_2) of hemoglobin indicates the portion of total oxygen-binding sites actually occupied by oxygen. The quantity of oxygen carried by hemoglobin is the product of the oxyhemoglobin saturation, the amount of hemoglobin per deciliter of blood, and the amount of oxygen each gram of hemoglobin can carry if fully saturated:

$$\text{Content of oxygen} = (1.34 \text{ mL} / \text{g})$$
$$\times \text{[Hemoglobin (g} / 100 \text{ mL)]} \times (SO_2)$$

The relationship between partial pressure of oxygen (PO_2) and percent saturation is alinear. The oxyhemoglobin dissociation curve is sigmoid shaped and provides a graphic representation of the affinity of hemoglobin for oxygen (Figure 1–9). The curve is relatively flat through the normal range of arterial blood so that moderate decreases in PaO_2 result in minimal decreases in percent saturation. Within the steep portion of the curve, a small change in PO_2 causes a large difference in saturation. The normal venous partial pressure of oxygen ($P\bar{v}O_2$) is within this range, allowing for adequate partial pressure of oxygen for diffusion to peripheral tissue, and opening binding sites for carbon dioxide on the hemoglobin molecule.

The relationship between PO_2 and SO_2 provides information about the relative affinity of hemoglobin for oxygen. This is described by the parameter P_{50}, the PO_2 associated with 50% saturation. Under usual condi-

tions the P_{50} is 27 mm Hg. A decrease in P_{50} reflects increased affinity of hemoglobin for oxygen or a shift in the curve to the left; an increase in P_{50} reflects decreased affinity or a shift in the curve to the right.

The affinity of hemoglobin for oxygen is altered by pH. When carbon dioxide is unloaded from blood into alveoli, the concentration of H^+ or PCO_2 decreases, the P_{50} decreases, and the curve shifts to the left. This aids loading oxygen in the pulmonary capillaries. When carbon dioxide is unloaded from peripheral tissue into blood, the concentration of H^+ or PCO_2 increases, the P_{50} increases, and the oxyhemoglobin dissociation curve shifts to the right. This promotes unloading of oxygen into tissue. Local changes in pH, PCO_2, and temperature in actively contracting muscles also favor unloading of oxygen. Similarly, an increase in 2,3-diphosphoglycerate (2,3-DPG), an intermediate metabolite in the red cell metabolic pathway, decreases hemoglobin–oxygen affinity by binding to hemoglobin. 2,3-DPG contributes physiologically to hemoglobin–oxygen affinity in conditions such as anemia, during acid–base abnormalities, and at altitude. Other factors that alter the affinity of hemoglobin for oxygen include carbon monoxide (which has an affinity for hemoglobin that is about 250 times greater than oxygen) and different types of hemoglobin. Human fetal hemoglobin has a P_{50} of 20 mm Hg. Affinity for oxygen may be increased or decreased in patients with hemoglobinopathies.

The quantity of oxygen dissolved in blood is much less than that bound by hemoglobin and is the product of the partial pressure of oxygen and its solubility constant (0.0031 mL/mm Hg $\times PO_2$). Total oxygen content of blood equals the sum of soluble and bound oxygen:

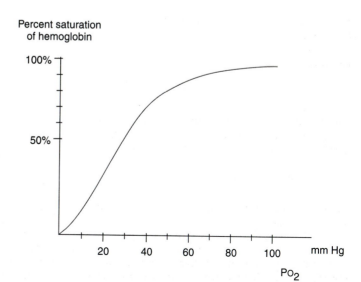

Figure 1–9. The oxyhemoglobin dissociation curve describes the relationship between hemoglobin saturation and the partial pressure of oxygen in blood.

Total content of oxygen $= (1.34 \text{ mL} / \text{g})$
$$\times [\text{Hemoglobin (g} / 100 \text{ mL})]$$
$$\times (S_{O_2}) + 0.0031 \text{ mL} / \text{Hg} \times P_{O_2}$$

Oxygen content of arterial (Ca_{O_2}) or venous ($C\bar{v}_{O_2}$) blood is calculated by substituting either arterial or mixed venous values of the partial pressure of oxygen and oxyhemoglobin saturation.

Delivery of oxygen (D_{O_2}) to peripheral tissue is a function of both the total content of oxygen in arterial blood and the cardiac output (CO):

$$D_{O_2} = Ca_{O_2} \times CO \times 10$$

where 10 is a factor to convert between liters and deciliters.

The shunt fraction can be calculated from the content of oxygen in arterial, mixed venous and capillary blood:

$$\dot{Q}s / \dot{Q}_T = (Cc_{O_2} - Ca_{O_2}) / (Cc_{O_2} - C\bar{v}_{O_2})$$

where $\dot{Q}s / \dot{Q}_T$ is the shunt fraction and Cc_{O_2} is the content of oxygen in capillary blood. The F_{IO_2} must be 100% to perform this calculation and a pulmonary artery catheter is required to obtain mixed venous blood samples. An increased shunt fraction occurs from structural abnormalities such as arteriovenous malformations, pathological processes such as lobar pneumonia or edema, or from intracardiac defects.

Carbon Dioxide Transport

Carbon dioxide is transported in blood as dissolved CO_2, carbaminohemoglobin, and bicarbonate. As with oxygen, the amount of carbon dioxide dissolved in blood is related to its partial pressure. However, the solubility of carbon dioxide is 20 times greater than that of oxygen. The relationship between Pa_{CO_2} and the amount of carbon dioxide dissolved is nonlinear. Carbon dioxide diffuses into erythrocytes and binds in part to proteins, primarily hemoglobin as carbaminohemoglobin. At normal Pa_{CO_2}, carbamino binding accounts for about 2.1 mL CO_2/100 mL blood, about 4% of the total carbon dioxide content. Most carbon dioxide is transported in blood as bicarbonate. Carbon dioxide binds with water to form carbonic acid. Carbonic acid dissociates, forming a hydrogen ion and a bicarbonate ion:

$$CO_2 + H_2O \leftrightarrow H_2CO_3 \leftrightarrow H^+ + HCO_3^-$$

Formation of bicarbonate in erythrocytes is rapid because of carbonic anhydrase. A high concentration of bicarbonate is formed in erythrocytes. As bicarbonate ions diffuse out of erythrocytes, chloride ions diffuse in to maintain electroneutrality. Extracellular formation of bicarbonate ion is much slower than intracellular because of the absence of carbonic anhydrase. Hydrogen ions formed in erythrocytes are buffered by hemoglobin, shifting the oxyhemoglobin dissociation curve to the right and facilitating the release of oxygen.

The interplay between oxygen, carbon dioxide, and hemoglobin promotes carbon dioxide loading and oxygen unloading in systemic capillaries and carbon dioxide unloading and oxygen loading in pulmonary capillaries. Hemoglobin is highly saturated in pulmonary capillaries and formation of carbaminohemoglobin is decreased, promoting unloading of carbon dioxide. This is known as the Haldane effect. As oxygen is released in systemic capillaries hemoglobin becomes less saturated and more carbon dioxide avid. This allows more carbon dioxide to bind; thus for any given Pa_{CO_2}, carbon dioxide content is increased. Even though carbamino makes up a small part of blood carbon dioxide storage, it undergoes a relatively large change between venous and arterial blood and accounts for over 25% of the carbon dioxide excreted through the lungs.

Henig NR, Pierson DJ: Mechanisms of hypoxemia. Respir Care Clin North Am 2000;6:501. [PMID: 11172576]. (This article is a thorough discussion of mechanisms of hypoxemia and tissue hypoxia.)

DEFENSE OF THE LUNGS

Thousands of liters of air are exchanged between alveoli and ambient air each day. Foreign substances (small particulate matter, microorganisms, noxious gases) enter with inhaled air through aspiration of oral and pharyngeal secretions. A variety of defense mechanisms protect the lungs from infection by these substances. These include anatomic defenses that promote deposition of particles in the upper airways and functional defenses that promote clearance of particles through actions such as cough, mucociliary activity, and cellular metabolism.

Particle deposition is an important phenomenon that prevents the majority of inhaled particles from reaching alveoli. Particle size and inspiratory flow rate are important determinants of particle deposition in upper airways. Deposition occurs in the nose and upper airways for particles of 10 µm or greater in diameter. Particles between 5 and 10 µm in diameter settle in the trachea, conducting airways, and alveoli. Particles 5 µm or less in diameter usually do not deposit in the lungs. Increase in the velocity of inspiratory flow also promotes deposition of particles by impaction in upper airways.

Particle clearance is promoted by mucociliary transport and cough. Cilia beat in a coordinated manner at frequencies of between 600 and 900 beats/min. Ciliary beating moves a blanket of mucus along the tracheobronchial tree in a cephalad direction. Two layers comprise the mucous blanket. The sol layer is adjacent to the cilia and a more viscous gel layer is located at the luminal surface. The gel layer consists of a complex polymer of mucopolysaccharides produced by goblet and mucus-secreting cells. Debris deposited on the mucous blanket move toward the oropharynx at a rate 6–20 mm/min.

Cough also facilitates clearance of airways. Cough is triggered by stimulation of irritant receptors found in the larynx, trachea, and major bronchi. These receptors are more common at points of bifurcation. The afferent pathway consists of the vagus, trigeminal, and glossopharyngeal nerves. The efferent pathway is via the recurrent laryngeal nerve, a branch of the vagus that controls the glottis, and the phrenic and spinal nerves that contract the diaphragm and expiratory muscles of the chest and abdominal walls. The initial phase of cough involves a deep inspiration. The glottis then closes and there is contraction of expiratory muscles. Intrathoracic pressures become extremely high during this phase. The glottis then opens and gas is exhaled at a high velocity. This high velocity imparts sufficient kinetic energy to the mucociliary blanket to cause dispersion and expectoration of mucus.

Several cellular defenses are triggered when particles deposit in alveoli. These include activation of phagocytic and inflammatory cells. Alveolar macrophages contain granules of digestive enzymes and are part of the mononuclear phagocyte system. They are 15–50 μm in diameter and develop from circulating monocytes. Macrophages scavenge organic and inorganic particles and process antigenic material. Foreign material encountered by macrophages attaches to the cell surface and is phagocytized. Opsonins, proteins that bind to extracellular material, increase adherence and facilitate engulfment and ingestion of particles. Intracellular digestion occurs via digestive enzymes. The foreign material is then either cleared via the mucociliary escalator or engulfed by the macrophage, which subsequently penetrates the epithelium and is transported by lymphatics to lymph nodes.

Cellular and humoral immune responses are vital in defending the lungs from infection. T-lymphocytes produce lymphokines and regulate immunoglobulin synthesis. B-lymphocytes transform into the plasma cells that produce antibodies. Lymphokines and immunoglobulins sensitize and activate cells of the defense system. Natural killer (NK) cells are lymphocytes that are capable of killing bacteria without prior sensitization. Immunoglobulin A (IgA) is a polypeptide–glycoprotein immunoglobulin complex found in the nasopharynx and upper airways. It binds to viruses and bacteria to prevent attachment and facilitate agglutination of the microorganisms. Organisms may be destroyed or detoxified by surface enzymes, lysozymes in leukocytes, and lactoferrin synthesized by polymorphonuclear cells. α_1-Antitrypsin inactivates proteolytic enzymes released from bacteria, neutrophils, and necrotic cells. Interferon is produced by macrophages and lymphocytes and has antiviral activity. Lymphocytes are found in the lymph nodes lining the trachea, carina, and at the hilum of each lung. There are some lymphocytes scattered in the parenchyma.

Welsh DA, Mason CM: Host defense in respiratory infections. Med Clin North Am 2001;85:1329. [PMID: 11680105]. (Review of the anatomic and cellular mechanisms that protect the lungs from infection.)

METABOLIC FUNCTIONS OF THE LUNGS

Although the main function of the lungs is gas exchange, the lungs have metabolic activities related to conversion or uptake of vasoactive substances, hormones, and mediators. The endothelium in the pulmonary circulation provides a large surface area for metabolism and removal of many substances. Prostaglandins E_1, E_2, and $F_2\alpha$ are removed during passage through the lungs. Bradykinin is inactivated and angiotensin I is converted to angiotensin II.

Type II alveolar epithelial cells synthesize and release surfactant; its secretion may be modulated by cyclic AMP, glucocorticoids, epidermal growth factor, and distention of the lungs. Substances involved in inflammation such as histamine, lysozomal enzymes, prostaglandins, leukotrienes, platelet-activating factor, serotonin, and chemotactic factors are released by cells in the lungs in response to pathological conditions. Some prostaglandins (E_2, $F_2\alpha$, G_2, H_2), bradykinins, histamine, and serotonin are produced and stored by cells in the lungs to be released later into the circulation.

The History & Physical Examination in Pulmonary Medicine

2

Michael E. Hanley, MD

ESSENTIALS OF DIAGNOSIS

- *Goals of the history are to develop a probable diagnosis or limited differential diagnosis and to assess severity of illness.*
- *Important features of symptoms include severity, chronicity, moderating and aggravating factors, and associated systemic symptoms.*
- *Risk factors for lung disease are identified in past medical, family, social, occupational, environmental, and drug histories.*
- *Physical examination should be directed to narrow the differential diagnosis or confirm a specific diagnosis.*
- *Pulmonary examination emphasizes assessing the quality of normal breath sounds as well as the presence and nature of adventitious sounds.*

General Considerations

Most patients present for pulmonary evaluation because they either have respiratory-related symptoms or signs or have a physical, radiographic, or physiological abnormality detected during routine health screening, evaluation of an unrelated medical problem, or through epidemiological surveys. This chapter describes the initial evaluation of these patients, focusing on interpretation of specific symptoms and physical findings. Evaluation begins with a thorough history and physical examination, with the goal of developing a specific diagnosis or narrowing the differential diagnosis. This is accomplished by characterizing the symptoms specific to the presenting illness and then searching for risk factors for the specific pulmonary conditions suggested by the history. Important qualities that help characterize presenting symptoms include their severity, chronology, aggravating or moderating factors, and associated systemic symptoms. Risk factors for pulmonary disease are sought through family, social, occupational, envi-

ronmental, and drug histories. Determining previous or concurrent nonpulmonary medical conditions that could impact the lungs is also important.

Performing a directed physical examination enhances the history and focuses the diagnostic process by searching for specific signs that either confirm the diagnosis or differentiate between various conditions that might explain the symptoms. Although the chest examination is primary, the importance of performing a complete examination cannot be overemphasized. Examination of nonpulmonary systems helps identify whether the symptoms originate from a primary pulmonary process or are pulmonary manifestations of nonpulmonary or systemic conditions such as cancer or connective tissue disorders. The physical examination also aids in assessing disease severity.

The history and physical examination are not always performed in a sequential fashion in a single interview. Although it is important to be systematic and complete in the diagnostic approach, the seasoned clinician learns to perform the directed examination as the history is obtained. Specific symptoms prompt an active search for physical findings while additional history is obtained. The evaluation also often takes place during several meetings. The first visit focuses on characterizing the history of the presenting illness, performing a broad search for risk factors, and completing a physical examination to identify the pathophysiology suggested by the history. Additional specific historical and physical clues are sought at subsequent interviews, directed by the results of tests ordered after the initial evaluation.

Medical History

A. CLINICAL MANIFESTATIONS

1. General considerations—Some patients referred for pulmonary evaluation are asymptomatic. They are referred because of abnormalities detected on chest radiograph or during assessment of nonpulmonary conditions. A discussion of the evaluation of these patients is beyond the scope of this chapter but may be found elsewhere in this book (Chapters 3, 22, 24, 41, and 42). Most symptomatic patients present with one of the four principal respiratory symptoms: dyspnea, cough with or without hemoptysis, chest pain, or wheezing.

2. Dyspnea—Under normal circumstances healthy people are not aware of their breathing. Dyspnea, or shortness of breath, is the sensation of difficult or labored breathing. Synonymous terms patients use to describe dyspnea include "breathlessness," "choking," "heavy breathing," "suffocating," and "tiredness." Occasionally patients describe dyspnea as chest tightness. In this situation the clinician must determine whether the symptom being described is truly dyspnea or chest pain.

Dyspnea results from an imbalance between ventilatory demand and capacity due to increased work of breathing, inability to perform the normal work of breathing, or a combination of these mechanisms. The perception of dyspnea is also influenced by the complex interaction of psychological factors and afferent signals from chemical and mechanical receptors. The components of work of breathing include total ventilatory demand (minute ventilation), work to overcome airway resistance, and work to overcome the elastance or stiffness of the respiratory system, which includes the lungs and thoracic cage. Ventilatory capacity depends on the mechanics of the respiratory system as well as neuromuscular performance. Increased total ventilatory demand by itself rarely causes dyspnea. For example, healthy persons increase their minute ventilation considerably during exercise but do not notice dyspnea until they near maximum exercise capacity. Psychological factors may have substantial impact on patients' perceptions of dyspnea. Because dyspnea is subjective there is significant individual variation in perception of this sensation. Most diseases cause dyspnea by multiple mechanisms, such as patients with asthma who have increased ventilatory demand due to dead space ventilation, increased work of breathing from abnormal airway resistance, and heightened awareness of breathing because of anxiety.

Diagnosing the cause of dyspnea is dependent on identifying the pattern of symptoms, in particular chronicity, circumstances in which it occurs, and associated symptoms. Specific types of dyspnea suggest certain diagnoses. Paroxysmal nocturnal dyspnea (PND) is dyspnea that awakens a patient from sleep. Patients typically describe a sensation of suffocation or air hunger one or more hours after falling asleep that is relieved within minutes of sitting up. Orthopnea is dyspnea that develops within minutes of assuming a recumbent position. PND and orthopnea are highly suggestive of a cardiac etiology, although they occur occasionally in patients with severe chronic obstructive pulmonary disease (COPD), asthma, gastroesophageal reflux, copious bronchial secretions, or aspiration. Additional history and signs of left ventricular failure help distinguish between these diagnoses. A history of cough with thick bronchial secretions, especially if purulent, suggests a primary pulmonary process. Patients with cardiac dysfunction may have cough, but it is generally dry. Heartburn suggests reflux. Caution must be exercised to avoid misinterpreting the significance of peripheral edema. Although edema suggests cardiac dysfunction, it may reflect right ventricular dysfunction secondary to cor pulmonale from a pulmonary disorder. Auscultation of the lungs is critical in making this distinction.

Other characteristics of dyspnea are associated with alternative diagnoses. Orthopnea that develops immediately upon lying down occurs in severely obese patients or patients with bilateral phrenic nerve paralysis or diaphragmatic disorders. Platypnea is dyspnea that develops or worsens in the upright position. It is nonspecific but is often associated with chronic liver disease or basilar pulmonary arteriovenous malformations. It is frequently accompanied by orthodeoxia, which is hypoxia that develops or worsens in the upright position.

Chronicity and timing are also important clues to the cause of dyspnea. Acute dyspnea is most commonly due to viral or bacterial pneumonia, asthma, pulmonary embolism, pneumothorax, pulmonary edema, aspiration, or mucous plugging of airways. Chronic, slowly progressive dyspnea is frequently caused by COPD, severe asthma refractory to bronchodilators, interstitial lung disease, or pulmonary vascular disease. Dyspnea that progresses during the work week with improvement during periods away from work suggests an occupational exposure. Seasonal variation or worsening of symptoms after exercise, exposure to cold dry air, pets, or nonspecific irritants may indicate reactive airways disease. A history of atopy or allergic symptoms also supports this diagnosis.

Evaluating dyspnea usually includes an assessment of severity. Although the degree of dyspnea rarely leads to a specific diagnosis, it does help in determining the severity of the underlying condition, monitoring responses to therapy, and in evaluation of disability. Dyspnea is graded based upon the amount of effort or work required to produce symptoms. There are, however, limitations to the usefulness of this approach. Psychological factors associated with the perception of distress make it difficult to standardize measures of dyspnea among different individuals. In addition, the degree of dyspnea reported is influenced by neurophysiological factors that can be affected by hypoxemia. Comorbidities, deconditioning, and coexistent symptoms also alter the degree of perceived dyspnea. For example, patients describe onset of dyspnea at lower levels of exercise when they also have leg pain. Finally, the metabolic demands of activity are determined by both total work performed and the rate at which work is performed.

Patients with dyspnea may reduce the rate of work performance and therefore their perception of dyspnea.

Several research scales have been developed in an effort to standardize assessment of the degree of dyspnea. These include the Oxygen Cost Diagram, Baseline Dyspnea Index, and University of California at San Diego Shortness of Breath Questionnaire. Although the reliability and validity of these scales have been documented, they remain self-assessments and their complexity limits their usefulness to practicing clinicians. Dyspnea may be more directly measured through assessment during supervised exertion such as the six-minute walk or bicycle ergometry, but these tests require referral to a specialty laboratory.

American Thoracic Society: Dyspnea. Mechanisms, assessment, and management: a consensus statement. Am J Respir Crit Care Med 1999;159:321. [PMID: 9872857]. (Comprehensive review of the pathophysiology, assessment, and management of dyspnea.)

Eakin EG et al: Validation of a new dyspnea measure: the UCSD Shortness of Breath Questionnaire. Chest 1998;113:619. [PMID: 9515834]. (Example of a dyspnea severity index questionnaire.)

Manning HL, Mahler DA: Pathophysiology of dyspnea. Monaldi Arch Chest Dis 2001;56:325. [PMID: 11770215]. (Brief review of mechanisms and assessment of dyspnea.)

Michelson E, Hollrah S: Evaluation of the patient with shortness of breath: an evidence based approach. Emerg Med Clin North Am 1999;17:221. [PMID: 10101348]. (Review of the emergency department evaluation of dyspnea with focus on causes other than reversible airway disease.)

3. Cough—Coughing protects the lungs from injury and infection by clearing large bronchial airways of accumulated secretions and foreign material. The cough reflex, which is mediated through motor nerves, results from signals transmitted in sensory nerves from irritant cough receptors to the central nervous system (CNS) cough center. Cough receptors are located throughout the respiratory tract and in extrapulmonary sites including the pleura and pericardium, auditory canals, paranasal sinuses, stomach, and diaphragm. Activation of this reflex occurs through receptor stimulation by inflammatory, mechanical, chemical, and thermal stimuli.

Chronicity is the most important characteristic to consider in evaluating cough. The most common causes of acute cough are viral or bacterial upper respiratory tract infections followed by pneumonia, aspiration, cardiogenic pulmonary edema, and rarely pulmonary embolism. Patients with viral upper respiratory tract infections rarely seek medical attention because their symptoms are self-limited and easily explained. The cause of acute cough is readily apparent in most other patients because of associated signs and symptoms of infection or heart failure. Patients who present with cough as the primary manifestation of pulmonary embolism represent a diagnostic challenge; potential clues to this diagnosis include unexplained tachycardia or hypoxia in the setting of a normal lung examination and chest radiograph.

Chronic cough is cough that lasts more than 3 weeks. The most common causes of chronic cough are tobacco-related chronic bronchitis followed by postnasal drip, occult asthma, and gastroesophageal reflux. More than 90% of patients who present for evaluation of chronic cough have one of these etiologies. Clues to these diagnoses include resolution of cough following cessation of smoking; nasal discharge, sinus tenderness, and secretions in the posterior pharynx; expiratory wheezing on lung auscultation; and regurgitation and heartburn. Less common causes include drugs (especially angiotensin-converting enzyme inhibitors and β-blockers), bronchogenic carcinoma, pneumoconioses, interstitial lung diseases, bronchiectasis, chronic infections, and nonpulmonary disorders such as cardiovascular disease and recurrent aspiration.

The medical history suggests a specific diagnosis in 70% of patients with chronic cough. Historical factors that should be considered are shown in Table 2–1. An algorithm for initial evaluation and management of chronic cough is shown in Figure 2–1.

Because most causes of cough are associated with some degree of sputum production, a history of sputum production does not limit the differential diagnosis. However, the nature and amount of sputa may be helpful. Sputum can be classified into five categories: clear and mucoid, purulent, putrid with three layers, rusty or blood-stained, and miscellaneous. Clear or mucoid sputum is usually caused by an inhaled irritant, is not the result of infection, and rarely requires antibiotic treatment. Purulent sputum suggests bacterial bronchitis or pneumonia and mandates antibiotic therapy in patients

Table 2–1. Historical clues important in the diagnosis of chronic cough.

Tobacco use
Recent change in the pattern or character of cough
Presence and quantity of sputum production
Hemoptysis
Heartburn
Improvement with antireflux therapy
Environmental and occupational inhaled exposures
Allergic and atopic histories
Nocturnal cough
Sinus symptoms
New drug exposure, especially angiotensin-converting enzyme (ACE) inhibitors and β-blocking agents
Substance abuse, especially crack cocaine

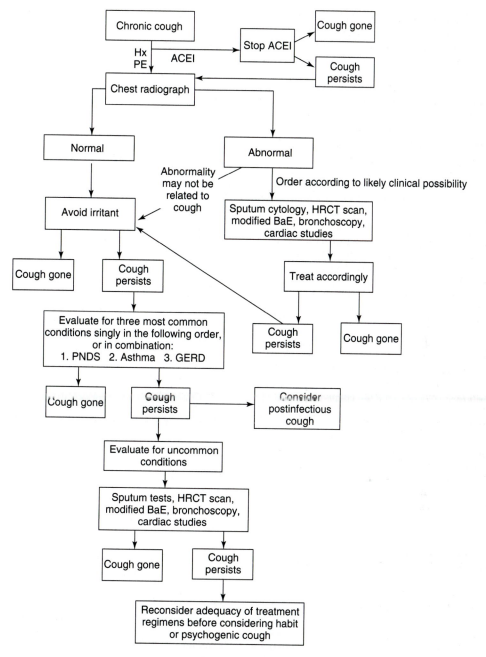

Figure 2–1. Algorithm for initial evaluation and management of patients with chronic cough. ACEI, angiotensin-converting enzyme inhibitor; BaE, barium esophagography; GERD, gastro-esophageal reflux disease; HRCT, high-resolution computed tomography; HX, history; PE, physical examination; PNDS, postnasal drip syndrome. (Reproduced, with permission from Irwin et al, Chest, 1998; 114:133S).

with exacerbations of COPD or with radiographic evidence of pneumonia. Copious putrid sputum implies an anaerobic infection such as lung abscess or necrotizing pneumonia. Severe bronchiectasis commonly is associated with production of copious amounts of purulent sputum that typically settles into three layers: a mucous layer above, a watery layer in the middle, and a purulent sediment below. Rusty or uniformly blood-stained sputum indicates the presence of red blood cells or hemoglobin. Cardiac causes and primary pulmonary inflammatory conditions should be considered. Two rare but characteristic sputa that suggest specific diagnoses are clear, golden-yellow sputum that accompanies biliary tract bronchial fistuli and copious watery sputum associated with alveolar cell carcinoma.

Evaluation of cough in tobacco users is especially challenging. For many smokers cough is due only to tobacco-related airway irritation and evaluation of the symptom in this setting results in unnecessary, expensive diagnostic tests. However, cough in this population may also be the first indication of a more serious problem such as chronic bronchitis, emphysema, or bronchogenic carcinoma. Clues that suggest one of these conditions include persistent, severe, or worsening cough, change in sputum production, hemoptysis, or constitutional symptoms such as weight loss and fatigue.

Cough is occasionally accompanied by hemoptysis, defined as expectoration of blood from the lower respiratory tract. Hemoptysis is categorized according to the amount of blood expectorated. Scant hemoptysis is characterized by blood streaking of sputa. Expectoration of less than 600 mL of blood but more than blood streaking is referred to as frank or gross hemoptysis. Massive hemoptysis is expectoration of more than 600 mL of blood in a 24-h period. Gross or massive hemoptysis warrants immediate evaluation. Initial evaluation should include careful examination of the nose and oropharynx to exclude pseudohemoptysis, which is expectoration of blood from a source other than the lower respiratory tract, such as aspirated blood from epistaxis or upper gastrointestinal hemorrhaging.

Although hemoptysis occasionally occurs because of abnormal hemostasis, it is most commonly due to disorders involving the airways, vasculature, or pulmonary parenchyma (Table 2–2). The differential diagnosis of hemoptysis depends on several factors, including amount and duration of bleeding, patient's age and smoking history, radiographic findings, and accompanying symptoms such as weight loss, chest pain, and fever. The volume of blood expectorated influences both the differential diagnosis and potential mortality. Massive hemoptysis is a medical emergency associated with significant mortality that requires monitoring in an intensive care unit. Acute bronchitis, the most com-

Table 2–2. Common causes of hemoptysis.

Systemic hemostasis
  Anticoagulant therapy
  Disseminated intravascular coagulation
  Thrombocytopenia

Airways disease
  Acute tracheobronchitis
  Bronchial adenoma
  Bronchiectasis
  Bronchogenic carcinoma
  Broncholithiasis
  Chronic bronchitis
  Cystic fibrosis
  Endobronchial metastasis
  Endobronchial tuberculosis
  Foreign body aspiration
  Tracheobronchial trauma

Parenchyma disease
  Aspergilloma
  Acute lupus pneumonitis
  Bacterial pneumonia
  Fungal pneumonia
  Goodpasture's syndrome
  Idiopathic pulmonary hemosiderosis
  Lung abscess
  Lung contusion
  Metastatic cancer
  Pulmonary tuberculosis
  Viral pneumonia
  Wegener's granulomatosis

Pathology in the vasculature
  Aortic aneurysm
  Congestive heart failure
  Mitral stenosis
  Pulmonary arteriovenous malformation
  Pulmonary embolism
  Schistosomiasis

mon cause of hemoptysis in the United States, is typically scant. It does not require extensive evaluation unless it is associated with an abnormal chest radiograph or is refractory to antibiotics. Bronchogenic carcinoma is uncommon in nonsmokers and patients under 35 years of age. Historical clues to this diagnosis include recent change in severity or character of cough and constitutional symptoms such as weight loss, fever, and anorexia.

Chronic cough is occasionally due to nonrespiratory tract disorders. Additional history for extrapulmonary or systemic diseases should be sought when symptoms do not suggest a pulmonary source. Heart disease associated with pulmonary venous hypertension such as cryptic mitral stenosis or left ventricular failure and neurological or gastrointestinal disorders that cause silent reflux or cryptic aspiration may present with cough. Occult aspiration can occasionally be detected by observing the patient swallow a glass of water. Immediate coughing suggests aspiration, with the rapidity and severity of the cough directly related to the size and severity of aspiration.

Hirshberg B et al: Hemoptysis: etiology, evaluation, and outcome in a tertiary referral hospital. Chest 1997;112:440. [PMID: 9266882]. (Retrospective analysis of etiology and outcome in 208 patients with hemoptysis.)

Irwin RS et al: Managing cough as a defense mechanism and as a symptom: a consensus panel report of the American College of Chest Physicians. Chest 1998;114:133S. [PMID: 9725800]. (Thorough review of pathophysiology, etiology, assessment, and management of chronic cough.)

Irwin RS: The diagnosis and treatment of cough. N Engl J Med 2000;343:1715. [PMID: 11106722]. (Concise review of evaluation of chronic cough.)

Irwin RS, Madison JM: Anatomic diagnostic protocol in evaluating chronic cough with specific reference to gastroesophageal reflux disease. Am J Med 2000;108:126S. [PMID: 10718465]. (Brief review of utility of a diagnostic protocol for chronic cough.)

Irwin RS, Madison JM: The persistently troublesome cough. Am J Respir Crit Care Med 2002;165:1469. [PMID: 12045118]. (Review of management of cough of greater than 2 months duration in immunocompetent adults.)

Jean-Baptiste E: Clinical assessment and management of massive hemoptysis. Crit Care Med 2000;28:1642. [PMID: 10834728]. (Review of evaluation and management of patients with massive hemoptysis, including discussion of the role of bronchial artery embolization.)

4. Chest pain—The differential diagnosis of chest pain is extensive. It may originate from any organ within the chest as well as the visceral and parietal pleura, diaphragm, chest wall, and overlying skin. The exception to this is the lung parenchyma, which is free of sensory fibers. Pathological pulmonary processes are associated with chest pain only when there is involvement of the adjacent pleura, chest wall, mediastinum, or diaphragm.

The cornerstone of the evaluation of chest pain is the nature of the pain. Critical characteristics include the quality, location, radiation, and duration of pain. Moderating or aggravating factors are also important. The severity of chest pain is rarely helpful in establishing a diagnosis. The quality and location of chest pain are related to the sensory innervation of the lesion that causes it. Chest pain can be classified into two main diagnostic categories by history: visceral cardiac and somatic pleuritic pain. The heart, pericardium, and mediastinal structures are innervated through autonomic pathways that travel through the vagus nerve. Pain associated with mediastinal and cardiac disease typically has a visceral pattern and is described as dull, heavy, pressure-like, or crushing. It is central in location, usually substernal or epigastric, and radiates to the arms and neck. Pain due to myocardial ischemia results from imbalance between supply and demand of myocardial oxygen. It is aggravated by activities that increase cardiac workload or induce coronary artery spasm, such as exertion, cold air, heavy meals, or emotional upset, and is relieved by rest. Persistent, intense pain of a cardiac quality that is not relieved by rest or vasodilating medications suggests myocardial infarction. Associated symptoms may include diaphoresis, palpitations, nausea, vomiting, and syncope.

Pericardial pain has both a cardiac and pleuritic quality because the adjacent visceral mediastinal and parietal chest wall pleura are often involved. Chest pain from pericarditis is constant and substernal in location. It is aggravated by breathing or lying in a recumbent position, especially on the left side, and is improved by sitting, leaning forward, or lying on the right side. The pain may radiate to the shoulder or neck if the adjacent diaphragmatic pleura is involved. Signs of cardiac tamponade should be sought if pericarditis is suspected. These include tachycardia, jugular venous distention, Kussmaul's sign (persistent or paradoxical increase of jugular venous distention during inspiration), pulsus paradoxus, and hypotension. Presence of these signs warrants emergent evaluation, including echocardiogram, right-sided heart catheterization, or pericardiocentesis.

Sensory innervation of the chest wall and diaphragmatic parietal pleural is through afferent fibers in the intercostal nerves. Chest pain from disease processes involving these structures is typically achy or sharp and well localized to the involved area. The pain is aggravated by coughing or deep breathing and is improved by shallow breathing or breath holding. Patients with pleuritic pain may complain of dyspnea because of pain-induced increased awareness of breathing and have evidence of chest wall splinting on physical examination. Pain originating from irritation of the diaphragmatic parietal pleura commonly radiates to the ipsilateral shoulder or side of the neck. Important additional clues in the evaluation of pleuritic chest pain include recent thoracic trauma or paroxysmal coughing, acuity of the pain, associated systemic symptoms, and localizing signs on physical examination. The acuity of pleurisy is determined by the rate of progression of the underlying disease. Pneumothorax, fractured ribs, or pulmonary embolism cause sudden, acute pain. Pleuritic pain from acute infectious causes such as viral or bacterial pneumonia is rapid in onset, progressive over several days, and associated with systemic inflammatory signs and symptoms such as fever, sweats, chills, myalgias, arthralgias, and malaise. In contrast, pain from chronic conditions such as tuberculous pleuritis, asbestos-induced pleural disease, metastatic cancer, and occasionally anaerobic pleuropulmonary infections has a more subtle onset and progresses over weeks to months. Examination of the involved chest wall area and adjacent structures, including the lung and upper abdomen, may lead to specific diagnoses. Point tenderness over a rib after trauma or coughing paroxysms suggests a rib fracture; point tenderness over one or more costochondral junctions, especially associated with localized warmth and erythema, indicates costochondritis or infectious costal arthritis.

Esophageal, upper gastrointestinal, and subdiaphragmatic diseases may cause chest pain that can be mistaken for cardiac or lung disease. Primary abdominal processes such as pancreatitis or cholecystitis should be considered in the differential diagnosis of lower chest pain, especially when unexplained pleural effusions exist. Esophagitis and esophageal spasm are usually associated with a history of heartburn, reflux, dysphagia, and odynophagia. If symptoms suggest an esophageal origin, a trial of an antacid/antireflux regimen should be administered before a more expensive and invasive evaluation is initiated.

Jouriles NJ: Atypical chest pain. Emerg Med Clin North Am 1998;16:717. [PMID: 9889737]. (Review of evaluation of chest pain with focus on noncardiac conditions.)

5. Wheezing, stridor, and snoring—Patients occasionally complain of audible sounds that can be heard without a stethoscope. The most frequent of these are wheezing, stridor, and snoring. These sounds occur from abnormal turbulent airflow at different sites in the respiratory tract. Snoring is easily distinguished from the others because it is a coarse, low-pitched sound that occurs only during sleep. It is associated with disorders involving the nasopharynx, oropharynx, and hypopharynx. Snoring is quite common, especially in men, and usually does not require evaluation. The most common pathological condition associated with it is obstructive sleep apnea. Clues to this diagnosis include daytime somnolence, morning headache, or unexplained erythrocytosis. Clinical manifestations of sleep-related breathing disorders are covered in detail in Chapter 28.

Discriminating stridor from audible wheezes can occasionally be difficult. Both are high-pitched, musical sounds that may occur during either phase of the respiratory cycle. However, wheezes are softer in quality and more likely to be heard during exhalation. They are discussed in more detail later in this chapter. Stridor is a harsh, loud sound of constant pitch. It is most commonly associated with disorders involving the larynx or trachea. Inspiratory stridor is usually laryngeal in origin whereas predominantly expiratory stridor suggests an intrathoracic cause. Stridor implies that critical narrowing of a major airway exists and represents a medical emergency with potential for complete airway obstruction and asphyxiation. The airway should be emergently evaluated with direct laryngoscopy, bronchoscopy, and/or soft tissue neck radiographs. Patients with stridor should be closely monitored in an intensive care unit and attended by personnel trained in airway management.

B. OTHER MEDICAL HISTORY

1. Past medical history—Pulmonary disease may represent only one manifestation of a systemic process. In addition, many chronic diseases follow cycles of remission and exacerbation. A thorough review of previous hospitalizations, medical evaluations, and history of other illnesses helps identify risk factors for specific pulmonary disorders and may uncover previously diagnosed dormant conditions that are again active. It also clarifies the chronicity of the current illness. Critical to this process is obtaining prior chest radiographs that can be reviewed.

2. Social and family history—Risk factors for lung disease can frequently be identified through a history of the patient's life-style and habits. Important areas to explore include sexual behavior, substance abuse, animal exposure, and hobbies. The history obtained may require confirmation through interviews with close associates. Risk factors associated with human immunodeficiency virus infection should be sought in patients presenting with opportunistic infections, pulmonary non-Hodgkin's lymphoma, or Kaposi's sarcoma. Clues to the diagnosis of atypical infections include travel to or residence in areas endemic for the infection or hobbies associated with exposure to sites or animals that are vectors for the infectious organism. A history of remote residence in endemic areas may be important in immunocompromised patients as active infection may initially present as dissemination of a previously acquired but dormant infection.

The family history is important for two reasons. First, it helps identify risk for genetically transmitted lung diseases. A number of lung diseases have a well-established genetic basis. These include cystic fibrosis, α_1-antiprotease deficiency, and hereditary telangiectasia. Other conditions, such as asthma and COPD, have a strong familial predisposition. A family history of these disorders should be sought where appropriate. The family history also helps identify illnesses related to common exposures, especially infections. Recent exposure to persons with transmittable infections such as influenza, varicella, and tuberculosis is an important clue to the diagnosis of these conditions. It is important to remember that the exposure for some infections, such as tuberculosis, may be quite remote in time.

3. Occupational and environmental history—Information about potential exposures through occupation or the environment is useful in evaluating patients with interstitial lung disease and asthma. Important clues are often based upon changes in the behavior of symptoms following exposure to or removal from various environments. Every dwelling in which the patient spends a significant period of time should be considered part of the home environment. Often overlooked are the homes of friends and life partners. Identification of specific agents that may contribute to illness requires specialized knowledge of workplace environments and may necessitate referral to an occupational medicine specialist. The occupational and environmental interview requires a detailed, systematic approach, as many exposure histories may be subtle or forgotten by the patient. For this reason, questionnaires that require the patient to systematically review his or her employment record, military service, hobbies and recreational activities, home environment, pets, and other potential exposures are helpful.

Pulmonary Physical Examination

A. GENERAL CONSIDERATIONS

Over the past few decades there has been increasing dependence on radiography at the expense of diminished clinical skills by providers. Although the chest radiograph is an indispensable tool in the diagnosis of lung disease it does have limitations. Plain radiography has little value in detecting thromboembolic disease and conditions that cause airflow obstruction, correlates poorly with the degree of physiological abnormalities, and is limited by significant interobserver variation in interpretation. Overdependence on chest radiographs, especially in monitoring patients, is wasteful and expensive, and leaves the clinician ill-prepared when practicing in a setting that lacks radiographic support. These limitations emphasize the need for care providers to maintain well-polished clinical skills and expertise in interpretation of physical findings. Physical evaluation of patients with respiratory symptoms should include both physical examination and chest radiography. The two techniques are complementary.

B. GENERAL EXAMINATION

Although the evaluation of patients with respiratory symptoms typically focuses on the chest examination, it is essential to assess nonpulmonary systems as well. Primary pulmonary disorders frequently have extrapulmonary manifestations and pulmonary symptoms often result from nonpulmonary conditions. This is especially true with regard to the cardiovascular system. Because of the complex interaction between the heart and lungs, dysfunction in one organ may in fact represent end-organ damage from a disease process originating in the other. A thorough cardiovascular examination including evaluation of neck veins, auscultation for murmurs, gallops, and adventitious heart sounds, palpation for heaves or lifts, and inspection for edema should be performed in all pulmonary patients. Special attention should be given to signs of pulmonary hypertension such as a tricuspid regurgitant murmur or an accentuated pulmonic heart sound (P_2).

Clubbing and cyanosis are also important extrapulmonary signs. Clubbing is nonspecific but quite common in many pulmonary diseases. It is distinctly uncommon in COPD and its detection in this disorder should prompt a search for bronchogenic carcinoma. True clubbing is characterized by an increased terminal tuft, increase in the angle between the nailbed and proximal skin to greater than 180 degrees, sponginess of the nailbed, and increased nail curvature. It must be differentiated from other nailbed abnormalities that mimic it in appearance. Cyanosis is a dark blue or bluish-gray discoloration of the skin, mucous membranes, and nailbeds associated with an increased percentage of reduced hemoglobin in the capillaries of these tissues. It can be very difficult or impossible to detect in patients with anemia or under fluorescent lighting. Cyanosis results from either inadequate oxygen saturation of arterial blood (central cyanosis), poor capillary perfusion (peripheral cyanosis), or both. It is frequently difficult to distinguish between central and peripheral cyanosis, although measurement of arterial oxygen saturation by pulse oximetry or arterial blood gases can be helpful.

C. CHEST EXAMINATION

Direct chest examination is based on four basic skills: inspection, palpation, percussion, and auscultation.

1. Inspection—Inspection includes an appraisal of the degree of respiratory distress, use of accessory muscles of respiration, and general examination of the thorax. Shape, symmetry, and movement of the thorax should be observed, including presence of kyphoscoliosis. The pattern of breathing should be noted. Commonly recognized abnormal patterns include tachypnea (rapid shallow breathing), hyperpnea (rapid deep breathing), bradypnea (slow breathing), and Cheyne–Stokes respirations (rhythmic waxing and waning in both rate and depth including apneic periods). The latter is common in small children and sleeping adults but also occasionally occurs with cardiac and neurological disorders. Hyperpnea in response to metabolic acidosis is termed

Kussmaul breathing. Rapid shallow breathing is an ominous sign. It is indicative of impending respiratory collapse when associated with very high respiratory rates (greater than 40 breaths/min in adults) or paradoxical thoracic/upper abdominal movement (inward abdominal retraction during inspiration). Emergent intubation may be required if the cause cannot be quickly reversed.

2. Palpation and percussion—Palpation and percussion have low sensitivity in identifying chest abnormalities. They therefore have limited value as screening techniques and do not need to be performed in every patient. Both techniques are helpful in clarifying the pathophysiology associated with abnormal auscultation. Dullness to percussion and decreased tactile fremitus suggest a pleural effusion or lobar atelectasis; dullness with increased fremitus occurs with lung consolidation. Hyperresonance associated with decreased fremitus suggests pneumothorax. Palpation is also useful in assessing chest wall pathology and movement. Important signs to search for include point tenderness in patients with chest pain or trauma, crepitus related to subcutaneous emphysema, and tumor masses arising from chest malignancies.

3. Auscultation—Auscultation of the lungs should be performed in a quiet environment free of distractions. The quality of lung sounds normally varies from region to region, necessitating systematic comparison of symmetrical lung regions. Auscultation should be performed over the anterior, midaxillary, and posterior chest regions; posterior auscultation proceeds from the apex to the base of the thorax. Lung sounds are assessed during quiet breathing followed by a deep breath, with special attention to the quality and intensity of normal breath sounds and presence of adventitious sounds.

The quality and intensity of normal breath sounds depend on the proximity of larger airways and the thickness of the underlying chest wall. Normal breath sounds include tracheal, bronchovesicular, and vesicular sounds. They are differentiated from one another based upon the duration of each phase of the respiratory cycle and their intensity and pitch. Tracheal sounds, which are normally heard during auscultation over the sternum, are relatively louder and higher pitched with an expiratory phase equal to or longer than inspiration. Vesicular sounds, which are normally heard during auscultation over the lung bases, are softer and relatively low-pitched. Vesicular sounds cannot be heard throughout the entire expiratory phase, resulting in the perception that the inspiratory phase is longer than expiration. Tracheal sounds heard over the lung periphery are called bronchial breath sounds. These result from enhanced transmission of sounds by pathological processes in the underlying lung and have a hollow or tubular character. They are commonly heard with lung consolidation and at the upper level of pleural effusions. Other signs of enhanced sound transmission heard in consolidated or atelectatic lung are egophony, bronchophony, and whispered pectoriloquy. Egophony is increased transmission of voice-generated sounds through the chest. When spoken words are transmitted clearly and distinctly, egophony is characterized as either bronchophony (if the words were spoken) or whispered pectoriloquy (if the words were whispered).

Adventitious lung sounds do not naturally occur in healthy persons. They originate from diseases in either the bronchopulmonary tree or pleura. Unfortunately there is significant confusion regarding the terminology used to describe adventitious sounds from the bronchopulmonary tree. Laennec originally referred to all adventitious sounds as rales, further classifying them as sibilant, sonorous, or crepitant, and used the term ronchus synonymously with rale. Unfortunately, the specificity of these terms was lost when his works were translated into English, resulting in confusion that has grown over the past 150 years. In 1985 The International Lung Sounds Association, in an effort to reduce confusion regarding these terms, recommended adoption of a standardized nomenclature system. Their schema, which is based on acoustic analysis of lung sounds, is now widely accepted. It limits descriptive terms to wet and dry crackles, wheezes, and rhonchi.

Crackles are discontinuous short, nonmusical, explosive sounds typically superimposed on underlying normal breath sounds. Although crackles may be subclassified as either fine or coarse, there is significant interobserver variation in making this distinction. Crackles are occasionally heard during expiration, but are more common in inspiration. They are associated with infiltrative lung diseases and conditions complicated by increased airway secretions.

Wheezes are continuous lung sounds that have a high-pitched, sibilant, musical quality. They may occur in either phase of the respiratory cycle but are more common during expiration, when airway caliber is smaller. The appearance of wheezes during a forced expiratory maneuver is common in healthy adults, limiting the clinical utility of this maneuver in the diagnosis of mild asthma. Wheezes can occur in any condition associated with bronchospasm, mucosal edema and congestion, intraluminal mucus accumulation, external airway compression, or dynamic airway narrowing, but are most commonly heard in patients with asthma and COPD. Wheezing that is localized to a specific part of the chest suggests focal obstruction of a larger bronchus by a neoplasm or foreign body.

Rhonchi are also continuous lung sounds but they have a low pitch and a tonal, sonorous quality. They are also associated with diseases characterized by airway narrowing.

Friction rubs are adventitious sounds that originate in the pleura. They are loud, coarse sounds that have a raspy or leathery quality. Rubs typically have an evanescent quality with variable intensity and may disappear altogether if a pleural effusion develops. Pleural rubs indicate thickening or inflammation of the pleura and are commonly associated with trauma, infections, neoplasm, or infarction.

Pasterkamp H, Kraman SS, Wodicka GR: Respiratory sounds. Advances beyond the stethoscope. Am J Respir Crit Care Med 1997;156:974. [PMID: 9310022]. (Thorough review of the scientific basis, acoustical analysis, and clinical significance of lung sounds.)

Diagnostic Imaging

Charles E. Ray, Jr., MD, & Linda M. Fielding, MD

General Considerations

There have been a number of discoveries over the past several decades that have changed the course of modern medicine. It is difficult to imagine, for instance, the practice of medicine without the use of antibiotics for infection and chemotherapeutic agents for neoplasms. The world in which medicine was practiced less than two generations ago, however, included neither of these types of agents. Other discoveries, often made serendipitously, have also significantly changed the way in which medicine is practiced. The discovery of the x-ray by Wilhelm Röntgen in 1895 is one such example.

Röntgen noticed a fluorescent glow arising from some barium-covered photographic plates while working on a Crooke's tube in his laboratory. Because the plates could obtain the phosphorescent glow only by being exposed to radiation and because no form of radiation known at the time had the ability to penetrate the black paper covering the plates, Röntgen proposed a mysterious new form of radiation that he called "x-rays." A few weeks later Röntgen presented his discovery at a physics conference and shortly thereafter in printed form as a brief 10-page paper. The first reports of the clinical utility of the new rays were published within the year; Röntgen had opened the way for a new field of medicine subsequently known as radiology. He was awarded the first Nobel Prize in physics for his discovery.

The clinical practice of radiology initially consisted solely of images obtained with a combination of x-rays and photographic film. The field now includes such diverse modalities as x-rays, nuclear medicine studies, angiography, computed tomography (CT), ultrasound (US), and magnetic resonance imaging (MRI). In addition, the realm of radiology has extended beyond the diagnostic arena into therapy; radiation therapy and interventional radiology are specialties within the field of radiology that are primarily concerned with treatment of patients.

The form of ionizing radiation that produces x-rays can, however, be detrimental. Case reports of radiation burns suffered as a result of working with x-rays appeared a few months following Röntgen's discovery; in 1896, 23 cases of radiodermatitis were reported. The Curie family, frequently credited with discovering natural radiation sources in the form of radium, suffered severely from radiation-induced disease. Marie Curie and her daughter Irene both died from leukemia, and Pierre had leukemia when he was killed in a carriage accident. It took many years for radiation safety to become standard in the field of radiology and many patients as well as practitioners suffered ill effects from what were once considered harmless rays.

Several modifications in the x-ray tube have made modern imaging modalities significantly safer than those around the start of the twentieth century. Proper shielding used on both x-ray tubes and patients significantly decreases exposure of patients and surrounding personnel. In addition, more homogeneous x-ray beams, leading to a decrease in the amount of harmful low-energy x-rays, has significantly decreased the risk to patients. Other developments, such as proper collimation of beams for plain x-rays and CT scanning, digital imaging, and MRI safety issues, have increased safety in medical imaging. Table 3–1 lists general radiation doses for commonly performed radiological procedures. To illustrate the actual risk of medical radiation exposure, if one million individuals received a lifetime whole-body dose of 1 rad, approximately 300 individuals (0.03%) would have some form of radiation-induced cancer. With the possible exception of some invasive examinations performed in interventional radiology and some early pregnancies, there are no instances in which a radiological procedure should not be performed due to fear of exposure to the radiation delivered.

Meyers MA: Glen W. Hartman Lecture. Science, creativity, and serendipity. AJR 1995;165:755. [PMID: 7676963]. (Interesting review of the discovery of x-rays.)

Normal Chest Radiograph Anatomy

Each of the various imaging modalities used to assess pulmonary pathology (radiography, CT, MRI, US, nuclear medicine studies, etc) has unique patterns of normal anatomy and pathology. Describing each of these modalities is beyond the scope of this chapter, however, a brief review of normal anatomy and methods of interpreting plain radiographs is presented below.

To understand pathological processes involving chest radiographs, normal anatomy and common variants on that anatomy that may involve chest structures must be completely understood. Although normal

Table 3–1. Doses of common radiological procedures.

Radiological Procedure	Whole-Body Dose (mrem)
Dental	2
Chest x-ray	10
Lumbar spine	130
CT head	200
Barium enema	1100
Ultrasound	0
MRI	0

Adapted from Paul and Juhl's *Essentials of Radiologic Imaging*, ed 5, Juhl JH, Crummy AB (editors). Lippincott, 1987, p 17.

anatomy is relatively easy to describe it is important to understand that "normal" actually encompasses a wide range of sizes and measurements. Slight variations in techniques such as minimal rotation of the patient and nominal changes in the degree of inspiratory effort may significantly change the appearance of the radiograph, all in the absence of real pathology.

As with the interpretation of any imaging study, only by having a systematic approach to interpretation of radiographs can the interpreter be certain that unexpected pathology is not missed. For instance, if a radiograph is obtained to confirm pneumonia and pneumoperitoneum or rib fracture is missed, the patient will likely be mismanaged regardless of the presence or absence of the suspected pneumonia.

A systematic approach can take many forms and the order in which all structures are assessed is simply the preference of the interpreter. The structures that must be assessed are listed in Table 3–2 and the order in which they are listed is the authors' own preference.

A. HEART

The cardiac silhouette can be evaluated on both the frontal and lateral views of the chest. Cardiomegaly is suggested by a cardiac silhouette that takes up slightly more than one-half of the thoracic diameter. In other words, if the heart is smaller than one of the lung fields, the patient does not have cardiomegaly.

Table 3–2. Structures to assess on CXR.

Heart
Pulmonary vascularity
Mediastinum
Pleura and pleural space
Lung parenchyma
Bones and soft tissues
Abdomen

Certain mediastinal structures are routinely visualized as projections off the mediastinal contour (Figure 3–1). Bulges along the lower right side of the heart on frontal radiographs typically are due to enlargement of the right atrium, whereas enlargement of the lower left side of the heart is associated with left ventricular enlargement. Left ventricular enlargement is particularly suspected if there is elevation of the apex of the heart off the left hemidiaphragm. Right ventricular and left atrial enlargement are generally best noted on lateral radiographs; the former is suspected when there is filling in of the retrosternal airspace (Figure 3–1) and the latter when soft tissue extends behind the lower margin of the heart.

B. PULMONARY VASCULARITY

Normal pulmonary vascularity is generally well defined and the vessels cannot be followed out to the edge of the lung fields on chest radiographs. Pulmonary vessels can usually be visualized to within approximately 2 cm of the pleural surface, except for the lung apices, where they can be visualized to approximately 3 cm. Pulmonary vessels become larger from the lung apices to the lung bases; vessels the same distance from the hilum going to upper lung fields are smaller than those going to lower lung fields. This is likely due to gravity and increased flow to the more capacious lower lobes of the lungs. "Cephalization" of the blood vessels occurs when this radiological finding is reversed; it is one of the early signs of congestive heart failure. Perivascular and interstitial edema due to congestive heart failure is also suspected when there are indistinct margins around vessels and the remainder of the structures are clear.

The main pulmonary arteries and veins make up the pulmonary hila. The size of the hilar silhouettes depends at least in part on variables such as the fluid status of the patient and inspiratory effort during film exposure. Central pulmonary vessels should have a smooth, tapered appearance as they progress to the lung periphery. Any abrupt change in contour is suggestive of underlying pathology, such as mediastinal adenopathy. In addition, if vessels are significantly larger centrally than they are peripherally ("pruned tree appearance"), the patient likely has underlying pulmonary arterial hypertension.

C. MEDIASTINUM

The mediastinal silhouette is composed of numerous vital structures. The mediastinum is generally separated into superior, anterior, middle, and posterior compartments. This separation facilitates formulating a differential diagnosis for abnormal processes. The mediastinum contains all of the vital structures of the chest except the pulmonary parenchyma. The superior mediastinum lies between the manubrium and thoracic vertebrae one through four. The anterior mediastinum is bounded by

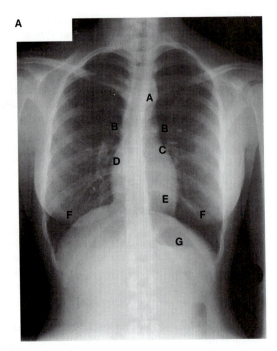
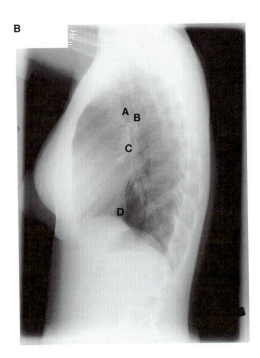

Figure 3-1. Normal CXR. Normal frontal (**A**) and lateral (**B**) radiographs of the chest demonstrating normal anatomy. **A:** A, aortic knob; B, pulmonary hilum; C, left atrial contour; D, right atrial contour; E, left ventricular contour; F, breast shadows; G, gastric air bubble. **B:** A, trachea; B, air in esophagus; C, pulmonary hilum; D, inferior vena cava/pericardial reflection.

the sternum anteriorly and pericardium posteriorly. The middle mediastinum consists of the heart and vascular structures noted on lateral radiograph; anything in the middle of the chest that is radiodense on lateral radiograph is within the middle mediastinum. The posterior mediastinum lies between the heart and the vertebral bodies. Vital structures contained within mediastinal compartments are listed in Table 3–3.

Normal mediastinal contours are shown in Figure 3–1. Prominences projecting off the normal mediastinal contour occasionally represent normal variations of anatomy rather than true pathology. A protuberance off the aortic arch, termed the aortic nipple, likely represents the left superior intercostal vein as it courses adjacent to the aorta. A widened superior mediastinum, which may be indicative of mediastinal hematoma in trauma patients, can commonly be seen on radiographs taken in the supine position with a poor inspiratory effort.

D. PLEURA AND PLEURAL SPACE

The pleura, which normally is a thin investiture of the lung surface, can be involved in a number of pathological processes. Pathology typically presents as either focal pleural thickening or as reactive pleural fluid.

Normal pleura can be visualized if the pleural surface is tangent to the x-ray beam. Certain pleural surfaces, or lines, are normal and should be assessed with each radiograph. The most important of these are the anterior and posterior junctional lines and the right paratracheal stripe. The junction lines, visualized as thin vertical white lines, represent the apposition of the pleural surfaces of the right and left upper lobes. The anterior junction line is usually projected over the trachea on frontal radiographs, and extends several centimeters inferiorly from the upper portion of the sternum. The posterior junctional line extends from the level of the thoracic inlet to the aortic arch. Both junctional lines should be less than 3 mm thick.

The right paratracheal stripe is a thin white vertical stripe that consists of the pleural surface of the right upper lobe and the lateral wall of the trachea. It should also measure 3–4 mm in diameter; thickening of the paratracheal stripe may be due to adjacent inflammatory or neoplastic changes.

E. LUNG PARENCHYMA

The majority of chest radiographs are obtained to evaluate the lung parenchyma. Assessing the lung fields can

Table 3–3. Mediastinal structures.

Anterior mediastinum
Lymph nodes
Thymus
Thyroid
Parathyroids
Internal mammary vessels

Middle mediastinum
Heart and pericardium
Ascending aorta
Superior vena cava
Azygous vein
Phrenic and vagus nerves
Trachea and main bronchi
Pulmonary arteries and veins
Lymph nodes

Posterior mediastinum
Descending aorta
Esophagus
Thoracic duct
Azygous and hemiazygous veins
Vagus nerves
Lymph nodes

Superior mediastinum
Aortic arch
Brachiocephalic and subclavian vessels
Trachea
Thymus
Thyroid
Esophagus

Adapted from Zylak CJ et al: Radiographics 1982;2:555.

be difficult, especially in the presence of underlying disease such as pulmonary vascular cephalization. A standard approach to assessing the lung fields must be undertaken every time radiographs are interpreted.

When assessing the lung fields, it is helpful to compare one hemithorax to the other in a step-by-step fashion. In other words, the lung underlying the first intercostal space on the right is compared to that on the left, followed by the second intercostal space, and so forth. It is vital not to forget to assess lung fields underlying superimposed ribs; small pulmonary nodules or other densities can be partially obscured by ribs. In the rare instance of bilaterally symmetric disease, comparison of the upper and lower lung fields of one hemithorax may also prove helpful.

Several pitfalls should be avoided when assessing the pulmonary parenchyma. Overlying shadows can mimic pathology and should be recognized as normal. In particular, in female patients overlying breast tissue gives the appearance of increased density within lower lung fields. As compared to lung pathology, overlying breast

tissue does not obscure any normal pulmonary structures, such as the pulmonary vasculature. With true air-space disease, such as pneumonia, adjacent vessels will be obscured. In addition to fatty breast tissue, nipples can also mimic well-defined pulmonary nodules. In some instances, particularly if the findings are not bilaterally symmetric, repeating the radiograph with radio-dense nipple markers helps to differentiate nipples from lung parenchymal disease.

One of the most common errors in reading radiographs is incompletely evaluating the lung parenchyma. There is a significant amount of pulmonary parenchyma behind the cardiac silhouette and behind the diaphragmatic reflections on the frontal view. These regions are visualized well on lateral projections. In the absence of a lateral radiograph, however, these areas should be carefully assessed on the frontal view. Looking at the margins of the underlying pulmonary vessels through the heart and diaphragm is a good way to assess these lung fields.

BONES

Although chest radiographs are rarely obtained to specifically evaluate osseous abnormalities, the bones should be thoroughly assessed. Visibility of bones will vary from patient to patient; bones in obese patients might be difficult to assess on routine radiographs due to different radiographic techniques. Dedicated radiographs of specific areas should be obtained to evaluate specific osseous structures such as the sternum, scapula, or shoulder. The technique used for chest radiographs is set to maximally visualize the lung parenchyma; the interpreter simply gets a "free look" at the bony thorax.

The best way to assess the osseous structures is by comparing one side to the other in a stepwise fashion. Ribs, clavicles, and shoulder girdles are all typically visualized bilaterally on routine chest radiographs. Although a full description of interpretation of bone radiographs is beyond the scope of this chapter, the overall bone density, cortical margins, focal abnormalities of density, and bony alignment should be assessed. Any suspicious finding on chest radiograph (CXR) should be followed by a clinical examination and/or dedicated radiographs of that region.

G. ABDOMEN

Radiographic techniques used to specifically assess the abdomen differ from those used when obtaining a chest radiograph. Abdominal structures noted on chest radiographs are underpenetrated and may be difficult to adequately visualize. In addition, the amount of the abdomen noted on chest radiographs varies from individual to individual depending upon the length of their thorax. In the majority of instances, however, at least a portion of the abdomen is visualized.

Two abdominal structures should always be inspected when looking at a chest radiograph. The first is the stomach bubble; most individuals have some gas in their stomach when a CXR is obtained. Gas should float to the top (fundus) of the stomach when the patient is standing and can be seen on both frontal and lateral projections. An air–fluid level is usually visualized, and should not be mistaken for intrathoracic abnormalities such as a pulmonary abscess. A hiatal hernia is occasionally noted as an abnormal air-containing structure or air–fluid level within the middle mediastinum. Displacement of the gastric gas bubble from the diaphragmatic shadow by more than approximately 3–4 cm suggests a subpulmonic effusion (fluid within the pleural space between the lung and the diaphragm).

The second abdominal structure is the diaphragm. The diaphragm cannot normally be visualized, however, the thin slip of diaphragm can be visualized when it is surrounded on both sides by gas, specifically air within the lungs on one side and free gas in the abdomen on the other. Therefore, if the diaphragm is distinctly visualized, pneumoperitoneum is likely. Upright chest radiographs are the most sensitive plain film projection for identifying pneumoperitoneum.

Interpretation pearls for chest radiographs are given in Table 3–4.

Imaging Modalities for the Chest

Many different imaging modalities are used to evaluate the chest. The most commonly ordered and least expensive is radiography (Figure 3–2). This test has high clinical utility for infectious diseases and screening patients at high risk for lung cancer. Chest radiographs can be obtained as posterior–anterior (PA, one view), PA and lateral (two view), or portable anterior–posterior (AP, one view) studies for initial evaluation. Specialized additional studies include lordotic (for apical masses), inspiratory and expiratory views (for pneumothoraces), and PA views with nipple markers (for evaluation of nodules in lower lung fields). Cost is low, especially for screening PA studies, which average under $100 U.S. Radiation exposure is also low, under 0.16 rad for a PA and lateral examination in an average size 20-year-old adult; the majority of this dose is from the lateral projection. Accessibility is high, even in an outpatient or nursing home setting, as portable x-ray units are readily available. Digital chest radiography will become more common in the future as image quality and acceptance improve.

Computed tomography (CT) is the next most commonly ordered procedure (Figure 3–3). The cost is generally believed high compared with radiography, but recent data dispute this. In one large tertiary care center, the actual cost of a hypothetical noncontrast CT examination was estimated at only $150 U.S. CT is usually used to provide further information about radiographic abnormalities first seen on plain films. This may change as numerous current trials are evaluating the cost effectiveness of thoracic CT in early detection of lung cancer. A more controversial use is the scoring of coronary artery calcification. CT can be performed both with and without the administration of intravenous contrast, and with processing to optimize visualization of lung, soft tissue, or bone. Radiation dose is slightly higher than in radiography. It is estimated at between 1 and 2 rads for older single slice nonhelical units, but is both lower and better collimated in newer multislice multidetector units. The radiation exposure level for CT is of some concern in children. The estimated lifetime cancer mortality risk has been documented to be an order

Table 3–4. CXR interpretation "pearls."

Lung fields behind the heart and diaphragm: A significant amount of pulmonary parenchyma is "hidden" by these structures. A lateral view will assess these areas. Carefully look at the pulmonary vascular shadows if only a frontal view is obtained.

Lung fields below rib shadows: Don't just look at the pulmonary parenchyma between the ribs. Compare lung parenchyma over the ribs from side to side as well.

Apical pleural reflections: There is relatively little pulmonary parenchyma in the lung apices compared to elsewhere in the thorax, whereas the amount of pleura is the same. The apices therefore are a good place to look for pleural-based diseases.

Breast shadows and nipples: Nipples can mimic solitary pulmonary nodules, and overlying breast tissue can mimic underlying pulmonary parenchymal disease. This can be especially misleading in a woman who has had a mastectomy.

Companion shadows above clavicles: The soft tissues lying on top of the clavicles are superimposed one upon the other to give the appearance of a soft tissue mass. These are called "companion shadows" and are normal. They should be symmetric from side to side.

Inspiratory effort: If the patient takes a small breath, the lung fields are inadequately filled to assess all the structures. The vessels appear crowded, and the mediastinal structures including the heart appear enlarged. A rule of thumb is that there should be at least 10 ribs visualized in a good inspiratory effort.

Correct exposure? Techniques for CXR vary from patient to patient. The correct technique should allow the interpreter to just visualize the spine through the mediastinal structures. Over- or underpenetrated films can make assessment of the lung fields difficult.

Abdomen and bones: Don't forget to assess all of the structures on the film!

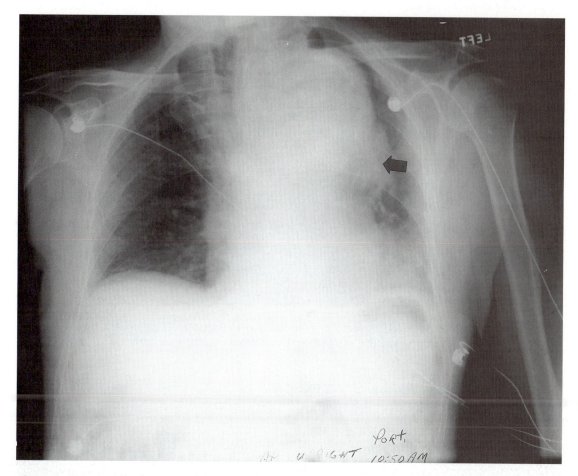

Figure 3–2. CXR demonstrating thoracic aortic dissection. Portable chest radiograph demonstrates thoracic aortic calcifications. The soft tissue density lateral to the calcified wall represents blood outside the vessel lumen, caused by a dissection.

of magnitude higher in CT studies of the head and abdomen in children when compared to adults. Methods are being developed to reduce helical CT radiation exposure by up to 45% with existing equipment.

Ultrasound is limited in chest disease due to the inability of medical sound wave technology to evaluate air-containing structures. External scanning (transthoracic) is useful for the peripheral lung parenchyma, pleura, and chest wall. Localizing fluid collections is a common indication, as well as evaluation of the heart and great vessels. Endoscopic ultrasound can be of great value in staging the extent of esophageal tumor and nodal spread. Ultrasound has no ionizing radiation exposure and the cost is moderate, usually around several hundred dollars. Useful results are more dependent on the skill and training of the operator performing the examination than in other radiological studies.

Nuclear imaging has many applications in the chest. One of the most common studies is the ventilation–perfusion ($\dot{V}/\dot{Q}$) scan for pulmonary embolism, although this is slowly being replaced by CT pulmonary angiography. ($\dot{V}/\dot{Q}$) imaging is also useful in preoperative assessment for resectable lung cancer by determining regional pulmonary reserve capacity when combined with function testing. Nuclear cardiology is also very important in providing information about cardiac vascularity and function. Positron emission tomography (PET) scanning allows metabolic activity to be imaged, identifying potential sites of cancer spread. It is cost effective in management of non-small-cell lung carcinoma (Figure 3–4); other cancers in which PET has clinical usefulness include colorectal, thyroid, melanoma, lymphoma, and breast. This technique also has potential use in clinical decisions about coronary

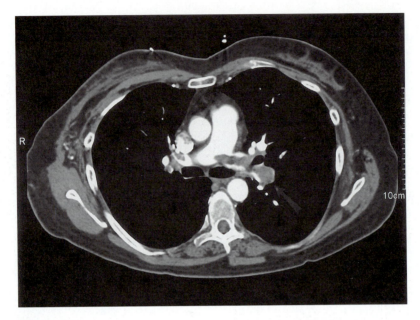

Figure 3–3. Computed tomographic pulmonary angiography. CT pulmonary angiogram demonstrating a large thrombus in the left main pulmonary artery.

revascularization by assessing myocardial viability. Other isotopes are occasionally used for thoracic imaging, including gallium for evaluation of lymphoma or sarcoidosis and sulfur colloid for esophageal dysmotility (Figure 3–5). Sulfur colloid lymphoscintigraphy is useful in identifying sentinel nodes for breast cancer biopsy. Cost can be moderate to high depending on the procedure and isotope. The radiation dose also varies.

Magnetic resonance imaging is useful in special circumstances. Recent improvements in gradients and imaging sequences are allowing assessment of cardiac function similar to nuclear medicine but with the added bonus of increased spatial resolution. Examination of the heart, aortic arch, and great vessels is possible without the complications of iodinated contrast. The lungs, however, still remain difficult to adequately evaluate by MRI, limiting it to a secondary role in cancer or parenchymal lung diseases. There is no ionizing radiation exposure, leading to considerable interest in pediatric use. Thermogenic effects from the radiofrequency field are the major physiological effect and are usually insignificant except in young infants or in pa-

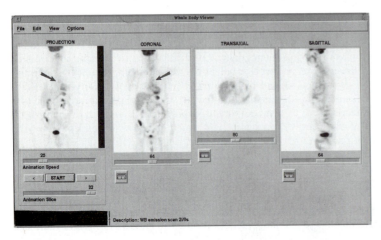

Figure 3–4. Whole-body positron emission tomography. Whole-body PET scan in a patient with non-small-cell lung carcinoma demonstrates a focus of increased activity in the mediastinum above the heart. This is indicative of nodal spread of the tumor.

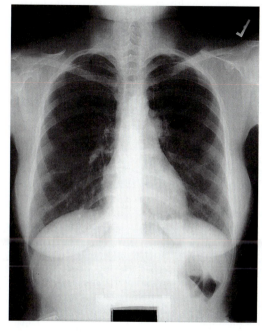

A

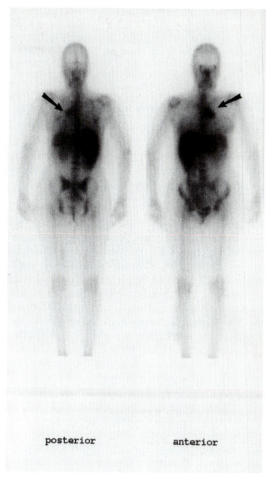

posterior   anterior

B

Figure 3–5. Radiograph and gallium scan in a patient with lymphoma. **A:** Frontal chest radiograph demonstrates a very subtle anterior mediastinal mass. **B:** Gallium scan demonstrates abnormal activity in the mediastinum, compatible with the biopsy-proven diagnosis of lymphoma.

tients with medical devices such as implants or braces. Other bioeffects include vertigo, metallic tastes, and possibly pain related to direct nerve and muscle stimulation at high electric field amplitudes. The cost can be extremely high and specialized equipment for vascular MRI is not commonly available. Patients must be screened for ferromagnetic materials, including older aneurysm clips and medical implants, such as pacemakers. Manufacturers of these devices can provide information about the safety of individual devices.

Angiography has a limited role in chest imaging. Pulmonary angiography remains the gold standard for assessment of embolism. Vascular malformations, such as arteriovenous malformations or sequestrations, can

be diagnosed and treated endovascularly. Cardiac angiography can be both diagnostic and therapeutic with stent or pacemaker insertion. These are very expensive and high radiation exposure examinations. Chest fluoroscopy is primarily used for line placement or image-guided percutaneous biopsy.

Chirikos TN et al: Screening for lung cancer with CT: a preliminary cost-effectiveness analysis. Chest 2002;121:1507. [PMID: 12006436]. (Analysis suggests screening is cost-effective if greater than 50% of detected cancers have localized stage.)

Geitung JT et al: Clinical utility of chest roentgenograms. Eur Radiol 1999;9:721. [PMID: 10354893]. (Prospective outcome analysis of the clinical utility of plain chest radiographs in a general practice.)

Slinger PD, Johnston MR: Preoperative assessment for pulmonary resection. Anesthesiol Clin North Am 2001;19:411. [PMID: 11571900]. (Nice review of a systematic approach to preoperative assessment of patients with resectable lung cancer.)

Pathological Processes Involving the Chest

Although a review of all the potential pathological processes involving the chest is beyond the scope of this chapter, a brief summary of common clinical entities and their radiological findings is presented below.

A. PERICARDIAL EFFUSION

There are several signs on chest radiography that may indirectly indicate the presence of a pericardial effusion. In the PA projection these include a "water-bottle" configuration of the heart, widening of the carinal angle, and density differences at the cardiac margin indicating the presence of fluid. A posteroinferior bulge from early fluid accumulation or a "stripe sign" related to displacement of the epicardial fat pad might be seen in the lateral projection. Small effusions, which can still cause tamponade, may not be easily identified on chest radiograph; in this case, lateral projections are superior to frontal radiographs. Fluid initially accumulates posteriorly within the pericardial sac but is usually identified first when anterior to the right ventricle. Echocardiography is frequently used to directly visualize suspected pericardial disease with the advantage of viewing cardiac motion in real time. This permits direct assessment of myocardial and valvular function. Transesophageal ultrasound is occasionally of value. Computed tomography images many different types of pericardial pathology including effusions, pericardial thickening, calcific pericarditis, neoplasms, and postoperative changes. CT is more sensitive for detection of pericardial masses than echocardiography, but the latter is preferred for effusions. Reflux of intravenous contrast into the azygous vein in the presence of a pericardial effusion has been reported as a CT indication of tamponade, whereas MRI may help differentiate pleural from pericardial effusions and characterize fluid type as a transudate or exudate.

B. PULMONARY EDEMA

Pulmonary edema may be divided into three types: cardiogenic, increased permeability, or hydrostatic/renal. Patients with pulmonary edema have enlarged hearts, vascular redistribution to the upper lobes with vessel engorgement, thickened septal (Kerley's) lines, peribronchial cuffing, and pleural effusions on chest radiograph. More severe edema may have parenchymal in-filtrates or consolidation. The type of edema may be difficult to determine when it is severe. A normal size heart and patchy pulmonary infiltrates are more indicative of permeability (acute respiratory distress syndrome, ARDS) edema, whereas cardiomegaly with septal lines is more indicative of a cardiogenic cause. Differentiating between hydrostatic and cardiogenic causes is difficult by current imaging methods. Measuring the vascular pedicle width has been proposed as a way to assess intravascular volume. Patients with a vascular pedicle width of greater than 70 mm coupled with a cardiothoracic ratio of greater than 0.55 are greater than three times more likely to have pulmonary venous pressures in excess of 18 mm Hg. This finding may indicate a hydrostatic cause in the presence of edema. CT can detect acinar infiltration, air-bronchograms, and microcystic transformation of the lungs in ARDS with greater sensitivity than chest radiography. MRI quantitative assessment of pulmonary edema and microvascular permeability is being studied but is still experimental.

C. INFECTIONS

The first imaging modality that should be used to evaluate pulmonary infections is chest radiographs, with CT reserved if radiography is inconclusive. Pneumonic processes can be alveolar, interstitial, or mixed in pattern. Alveolar infiltrates in children, especially if lobar in nature, indicate a bacterial infection. Interstitial infiltrates can be either bacterial or viral. Streptococcal pneumonia is the most common cause of community-acquired pneumonia requiring hospitalization in adults. The radiographic pattern is typically lobar, with cavitation uncommon. High-resolution CT (HRCT) may be useful in distinguishing bacterial from atypical pneumonias. Bacterial pneumonia is typically characterized by segmental airspace consolidation at the outer lung surface, whereas atypical pneumonias tend to show centrilobular shadows, a ground-glass appearance, and central lung involvement. Bacterial infection is the most common cause of lobar or segmental infiltrates in human immunodeficiency virus (HIV)-infected persons, but upper lobe consolidation suggests *Pneumocystis carinii* in the differential diagnosis. Unfortunately, there is a great degree of overlap in the appearance of various bacterial and viral pulmonary infections, and precise identification by imaging is often impossible.

Circular infectious infiltrates in the lungs, termed round pneumonias, can mimic tumors. They are seen more commonly in children than adults and radiographically often show signs of atelectasis. Adult round pneumonias are uncommon, but a history of cough and fevers in the setting of a recent normal chest radiograph suggests the diagnosis. Confirmation depends upon response to a course of antibiotic therapy and resolution on a repeat chest radiograph in 2–3 weeks. Any persistent or growing pulmonary mass should be assessed as a potential cancer, since postobstructive pneumonitis commonly occurs with endobronchial lesions.

Tuberculosis has multiple radiological findings. The most common pattern in primary tuberculosis is parenchymal infiltrates and adenopathy. Apical, posterior upper lobe, and superior segment cavitary lesions are seen in postprimary tuberculosis. The biological activity of postprimary disease is based in part on imaging stability for at least 6 months. There is, however, a wide range of variance, and infiltrates in basal lung zones or pleural effusions should not exclude the diagnosis. Cases of enlarged lymph nodes without pulmonary infiltrates mimicking lymphoma can occur in tuberculosis, although this is more common in children than adults. Calcified nodules in the lung parenchyma or mediastinum can indicate postprimary tuberculosis, but may also be related to other prior infections, metabolic disorders, neoplasms, or occupational exposures. In HIV patients, mediastinal adenopathy, miliary disease, and pleural effusions are more common than in the general tuberculous population. In diabetics, the frequency of lower lung lesions increases with age whereas the proportion of cavitation decreases; the latter is likely related to increased alveolar oxygen pressure in the lower lobes.

The most commonly encountered pulmonary fungal infections are *Aspergillus*, followed by *Cryptococcus* and *Candida*. Pulmonary manifestations of aspergillosis depend on the patient's preexisting pulmonary and immune status. Inhalation of spores can cause allergic alveolitis, whereas bronchopulmonary aspergillosis occurs in patients with asthma or cystic fibrosis. Mycetomas (fungus balls) (Figure 3–6) develop from secondary invasion of lung cavities, and invasive aspergillosis occurs in immunosuppressed individuals. Thick-walled cavitary lesions indicative of abscess formation and angioinvasion are common in acquired immunodeficiency syndrome (AIDS) and are better defined on CT than on plain radiographs. *Cryptococcus neoformans* and *Candida* infections are less specific, although the presence of miliary nodules may have some association with pulmonary *Cryptococcus*.

Empyemas are usually followed by chest radiographs, but both ultrasound and CT are useful in management. They often have an effusion adjacent to areas of dense pulmonary consolidation on plain radiographs. Postdrainage films may show hydropneumothorax, but this finding predrainage or excessive loculation can indicate the development of bronchopulmonary fistulas.

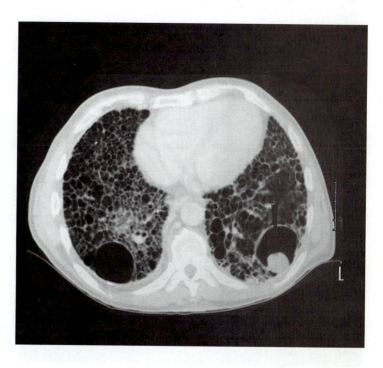

Figure 3–6. Aspergilloma. High-resolution CT demonstrates an aspergilloma in a left lower lobe cavity.

D. TRAUMA

Chest trauma can be blunt or penetrating. Blunt impact to the chest can cause fractures, lung contusion, or injury to mediastinal structures. Chest radiographs remain the initial imaging modality to rapidly screen patients, although spiral CT is more sensitive and specific. Findings range from mediastinal widening, indicative of hematoma or vascular dissection, to pulmonary contusions with consolidation. Pneumothoraces are often associated with rib fractures; subcutaneous air may also indicate airway or lung injury. Only 15% of patients with penetrating thoracic trauma need a therapeutic operative procedure, but life-threatening conditions do occur in this group. Newer diagnostic modalities including echocardiography and CT are useful in evaluating potential injuries to the heart, major vessels, and other visceral structures. Aortography still remains the standard of reference for studying the thoracic aorta or brachiocephalic vessels in blunt trauma as injuries can be subtle. MRI imaging with MR angiography is not a primary study for either blunt or penetrating injuries, but may be useful if other studies are equivocal or there is contraindication to iodinated contrast.

E. PNEUMOTHORAX

Pneumothoraces can develop spontaneously or from trauma or iatrogenic injury. Chest radiographs with inspiratory and expiratory views may reveal subtle pneumothoraces because the pneumothorax will not compress with expiration. Attempts have been made to estimate the size of the pneumothorax by inspiratory PA radiographs. Because the air collection that surrounds the lung is a sphere overlying a sphere, the true size of the pneumothorax is larger than it appears on the film. The percentage of the pneumothorax may be estimated by various formulas using measurements of intrapleural distance.

Tension pneumothorax deviates the mediastinum to the contralateral side. Patients with AIDS are at an increased risk of pneumothorax, usually in the setting of *Pneumocystis carinii* pneumonia. Two view chest radiographs or CT best determine thoracostomy tube position, but these are not necessary or readily available for all patients. Intralobar positioning of the tube can be suspected on a frontal radiograph if the catheter is straight at the insertion site and terminates at the hilum. A curving chest drain is more likely to be located either anteriorly or posteriorly with respect to the lung. Critically ill patients with complicated pleural collections and chest tubes may require evaluation with CT.

F. CHRONIC INFLAMMATORY LUNG DISEASE

Many chronic lung diseases are evaluated by HRCT of the chest. Pneumoconioses are diseases resulting from accumulation of dust in the lungs. Examples include as-

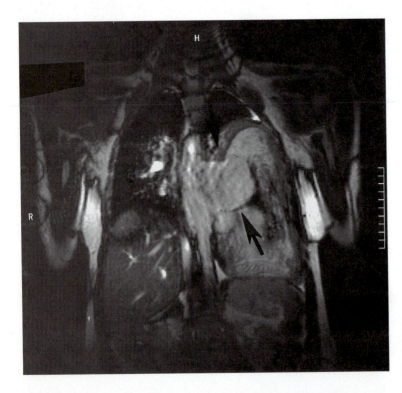

Figure 3–7. Liposarcoma. Coronal MRI of a mediastinal liposarcoma with extension into the left hemithorax.

bestosis, silicosis, and berylliosis. Asbestosis demonstrates pleural fibrosis and plaques that may calcify. Silicosis produces nodules and adenopathy with "eggshell calcification." CT may show emphysema associated with silicosis, but this is usually not seen by chest radiograph. Beryllium disease produces small nodules with lower lobe distribution. Chemical pneumonitis initially produces edema typical of permeability edema, but may progress to chronic bronchiolitis obliterans. Extrinsic allergic alveolitis may have a diffuse ground-glass appearance by CT in the subacute phase, with air trapping and a diffuse reticulonodular pattern evident late in the disease process.

HRCT can help differentiate different types of idiopathic interstitial lung disease. Usual interstitial pneumonitis (UIP) is characterized by honeycombing, patchy subpleural opacities, and irregular lines. Acute interstitial pneumonitis (AIP) presents with a bilateral extensive ground-glass appearance indicative of airspace disease, whereas desquamative interstitial pneumonitis (DIP) displays patchy subpleural opacities in the mid and lower lung zones. The major radiographic findings of smoking-related respiratory bronchiolitis are bronchial wall thickening, centrilobular nodules, and ground-glass opacity with centrilobular emphysema.

The imaging findings of other types of interstitial lung disease are less specific. Sarcoidosis has a more specific chest radiographic appearance with hilar adenopathy and linear opacities. Disease activity in sarcoidosis has been quantitated with gallium-67 isotope scanning.

G. NEOPLASMS

Primary lung tumors range from small "coin" lesions to large central endobronchial masses. Adenopathy, mediastinal invasion, or secondary sites of disease are important in staging and treatment (Figure 3–7). All radiological modalities are used in the evaluation of suspected lung cancers. Early detection trials using CT in high-risk populations are ongoing. Bronchoalveolar cancer mimics the appearance of an inflammatory process due to its peripheral location. Tumors with a distinct mass rather than infiltrative lesions by radiogra-

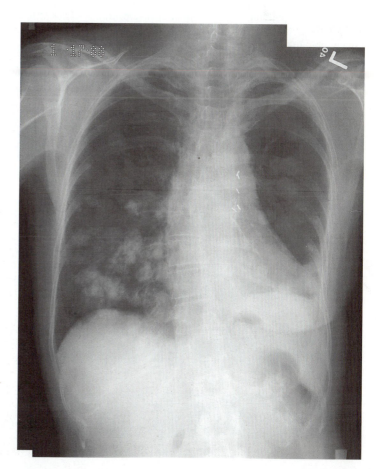

Figure 3–8. Metastatic lung carcinoma. Frontal chest radiograph in a patient after lobectomy for primary lung carcinoma. Multiple bilateral pulmonary nodules are noted, compatible with recurrent metastatic lung cancer.

phy tend to have nonmucinous and sclerosing histological features indicative of better survival.

Other primary tumors can involve the chest, including sarcomas and breast cancer. Mediastinal tumors include thymoma, teratoma, and lymphoma. These often present as mediastinal masses on chest radiographs. Thymomas are associated with myasthenia gravis; CT is recommended in adults with this condition. CT may also be useful in distinguishing malignant from benign thymic tumors when there is an irregular contour, areas of low attenuation, and multifocal calcification, and can help determine invasiveness. CT can preoperatively evaluate teratomas for rupture or calcification. Occasionally, MRI may be useful in distinguishing intralesional fat or fluid. Lymphoma can present both nodally and as visceral lung consolidation. CT is more reliable than chest radiography in staging mediastinal adenopathy in lymphoma. Primary large B cell lymphomas typically present as bulky anterior mediastinal masses with areas of necrosis. B cell lymphoma of bronchus-associated lymphoid tissue (BALT) usually appears as airspace consolidation or nodules. Hodgkin's disease is usually nodal but can present with a combination of both nodal and pulmonary parenchymal involvement.

Metastatic disease frequently affects the lungs. It usually presents as small peripheral pulmonary nodules but lymphangitic spread is sometimes seen, especially in breast or lung cancers (Figure 3–8).

Broderick LS et al: Imaging of lung cancer: old and new. Semin Oncol 1997;24:411. [PMID: 9280220]. (Discussion of the merits of various imaging modalities and their role in evaluating lung cancer.)

Ely EW, Haponik EF: Using the chest radiograph to determine intravascular volume status: the role of vascular pedicle width. Chest 2002;121:942. [PMID: 11888980]. (Thorough discussion of the value of vascular pedicle width in estimating intravascular volume.)

Franquet T: Imaging of pneumonia: trends and algorithms. Eur Respir J 2001;18:196. [PMID: 11510793]. (Discussion of the different imaging methods used in the diagnosis and management of pulmonary infections.)

Gotway MB et al: The radiologic spectrum of pulmonary Aspergillus infections. J Comput Assist Tomogr 2002;26:159. [PMID: 11884768]. (Nice review of the different radiological patterns associated with various forms of pulmonary aspergillosis.)

Hwang JH et al: Recent advances in radiology of the interstitial lung disease. Curr Opin Pulmon Med 1998;4:281. [PMID: 10813203]. (Review of radiographic findings in various forms of idiopathic interstitial lung disease.)

Karia DH et al: Recent role of imaging in the diagnosis of pericardial disease. Curr Cardiol Rep 2002;4:33. [PMID: 11743920]. (Nice review of the value of different radiological modalities in evaluating pericardial disease.)

Laboratory Evaluation

4

Robert A. Winn, MD, Edward D. Chan, MD, Sarah McKinley, MD, & Mark Geraci, MD

■ PULMONARY FUNCTION TESTING

Robert A. Winn, MD, & Edward D. Chan, MD

 ### ESSENTIALS OF DIAGNOSIS

- *In most instances spirometry is adequate to diagnose the presence of lung disease, although a specific diagnosis cannot be made with spirometry alone; patient history is needed.*
- *Categorization of the physiology of lung disease into either obstructive or restrictive allows development of a differential diagnosis.*
- *Lung volumes and diffusion refine the diagnosis.*
- *Testing of muscle strength and bronchial provocation aid in difficult cases.*

General Considerations

Pulmonary function tests (PFTs) evaluate airflow obstruction, bronchodilator response, lung volumes, and gas exchange (diffusion capacity). Indications for pulmonary function testing are broad and include (1) evaluation of pulmonary symptoms to detect impairment and assess its severity, (2) classification of obstructive, restrictive, or mixed patterns of disease, (3) evaluation of response to various treatments including bronchodilators for asthma and corticosteroids for interstitial lung disease, and (4) monitoring pulmonary side effects of treatment (eg, methotrexate, amiodarone). Less commonly, PFTs are used for evaluation of disability in symptomatic patients and for preoperative evaluation. The latter includes operative risk for general surgery, transplant risk of postoperative pulmonary complications, and evaluation of the postoperative function for patients scheduled to undergo lung resection. Pulmonary function testing can also help define disease prognosis, eg, forced expiratory volume in 1 s (FEV_1) has a relatively high correlation with the presence of chronic obstructive pulmonary disease (COPD), lung cancer, coronary artery disease, and stroke. For persons with occupational exposures, serial tracking may determine onset of disease and need for removal from the exposure. Many conditions causing obstructive or restrictive lung disease will be discussed in this chapter. Treatments for these numerous conditions are discussed in the respective disease-focused chapters in this volume.

It is important to understand that PFT values vary in healthy people. Unlike other tests that have a narrow normal range (eg, electrolytes, arterial blood gas, cholesterol panel), PFTs have a wide range of normal. In fact, the results obtained from PFTs are greatly influenced by the individual's height, weight, age (few normal values have been generated for those less than 20 or greater than 70 years of age), sex (some normal values are based on males only), and race (predicted values for Hispanic, African-American, and Asian ethnicity are often 10–15% lower than for whites). It is clear that spirometry is highly effort dependent. Therefore, obtaining accurate measurements depends on cooperation and maximum patient effort, correctly calibrated equipment, and the use of trained respiratory personnel to conduct all tests. Furthermore, when interpreting the results of PFTs, it is imperative to consider the clinical context in which the test was ordered.

It is appropriate to order the components of PFTs (airflow/spirometry, lung volumes, diffusion capacity) based on specific symptoms and physical examination of the patient. Simple spirometry measures airflow, whereas full PFTs include, in addition to the spirometry, the measurement and calculation of lung volume and diffusion capacity. Measuring diffusion capacity of the lung for carbon monoxide (DL_{CO}) in patients with a clear history and presentation for asthma is generally neither necessary nor cost effective. On the other hand, obtaining full PFTs in patients with a history of significant occupational exposure or suspicion for interstitial lung disease is appropriate.

Evaluation of Airflow

Spirometry is measured by a volume displacement instrument called a spirometer, with volume as the measured variable and expiratory flow rates obtained by dividing volume into timed segments. Spirometry measures forced vital capacity (FVC), slow vital capacity (SVC), inspiratory capacity (IC), and expiratory reserve volume (ERV). Basic spirometry readings include the FVC, FEV_1 (the volume exhaled in the first second of the FVC), and the FEV_1/FVC ratio. These are reproducible, inexpensive, and widely available. Spirometry is helpful in detecting airflow limitation and obstructive lung disease, as well as in suggesting restrictive lung disease.

When the FEV_1 is decreased out of proportion to the FVC, an obstructive pattern is present. The flow–volume loop often has a concave shape (Figure 4–1). A normal percent predicted FEV_1 is between 80% and 120%. An FEV_1 value of 70–79% of predicted is considered mild airflow limitation. Moderate airflow limitation is defined as 51–69% of predicted and severe as <50% of predicted.

The normal FEV_1/FVC ratio is greater than 0.75 for those 60 years of age or younger and greater than 0.70 for those older than 60 years. A ratio greater than 0.80 (a relative increase in airflow) suggests the possibility of restrictive lung disease. In contrast, if the values are clearly below those expected for the predicted ratio based on age, obstructive lung disease is likely. However, a value lower than the expected ratio does not exclude a restrictive lung process. In this instance, lung volumes can be helpful in differentiating obstructive from restrictive causes of a reduced FEV_1/FVC ratio.

Bronchodilator Response

Assessing for a bronchodilator response is important in determining the reversibility of obstructive lung disease. In mild airflow limitation, a significant bronchodilator response may be the only indication of obstructive lung disease. The American Thoracic and European Respiratory Societies have defined a bronchodilator response as

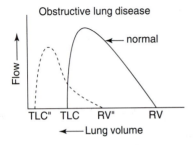

Figure 4–1. Obstructive lung disease, increased lung volume [shown by increased residual volume (RV) and total lung capacity (TLC)], and increased RV illustrating air trapping and decreased airflow compared to normal.

an FEV_1 or FVC increase from baseline > 12% and at least 200 mL. Thus, a positive bronchodilator response is indicated when any of the following is present: (1) an increase in FEV_1 or FVC of ≥12% and an absolute increase of ≥200 mL, (2) a significant isovolume shift defined as a decrease in total lung capacity (TLC) or thoracic gas volume (TGV) by at least 500 mL or ≥15%, or (3) evidence of dynamic air trapping due to collapsible airways during a forced expiratory maneuver. Collapsible airways are often indicated by an SVC that is at least 500 mL larger than the FVC.

To determine a bronchodilator response, the patient's bronchodilators should be discontinued prior to testing, if clinically possible. Short-acting β-agonists should be stopped 4–6 h prior to testing; long-acting β-agonists, cromolyn, ipratropium, and short-acting theophyllines should be stopped 12 h prior to testing; and long-acting theophyllines should be stopped 24 h prior to testing. Next, a baseline spirometry is performed in the absence of a bronchodilator. Then, a short-acting bronchodilator such as albuterol is given and the changes in FVC, FEV_1, and the FEV_1/FVC ratio are evaluated by repeating the spirometry. Although the presence of a bronchodilator response confirms airway reactivity, the absence of a response measured by spirometry does not necessarily indicate a lack of "effectiveness" of bronchodilators. Patients may have continued their medications or the response may be improvement in hyperinflation with an isovolume flow shift and lessening of dyspnea (see above) rather than a change in the FEV_1. The most reproducible marker of the effectiveness of a bronchodilator is improvement in ambulation distance during the 6-min walk test.

Lung Volumes

Determination of lung volume assesses for restrictive lung disease, provides evidence of hyperinflation in obstructive lung disease, and is needed for interpreting DL_{CO} measurements. Lung volumes are composed of the residual volume (RV), expiratory reserve volume (ERV), tidal volume (V_T), and inspiratory reserve volume (IRV). Lung capacities are made up of a combination of two or more of these lung volumes. The relationships between the different lung volumes and capacities are illustrated in Figure 4–2. These include inspiratory reserve capacity (IRC = V_T + IRV), vital capacity (VC = ERV + IRC), functional residual capacity (FRC = RV + ERV), and total lung capacity (TLC = RV + ERV + V_T + IRV or VC + RV or FRC + IRC). FRC is referred to as the thoracic gas volume (TGV) when measured by body plethysmography. FRC (or TGV) is effort independent and represents a position of equilibrium between the elastic recoil of the lungs and the expansion of the chest wall. All other lung volumes

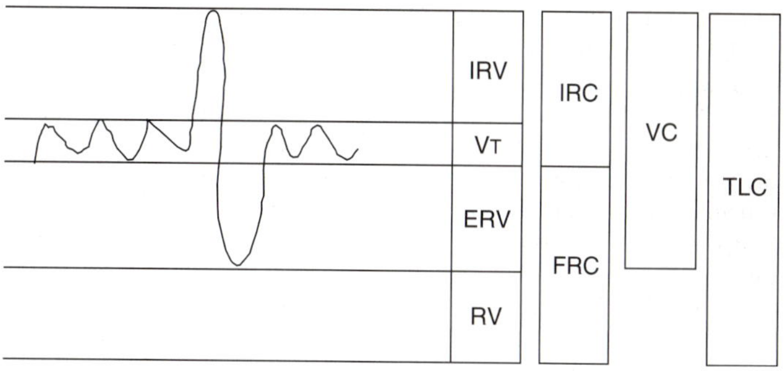

Figure 4–2. Static lung volumes. IRV, inspiratory reserve volume; V_T, tidal volume; ERV, expiratory reserve volume; RV, residual volume; IRC, inspiratory reserve capacity; FRC, functional reserve capacity; VC, vital capacity; TLC, total lung capacity.

are effort dependent as they rely on the measurement of SVC.

To determine lung volumes, the FRC or TGV is measured, and the other lung volumes (TLC, RV) are then calculated by the addition or subtraction of the spirometrically determined IC and ERV, respectively. Either one of two general methods is used to determine FRC: a gas dilution technique (helium equilibration or nitrogen washout) and body plethysmography (body box). In the helium dilution method, the patient rebreathes helium in a closed circuit of known volume and initial helium concentration until equilibration occurs. The nitrogen washout technique takes advantage of the 79% nitrogen in the atmosphere. By breathing 100% O_2, the lung is washed free of nitrogen, and the exhaled gas is collected. Because little nitrogen diffuses into the lungs, the volume of nitrogen collected in exhaled air after several minutes is used to estimate lung volume.

When volumes are measured with the body box, the FRC is referred to as TGV. Plethysmography is performed to calculate the change in box volume during a panting maneuver. For this, the patient sits inside a large closed box. The relation between mouth pressure and box pressure is plotted and the change in lung volume is calculated to give TGV, taking advantage of Boyle's law, which states that the product of pressure and volume is constant in a closed system. The box measurements are more reproducible than dilution techniques. The other advantage of body plethysmography is that unlike the gas distribution methods, it measures gas volume that does not communicate freely with the central airways and provides a more accurate reflection of volume for patients with bullous emphysema.

The normal predicted ranges for lung volumes are TLC 80–120%, FRC 75–120%, and RV 75–120% of predicted values. Increased lung volumes are typically seen with obstructive lung disease (Figure 4–1) with TLC or FRC (TGV) ≥120% of predicted. Air trapping and hyperinflation are also characteristic of obstructive lung disease. Air trapping is defined by an increase in RV to > 120% of predicted. Hyperinflation is defined

as a TLC and TGV > 120% of predicted and an RV > 140% of predicted.

Obstructive lung disease is most often caused by asthma, COPD, or bronchiectasis. A more detailed differential diagnosis of obstructive lung disease includes reactive airway dysfunction syndrome (RADS) due to toxin or viral exposure, chronic bronchitis, emphysema, bronchopulmonary dysplasia, bronchiolitis, and sarcoidosis.

Restrictive lung disease is defined as a reduction in all volumes and capacities. The classic findings in restrictive lung disease are a TLC or FRC < 75% of predicted, reduced RV and VC, and a normal to high FEV_1/FVC ratio. The degree of restriction is based on percent of predicted TLC: mild is 70–75% of predicted, moderate is 50–69% of predicted, and severe is <50% of predicted. Restriction may also be detected from the flow–volume loop as seen by a rightward shift of volumes (Figure 4–3). Although the volumes are low compared to the predicted curve, the flows are supranormal compared to the predicted curve (see Figure 4–3). The obstructive and restrictive findings for spirometry and lung volumes are contrasted in Table 4–1.

Restriction may be from either intrinsic lung disorders (eg, pulmonary fibrosis, interstitial and infiltrative disease, or diffuse alveolar disease) or extrinsic causes such as chest wall restriction (eg, pleural or skeletal), neuromuscular disease, abdominal splinting, or obesity. The different PFT patterns of restriction from interstitial disease, neuromuscular disease, and chest wall problems are shown in Table 4–2.

Mixed Restrictive–Obstructive Disease

Mixed disease is often associated with a normal FRC, decreased TLC, and increased RV (Figure 4–4). Diffuse interstitial or infiltrative lung diseases typically cause restrictive patterns with normal or high FEV_1/FVC and reduced lung volumes (TLC, FRC/TGV, and RV). Airflow limitation defects are often seen in end-stage interstitial lung disease and sarcoidosis (Figure 4–4).

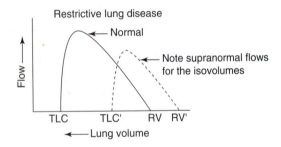

Figure 4–3. Restrictive lung disease demonstrated by supranormal airflow and decreased lung volumes [total lung capacity (TLC) and residual volume (RV)] compared to normal.

Bronchiectasis, although usually obstructive, can also cause reduced expiratory flow rates due to airway obliteration. The reduced volumes (eg, TLC) are due primarily to fibrosis of lung distal to the narrowed bronchiectatic lung segments. Constrictive bronchiolitis and panbronchiolitis are more commonly associated with an obstructive pattern with hyperinflation. Although bronchiolitis is primarily an airway disease, it can have a restrictive lung pattern as in bronchiolitis obliterans organizing pneumonia (BOOP). In summary, interstitial lung diseases that are most often restricted but can be associated with airflow limitation include neurofibromatosis, lymphangioleiomyomatosis, tuberous sclerosis, chronic hypersensitivity pneumonitis, sarcoidosis, eosinophilic granuloma, and the combination of interstitial lung disease superimposed on COPD.

Table 4–1. Diagnosis of ventilatory impairment: obstructive versus restrictive disease.

Parameter[1]	Obstructive	Restrictive
FEV$_1$	Decreased	Normal or decreased
FVC	Normal or decreased	Decreased
% FEV$_1$	Decreased	Normal or increased
RV	Normal or increased	Decreased
FRC (TGV)	Increased	Decreased
TLC	Normal or increased	Decreased

[1]FEV$_1$, forced expiratory volume in 1 s; FVC, forced vital capacity; RV, residual volume; FRC, functional residual capacity; TGV, thoracic gas volume; TLC, total lung capacity.

Diffusion Capacity (D$_{LCO}$) to Assess Gas Exchange

The single breath D$_{LCO}$ measures the ability of the lung to transfer gas and saturate the hemoglobin in red blood cells. Because CO is so avidly bound to hemoglobin, it is an ideal gas for assessing the ability of the lung to transfer gas. It is used as a surrogate for oxygen transfer. D$_{LCO}$ is considered to be the flow rate (mL/min) of CO gas per mm Hg of CO pressure gradient from alveolus to capillary blood. Ventilation–perfusion matching and the surface area of blood flowing by ventilating alveoli affect diffusion.

The diffusion measurement technique involves inhaling a single breath of gas enriched for helium and CO, with subsequent measurement, often by chromatography, of the expired gas. When the lungs work well, very little CO is collected in the expired gas. When the lung is diseased, less CO diffuses into the lungs and higher levels are measured in the expired gas.

The normal predicted range for D$_{LCO}$ is 75–120%. An increased D$_{LCO}$ (>120% of predicted) may be caused by increased recruitment of the pulmonary vascular bed (exercise, left to right intracardiac shunts), asthma (increased pulmonary blood volumes due to more negative intrathoracic pressure), extremely high altitudes, early congestive heart failure, or increased hemoglobin (polycythemia, pulmonary hemorrhage) that binds CO.

In contrast, D$_{LCO}$ is decreased (<80% of predicted) in conditions that disrupt the alveolar-capillary surface for gas transfer. A simplified schema shows ways in which diffusion capacity is altered with disease (Figure 4–5). Disorders can impair gas exchange/diffusion by destruction of alveoli and adjacent capillary networks (emphysema), alveolar filling with fluid or pus (pulmonary edema or pneumonia), causing atelectasis (lung tumor), increased tissue in the interstitial space (interstitial lung disease), or decreasing blood flow past ventilating alveoli (pulmonary embolism). D$_{LCO}$ is clinically most useful in distinguishing emphysema from asthma or assessing interstitial lung disease. An isolated reduction in diffusion capacity suggests pulmonary vascular disease such as primary or thromboembolic pulmonary hypertension. Patients with anemia also have lower measured D$_{LCO}$. Thus D$_{LCO}$ is usually adjusted for hemoglobin level.

Bronchial Provocation Challenge Tests

Bronchoprovocation maneuvers are used to evaluate airway hyperresponsiveness or reactivity. Hyperresponsiveness is not the same as obstruction, although it is usually seen in patients with asthma, and can be seen with normal spirometry. Conditions inducing airway hyperresponsiveness in addition to asthma include al-

Table 4–2. Lung volume patterns in restrictive disease.

Parameter[1]	Pulmonary Fibrosis	Neuromuscular Disease	Chest Wall Restriction (Chest Strapping or Pleural Disease)
TLC, RV, FRC	Decreased	TLC is decreased, RV is usually high, FRC is usually normal	Decreased
Maximal static recoil pressure	Increased	Decreased	Decreased
PI$_{max}$, PE$_{max}$	Unchanged	Decreased	
RV/TLC	Unchanged	Decreased	Increased because RV is minimally affected, whereas the ability to expand the chest is markedly decreased

[1]TLC, total lung capacity; RV, residual volume; FRC, functional residual capacity; PI$_{max}$, maximum inspiratory pressure; PE$_{max}$, maximum expiratory pressure.

lergic rhinitis, viral upper respiratory infections, and exposure to airway toxins, such as phosgene or chlorine gas, and exposure to inhaled occupational chemicals, such as toluene diisocyanate. Bronchoprovocation testing should be considered for patients who have normal PFTs, but also have symptoms consistent with asthma, and in whom a laboratory-based diagnosis is required for definitive diagnosis. The tests are sensitive for asthma, but nonspecific. A negative study is useful in that it all but excludes asthma. There are several accepted ways of performing a bronchial provocation test: exercise, chemical, or isocapnic hyperventilation. In specific cases, an allergen may be administered, but use of this is risky and is rarely indicated.

The first and often easiest bronchoprovocation method is exercise-induced bronchoconstriction. Ambient room air should be dry and cool; supplemental cool dry air may also be provided in the laboratory. In general, FEV$_1$ should increase with exercise but drops after exercise for the hyperreactive patient with asthma. FEV$_1$ is measured at baseline and then 1, 3, 5, 10, 15,

and 20 min after exercise. If FEV$_1$ decreases by $\geq$15% with exercise, exercise-induced bronchoconstriction is present. Patients who have difficulty breathing should be treated with a bronchodilator and the FEV$_1$ response to the bronchodilator should be remeasured. Otherwise, the bronchodilator is administered at the end of the 20-min evaluation period.

The second and most accurate method to assess hyperreactivity is by the methacholine (or histamine) provocation test. A positive (abnormal) test is indicated when FEV$_1$ falls by 20% from baseline at a methacholine concentration of $\leq$8 mg/mL. The FEV$_1$/FVC ratio should also fall for a positive methacholine challenge test. An FEV$_1$/FVC ratio that does not drop or that increases during the test despite decreases in FEV$_1$ suggests poor effort and/or variable extrathoracic obstruction. If this occurs, the test is repeated in a separate encounter beginning at a methacholine dose at the level at which the FEV$_1$ fell to 20%. Truncating the test duration helps determine if true airway hyperresponsiveness is present, eg, if the fall in FEV$_1$ was related to a suboptimal effort, then no fall should occur by beginning at this dose. Also, inspection of the inspiratory loops may detect variable extrathoracic obstruction such as vocal cord dysfunction.

Lastly, isocapnic hyperventilation may also help in detecting hyperresponsive airways disease. Minute ventilation is increased by deep breathing to a target of 80% maximum voluntary ventilation for 5 min. A decrease in FEV$_1$ by $\geq$10% from baseline is diagnostic of hyperresponsive airways disease.

Upper Airway Obstruction

Upper airway obstruction is rare but has characteristic patterns on pulmonary function testing. It may be fixed or variable (Figure 4–6). Fixed airway obstruction,

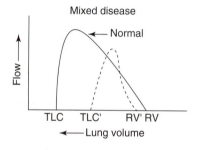

Figure 4–4. Characteristic curve of restrictive and obstructive lung disease. TLC, total lung capacity; RV, residual volume.

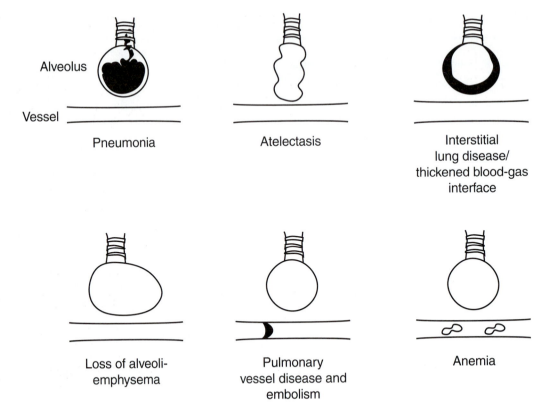

Figure 4–5. Causes of impaired diffusion capacity.

whether it is intrathoracic or extrathoracic, causes truncation of both the inspiratory and expiratory loops. Variable obstruction may have abnormalities of either the expiratory loop (intrathoracic obstruction) or the inspiratory limb (extrathoracic obstruction) (Figure 4–6). Examples of fixed and variable obstructions include variable intrathoracic obstruction (some large airway tumors), variable extrathoracic obstruction (VCD, unilateral vocal cord paralysis), and obstruction fixed throughout the respiratory cycle (subglottic stenosis, tracheal tumors).

Respiratory Muscle Weakness

Respiratory muscle weakness should be considered in any individual who presents with dyspnea, hypercarbia, and hypoxemia, as well as in the difficult-to-wean patient. Causes include primary disorders that involve neuromuscular weakness, diseases in which muscle or neuromuscular weakness is only a component, or drug-induced muscle or neuromuscular weakness. Respira-

tory muscle weakness may present insidiously or in a fulminant fashion; the presentation has been described as a "wolf in sheep's clothing" because the underlying potentially lethal condition is clouded by vague symptoms of weakness. The pulmonary function testing and gas-exchange abnormalities associated with muscle weakness include low FEV_1 and low FVC, with a normal FEV_1/FVC ratio, low maximum inspiratory pressure (MIP) and maximum expiratory pressure (MEP), maximal voluntary ventilation (MVV) < $FEV_1 \times 40$, low TLC, high RV, and normal FRC. There may be an increased A–aO_2 gradient due to atelectasis that improves with deep breaths or exercise.

Diseases associated with muscle weakness include acid-maltase deficiency (an autosomal recessive glycogen storage disease resulting in muscle glycogen accumulation), Guillain–Barré syndrome, myasthenia gravis, amyotrophic lateral sclerosis, and polymyositis with intercostal muscle and diaphragmatic weakness. Disorders associated with muscle weakness as a component of other primary disorders include hyperthyroidism, hy-

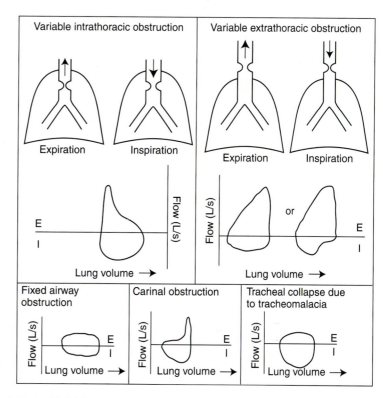

Figure 4–6. Various causes of airway obstruction.

pothyroidism, and systemic lupus erythematosis. Hyperthyroidism causes a proximal and distal myopathy and is associated with both inspiratory and expiratory muscle weakness. Hypothyroidism causes inspiratory and expiratory muscle weakness, reduced ventilatory drive, and upper airway obstruction. Systemic lupus erythematosis sometimes causes a syndrome known as "shrinking lung," which is attributed to diaphragm and/or intercostal muscle weakness. For drug-induced respiratory muscle weakness, the drugs in many instances exacerbate an underlying muscle or neuromuscular disorder. Examples include aminoglycoside-induced neuromuscular weakness, hypokalemia, or hypophosphatemia in a person with amyotrophic lateral sclerosis.

ATS/ERS: Statement on respiratory muscle testing. Am J Respir Crit Care Med 2002;166:518. [PMID: 12186831]. (An official statement of the European Respiratory Society offering guidelines based on a literature review of respiratory muscle testing.)

Coates AL et al: Sources of variation of FEV$_1$. Am J Respir Crit Care Med 1994;149:439. [PMID: 8306042]. (A review of variations associated with the measurement of FEV$_1$.)

Crapo RO et al: American Thoracic Society statement: guidelines for methacholine and exercise challenge testing—1999. Am J Respir Crit Care Med 2000;161:309. [PMID: 10619836]. (An official statement of the American Thoracic Society including general guidelines based on a review of the most current literature.)

Crapo RO, Jensen RL, Wanger JS: Single breath carbon monoxide diffusing capacity. Clin Chest Med 2001;22:637. [PMID: 11787656]. (An update and recommendations for a standard technique.)

Hankinson JI, Odencrantz JR, Fedan KB: Spirometric reference values from a sample of the general U.S. population. Am J Respir Crit Care Med 1999;159:179. [PMID: 9872837]. (A general review of reference values and variations in pulmonary function testing in the U.S. population.)

Leith DE, Brown R: ERS/ATS Workshop Series: Human lung volumes and the mechanisms that set them. Eur Respir J 1999;13:468. [PMID: 10065702]. (An update and a review of measuring human lung volumes and the mechanisms involved in that process.)

Mahler DA: The pulmonary function laboratory. Clin Chest Med 1989;10:129. [PMID: 2661113]. (A general review of pulmonary function tests.)

Salzman SH: Pulmonary function testing: tips on how to interpret the results. J Respir Dis 1999;20:809. (A review of the general topic of pulmonary function testing.)

Stocks J, Quanjer PH: Reference values for residual volume, functional residual capacity, and total lung capacity. ATS/ERS statement. Eur Respir J 1995;8:492. [PMID: 7789503]. (A report on reference values used in standard pulmonary function testing.)

■ INTERPRETATION OF ACID–BASE STATUS

Robert A. Winn, MD

 ESSENTIALS OF DIAGNOSIS

- *Arterial blood gases are easy to obtain and provide a wealth of clinical information.*
- *It is important to interpret results in conjunction with serum bicarbonate levels and within the clinical context.*
- *Use the anion gap for assessment of metabolic acidosis.*
- *The excess anion gap or delta gap can pinpoint the hidden parts of a mixed acid–base disorder.*

Acid–Base Interpretation

An appropriate understanding of acid–base disturbances mandates a systematic approach including taking a detailed history, verifying the accuracy of the acid–base data by checking it with the Henderson–Hasselbalch equation (Table 4–3), identifying the primary acid–base

Table 4–3. Values for pH and corresponding [H$^+$].

pH	[H$^+$] (mEq/L)
7.80	16
7.75	18
7.70	20
7.65	22
7.60	25
7.55	28
7.50	32
7.45	35
7.40	40
7.35	45
7.30	50
7.25	56
7.20	63
7.15	71
7.10	79
7.05	89
7.0	100

disorder, and evaluating whether it is a simple or mixed acid–base disorder. Furthermore, knowledge of the compensatory responses, accurate interpretation of plasma electrolytes and arterial blood gases, as well as the ability to calculate both a serum and urine anion gap will also help to interpret acid–base status.

The development of acid–base disturbances is primarily determined by changes in the levels of bicarbonate concentration or by changes in the arterial CO_2 tension/pressure ($PaCO_2$). The major organs involved in this process are the kidneys and lungs. In humans, the chief buffer to this is the carbonic–bicarbonate pair. The Henderson–Hasselbalch equation shows the interrelationship between hydrogen concentration, bicarbonate, and $PaCO_2$:

$$pH = 6.1 + \log([HCO_3^-]/(0.03 \times PaCO_2))$$

or the Henderson equation:

$$[H^+] = 24 \times PaCO_2 / [HCO_3^-]$$

Acidemia is defined as an increase in the concentration of the hydrogen ion and the resultant decrease in the arterial pH. Acidosis, on the other hand, is the process that leads to a lower pH if there is no correction or compensation. Although it is counterintuitive, a patient may have acidosis with a normal or high pH if there is a second process causing alkalemia.

Alkalemia is defined as a decrease in the concentration of hydrogen ion and the resultant increase in arterial pH. Alkalosis is the process that leads to a higher pH if there is no correction or compensation. A patient may have alkalosis with a normal or low pH.

A. IMPORTANCE OF HISTORY AND PHYSICAL EXAMINATION

Taking a detailed history and performing a thorough physical examination are important in determining various acid–base abnormalities. In fact, a given set of acid–base parameters is never in and of itself diagnostic of a specific acid–base disorder, but can be associated with a variety of acid–base abnormalities. A cursory interpretation of an arterial blood gas may appear to show a simple acid–base abnormality, but upon further investigation of the history may actually represent a more complex interplay of coexisting acid–base disturbances not discovered by interpretation of the arterial blood gas alone. A careful history and physical examination will often provide important clues to the prevailing acid–base status and can aid in narrowing the differential diagnosis. This is especially important for patients with drug ingestions, vomiting, diarrhea, and diabetes mellitus.

B. Verifying the Accuracy of the Data

The components of the HCO_3–CO_2 system should always be in equilibrium in the blood. Therefore, the pH, Pa_{CO_2}, and serum HCO_3 must be consistent with the Henderson–Hasselbalch equation. Not uncommonly, arterial blood gas interpretations that lead to confusion or defy conventional interpretation are associated with a lack of internal consistency.

Errors in valid evaluation of acid–base status can begin as early as the time of collection of specimen or be introduced subsequently during the measurement of the individual parameters (pH, Pa_{CO_2}, HCO_3). The most common error occurs in the chemical determination of bicarbonate, HCO_3. Use of the Henderson–Hasselbalch equation verifies the accuracy of the acid–base data. If the measurements of pH, Pa_{CO_2}, and serum HCO_3 do not fit reasonably well into these equations of the HCO_3–CO_2 system, an error in one or more of the values has likely occurred, and a repeat arterial blood gas and serum bicarbonate value should be performed. Table 4–3 provides the consistent pH and hydrogen ion concentration correlations to check this.

The following can be used to determine if the data are internally valid:

1. Check the Henderson or Henderson–Hasselbalch equation:

    $$[H^+] = 24 \times Pa_{CO_2} / [HCO_3^-]$$

    or

    $$pH = 6.1 \log + ([HCO_3^-] / (0.03 \times Pa_{CO_2}))$$

2. Next, for each 0.01 unit change in pH from 7.4, the $[H^+]$ changes by 1 mmol/L in an inverse fashion, ie,

    $$[H^+] = 40 + (\Delta pH)(1 \text{ mEq}/L) / (0.01)$$

3. For example, for a pH of 7.32, Pa_{CO_2} of 24, Po_2 of 104, fraction of inspired oxygen (Fio_2) of 0.21, and HCO_3 of 23

    $$[H^+] = (24) \times (24) / (23)$$

ie, the Henderson equation would equal 25. But for a pH of 7.32, the expected $[H^+]$ would be

$$[H^+] = 40 + (0.08)(1 \text{ mEq}/L) / 0.01 = 48$$

(check Table 4–3). Thus, the data are not internally consistent. For a pH of 7.32 with a Pa_{CO_2} of 24 the $[H^+]$ should be 48 and not 25. The HCO_3 should also be lower than 23.

Determining the Serum Anion Gap

The anion gap is the difference between the unmeasured anions (negatively charged molecules) and the unmeasured cations (positively charged particles) in the serum. It reflects primarily the negative charge of the circulating proteins in the serum. Thus the difference $[Na] - ([Cl] + [HCO_3])$ determines the anion gap. A normal anion gap is defined as a value of 10 ± 4 mEq/L in most laboratories. There are multiple factors that influence the measurement of the anion gap. Hypoalbuminemia, hyponatremia, paraproteinemia, and increased $[K]$, $[Mg]$, $[Ca]$, and $[NH_4]$ may all lower the calculated anion gap measurement. In fact, a decrease of 50% or greater in serum albumin can decrease the measured anion gap by 5 mEq/L.

The delta (Δ) gap is a measurement of the difference between the observed serum anion gap (AG) and the adjusted normal value. It can reveal a high AG metabolic acidosis where acidified anions are retained in the serum but the acidosis is obscured by other acid–base disorders. A normal Δ gap is 0. A positive Δ gap may be the first clue that a high AG metabolic acidosis coexists with a simultaneous metabolic alkalosis or a respiratory acidosis. Delta gap is calculated by subtracting the normal value for an AG from the calculated serum AG minus the difference between the normal value for $[HCO_3]$ and the measured serum bicarbonate, ie,

$$\Delta \text{ gap} = (\text{calculated AG} - \text{normal AG}) -$$
$$(\text{normal HCO}_3 - \text{measured HCO}_3)$$
$$\text{or (calculated AG} - 12) - (24 - \text{measured HCO}_3)$$

Determining the Osmolal Gap

The osmolal gap is used to detect the presence of ingested toxins such as ethylene glycol or methanol, for example. These toxins often cause an increased anion gap acidosis. The osmolal gap is the difference between the measured osmolality and the calculated osmolality. The calculated osmolality is determined by $[2 [Na] +$ serum glucose/18 + blood urea nitrogen (BUN)/2.8]. A normal osmolal gap (ie, calculated osmolality – serum osmolality) value should be < 10 mOsm. A calculated osmolality >10 mOsm more than the serum osmolality suggests the presence of an ingested toxin as a contributor to an anion gap acidosis.

Simple Acid–Base Abnormalities

The term simple acid–base disorder denotes the presence of a single abnormality associated with an expected compensatory response (Table 4–4). The four simple acid–base disturbances are metabolic acidosis, metabolic

Table 4–4. Compensation in simple acid–base disorders.

Metabolic acidosis
  $Paco_2 = (1.5 \times HCO_3^-) + 8 \pm 2$
Metabolic alkalosis
  $Paco_2 = (0.7 \times HCO_3^-) + 21 \pm 1.5^1$
Respiratory acidosis
  Acute: $HCO_3^- = [(Paco_2 - 40)/10] + 24$
  Chronic: $HCO_3^- = [(Paco_2 - 40)/3] + 24$
Respiratory alkalosis
  Acute: $HCO_3^- = [(40 - Paco_2)/5] + 24$
  Chronic: $HCO_3^- = [(40 - Paco_2)/2] + 24$

---

[1]For a bicarbonate (HCO_3^-) level greater than 40, the formula to be used is $Paco_2 = (0.75 \times HCO_3^-) + 19 \pm 7.5$.
From Madias NE: Acid-base. Combined Critical Care Course (SCCM/ACCP), 2002.

alkalosis, respiratory acidosis, and respiratory alkalosis. In metabolic acidosis, the primary change is a decrease in serum HCO_3, with the resultant compensatory response of hyperventilation, which decreases the $Paco_2$. The primary disturbance in metabolic alkalosis is an increase in serum HCO_3, which results in a hypoventilation response with a resultant rise in $Paco_2$. In respiratory acidosis the primary disorder is an increase in $Paco_2$, with a secondary increase in serum HCO_3. This is achieved by a transient increase in acid excretion and a sustained increase in the HCO_3 produced by the kidney. The primary change in respiratory alkalosis is a decrease in $Paco_2$; the secondary response is a decrease in serum HCO_3 resulting from a transient decrease in acid excretion and a sustained decrease in HCO_3 reabsorption by the kidney. Assuming that a steady state is present, an accurate set of acid–base data that does not meet the expected limits for each simple acid–base disorder may indicate a mixed acid–base disturbance. The process of how to envision each simple acid–base disorder is outlined below. An alternative strategy is to use a standard nomogram to plot results and detect the outliers.

A. METABOLIC ACIDOSIS

Metabolic acidosis is the accumulation of increased acid or decreased extracellular HCO_3. It occurs secondary to increased endogenous production of acid that the kidney cannot fully excrete (eg, diabetic ketoacidosis), exogenous acid sources (eg, drug ingestion), loss of endogenous HCO_3 (eg, severe diarrhea), or decreased renal excretion of acid (eg, chronic renal failure) (Table 4–5). Clinical signs and symptoms of metabolic acidosis include Kussmaul respirations, which are rapid deep breaths. Patients may have increased pulmonary vascular resistance, suppressed myocardial contractility, arrhythmias, right shift of the oxyhemoglobin dissocia-

Table 4–5. Classification of metabolic acidosis by presence or absence of an anion gap.

Increased anion gap
  Lactic acidosis
  Ketoacidosis
    Diabetes
    Alcohol-induced
    Starvation
  Renal failure
  Toxin ingestion
    Salicylates
    Methanol
    Ethylene glycol
    Paraldehyde
Normal anion gap (hyperchloremic)
  Gastrointestinal loss of HCO_3
    Ureteral diversion
    Diarrhea
    Ileostomy
    Proximal colostomy
  Renal loss of HCO_3
    Proximal renal tubular acidosis
    Carbonic anhydrase inhibitor
  Renal tubular disease
    Acute tubular necrosis
    Chronic tubulointerstitial disease
    Distal renal tubular acidosis (types I and IV)
    Hypoaldosteronism, aldosterone inhibitors
  Pharmacological
    Ammonium chloride
    Hyperalimentation
    Dilutional acidosis

From Zimmerman J: Acid-base disorders. ACCP Pulmonary Board Review, 2001.

tion curve resulting in increased release of oxygen to tissue, hyperkalemia, increased protein catabolism, and increased insulin resistance.

Use of a simple consistent evaluation is invaluable in the interpretation of metabolic acidosis. First, determine if the pH is lower than 7.4. If so, this is clearly a primary acidosis. Next, determine if there is an anion gap. In an uncomplicated AG acidosis, every increase of 1 mmol/L in the AG should result in a decrease of 1 mmol/L HCO_3. An alternative way to look at this is the "Winter" equation showing the $Paco_2$–HCO_3 relationship for simple metabolic acidosis (Table 4–4). Deviation from this association suggests a mixed acid–base disorder.

Because of the relationship between the AG and HCO_3, the Δ gap can be determined by taking the difference between both values. Thus, Δ gap = (deviation of AG from normal gap) − (deviation of HCO_3 from normal level of serum HCO_3) or (calculated AG − 12) −

(24 − measured HCO_3). The normal Δ gap is 0. A Δ gap that is positive, especially if the value is higher than 6, indicates a coexisting metabolic alkalosis or a respiratory acidosis. Thus, a Δ gap of zero would indicate a simple high AG acidosis. A Δ gap greater than zero would show a mixed metabolic acidosis plus a primary metabolic alkalosis, or a mixed high AG metabolic acidosis plus chronic respiratory alkalosis with metabolic compensation. A Δ gap less than zero would indicate a mixed AG metabolic acidosis plus non-AG metabolic acidosis, a mixed high AG metabolic acidosis plus chronic respiratory alkalosis with compensatory non-AG metabolic acidosis, or a mixed high AG metabolic acidosis plus low AG metabolic acidosis.

B. METABOLIC ALKALOSIS

The primary disturbance in metabolic alkalosis is an increase of HCO_3 or the loss of acid. The compensatory respiratory response to metabolic alkalosis is a rise of $PaCO_2$ due to hypoventilation. The respiratory response is limited to a maximum compensation of a $PaCO_2$ of 50–55 mm Hg (Table 4–4).

There are two categories of metabolic alkalosis (Table 4–6). Metabolic alkalosis is associated with hypovolemic

Table 4–6. Classification and etiology of metabolic alkalosis.

Hypovolemic, Cl⁻ depleted
  Gastrointestinal loss of H^+
    Vomiting
    Gastric suction
    Cl⁻ rich diarrhea
    Villous adenoma
  Renal loss of H^+
  Diuretics
  Posthypercapnia
  High-dose carbenicillin
Hypervolemic, Cl⁻ expanded
  Renal loss of H^+
    Primary hyperaldosteronism
    Primary hypercortisolism
    Adrenocorticotropic hormone excess
  Pharmacological hydrocortisone/mineralocorticoid excess
  Renal artery stenosis with right-ventricular hypertension
  Renin-secreting tumor
  Hypokalemia
  Bicarbonate overdose
    Pharmacological overdose of $NaHCO_3$
    Milk–alkali syndrome
    Massive blood transfusion

From Zimmerman J: Acid-base disorders. ACCP Pulmonary Board Review, 2001.

chloride depletion (saline responsive) in the first and with hypervolemic chloride expansion (saline resistant) in the second. The etiology of the hypovolemic chloride depletion form includes loss of $[H^+]$ from the gastrointestinal tract, loss of $[H^+]$ from the kidney, use of diuretics or carbenicillin, and a response to recent hypercapnia that has resolved. The causes of hypervolemic chloride expansion alkalosis include bicarbonate overdose, loss of $[H^+]$ from the kidney, hypokalemia, a renin-secreting tumor, mineralocorticoid excess, renal artery stenosis, excessive mineralocorticoid, and primary hyperaldosteronism. Both the history and the measurement of urine chloride can be helpful in distinguishing the two categories. Urine chloride is <20 mmol/L in the chloride depletion form and >20 mmol/L in the chloride expansion form of metabolic alkalosis. Hypokalemia is associated with both types of metabolic alkalosis.

Clinical signs and symptoms of metabolic alkalosis include tachycardia, arrhythmias, and an obtunded mental status. There is an increased risk of seizures, decreased cerebral blood flow, hypocalcemia, and hypokalemia.

C. RESPIRATORY ACIDOSIS

The major disturbance in respiratory acidosis is ineffective ventilation and increased CO_2 production due to either ventilatory failure or disordered central control of ventilation. The compensatory response is an increase in the concentration of $[HCO_3]$.

The normal respiratory response to hypercapnia is an increase in alveolar ventilation. The drive to increase the respiratory ventilation is determined by changes in the $[H^+]$ concentration of the cerebrospinal fluid (CSF), which then influences the chemoreceptors of the medulla. Furthermore, because the CSF is relatively free of nonbicarbonate buffers, the CO_2 that readily diffuses across the blood–brain barrier contributes to a significant increase in the CSF $[H^+]$. The CSF pH is then corrected by a slower rise in CSF $[HCO_3]$ that results from transfer of cerebral or blood bicarbonate. Acute increases in $PaCO_2$ will lead to increases of the serum HCO_3. For each increase of 10 mm Hg in $PaCO_2$, the HCO_3 increases by 1 mmol/L. In acute respiratory acidosis the pH decreases 0.08 units for each increase of 10 mm Hg in $PaCO_2$. In contrast, for chronic respiratory acidosis, the pH decreases 0.03 units for each increase of 10 mm Hg in $PaCO_2$.

The causes of respiratory acidosis include airway obstruction, depression of the respiratory center (brain injury, drugs), increased CO_2 production (malignant hyperthermia, hypermetabolism, high carbohydrate diet), neuromuscular diseases, and pulmonary disorder [obstructive, restrictive, hemothorax/pneumothorax, acute respiratory distress syndrome (ARDS)/acute lung injury, obesity hypoventilation syndrome, and flail chest]. Clinical signs and symptoms include somnolence, confusion, tremors, headaches, asterixis, tachycardia, and hypertension. Arrhythmias and peripheral vasodilation are often detected.

The kidney plays only a nominal role in the acute setting of respiratory acidosis. This is due to the slow reabsorption of HCO_3 by the kidney. In chronic respiratory acidosis, however, the kidney compensates by proximal reabsorption of HCO_3, which is accompanied by the loss of $[Cl]$, and distal tubule secretion of $[H^+]$, which is then trapped by $[NH_4]$ and excreted. Although adequate compensation is achieved by kidney reabsorption of HCO_3, it does not result in complete compensation. The limit of renal compensation in chronic respiratory acidosis is an HCO_3 of 45 mmol/L. If the levels of HCO_3 are higher, there must also be a secondary metabolic alkalosis (Table 4–4).

D. RESPIRATORY ALKALOSIS

The primary problem in respiratory alkalosis is hyperventilation, or breathing too much. Alveolar ventilation is affected by chemoreceptors in the medulla and great vessels, cortical input, and pulmonary chemoreceptors and stretch receptors. The HCO_3 decreases 2 mmol/L for each decrease of 10 mm Hg in $PaCO_2$ in acute respiratory alkalosis. A pH increase of 0.08 units is associated with a decrease of 10 mm Hg in $PaCO_2$. In chronic respiratory alkalosis an increase of 0.03 units in pH is associated with a decrease of 10 mm Hg in $PaCO_2$ (Table 4–4). Common causes of respiratory alkalosis are hypoxia (pulmonary edema, right-to-left cardiac shunts, and high altitude), acute or chronic pulmonary disease (pulmonary emboli, pulmonary edema, and COPD), and overstimulation of the respiratory center (sepsis, pregnancy, liver disease, progesterone, salicylates, pain, and organic brain diseases). The clinical signs and symptoms of respiratory alkalosis include changes in mental status (eg, confusion, seizures), paresthesias, arrhythmias, muscle cramps, hypokalemia, hypophosphatemia, and hypocalcemia.

Mixed Acid–Base Abnormality

Assuming that a steady state of acid–base is present, an accurate set of acid–base data that does not meet the expected limits for each simple acid–base disorder may indicate a mixed acid–base disturbance. For example, a patient may have an acid–base disorder that has an anion gap metabolic acidosis, a metabolic alkalosis, and a superimposed primary respiratory acidosis (triple acid–base disorder) (Table 4–7). This can be seen in patients with a preexisting chronic acid–base disorder who subsequently develop an acute acid–base process. Hallmarks of a mixed acid–base disturbance are a normal pH, $PaCO_2$, and HCO_3 deviating in directions opposite from that expected (ie, high $PaCO_2$ and high HCO_3 or low $PaCO_2$

and low HCO_3), and a pH that changes in the opposite direction for a known primary disorder. Common mixed acid–base disorder situations are outlined in Table 4–7.

To assess the presence of a mixed acid–base disorder accurately, an organized and systematic approach is required. First, determine the pH. Is there an acidosis or alkalosis? Whichever side of 7.40 the pH is on, the process that caused it to shift to that direction is the primary abnormality. Next, determine if the primary process is metabolic or respiratory. If a primary respiratory disturbance is present, determine if it is acute or chronic. If a primary metabolic acidosis disorder exists, determine if an AG is present. Next, check for an appropriate respiratory compensation by checking the Winter equation (serum $HCO_3 \times 1.5 + 8 \pm 2$). If there is an AG metabolic acidosis, calculate the Δ gap to see if other metabolic or respiratory disorders are present. Lastly, check the lactic acid level and calculate the osmolal gap to evaluate for the presence of ingested toxins such as methanol.

As an example, a previously healthy patient presents with the following laboratory data: pH 7.44, $PaCO_2$ 12, and PO_2 108 on room air and the following electrolytes: Na 136, K 5.5, Cl 106, HCO_3 8, BUN 100, and creatinine (Cr) 7.1.

1. Are the data internally consistent? $24 \times PaCO_2/HCO_3 = 24 \times 12/8 = 36$. An $[H^+]$ of 36 mEq/L corresponds to a pH of ~7.44 (see Table 4–3). The data are internally consistent.

2. The overall pH is within the normal range at 7.44.

3. There appears to be both a metabolic and respiratory component, ie, the serum HCO_3 is < 24 and the $PaCO_2$ is < 40.

4. Check the metabolic anion gap: 136 [Na] – (106 [Cl] + 8 [HCO_3]) = 22. Therefore there is a metabolic anion gap acidosis.

5. Is there an appropriate respiratory compensatory response? The Winter equation should be used to evaluate this question: serum $HCO_3 \times 1.5 + 8 \pm 2$, thus $8 \times 1.5 + 8 \pm 2 = 20$, which is within the range of 18–22. The $PaCO_2$ of our patient is outside of the range at 12, thus there is also a primary respiratory alkalosis disturbance. Given the acute nature of this patient's presentation, the respiratory abnormality is most likely an acute disorder.

6. Check the Δ gap: (calculated AG – normal AG) – (normal serum HCO_3 – measured serum HCO_3); thus $(22 - 12) - (24 - 8) = -4$. With these results, this patient could have a mixed AG metabolic acidosis plus a non-AG metabolic acidosis, a mixed AG metabolic acidosis plus a chronic respiratory alkalosis with compensatory

Table 4–7. Common clinical syndromes associated with mixed acid–base disorders.

Respiratory acidosis and metabolic acidosis	ACID–BASE CALCULATIONS[1]	
Cardiopulmonary arrest		
Lactic acidosis with COPD exacerbation	(Acute) respiratory acidosis	Decrease in pH =
Diabetic ketoacidosis		$0.08 \times \dfrac{(Paco_2 - 40)}{10}$
Profound hypophosphatemia		
Respiratory failure with one of the following		Increase in $[HCO_3^-]$ =
Renal failure		$\dfrac{\Delta Paco_2}{10} \pm 3$
Diarrhea		
Intoxication with ethylene glycol, methanol, or ethanol	(Chronic) respiratory acidosis	Decrease in pH =
Respiratory alkalosis and metabolic alkalosis		$0.03 \times \dfrac{(Paco_2 - 40)}{10}$
Overventilation in a mechanically ventilated patient with a COPD exacerbation		Increase in $[HCO_3^-]$ =
Hyperemesis in pregnancy		$3.5 \times \dfrac{\Delta Paco_2}{10}$
Liver disease (eg, cirrhosis) with diuretic use or emesis		
Respiratory acidosis and metabolic alkalosis	(Acute) respiratory alkalosis	Increase in pH =
Severe hypokalemia		$0.08 \times \dfrac{(40 - Paco_2)}{10}$
COPD exacerbation with emesis, gastric suctioning, or diuretics		Decrease in $[HCO_3^-]$ =
Respiratory alkalosis and metabolic acidosis		$2 \times \dfrac{\Delta Paco_2}{10}$
Salicylate intoxication		
Sepsis	(Chronic) respiratory alkalosis	Increase in pH =
Liver disease with lactic acidosis		$0.03 \times \dfrac{(40 - Paco_2)}{10}$
Renal insufficiency with congestive heart failure or pneumonia		Decrease in $[HCO_3^-]$ =
Metabolic acidosis and metabolic alkalosis		$5 \times \dfrac{\Delta Paco_2}{10}$
Ketoacidosis with emesis, diuretics, or gastric suctioning	Metabolic alkalosis	Increase in $Paco_2$ = $0.6 \times \Delta[HCO_3^-]$
Uremia with emesis, diuretics, or gastric suctioning	Metabolic acidosis	$AG = [Na] - ([Cl^-] + [HCO_3^-])$ Estimated $PaCO_2 = 1.5 \times [HCO_3^-] + 8 \pm 2$ $\Delta gap = (AG - 12) - (24 - HCO_3^-)$

[1]AG, anion gap; Δ, delta or change.

non-AG metabolic acidosis, or a mixed AG metabolic acidosis plus a non-AG metabolic acidosis. In this patient's case a high AG metabolic acidosis plus a non-AG metabolic acidosis is most likely.

Adrogue HJ, Madias NE: Management of life threatening acid–base disorders: first of two parts. N Engl J Med 1998;338:26. [PMID: 9414329]. (Details on treatment of acid–base disorders.)

Adrogue HJ, Madias NE: Management of life threatening acid–base disorders: second of two parts. N Engl J Med 1998;338:107. [PMID: 9420343]. (Further details on treatment of acid–base disorders.)

Breen P: Arterial blood gas and pH analysis. Clinical approach and interpretation. Anesthesiol Clin North Am 2001;19(4):885. [PMID: 11778384]. (A comprehensive outline of arterial blood gas analysis.)

Wilson WC: Clinical approach to acid–base analysis. Importance of the anion gap. Anesthesiol Clin North Am 2001;19(4):907. [PMID: 11778385]. (Further details on arterial blood gas analysis.)

Wrenn K: The delta gap: an approach to mixed acid–base disorders. Ann Emerg Med 1990;19:1310. [PMID: 2240729]. (An outline of a highly useful clinical tool, the delta gap.)

GENETIC EVALUATION IN LUNG DISEASE

Sarah McKinley, MD, & Mark Geraci, MD

 ESSENTIALS OF DIAGNOSIS

- Genetic testing can provide information useful for disease prevention, treatment, prognosis, and family counseling.
- Genetic testing should include consideration of the emotional, financial, and social impact of positive test results on patients and families.
- The majority of genetic testing currently performed in pulmonary medicine is for cystic fibrosis and α₁-antitrypsin deficiency.
- Genetic testing will become increasingly important as knowledge of the genetic basis of other diseases grows.

General Considerations

The Human Genome Project has changed the face of medical genetics. The goal of this project is to provide a detailed map of the 24 human chromosomes including the base sequences of all human genes. This map provides information essential in identifying specific mutations associated with various diseases. This has resulted in an explosion of knowledge regarding the contribution of individual genes to the pathophysiology of disease, including some pulmonary conditions.

Few disorders in pulmonary medicine currently mandate specific DNA tests for definitive diagnosis. The role of genetic evaluation in pulmonary disease before the Human Genome Project was primarily limited to single-gene (also known as Mendelian) disorders, such as cystic fibrosis and α₁-antitrypsin deficiency. The project, however, has provided insight into genes that although not directly causative, alter disease susceptibility and contribute to pathogenesis. Genes are now known to play a role in many diseases once thought to be caused solely by environment. For example, observations of higher rates of asthma within families and greater concordance of asthma between monozygotic than dizygotic twins have suggested a genetic component to this disease. However, pedigree analysis does not reveal a pattern consistent with mutations in a single gene. This has led to the hypothesis that asthma is caused by interactions of multiple genes (polygenic) that increase susceptibility rather than single gene mutations (monogenic or Mendelian). The map created by the Human Genome Project is providing tools necessary to help identify these susceptibility genes. As understanding of complicated genetic conditions grows, genetic testing will become more important in elucidating the pathogenesis of non-Mendelian diseases and guiding their treatment.

The goal of this section of the chapter is to briefly review issues regarding genetic evaluation of lung disease and currently available testing. Genetic evaluation of hypercoagulable states is not discussed here but is reviewed in Chapter 19.

Suspecting Genetic Lung Disease

Diagnosis of genetic lung disease requires a high degree of clinical suspicion. Careful history taking, including a review of childhood illness and family history of disease, can provide clues to a genetic origin of disease (Table 4–8). Characteristics of disease presentation, such as anatomic distribution of disease, may also suggest a genetic etiology. For example, basal rather than apical-predominant bullous emphysema should prompt consideration of α₁-antitrypsin deficiency. Pulmonary arteriovenous malformations are sufficiently rare that their presence should elicit further evaluation for hereditary hemorrhagic telangiectasia. Other diseases with familial predisposition include idiopathic pulmonary fibrosis, primary pulmonary hypertension, and asthma. The role of genetic evaluation in these diseases is under investigation.

Genetic Testing in Cystic Fibrosis

Cystic fibrosis (CF) is the most common inherited pulmonary disease. Given a carrier rate in white popula-

Table 4–8. Historical elements that suggest inherited lung disease.

General
  Symptoms present since childhood
  Disease presenting at an age younger than expected
  History of similar respiratory disease in family members
Disease specific
  Symptoms of recurrent cough, sputum production, or respiratory tract infections (including otitis and sinusitis)
  Sterility in patient or family members
  Pancreatic insufficiency in patient or family members
  Presence of or family history of pulmonary arteriovenous malformations
  Idiopathic cirrhosis in patient or family members

tions of 1 in 20 persons, the United States has 7 million carriers (heterozygotes) of the CF gene. CF is marked by recurrent pulmonary infections with development of bronchiectasis and fibrotic lung disease. A more detailed discussion of this disease and its clinical manifestations can be found in Chapter 8.

The autosomal recessive inheritance pattern of CF was recognized in 1946 via the study of pedigrees of affected families. Based on Mendelian genetics, the pattern of inheritance identified implied that CF was caused by a defect of a gene at a single locus. This locus, which encodes a protein called the cystic fibrosis transmembrane conductance regulator (CFTR), was discovered in 1989 on the long arm of chromosome 7. Defects in both copies of the CFTR gene are required to produce classic CF.

More than 800 mutations of the CFTR gene that produce the CF phenotype have been described. These defects have been divided into five broad classes based on their impact on the final CFTR molecule (Table 4–9). The ΔF508 mutation is the most common defect. Its name is descriptive of the defect: Δ signifies deletion, F signifies the amino acid phenylalanine, and 508 signifies the position of this amino acid in the normal CFTR protein product. The ΔF508 mutation is responsible for two-thirds of all CFTR mutations worldwide, but causes up to 90% of CF in persons of Northern European descent.

Although sweat testing remains the gold standard of CF diagnosis, DNA testing can also be used to confirm a diagnosis in suspected cases. The Cystic Fibrosis Foundation Consensus Statement in 1998 included a new diagnostic criterion involving the identification of mutations known to cause CF in both CFTR genes in patients with a characteristic phenotype.

Table 4–9. Classification of genetic mutations causing cystic fibrosis.

Class	Nature of Defect	Effect on CFTR Protein
I	Defective protein synthesis	Absence of CFTR
II	Production of abnormal protein (includes ΔF508)	CFTR unable to reach cell membrane
III	Disrupted activation and regulation	Decreased CFTR activity
IV	Altered chloride conductance	Decreased CFTR activity (mild disease)
V	Defective splicing	Decreased amount of protein (mild disease)

Testing is usually performed in specialized laboratories. Blood samples or buccal swabs are collected for DNA analysis and comparison to known mutations. Current testing identifies about 80 of the more than 700 known mutations associated with CF, including the ΔF508 mutation.

Identification of only one defective CFTR gene, although insufficient for definitive diagnosis of CF, does not rule out the diagnosis and should prompt further testing. The allele that is "normal" by genetic testing in such situations may in fact represent a mutation not yet included in the limited test panel. Further evaluation for CF, such as by nasal epithelial ion transport or repeat sweat testing, should be pursued.

A mutation in only one CFTR allele, although not sufficient to cause classic CF, may predispose patients to other diseases. These conditions, termed CFTR-related diseases, include pulmonary conditions such as asthma, allergic bronchopulmonary aspergillosis, and disseminated bronchiectasis. Other organ systems may also be affected by single CFTR mutations, causing conditions such as congenital bilateral absence of the vas deferens or chronic pancreatitis.

Genetic Testing in α₁-Antitrypsin Deficiency

A minority of cases of emphysema in the United States is due to α₁-antitrypsin (α₁-AT) deficiency. This disorder is caused by insufficient or dysfunctional α₁-AT. α₁-AT is vital in preserving lung structure because it inhibits proteinases that are released during inflammation and exposure to cigarette smoke. The production of this protein is controlled by the α₁-AT gene locus on the long arm of chromosome 14. The two alleles of α₁-AT are codominantly expressed, meaning each allele in a normal person produces half of the total α₁-AT. Alleles are named for the characteristic bands they produce by protein electrophoresis. The most common allele is the M allele. Most people are homozygous for the M allele (symbolized *PiMM*). Two other alleles recognized are the S and Z alleles. The S allele produces α₁-AT levels that are 60% of the M allele level. Because these proteinase levels are relatively preserved, patients with one or two S alleles have adequate α₁-AT levels and do not have increased rates of pulmonary disease. The Z allele, however, results in an abnormal α₁-AT structure with a single amino acid substitution that causes the protein to fold abnormally. The protein becomes trapped within the hepatocytes where it was synthesized. Persons homozygous for the Z allele (*PiZZ*) produce serum α₁-AT levels that are only 20% of those produced by persons homozygous for the M allele (*PiMM*). These patients have an accelerated rate of decline in lung function even in the absence of smoking.

The *PiZZ* phenotype is found in one in 1500 to one in 5000 births and is responsible for 1–10% of cases of emphysema diagnosed in the United States. Patients who have homozygous *PiZZ* α_1-AT deficiency have a 50–80% chance of developing clinically significant emphysema. Cigarette smoking produces emphysema in these patients at a younger age, typically in the third or fourth decade of life. Heterozygotes with one Z allele and one M allele (*PiMZ*) may have low or low normal α_1-AT levels but rarely have clinical disease. Patients with the *PiSZ* genotype may develop emphysema but it is generally milder than in *PiZZ* patients and develops only in those who smoke.

α_1-AT deficiency is usually diagnosed via phenotypic analysis of the protein products themselves rather than via gene analysis. However, gene analysis via polymerase chain reaction (PCR) can be performed on dried blood spot specimens. The World Health Organization in 1997 advocated screening patients who have chronic obstructive pulmonary disease (COPD) and asthma for α_1-AT deficiency with protein testing. DNA testing should be considered in those with abnormal protein screening results. Testing should also be considered in patients with a personal or family history of α_1-AT deficiency who are contemplating having children. Neonatal testing with heel stick blood sample analysis can also be considered in this context.

Patients present on rare occasions with decreased levels of α_1-AT but with either normal band patterns or patterns inconsistent with S or Z. A gene frequently responsible for this presentation is the "null gene" for α_1-AT. The null gene fails to produce any α_1-AT, so abnormal protein is not detectable by protein screening. Other genes exist that produce protein that is nonfunctional but indistinguishable from normal α_1-AT on protein electrophoresis. These diagnoses should be considered in patients with typical disease who have a low to normal α_1-AT level but a normal electrophoresis pattern. The diagnosis of α_1-AT deficiency due to these genetic defects can be confirmed via genotyping by PCR.

Genetic Testing in Primary Pulmonary Hypertension

Primary pulmonary hypertension (PPH) is a rare, severe disease marked by a progressive increase in pulmonary vascular pressures without apparent cause. PPH ultimately results in right heart failure if it is untreated. It predominantly affects women of childbearing age. One to two persons per million are affected each year in the United States. PPH progresses rapidly without therapy, with a mean survival of less than 3 years. Early therapy improves survival and quality of life, although treatment must be life-long.

PPH usually occurs sporadically, but 6% of patients with PPH have a family history of pulmonary hypertension. Familial primary pulmonary hypertension (FPPH) is clinically indistinguishable from sporadic PPH (SPPH). However, genetic anticipation appears to occur in affected families, meaning disease occurs at a younger age in subsequent generations of affected family members.

Review of familial cases suggests that FPPH follows an autosomal dominant transmission pattern with incomplete penetrance. More females appear to have the gene and develop disease than males, but examples of direct father to son transmission rule out X-linkage. Affected members and carriers are more likely to have female children, suggesting the genetic defect of FPPH may play a role in fetal development and cause increased intrauterine loss of male offspring.

Linkage analysis has been performed to try to identify a responsible gene. This technique involves a review of known polymorphisms, or normal highly variable genes, in individuals and families affected by FPPH to detect patterns in genes that correlate with presence of disease. This technique localized a potential gene to chromosome 2q. The specific gene was identified when mutation of the bone morphogenetic protein receptor (BMPR)-2 on chromosome 2q was shown to produce FPPH. Of patients with FPPH 50% have a heterozygous mutation in BMPR-2.

Despite the identification of a genetic defect responsible for many cases of FPPH and SPPH, understanding how this defect produces disease remains in its infancy. BMPR-2 is a receptor in the transforming growth factor (TGF)-β family. BMPR-2 is a receptor expressed throughout human tissues for growth factors known as bone morphogenetic proteins. These proteins are key growth factors in embryonic development (homozygous mutation of BMPR-2 results in fetal loss), although their role in adults is poorly understood and currently is the subject of scientific scrutiny. Why mutation of such a ubiquitous receptor produces disease isolated to the lung is unknown. Description of the functional impacts of BMPR-2 receptor mutations, such as effects of gene mutations on the amount or function of receptor produced, is vital to understanding this disease. Low penetrance of FPPH suggests other genetic or environmental factors must be present in addition to the BMPR-2 mutation to produce clinical disease.

Studies of patients with sporadic PPH suggest BMPR-2 mutations also contribute to that condition. At least 26% of patients with SPPH have BMPR-2 mutations, although none of more than 350 normal persons had a similar mutation.

Forty-six different mutations of the BMPR-2 gene have been identified in patients with FPPH and SPPH.

BMPR-2 mutations are not detectable in 50% of patients with FPPH.

The role for genetic testing in PPH remains uncertain. Although testing can identify some individuals who are at risk, heterozygous mutation does not predict disease development as heritability of the disorder exhibits incomplete penetrance. In addition, the majority of patients with SPPH and up to 50% with FPPH do not demonstrate BMPR-2 mutations.

Genetic Testing in Hereditary Hemorrhagic Telangiectasia

Hereditary hemorrhagic telangiectasia, also known as Osler–Weber–Rendu, is a heritable systemic disorder marked by mucocutaneous telangiectasias with predilection to develop arteriovenous malformations in many organs including the lung, liver, and brain. The incidence of this disorder is as high as one per 10,000 persons. It follows an autosomal dominant heritance pattern with age-related penetrance (increase in clinical disease develops with advancing age). Mutations in two genes have been identified in families with hereditary hemorrhagic telangiectasia: activin receptor-like kinase (ALK)-1 on chromosome 12 and endoglin on chromosome 9. Both are proteins involved in TGF-β superfamily receptor complexes, similar to the BMPR-2 protein associated with primary pulmonary hypertension. Most cases involve a heterozygous mutation in one of these proteins, although a few reports of homozygous defects exist. This disease is believed to arise from these mutations due to TGF-β effects on vasculogenesis, although the mechanisms by which this occurs are only speculative. Identifying the genes responsible for this disease is providing insight into pathogenesis and possibly future treatments. The disease is usually diagnosed via radiographic and physiological testing, but genetic testing can provide information for families at risk. As this disease can vary from asymptomatic minor telangiectasias to life-threatening arteriovenous malformations, genetic testing provides information only regarding relative risk, not severity of disease.

Pharmacogenetics

Pharmacogenetics is the study of how gene expression influences responses to medications. One of the best-studied examples of this phenomenon is response to β_2-receptor agonist medications. These medications have therapeutic effects via cell surface receptors called ADRB2. Some individuals experience significant down-regulation of these receptors after exposure to β_2-receptor agonist therapy, leading to decreasing effect of subsequent doses of medication. The process of receptor down-regulation resulting in decreased thera-

peutic effect is called desensitization. Different genes that produce the ADRB2 receptor (polymorphisms) are associated with different degrees of receptor down-regulation. Some polymorphisms show little down-regulation; these patients experience very little desensitization in response to β_2-receptor agonist therapy. Patients with higher degrees of desensitization may require less frequent dosing of medication to maintain adequate response. More studies are under way to better delineate which polymorphisms are present in populations and what effects they have on medication response. Pharmacogenetics may eventually play an important role in management of many diseases, such as predicting response to therapy in lung cancer or interstitial lung disease guiding choices of medications or administration regimens.

Types of Genetic Tests

Genetic testing is not synonymous with DNA testing. Many tests provide information about a patient's genotype, such as protein electrophoresis in patients with α_1-AT deficiency, without involving DNA analysis. DNA testing is also available and provides specific information regarding an individual's genetic code. DNA tests can be performed on many different samples including buccal swabs or small samples of blood, such as from heel stick specimens in neonates.

The type of genetic test performed depends on the suspected diagnosis. DNA analysis by polymerase chain reaction is most commonly used for diseases in which the responsible gene and mutation are known. The polymerase chain reaction technique involves accurate amplification of small quantities of DNA, such as from a buccal swab. The DNA can then be compared to known mutations. One example of this type of testing is in CF, where DNA collected from a patient is compared to known mutations, such as ΔF508. The number of mutations that can be tested for is rapidly growing. Internet-based databases, such as Genetest (www.genetest.org), provide clinicians with a searchable database of available tests and laboratories that perform them.

Specialists in medical genetics can also perform testing for suspected genetic diseases where neither the specific mutation nor the causative gene is known. This is done through linkage analysis. A thorough family history is performed to identify affected family members. Markers present on all genes are then used to determine which markers appear to travel with disease in the affected family. DNA must be obtained from multiple family members to perform this testing. Linkage analysis allows medical geneticists to localize unknown genes to a specific region of one chromosome and identify other family members who may be affected.

Neonatal Screening of Cystic Fibrosis

Population-based genetic screening for CF is feasible because many of the mutations responsible for it have been identified. DNA microarray technology facilitates rapid screening for multiple mutations. Studies are ongoing to determine the long-term clinical benefits and social effects of such screening on patients and their families. Short-term analysis suggests that neonatal screening for CF may result in better nutrition and lung function. Despite this short-term evidence, the National Institutes of Health does not currently recommend routine neonatal screening of the general population for CF.

Neonatal screening in families with an increased likelihood of having children with CF is common. Fifty to 90% of families at risk are considering or have had genetic testing. Of these families 17–84% report they would terminate a pregnancy for a finding of CF.

Ethical Considerations

Because genetic testing has many implications for patients and family members, genetic counseling should precede most testing. Although a complete discussion of the emotional, social, and ethical implications of testing is beyond the scope of this text, clinicians should consider the impact testing can have on patients and their families. Positive tests can affect reproductive decisions, insurability, or employment. Confidentiality is also an issue when a test necessitates testing of family members. Consultation with a medical geneticist may be appropriate to assist with informed consent, interpretation of test results, and family and reproductive counseling.

Burke W: Genomic medicine: genetic testing. N Engl J Med 2002;347:1867. [PMID: 12466512]. (Concise review of issues regarding genetic testing in clinical medicine.)

Guttmacher AE, Collins FS: Genomic medicine—a primer. N Engl J Med 2002;347:1512. [PMID: 12421895]. (Basic review of the application of genetics to clinical medicine.)

Joos LJ, Sandford AJ: Genotype predictors of response to asthma medications. Curr Opin Pulm Med 2002;8:9. [PMID: 11753118]. (Example of pharmacogenetics in clinical medicine.)

Kimyai-Asadi A, Terry PB: Ethical considerations in pulmonary genetic testing and gene therapy. Am J Respir Crit Care Med 1997;155:3. [PMID: 9001280]. (In-depth discussion of the ethics of genetic testing in pulmonary medicine.)

Mahadeva R, Lomas DA: Alpha$_1$-antitrypsin deficiency, cirrhosis, and emphysema. Thorax 1998;53:501. [PMID: 9713452]. (Review of genetics and molecular biology of α_1-antitrypsin deficiency.)

Sandford AJ, Paráe PD: The genetics of asthma. Am J Respir Crit Care Med 2000;161:S202. [PMID: 10712375]. (Overview of current knowledge and future investigations in genetics of asthma.)

Stuhrmann M et al: Mutation screening for prenatal and presymptomatic diagnosis: cystic fibrosis and hemochromatosis. Eur J Pediatr 2000;159:S186. [PMID: 11216897]. (Review of issues in genetic screening, including detection rates and ethics.)

Relevant Web Sites

http://www.cff.org
Cystic Fibrosis Foundation
http://www.genet.sickkids.on.ca
Cystic Fibrosis Mutation Database
http://www.genetests.org
GENETEST homesite (search engine of currently available genetic tests)
http://www.ornl.gov/hgmis
Human Genome Project Homesite

Procedures in Pulmonary Medicine

Joseph T. Crossno, Jr., MD, PhD

Several procedures may be required for either diagnostic or therapeutic evaluation of pulmonary disease. Some procedures can be performed by experienced primary care physicians; however, more invasive procedures are more safely performed by a specialist. This chapter will discuss the indications, contraindications, risks, complications, and potential diagnostic yield of each procedure.

GENERAL CONSIDERATIONS

A complete history should be obtained and physical examination performed prior to any procedure. Particular attention should be paid to a history of bleeding diathesis or coagulopathy, current use of anticoagulant medications, and allergic or adverse reactions to anesthetic agents. Performing a safe procedure with limited morbidity is determined by properly positioning the patient and operator as well as familiarity and experience with the procedure and necessary equipment. Informed consent must be obtained and universal precautions practiced. In addition, aerosol and respiratory droplet isolation may be required depending on the clinical context.

PLEURAL PROCEDURES

The majority of pleural procedures are directed at determining the etiology of a pleural effusion. Pleural effusions complicate many different thoracic and extrathoracic diseases; the chest radiograph is often the only clue to their presence. In general, the nature and etiology of a pleural effusion should be determined whenever the distance between the inside of the thoracic cavity and the outside of the lung parenchyma is greater than 10 mm on a decubitus chest radiograph.

Thoracentesis

Thoracentesis is aspiration of fluid from the pleural space by percutaneous insertion of a small bore needle or catheter through the chest wall.

A. INDICATIONS

The most common indication is evaluation of a pleural effusion of unknown etiology; this generally begins with determining whether it is transudative or exudative. Thoracentesis can be either diagnostic, therapeutic, or both, and helps determine whether further drainage procedures are necessary.

B. CONTRAINDICATIONS

There are no absolute contraindications to thoracentesis; however coagulopathy, bleeding diathesis, small size, presence of loculations, an obliterated pleural space, significant respiratory impairment in the contralateral lung, poorly defined anatomical landmarks, or an uncooperative patient are relative contraindications. In these circumstances, an experienced operator should perform the procedure. Ultrasound guidance is particularly useful in localizing effusions that are small, loculated, or in mechanically ventilated patients.

C. PROCEDURE

1. Seat the patient comfortably upright and preferably leaning slightly forward on a support.
2. Perform percussion of the posterior chest wall to determine the level of the effusion and palpation to identify posterior lateral anatomical landmarks.
3. A sterile technique is used to prepare the skin with providone-iodine paint and sterile drapes.
4. The skin is anesthetized with 1% or 2% lidocaine by making a subcutaneous wheal at the appropriate intercostal space. A larger needle is used to anesthetize the deeper intercostal structures by carefully advancing through the inferior margin of the intercostal space immediately over the inferior rib, thus avoiding injury to the neurovascular bundle that lies superiorly in the intercostal space.
5. Once pleural fluid is localized, diagnostic samples are obtained for analysis and culture. Flexible plastic tubing and vacuum bottles should be employed at this time if a therapeutic thoracentesis is being performed. Generally, no more than 1000 mL of fluid should be removed at one time to minimize the risk of reexpansion pulmonary edema. Larger volumes of fluid may be removed if done slowly, but the procedure should be halted if the patient begins to cough, experience chest pain, or demonstrate other signs of increasing negative pleural pressure.

6. The needle or catheter is removed and the site bandaged after pleural fluid aspiration is completed. An upright expiratory chest radiograph should then be obtained to screen for a pneumothorax.

D. SAMPLE ANALYSIS

Analysis of the thoracentesis specimen is critical to determining the etiology of the effusion. The clinical context in which the pleural effusion is discovered dictates which laboratory studies should be performed and the extent to which diagnosis of a particular disease is pursued. Evaluation of pleural fluid is reviewed in detail in Chapter 22.

1. Appearance—The appearance of the pleural fluid should be examined directly. Frank pus with a putrid odor suggests empyema; grossly bloody fluid suggests hemothorax or malignancy. Cloudy pleural effusions are consistent with either chylothorax or empyema, but clear straw-colored fluid suggests a transudate.

2. Chemistry—Pleural fluid protein and lactate dehydrogenase (LDH) should always be obtained to differentiate between transudative and exudative effusions. Glucose, pH, amylase, triglycerides, and cholesterol may be ordered as dictated by the clinical setting.

3. Cell counts and cytology—Complete and differential cell counts are particularly helpful in limiting the diagnosis. Cytological analysis of concentrated pleural fluid is diagnostic in 40–90% of malignant pleural effusions depending on sample volume and number of repeated samplings.

4. Microbiological stains and cultures—All thoracentesis samples, but particularly exudative pleural effusions, should be Gram- and acid-fast-stained. In addition, culture for aerobic/anaerobic bacteria and mycobacterial organisms should be performed.

E. RISKS AND COMPLICATIONS

Pneumothorax is the most common complication from thoracentesis, occurring in approximately 10% of cases. Risk factors for pneumothorax include small or loculated effusions, thick chest wall, and an uncooperative patient.

   Hemothorax and pulmonary parenchymal laceration are rare complications. Hemothorax usually results from laceration of an intercostal vessel in coagulopathic patients, whereas parenchymal lacerations are related to poor operator skill.

   Reexpansion pulmonary edema may be more common following removal of greater than 1000 mL of pleural fluid. The etiology of this complication is unknown; various patient series suggest it may or may not be more common than previously thought.

Infections of the chest wall or pleural space occur but are extremely rare.

Colt HG, Brewer N, Barbur E: Evaluation of patient-related and procedure-related factors contributing to pneumothorax following thoracentesis. Chest 1999;116:134. [PMID: 10424516]. (Study of factors associated with development of pneumothorax after thoracentesis.)

Closed Needle Pleural Biopsy

Small parietal pleural samples can be obtained with a closed needle biopsy. Needle pleural biopsy should be performed as part of the initial thoracentesis if malignancy or granulomatous disease is suspected.

A. INDICATIONS

An aggressive approach is warranted for any undiagnosed exudative pleural effusion with a progressive clinical course or with increasing pleural fluid LDH levels obtained during serial thoracentesis.

B. CONTRAINDICATIONS

The contraindications for closed biopsy are identical to those for thoracentesis.

C. PROCEDURE

1. Biopsies may be done with Cope, Abrams, or Tru-Cut needles. Patient preparation is identical for each needle and is the same as for thoracentesis.

2. After the appropriate intercostal space of the posterior thorax is identified and prepared in a sterile fashion, a large volume (10–15 mL) of 1% or 2% lidocaine is administered via multiple radial injections to anesthetize a large area of parietal pleura and rib periosteum in the inferior intercostal space.

3. A 0.5-cm skin incision is made with a #11 scalpel to allow free passage of the blunt biopsy needle through the skin and subcutaneous tissues. The biopsy needle is then inserted with the cutting edge positioned inferiorly to avoid the neurovascular bundle.

4. Pleural fluid may be aspirated for analysis through the biopsy needle into a syringe or vacuum bottle. Multiple tissue samples (5–10) are then obtained with the closed cutting needle. The biopsy needle is removed from the thorax, the incision site is closed with suture material, and a sterile dressing is applied. A chest radiograph should then be obtained to screen for a pneumothorax.

D. SAMPLE ANALYSIS

Pleural fluid is sent for laboratory analysis as described under "thoracentesis." Several pleural biopsy samples should be placed in 0.9% saline for culture and the majority of samples should be placed in 10% formalin for histological evaluation.

E. DIAGNOSTIC YIELD

Parietal pleural biopsy is positive in 40–60% of patients with malignant pleural disease. The combination of pleural fluid cytology and pleural biopsy histopathology increases the sensitivity to greater than 65%. Closed needle pleural biopsy, however, is most valuable in diagnosing tuberculous pleuritis; the presence of pleural granulomas is virtually diagnostic of this condition. Although pleural fluid culture is only 25% sensitive, biopsy is positive for granulomas in 50–80% of patients with tuberculosis. If initial biopsies are nondiagnositic, repeat biopsy is positive in 10–40% of cases. Combining histopathological examination with biopsy culture is diagnostic in 95% of cases.

F. RISKS AND COMPLICATIONS

The two major complications of closed needle pleural biopsy are pneumothorax and hemorrhage. Pneumothoraces large enough to require chest tube evacuation occur in only 1% of pleural biopsies. Most pneumothoraces develop due to leakage of air through the biopsy needle rather than puncture of lung parenchyma. Overall bleeding complications are rare, but hemorrhage can result from either intercostal vessel laceration or biopsy needle insertion into another organ (eg, kidney, spleen, or liver). A final complication in malignant pleural disease is seeding of malignant cells along the needle biopsy tract.

Escudero Bueno C et al: Cytologic and bacteriologic analysis of fluid and pleural biopsy specimens with Cope's needle: study of 414 patients. Arch Intern Med 1990;150:1190. [PMID: 2353852]. (Article describes yield of thoracentesis and Cope needle biopsy in 414 patients with pleural effusion.)

Thoracoscopic Pleural Biopsy

A. INDICATIONS

Thoracoscopy is indicated to evaluate pleural effusions that remain unexplained after pleural fluid analysis and closed needle biopsy. Thoracoscopy is safe and may eventually supplant closed needle biopsy because it has greater diagnostic yield and allows direct visualization of pleural surfaces.

B. CONTRAINDICATIONS

The only absolute contraindication to thoracoscopy is lack of free pleural space in which to enter and maneuver the thoracoscope. Relative contraindications include cough, hypoxemia, hypocoagulability, and cardiac abnormalities.

C. PROCEDURE

Thoracoscopy can be performed by pulmonologists through a single access site under local and conscious sedation with patients ventilating spontaneously. Operator experience is a key consideration; if more extensive intervention or greater access to the pleura and lung surfaces are required the procedure should be deferred to a thoracic surgeon. After a pneumothorax is induced, the thoracoscope is introduced through the chest wall into the pleural space. Thoracoscopy permits direct visualization of the pleura and external surface of the lung. It facilitates sampling of pleural fluid, biopsy of both pleura and peripheral lung parenchyma, lysis of adhesions, and pleurodesis. A chest tube(s) is inserted after completion of the procedure to evacuate the pneumothorax. The chest tube can be removed after the lung has reexpanded and the patient is discharged the same day if there is no bronchopleural fistula.

D. SAMPLE ANALYSIS AND DIAGNOSTIC YIELD

The advantage of thoracoscopy is its ability to achieve early diagnosis when pleural fluid cytology and needle biopsy have failed. Thoracoscopy reveals gross features suggestive of cancer in 85% of patients ultimately diagnosed with malignancy. Macroscopic diagnosis must always be confirmed by histological examination however, because some malignancies appear similar to nonspecific inflammation and inflammatory lesions can phenotypically mimic malignant tumors. The diagnostic sensitivity of this procedure is 93–97% in patients with tuberculous or malignant pleural disease.

E. COMPLICATIONS

Thoracoscopy is a safe procedure, with a mortality rate of less than 0.01%. Subcutaneous emphysema occurs in 0.5% of patients. Oxygen desaturation during the procedure, hemorrhage, infection, cardiac arrhythmias, and persistent postoperative air leak with chronic pneumothorax occur in fewer that 2% of cases. Fifteen percent of patients experience hyperthermia lasting 12 to 24 h.

Boutin C, Astoul P: Diagnostic thoracoscopy. Clin Chest Med 1998;19:295. [PMID: 9646982]. (Review of technique, indications, and results of medical thoracoscopy.)

Loddenkemper R: Thoracoscopy—state-of-the-art. Eur Respir J 1998;11:213. [PMID: 9543295]. (Comprehensive review of medical thoracoscopy, including indications and diagnostic yield.)

Open Biopsy of the Pleura

A. INDICATIONS

Open pleural biopsy is indicated in progressive pleural disease undiagnosed by conservative procedures or not amenable to thoracoscopy.

B. CONTRAINDICATIONS

The contraindications of open pleural biopsy are the same as those for thoracoscopic pleural biopsy.

C. PROCEDURE

Pleural biopsy is performed under general anesthesia via open thoracotomy. The pleural surfaces are directly visualized to obtain samples for culture and histology.

D. DIAGNOSTIC YIELD

Most patients who undergo open pleural biopsy have been previously evaluated by thoracentesis, closed pleural biopsy, and/or thoracoscopy. This results in selection bias regarding the yield of and diagnoses obtainable by open biopsy. A specific diagnosis is identified in 40–60% of patients undergoing the procedure; the most common diagnoses are malignancy and tuberculosis. The age of the patient, incidence of various diseases in the population of patients being studied, and extent of previous evaluation influence the yield.

E. COMPLICATIONS

Complications of open pleural biopsy are those associated with thoracotomy and include atelectasis, pleural hemorrhage, and postoperative pneumonia. These are rare in the absence of significant underlying lung disease or a simultaneous parenchymal lung biopsy.

BRONCHOSCOPY

Flexible Fiberoptic Bronchoscopy (FOB)

Developed in 1964 by Ikeda, flexible fiberoptic bronchoscopy (FOB) has largely replaced rigid bronchoscopy in the diagnosis of infectious, inflammatory, and malignant disease of the chest. Advantages of flexible FOB include (1) a more extensive view of the tracheobronchial tree, (2) ease of performance with excellent patient tolerance, and (3) no requirement for endotracheal intubation and general anesthesia.

A. INDICATIONS

Diagnostic and therapeutic indications for FOB are listed in Table 5–1.

B. CONTRAINDICATIONS

Absolute contraindications to bronchoscopy include lack of patient consent, an inexperienced operator, and lack of facilities available to handle potential complications of the procedure. Relative contraindications that increase the risk of complications include angina or recent myocardial infarction, unstable cardiac arrhythmia, unstable bronchial asthma, respiratory insufficiency with hypoxemia and/or hypercarbia, pulmonary

Table 5–1. Indications for fiberoptic bronchoscopy.

Diagnostic indications
  Investigate
    Airway patency
    Vocal cord paralysis
    Persistent cough
    Localized wheeze/stridor
    Paralyzed hemidiaphragm
    Atelectasis
    Hemoptysis
    Abnormal sputum cytology
  Evaluate
    Abnormalities on chest radiograph
      Mass lesions
      Diffuse and focal infiltrates
    Nonresolving pneumonia
    Tracheobronchial injury in thoracic trauma
    Tracheoesophageal fistula
    Airway injury from inhalational injury and burns
    Staging and evaluation of lung cancer
    Obtain specimens for microbiological studies
    Posttracheostomy airway complications
Therapeutic indications
  Removal of retained secretions
  Removal of foreign bodies
  Perform difficult endotracheal intubations
  Laser therapy of obstructive airway lesions
  Stenting of obstructing endobronchial lesions
  Dilation of airway stenosis
  Placement of endobronchial radiation therapy (brachytherapy)
  Therapeutic lung lavage for pulmonary alveolar proteinosis

hypertension, coagulopathy, uremia, and poor patient compliance.

C. PROCEDURE

1. Patient preparation prior to the procedure includes (a) informed consent, (b) minimum 8-h fast to reduce the risk of aspiration, (c) topical anesthesia, and (d) optional premedication. Use of intravenous benzodiazepines and/or narcotics for conscious sedation, amnesia, and cough suppression without impairment of ventilation, oxygenation, or cooperation are controversial. Many side effects of this procedure are secondary to these premedications. Regardless, patients should always be accompanied to and from the procedure by an adult in anticipation of the possible administration of sedation.

2. Routine intraoperative monitoring includes continuous heart rate, blood pressure, electrocardio-

gram, and pulse oximetry. All patients should receive supplemental oxygen during and after the procedure.

3. Three approaches are available for passage of the bronchoscope. Transnasal and transoral routes may be used in nonintubated patients; mechanically ventilated patients require passage through the endotracheal tube. The transnasal approach provides the greatest patient comfort; the transoral approach is reserved for patients with bleeding disorders or difficult nasal anatomy.

4. The bronchoscope is inserted and advanced to the level of the pharynx and larynx. A complete examination of the airways above the trachea is performed and vocal cord anatomy and mobility are evaluated. The scope is then passed through the cords. After inspection of the trachea, all carinae and segmental bronchial orifices are examined for sharpness, position, texture, color, size, and patency. The bronchial mucosa is also inspected for the presence of submucosal infiltration, inflammation, and secretions.

D. Sample Analysis and Diagnostic Yield

Bronchoscopy provides specimens for microbiological, histological, and cytological analysis. Specimens are collected using a variety of techniques, including bronchial washing, bronchial brushing, bronchoalveolar lavage (BAL), endobronchial or transbronchial forceps biopsy (TBBx), and endobronchial or transbronchial needle aspiration (TBNA). Diagnostic yield is influenced by specimen size and number, distribution of the disease process, and biopsy specimen crush artifact, which make histological pattern recognition difficult. The diagnostic yield for endoscopically visible lesions when using a variety of sampling techniques is approximately 70–95%. The diagnostic yield of transbronchial procedures for peripheral nodules depends on the size of the lesion and the number of specimens obtained. Yield for nonendoscopically visible peripheral parenchymal lesions greater than 3 cm in diameter is greater than 80% (range 44–85%). However, the yield for peripheral lesions less than 2 cm in diameter is as low as 20% (range 23–58%). The addition of washings, brushings, BAL, and TBNA increases the yield to approximately 60%. The yield of TBNA in evaluating mediastinal nodes in patients with lung cancer is 10–50% and depends on detection of mediastinal lymphadenopathy by chest computed tomography (CT) scanning. In general, disease processes with a peribronchial distribution are more likely to be diagnosed by TBBx than are other diffuse processes.

E. Complications

FOB is safe in the hands of experienced operators. Major complications have been reported in 0.08–5% of procedures, with a mortality of 0.01–0.5%. The risk of major complications is highest in those with active ischemic heart disease and advanced pulmonary disease. Major complications include pneumothorax, pulmonary hemorrhage, and respiratory failure. Other complications include sedation-induced hypoventilation, hypoxemia, cardiac dysrhythmias, cardiac ischemia, bronchospasm, fever, and rarely bacteremia.

Baaklini WA et al: The diagnostic yield of fiberoptic bronchoscopy in evaluating solitary pulmonary nodules. Chest 2000;117: 1049. [PMID: 10767238]. (Four-year retrospective review of yield of FOB in 177 patients.)

Chechani V: Bronchoscopic diagnosis of solitary pulmonary nodules and lung masses in the absence of endobronchial abnormality. Chest 1996;109:620. [PMID: 8617067]. (Study comparing diagnostic yield and complications of bronchial washing, transbronchial biopsy, bronchial brushing, and transbronchial needle aspiration of lung nodules and masses.)

Rigid Bronchoscopy

A. Indications

Rigid bronchoscopy is indicated in patients with large airway obstruction in whom flexible FOB is not feasible. Other common indications for rigid bronchoscopy include massive hemoptysis, foreign body aspiration, laser therapy of obstructive lesions, dilation or stenting of tracheobronchial obstructions, broncholithiasis, and removal of thick, copious impacted secretions.

B. Contraindications

The contraindications of rigid bronchoscopy are the same as those for flexible FOB.

C. Procedure

Rigid bronchoscopy is performed with the patient under general anesthesia. It should be performed by an experienced bronchoscopist in an operating room.

D. Diagnostic Yield

Rigid bronchoscopy is primarily a therapeutic modality and is rarely used for diagnostic purposes. The advantage of the procedure is that the central lumen of the instrument provides access for a variety of instruments while maintaining maximal central airway patency.

E. Risks and Complications

The major risks of this procedure are those associated with general anesthesia. In addition, cervical spine, mandible, or skull injuries may be aggravated due to manipulation during the procedure. Limitations of rigid bronchoscopy include inability to evaluate distal airways or to perform it on mechanically ventilated patients.

Miller JI Jr: Rigid bronchoscopy. Chest Surg Clin North Am 1996;6:161. [PMID: 8724272]. (General review of indications and techniques of rigid bronchoscopy.)

PARENCHYMAL LUNG BIOPSY

Initial attempts to sample lung tissue are usually accomplished by FOB with TBBx. However, these small tissue specimens are frequently of insufficient size to diagnose some diffuse lung diseases, necessitating more invasive techniques.

Video-Assisted Thoracoscopic Surgery (VATS)

Thoracoscopy and thoracoscopic surgery are in the midst of a revival as a result of advances in video imaging and instrumentation. Video-assisted thoracoscopic surgery lung biopsy (VATS-LB) specimens are wedge resections of lung parenchyma obtained using a stapler mechanism. Biopsy samples are of a size (3–6 cm) similar to those obtained during thoracotomy. The advantage of VATS-LB is comparable diagnostic yield to open lung biopsy with lower duration of hospitalization and patient morbidity.

A. INDICATIONS

The list of diagnostic and therapeutic indications for VATS continues to grow. Although no prospective, randomized trials comparing conventional and thoracoscopic procedures exist, growing clinical experience supports the use of thoracoscopic techniques for certain clinical situations. These are listed in Table 5–2.

B. CONTRAINDICATIONS

Absolute and relative contraindications for VATS are the same as those for thoracoscopic pleural biopsy. Contraindications for pulmonary biopsy include mean pulmonary arterial pressure greater than 35 mm Hg, end-stage interstitial fibrosis, arteriovenous aneurysm, hydatid cyst, and vascular tumor.

Table 5–2. Indications for VATS.

Lung biopsy for diffuse pulmonary infiltrates
Pleural biopsy of pleural effusions
Pleurectomy/pleurodesis
Decortication of hemothorax or empyema
Lobectomy
Blebectomy/bullectomy
Spontaneous or secondary pneumothorax with persistent air leak
Lung volume reduction surgery
Biopsy or excision of mediastinal lesions
Pulmonary resection for bronchogenic carcinoma

C. PROCEDURE

VATS is performed by thoracic surgeons in an operating room utilizing local and generalized anesthesia and single-lung ventilation via double-lumen endotracheal tube intubation. After intubation and bronchoscopic confirmation of tube placement, patients are positioned in the lateral decubitus position with the ventilated lung down. Ventilation is isolated to the dependent lung. The nondependent lung is collapsed by suction or positive pressure introduced into the pleural cavity. Although some procedures can be performed using single or dual access sites, most therapeutic procedures require three incisions in the lateral chest wall. These incisions are less than 2 cm in length if the procedure is performed purely with a thoracoscope. If more extensive exposure is required an extended thoracoscopy or limited minithoracotomy is performed. Access should provide sufficient working space within the chest cavity and allow the thoracoscopist sufficient space for mobilization of endoscopic stapling devices and graspers around anatomic structures. One or more chest tubes are inserted at the end of the procedure for evacuation of air and fluid. Chest tubes are attached to a negative suction drainage device and surgical incisions are closed in layers. Pleural drainage should be continued until the lung is reexpanded, bronchopleural fistulas have resolved, and chest tube drainage is less than 100 mL/day.

D. SAMPLE ANALYSIS AND DIAGNOSTIC YIELD

VATS-LB samples can be obtained for microbiological and histological analysis. The sensitivity of VATS-LB in diffuse malignant lung disease is 90%; in fibrotic lung disease it is 86%. However, sensitivity for a wide variety of diffuse lung diseases ranges between 42% and 81%. Results of therapeutic VATS procedures vary depending on the disease process. A recent survey of thoracic surgeons revealed that VATS is thought to be an acceptable technique for diagnosis of indeterminate pulmonary nodules and anterior and posterior mediastinal masses as well as for management of clotted hemothorax, early empyema, secondary pneumothorax, and limited cancer. Whether these procedures should replace or augment conventional open procedures is currently being addressed.

E. RISKS AND COMPLICATIONS

Thoracoscopy and VATS-LB are safe procedures with low morbidity. Many complications can be avoided with routine surgical precautions. Complications from therapeutic thoracoscopy are anesthesia, instrument, or procedure related. Mortality rates range from 0.3–1% with a morbidity up to 15% depending on patients' age, underlying lung function, and performance status. Complications include persistent bronchopleural fistula lasting more than 7 days, conversion to open thoracotomy, postoperative bleeding requiring intervention, wound infection, and equipment failure.

Colt HG: Therapeutic thoracoscopy. Clin Chest Med 1998;19: 383. [PMID: 9646989]. (Review of indications and techniques of therapeutic thoracoscopy.)

Open Lung Biopsy

A. INDICATIONS

Open lung biopsy (OLB) is the gold standard, other than autopsy, against which all other diagnostic procedures for intrathoracic diseases are compared. OLB may be required as a result of contraindications to other less invasive procedures or technical difficulties limiting VATS procedures. The major indication for OLB is the clinical judgment that diagnostic information critical to patient management cannot be obtained in any other way.

B. CONTRAINDICATIONS

There are no specific contraindications to OLB. The therapeutic benefit from the information likely to be gained must be weighed in each patient against the morbidity and mortality associated with a thoracotomy. In this regard OLB is controversial in certain settings. For example, OLB provides a specific diagnosis that alters therapy in 70% of patients with acute respiratory failure and diffuse pulmonary infiltrates. Unfortunately, information obtained from OLB has little effect on subsequent hospital (30%) or 1-year (10%) survival.

C. PROCEDURE

OLB is performed under general anesthesia and positive pressure ventilation. The site chosen for the thoracotomy and extent of incision depend on underlying pathology, need for multiple biopsy samples, and expectations regarding whether a major surgical resection will be required.

D. DIAGNOSTIC YIELD

Diagnostic yield depends on whether the most radiographically involved lobe is sampled. Usually at least two separate specimens are obtained as determined by chest CT scans. An advantage of OLB is the ability to directly palpate and visualize thoracic structures. This results in a higher degree of diagnostic sensitivity and a specificity of up to 95%.

E. COMPLICATIONS

Complications of OLB are those inherent to thoracotomy in patients with pulmonary disease. These complications involve the thoracotomy incision, pleural space, and adjacent cardiothoracic structures. Transient atelectasis and pneumonitis are common secondary to chest wall and diaphragmatic splinting. Pleural space complications include bronchopleural fistula, serous effusions, empyema, and hemorrhage. One advantage of OLB is that pleural space drainage time is reduced because surgical defects can be closed with a primary suture. These procedural complications are relatively uncommon when principles of pulmonary surgery, pleural space drainage, and antibiotic administration are employed. The mortality rate for OLB averages 1.5%.

Hunninghake GW et al: Utility of a lung biopsy for the diagnosis of idiopathic pulmonary fibrosis. Am J Respir Crit Care Med 2001;164:193. [PMID: 11463586]. (Prospective study comparing clinical diagnosis to surgical lung biopsy in interstitial lung disease.)

Qureshi RA et al: Does lung biopsy help patients with interstitial lung disease? Eur J Cardiothorac Surg 2002;21:621. [PMID: 11932157]. (Study of factors that determine the yield of surgical lung biopsy in interstitial lung disease.)

Temes RT et al: The lingula is an appropriate site for lung biopsy. Ann Thorac Surg 2000;69:1016. [PMID: 10800786]. (Retrospective review of yield of surgical lung biopsy based on biopsy site.)

PULMONARY ARTERY CATHETERIZATION

Pulmonary artery catheterization (PAC) is insertion of a catheter through the right-sided chambers of the heart into the pulmonary artery (PA) to measure hemodynamic parameters.

A. INDICATIONS

Table 5–3 lists the conditions for which PAC should be considered. The decision to proceed with invasive hemodynamic monitoring is influenced by a variety of factors, including procedural risk versus risk of therapy based on a noninvasive approach. More precise determination of the underlying physiology is required when potential consequences of empirical management on gas exchange, cardiac function, or renal function are overly worrisome.

B. CONTRAINDICATIONS

Patients who are anticoagulated or receiving thrombolytic therapy should undergo central venous catheterization and PAC only from sites accessible to direct pressure. Patients with preexisting left bundle branch block should undergo PAC only if external or transvenous pacemaker equipment is available. This is due to the risk of a right bundle branch block developing, resulting in complete heart block.

C. PROCEDURE

PAC should be performed only by trained individuals who frequently perform the procedure and have the knowledge to recognize and correct its complications.

Table 5–3. Indications for pulmonary artery catheterization.

Evaluate etiology of hypotension
  Hypovolemic
  Cardiogenic
  Septic
Evaluate cardiac function/hemodynamic status
  Acute myocardial infarction
  Left ventricular/right ventricular failure
  Ventricular septal rupture
  Acute mitral regurgitation
  Tricuspid regurgitation
  Valvular heart disease
  Pericardial tamponade
  Constrictive pericarditis
  Undiagnosed tachyarrhythmias
  Pulmonary hypertension (primary or secondary)
Evaluate etiology of respiratory distress
  Cardiac pulmonary edema
  Noncardiac pulmonary edema
Evaluate fluid status
  Oliguric renal failure
  Sepsis
Monitor therapeutic interventions
  Volume resuscitation
  Vasopressor therapy
  Vasodilator therapy
  Inotropic therapy

1. A percutaneous 8 French sheath catheter is inserted into an internal jugular, subclavian, or femoral vein using sterile technique.

2. The pulmonary artery catheter is then visually inspected to assess balloon inflation. The balloon should not leak and should extend beyond the catheter tip. This prevents endovascular damage during flow-directed passage through the right ventricle.

3. The catheter is then flushed with sterile saline solution to remove air and prevent air embolism. The PAC pressure tracing monitor should be placed on the appropriate scale and the catheter physically shaken to ensure that a pressure tracing is demonstrated.

4. The catheter is then placed through the venous introducer sheath. The balloon is inflated after the catheter is advanced about 15 cm. The catheter is then advanced until right atrial (RA) and then right ventricular (RV) tracings appear (Figure 5–1). It is then advanced again until the diastolic pressure rises above RV diastolic pressure. This is a pulmonary artery (PA) tracing. The pulmonary capillary wedge pressure (PCWP) waveform appears as the pressure falls when the catheter is advanced slightly farther into the PA.

5. Deflation of the balloon should result in a PA waveform tracing. If the PA tracing does not reappear the balloon is deflated and the catheter is pulled back into the PA. No more than two-thirds of the balloon volume should be necessary to produce a PCWP tracing. Less volume suggests the catheter is too distal, placing the patient at risk for pulmonary infarction.

6. The catheter is then sutured into place and a sterile sleeve is secured.

7. The balloon should remain deflated at all times except for intermittent PCWP readings.

8. A chest radiograph is necessary to confirm that the catheter tip is in position (within 3–5 cm of the midline) and daily radiographs should be obtained to ensure the catheter has not migrated distally.

9. Continuous waveform monitoring ensures that the catheter neither retracts into the RV nor advances into a PCWP position.

D. DIAGNOSTIC YIELD

See Table 5–4.

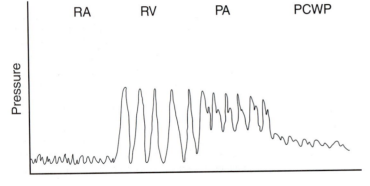

Figure 5–1. Pressure wave tracings encountered during pulmonary artery catheterization.

Table 5–4. Analysis of pulmonary artery catheterization hemodynamics.[1]

Disease State	RA	RV	PA	PCWP	CO	SVR	MAP
Cardiogenic shock	↑	↑	↑	↑	↓	↑	↓
Hypovolemic shock	↓	↓	↓	↓	↓	↑	↓
Cardiac tamponade	↑	↑	↑	↑	↓	↑	↓
Congestive heart failure (biventricular)	↑	↑	↑	↑	↓	↑	↓
Primary RV failure	↑	↑	↓	↓	↓	↑	↓
LV failure	↑	↑	↑	↑	↓	↑	↓
Septic shock	N or ↓	N or ↓	N or ↓	N or ↓	↑	↓	↓
ARDS	N or ↑	N or ↑	N or ↑	N or ↓	N,↑,↓	N,↑,↓	N,↑,↓
Acute pulmonary embolism	↑	↑	↑	↓	↓	↑	↓
Ventricular septal defect	↑	↑	↑	↑	↓	↑	↓
COPD	↑	↑	↑	N	↓	↑	↓
Constrictive pericarditis	↑	↑	↑	↑	↓	↑	↓
Restrictive pericarditis	↑	↑	↑	↑	↓	↑	↓
Primary pulmonary hypertension	↑	↑	↑	N	↓	N	↓

[1]RA, Right atrial pressure; RV, right ventricular pressure; PA, pulmonary artery pressure; PCWP, pulmonary capillary wedge pressure; CO, cardiac output; SVR, systemic vascular resistance; MAP, mean arterial pressure; ↑, increased; ↓, decreased; N, normal; ARDS, acute respiratory distress syndrome, COPD, chronic obstructive pulmonary disease.

1. Pressure. All pressures should be measured at end expiration.

   a. Right atrium (RA): Normal pressure is 0–6 mm Hg.

   b. Right ventricle (RV): Normal pressure is 17–30/0–6 mm Hg. The RV systolic pressure should equal the PA systolic pressure.

   c. Pulmonary artery (PA): Normal pressure is 15–30/5–15 mm Hg.

   d. Pulmonary capillary wedge (PCWP): Normal pressure is 2–12 mm Hg. It correlates well with left ventricular end-diastolic pressure, provided the patient has normal mitral valve and left ventricular function.

2. Cardiac output (CO) is measured by the thermodilution technique. A known amount of cold solution is injected into the RA port; a thermistor 4 cm from the tip of the catheter measures the temperature change allowing calculation of CO using the thermodilution principle. Measurements are inaccurate in low cardiac output states, with tricuspid regurgitation, and with atrial or ventricular septal defects.

3. Mixed venous blood oxygen saturation obtained from the distal port of a nonwedged catheter can be used as an indirect measure of CO but should be interpreted with caution as several conditions alter its reliability.

4. Despite its widespread use the role of PAC in managing critically ill patients is controversial. There has been significant criticism in recent medical literature regarding the safety and utility of PAC in critically ill patients. The Society of Critical Care Medicine has suggested a multicenter study to evaluate the effectiveness of the device. However, some authorities believe that the hemodynamic information obtained from PAC is of considerable value in guiding therapy of critically ill patients, especially when empiric therapeutic trials have proven unsuccessful or are potentially hazardous. Implicit in this point of view is that the physician using PAC hemodynamic data must understand the principles of cardiopulmonary pathophysiology and recognize the pitfalls associated with obtaining and interpreting data. Table 5–4 demonstrates only the common patterns associated with certain pathophysiologi-

cal conditions. Faulty clinical decisions based on inaccurate or misleading data are likely a greater threat to patient morbidity than are the risks of pulmonary artery catheter placement.

E. COMPLICATIONS

Complications common to PAC include those related to obtaining vascular access and those due to the catheter itself. Complications related to central venous cannulation include pneumothorax, hemorrhage, infection, thrombosis, venous air embolism, arterial puncture, thoracic duct injury, and neurological complications. Complications related to the catheter include tachyarrhythmias, right bundle branch block, complete heart block, cardiac perforation, thrombosis, pulmonary infarction, pulmonary artery rupture, knotting of the catheter, endocarditis, pulmonic valve insufficiency, and balloon fragmentation and/or rupture with embolization.

Conners AF et al: The effectiveness of right heart catheterization in the initial care of critically ill patients. SUPPORT Investigators JAMA 1996;276:889. [PMID: 8782638]. (Five-year observational study that suggests early right heart catheterization is associated with increased mortality.)

Coulter TD, Wiedemann HP: Complications of hemodynamic monitoring. Clin Chest Med 1999;20:249. [PMID: 10386255]. (Review of complications associated with PAC.)

Layon AJ: The pulmonary artery catheter: nonexistential entity or occasionally useful tool? Chest 1999;115:859. [PMID: 10084503]. (Good discussion regarding the controversy surrounding safety and efficacy of PAC.)

Pulmonary Artery Catheter Consensus Conference: Consensus statement. Crit Care Med 1997;25:910. [PMID: 9201042]. (Consensus statement regarding indications and safety of PAC.)

SECTION II
Diseases of the Airways

<table>
<tr><td>Asthma</td><td>6</td></tr>
</table>

David A. Kaminsky, MD

ESSENTIALS OF DIAGNOSIS

- *Cough, shortness of breath, wheezing, and chest discomfort, often in association with triggering factors.*
- *Wheezing, diminished breath sounds, hyperinflated lung fields, hyperresonance to percussion; examination can be normal.*
- *Variable degrees of airflow limitation, improvement in airflow following bronchodilator therapy, airtrapping, and airways hyperresponsiveness.*

General Considerations

Asthma is a chronic inflammatory condition of the lungs. It has no known distinct etiology, and there are many different clinical manifestations, making asthma a syndrome rather than a specific disease. Asthma affects approximately 7% of the U.S. population, both adults and children, resulting in 17 million people with asthma in the United States, and over 100 million worldwide. The socioeconomic burden of asthma is high, with over 11 billion dollars spent in total costs in 1998, including billions of dollars in indirect costs from lost productivity. The prevalence of asthma is increasing worldwide, having risen approximately 75% over the years 1980–1994 in the United States. The reasons for this increase are likely due, in part, to increased exposure of susceptible individuals to indoor air pollutants or allergens, and perhaps also to a changing microbiological environment that impacts immune system development. The National Institutes of Health (NIH) and World Health Organization (WHO) have issued disease management guidelines to assist in the consis-

tent diagnosis and treatment of asthma, but dissemination of these guidelines to the medical community is incomplete.

Pathogenesis

The inflammation involved in asthma extends throughout the respiratory tree (Figure 6–1). The clinical manifestations of asthma are a consequence of the effects of this inflammation on the airways and surrounding lung parenchyma, resulting in airway narrowing, airflow limitation, and alterations in lung mechanics.

Many patients with asthma exhibit a two-phase response when exposed to allergen, and this response pattern serves as a useful paradigm to characterize the inflammatory events that are thought to occur. Initially, upon exposure to a sensitizing stimulus in a susceptible individual, mast cells and epithelial cells within the airway are activated and release histamine, leukotrienes, tryptase, and other mediators, which together cause airway smooth muscle constriction, vasodilation, airway edema, and mucus secretion. These events lead to acute wheezing, cough, and shortness of breath from airway narrowing and edema. This is the so-called early asthmatic response that typically occurs within minutes of exposure, and lasts approximately 1 h. The early asthmatic response is best treated with β-agonists that relax airway smooth muscle, and may be prevented by pretreatment with β-agonists, antileukotrienes, and nedocromil or cromolyn. Steroid treatment does not appear to substantially affect this early phase.

Leukotrienes, cytokines, and growth factors released by mast cells, as well as other mediators, may then initiate a cascade of inflammation by calling additional cells into the airway, such as eosinophils, T-lymphocytes, and neutrophils. These cells are then activated to release further chemokines, cytokines, and other mediators, resulting in additional inflammatory cell recruitment and

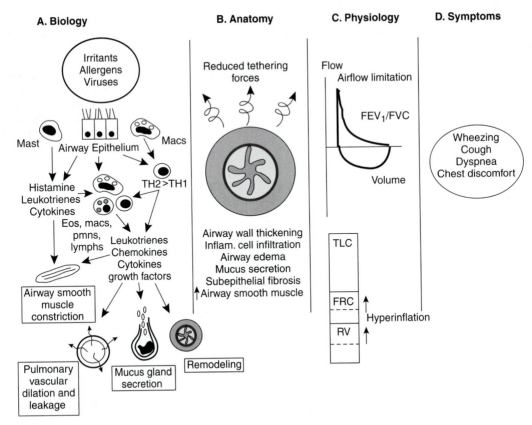

A. Biology   **B. Anatomy**   **C. Physiology**   **D. Symptoms**

Figure 6–1. Overview of asthma pathophysiology. *A:* Biology. The biology of asthma involves the release of mediators, cytokines, and other signals from activated inflammatory cells, resulting in airway smooth muscle constriction, pulmonary vascular dilation and leakage, and mucous gland secretion. Over time, these processes result in airway remodeling. Macs, macrophages; eos, eosinophils; pmns, polymorphonuclear leukocytes; lymphs, lymphocytes; TH1, TH2, T-helper cell type 1, 2. See text for details. *B:* Anatomy. Airway remodeling is seen by airway wall thickening from inflammatory cell infiltration, airway edema, increased mucus secretion, subepithelial fibrosis and increased smooth muscle mass. In addition, there may be a loss of the linkage between the airway wall and surrounding tethering elements of the alveoli. *C:* Physiology. The physiological effects of the narrowed, thickened airways are airflow limitation and gas trapping, resulting in hyperinflation. *D:* Symptoms. The symptoms arising from these underlying pathophysiological changes include wheezing, cough, dyspnea, and chest discomfort.

further airway smooth muscle constriction, airway edema, and mucus secretion. A specific type of T-lymphocyte, the TH2 helper cell, appears to be more common in asthma based on the pattern of cytokines [interleukin (IL)-4, 5, 9, and 13, granulocyte-macrophage colony-stimulating factor (GM-CSF)] found in the syndrome. This TH2 phenotype is involved in allergic inflammation and defense against parasites, whereas the TH1-type cell (associated with interferon-γ and IL-12) is involved in antibody-mediated immunity in response to viruses and bacteria. A shift of TH1 to TH2 cells appears to be an important component of allergic airway

inflammation, and may result from a skewing of immune responses that occurs early in life. In individuals exposed to orofecal infections, mycobacteria, and other organisms, a TH1-predominant phenotype results, and allergic asthma is less prevalent. In environments such as those associated with enhanced hygiene, where there are fewer exposures to infectious organisms and more widespread use of antibiotics, TH1 responses are less prevalent and a TH2-type immune response may become more important. This is the basis of the so-called "hygiene hypothesis" of asthma, which attempts to explain this skewed TH2 response and subsequent increased propensity to development of allergic airway inflammation. However, this paradigm of TH2 predominance in asthma cannot fully explain all of the pathogenesis of asthma, because, among other reasons, asthma and allergies need not coexist.

Because of the influx of inflammatory cells that results following the early response, a second wave of inflammation becomes clinically manifest 4–6 h after the initial exposure. At this time, the patient may develop repeated or worsening shortness of breath, cough, or wheezing. This second wave of symptoms is called the late asthmatic response, and can be demonstrated in about 50% of individuals with asthma. The events of the late asthmatic response are thought to be similar to those that occur on a chronic basis in all patients with persistent asthma symptoms. These events include additional inflammatory cell recruitment and activation, with ongoing airway inflammation and bronchoconstriction. Steroid treatment is the mainstay of therapy for this ongoing inflammatory phase, although long-acting bronchodilators are also used to combat the persistent bronchoconstriction.

Ongoing inflammation associated with persistent symptoms may result in permanent remodeling of the airway and chronic, persistent airflow limitation. This airway remodeling has been demonstrated in experimental animals and in humans as airway wall thickening associated with increased deposition of collagen in the subepithelial reticular basement membrane, increased smooth muscle mass and inflammatory cell infiltration, and mucous gland hyperplasia. Such remodeling results in an airway that remains narrowed and is more susceptible to enhanced narrowing during smooth muscle constriction. Clinically, with long-standing asthma, there is an accelerated rate of loss of lung function as measured by forced expiratory volume (FEV_1), with persistent airflow limitation despite maximum treatment, and failure of significant bronchodilation following β-agonists. Attenuating this potential, long-term consequence of inadequately controlled and treated asthma is a primary goal of asthma care.

The inflammation involved in asthma is known to exist throughout the airway tree, and even extends into the lung parenchyma. The functional consequences of this extent of inflammation are significant hyperinflation due to gas trapping and gas maldistribution that is typically seen in subjects with persistent asthma. Such hyperinflation and maldistribution result in increased work of breathing and dyspnea, due to both the mechanical disadvantage of the elongated muscles of respiration and the increased inefficiency of breathing from mismatching of ventilation and perfusion.

More detailed abnormalities in the lung periphery have recently been shown in studies that have measured increased resistance in the small, distal airways, increased apparent stiffness of the lung tissue (elastance), and increased responsiveness of the lung periphery to bronchoconstrictive agents. All of these effects may result in increased airflow limitation and work of breathing, as well as aberrant gas exchange. In addition, inflammation of the lung parenchyma, together with remodeling of the airway wall, may reduce the ability of the lung parenchyma to tether open the airways. This effect may result in enhanced airway narrowing for a given degree of airway smooth muscle constriction. In addition, this effect may partly explain the failure of patients with asthma to bronchodilate their airways following a deep inhalation, a response that is seen in healthy subjects. This bronchodilatory effect may play an important role in maintaining a relatively flaccid state of airway smooth muscle tone, preventing such muscle from becoming chronically contracted. Thus, patients with asthma may lack an essential protective effect of periodic deep breathing that helps maintain patency.

Busse WE, Lemanske RF, Jr: Asthma. N Engl J Med 2001;344: 350. [PMID: 11172618]. (A general review of asthma, with particular emphasis on pathogenesis.)

Fish JE, Peters SP: Airway remodeling and persistent airway obstruction in asthma. J Allergy Clin Immunol 1999;104:509. [PMID: 10482819]. (A review of current concepts of airway remodeling and its functional consequences in asthma.)

Fredberg JJ: Airway obstruction in asthma: does the response to deep inspiration matter? Respir Res 2001;2:273. [PMID: 11686895]. (An overview of the phenomenon of response of airway function to deep inspiration in asthma, with proposed mechanisms.)

Lange P et al: A 15-year follow-up study of ventilatory function in adults with asthma. N Engl J Med 1998;339:1194. [PMID: 9780339]. (A study documenting the accelerated rate of decline in lung function in chronic asthma.)

Maddox L, Schwartz DA: The pathophysiology of asthma. Annu Rev 2002;53:477. [PMID: 11818486]. (A different approach to discussing asthma pathogenesis, with emphasis on molecular mechanisms and genetics.)

Tulic MK, Christodoulopoulos P, Hamid Q: Small airway inflammation in asthma. Respir Res 2001;2:333. [PMID: 11737932]. (A general review of evidence favoring small airway involvement in asthma.)

Clinical Manifestations

A. SYMPTOMS AND SIGNS

The classic symptoms of asthma are wheezing, cough, shortness of breath, and chest discomfort. Each can be explained on the basis of the underlying pathophysiological events involved in asthma. Airway narrowing results in diffuse wheezing; airway wall and parenchymal inflammation result in stimulation of irritant receptors and cough; shortness of breath and chest discomfort both arise from the increased work of breathing necessary to overcome the increased resistance of the airways and elastance of the lung tissue, as well as from hyperinflation and ventilation–perfusion mismatching.

The classic signs of mild asthma may include wheezing and increased chest wall dimensions, with hyperresonance due to hyperinflation. However, the physical examination may also be entirely normal, especially during times of disease inactivity. With worsening airway narrowing and airflow limitation, wheezing typically becomes more apparent, but, as airflow limitation becomes even more severe, less air is transported through narrowed airways and wheezing may actually diminish. The increased work of breathing may cause tachypnea, diaphoresis, and use of accessory muscles, with the patient assuming an upright position and being unable to lie down. The increased work of breathing may also result in an increased pulsus paradoxus. With impending respiratory failure, the chest may be silent, the patient unable to speak in full sentences, and respiratory muscle fatigue may be seen by a paradoxical breathing pattern, reduced pulsus paradoxus, and inability to stay upright. Signs of cyanosis and shock may ultimately ensue.

B. PULMONARY FUNCTION STUDIES

Pulmonary function studies in asthma (Table 6–1) classically show a reduced FEV_1 and FEV_1/forced vital capacity (FVC) ratio, indicative of airflow limitation. Typically, the FEV_1 or FVC improve by at least 200 mL and 12% following administration of short-acting bronchodilator, indicative of reversibility. However, not all patients with asthma have abnormal spirometry.

Lung volumes typically reveal a normal total lung capacity (TLC), but a variably elevated functional residual capacity (FRC) and a more commonly elevated residual volume (RV), indicative of hyperinflation from gas trapping. Elevated FRC and RV may fall after administration of a bronchodilator, indicating reduced gas trapping from improved airflow. Such reductions should be at least 15–20% to be deemed significant. Of note, FRC measured by gas dilution techniques may be falsely low because of poorly communicating regions of lung. On the other hand, thoracic gas volume (FRC) measured by body plethysmography may be overestimated because of an underestimation of alveolar pressure by the directly measured mouth pressure.

Airway resistance in asthma is usually elevated, as seen by a reduced specific airway conductance (sGaw). A significant improvement in conductance following bronchodilator is considered at least 25%.

Diffusion is usually normal, or slightly elevated, in asthma. The reason for the elevation of the diffusing capacity may be increased perfusion relative to ventilation in less gravity-dependent lung regions and increased pulmonary capillary volume. Both of these effects are likely a result of the increased negative intrathoracic pressure that develops in asthma during normal breathing, which is necessary to overcome the increased work

Table 6–1. Pulmonary function abnormalities in asthma.[1]

Test	Findings	Comments
Spirometry		
FEV_1	NL/↓	↑ ≥ 12% and 200 mL after BD
FVC	NL/↓	↑ ≥ 12% and 200 mL after BD
FEV_1/FVC	NL/↓	
FV Loop	NL/expiratory flow limitation	
Lung volumes		
TLC	NL/↑	
FRC	NL/↑	↓ ≥ 15–20% after BD
RV	NL/↑↑	↓ ≥ 15–20% after BD
Diffusion		
DL_{CO}	NL/↑	
Airway resistance	NL/↑	sGaw may be NL/↓
Bronchial challenge		
Methacholine	PC_{20} FEV_1	< 8 mg/mL, PC_{40} sGaw < 8 mg/mL
Exercise	↓ FEV_1	≥ 10–15% after exercise
Pressure–volume curve	NL/shifted upward, possibly with increased slope (compliance)	

[1]NL, normal; BD, bronchodilator; ↑, increased; ↓, decreased; DL_{CO}, diffusing capacity of the lung for CO; PC_{20} FEV_1, provocative concentration causing a 20% fall from baseline in FEV_1; PC_{40} sGaw, provocative concentration causing a 40% fall from baseline in sGaw, specific airway conductance.

of breathing. Because of gas maldistribution, the single-breath alveolar volume may underestimate the true TLC as measured either by the inert gas technique or body plethysmography.

Bronchial challenge studies to elicit bronchospasm, in response to methacholine or exercise, are a key component of pulmonary function testing. The physiological manifestations of asthma include not only variable airflow limitation, which is reversible with bronchodilators, but also airways hyperresponsiveness. The definition of airways hyperresponsiveness is seen by a leftward shift of the dose–response curve to methacholine. Such a shift indicates that patients not only respond with a more maximal response than normal subjects, but also are more sensitive to this irritant, responding to lower doses. A patient with asthma may have normal pulmonary function at baseline, including no response to bronchodilator, but still demonstrate airways hyperresponsiveness (see Table 6–1).

Pressure–volume studies in patients with asthma usually show a curve shifted upward compared to normal, due to hyperinflation and increased lung volumes. In contrast to emphysema, the curve typically has a normal slope, indicating normal compliance. However, some patients with chronic asthma have been shown to have a reduced compliance without evidence of emphysema. Such a pattern is of concern because a loss of elastic recoil (increase in compliance) could result in enhanced airway narrowing due to a loss of the tethering effect of the surrounding lung parenchyma on the airways. The cause of such a loss of recoil remains unexplained.

C. Other Tests

Arterial blood gases in mild asthma are usually normal, but as severity increases, a respiratory alkalosis and widened alveolar–arterial oxygen gradient develop, reflecting increased ventilation due to worsening efficiency of ventilation and ventilation–perfusion mismatch, respectively. When $PaCO_2$ begins to normalize in a patient with persistent severe asthma, this indicates not that the patient is improving, but rather that the patient is fatiguing, and may signal impending respiratory failure.

Chest x-rays in subjects with asthma may be normal, or may show signs of hyperinflation with increased lung volumes, hyperluceny, depressed diaphragms, and increased retrosternal airspace. Signs of barotrauma including pneumomediastinum, pneumothorax, or subcutaneous emphysema may also be seen. Airway wall thickening may also be present. Lung infiltrates indicate underlying pneumonia, but may also represent focal atelectasis from mucus plugging of airways.

The electrocardiogram in asthma may be normal, or may show tachycardia with signs of right ventricular strain from elevated pulmonary artery pressures, including rightward axis, right bundle branch block, or persistent S waves in the lateral precordial leads.

Irvin CG, Cherniack RM: Pathophysiology and physiologic assessment of the asthmatic patient. Semin Respir Med 1987;8:201. (A classic review of the physiological abnormalities in asthma.)

Differential Diagnosis

In 1934, Chevalier Jackson stated "Not all that wheezes is bronchial asthma." This statement is as true today as it was then. Wheezing is a nonspecific sign of airway narrowing, and hence any process that results in airway narrowing may cause wheezing (Table 6–2). The most common and important causes are chronic bronchitis and emphysema, congestive heart failure, pneumonia, and pulmonary embolism, but foreign bodies, airway tumors, airway compression from tumor or scarring, or airway involvement from sarcoidosis or bronchiectasis should all also be considered. Wheezing may also emanate from the supraglottic airways, so vocal cord pathologies, and vocal cord dysfunction in particular (see below), are in the differential diagnosis. Coughing and shortness of breath are also nonspecific symptoms, so common conditions such as postnasal drip from sinus disease, gastroesophageal reflux disease, and interstitial lung disease should all be considered. A careful history, physical examination, chest x-ray, and pulmonary function tests are usually able to narrow the differential.

Table 6–2. Differential diagnosis of asthma.

Upper airway narrowing
 Vocal cord polyp, tumor
 Vocal cord dysfunction (paralysis or functional)
 Tracheal stenosis or compression
Lower airway narrowing
 Chronic bronchitis
 Emphysema
 Airway tumor
 Airway compression (eg, tumor, mass, enlarged vessel)
 Airway stricture (eg, stenosis)
 Airway foreign body
 Airway inflammation (eg, sarcoidosis, bronchiectasis)
 Airway edema (eg, heart failure, pulmonary edema)
 Bronchoconstriction (eg, pulmonary embolism, anaphylaxis, postviral, toxic/irritant inhalation)
 Low lung volume (eg, obesity)

Treatment

Because asthma is an inflammatory lung disease, treatment with antiinflammatory agents is the mainstay of therapy. Indeed, the use of antiinflammatory agents, primarily inhaled corticosteroids, with the addition of long-acting bronchodilators for moderate-to-severe symptoms, is considered the best form of treatment for persistent asthma. Short-acting bronchodilators are used only to relieve acute symptoms.

A. PHARMACOKINETICS OF INHALED MEDICATIONS

Treating asthma with inhaled medications entails its own set of unique principles. Providing a drug to treat the lungs by inhalation makes sense, since the drug is delivered directly to the target organ and not to the entire body. However, current methods of drug delivery, by metered-dose inhaler (MDI) or dry powder inhaler, deliver only 10–15% of dispensed medication to the lung. The reason for this is due to particle size and mode of delivery. Upon release from an MDI, particles are relatively large and travel at high velocity, resulting in their impaction on the mucous membranes of the oropharynx. This fraction of medication is either absorbed systemically from the mucous membranes or swallowed, where it can gain access to the central circulation after first traveling through the portohepatic circulation. Drugs with high first-pass metabolism are ideally indicated to reduce the amount of active drug swallowed from reaching the systemic circulation. To reduce oropharyngeal deposition, spacer devices should be used in conjunction with MDIs, which puts physical distance between the device and the mouth thereby allowing particles to slow down and become smaller in size.

Patients should inhale slowly and deeply and hold their breath following drug inhalation to reduce impaction in the upper airway and allow maximal time for deposition in the lower airway. Particles the size of 1–5 μm are best for deposition in the lower airway. Hydrofluoroalkane propellants, which are chlorfluorocarbon free, allow generation of much smaller particles from MDIs with resultant improved deposition within the lung periphery. Because asthmatic inflammation and airway narrowing are known to extend to the distal regions of the lung, such distal deposition would appear to improve a drug's efficacy, but this is unproven.

B. INHALED CORTICOSTEROIDS AND OTHER ANTIINFLAMMATORY DRUGS

There are many forms of inhaled antiinflammatory agents, and the most important of these are the inhaled corticosteroids (Table 6–3). All corticosteroids work by the same mechanism, which involves binding to an intracellular receptor that is translocated to the nucleus and acts as a transcription factor, influencing gene expression. In this way, steroids work by shutting down inflammatory genes and promoting expression of antiinflammatory genes. Thus, the different formulations differ only by their pharmacokinetic parameters.

Corticosteroids have been shown to attenuate the inflammation associated with asthma, as indicated by decreased levels of mediators, cytokines, inflammatory cells, and other markers. Recent studies have also shown that inhaled corticosteroids lead to short-term reduction in subepithelial basement membrane thickening, implying that they may have a disease-modifying effect. Indeed, some studies have shown a reduction in the accelerated rate of decline of lung function in patients treated with inhaled steroids, although this point remains unproven. Pulmonary function, including airways hyperresponsiveness, is also improved.

Clinically, steroids improve asthma symptoms and sustained control, resulting in less use of β-agonists, fewer exacerbations associated with days lost from school and work, less nighttime awakening, fewer office and emergency room visits, and overall improved quality of life. Side effects of inhaled corticosteroids include local oropharyngeal irritation and thrush, and systemic cortisol suppression. The clinical effects of cortisol suppression do not appear to be significant, although case reports of hypoglycemia associated with adrenal suppression in children taking high doses of inhaled steroids have appeared. Other side effects of inhaled corticosteroids may include transient reduction in growth velocity in children and increased risk of cataracts. All of these can be minimized by using the lowest dose possible, rinsing the mouth following administration, and using a spacer with any form of MDI steroid.

Other forms of antiinflammatory therapy are also available (Table 6–4), but none compares to the importance of the corticosteroids. Cromolyn and nedocromil are inhaled drugs that modify inflammation at the level of controlling mast cell activation and inhibiting sensory nerve activation. Both drugs are used commonly in children, but the recently published CAMP trial demonstrated that inhaled budesonide was superior to inhaled nedocromil in improving airway hyperresponsiveness and asthma control. Theophylline has been shown to have antiinflammatory properties in addition to its classically known bronchodilatory effects, and may serve as an important adjunct to inhaled steroids. Unfortunately, theophylline has a narrow therapeutic window when dosed in a conventional manner. However, even low doses of theophylline have some clinical benefit as add-on therapy, possibly from antiinflammatory activity. Antileukotrienes have antiinflammatory properties as seen by their association with lower eosinophil and exhaled nitric oxide levels. Antihistamines are antiinflammatory in the sense that they attenuate the effects of histamine release.

Table 6–3. Usual dosage for long-term-control medication.

Medication	Dosage form	Adult dose	Child dose
Inhaled corticosteroids (see estimated comparative daily dosages for inhaled corticosteroids)			
Systemic corticosteroids (applies to all three corticosteroids)			
Methylprednisolone	2, 4, 8, 16, 32 mg tablets	7.5–60 mg daily in a single dose in AM or every other day as needed for control	0.25–2 mg/kg daily in single dose in AM or every other day as needed for control
Prednisolone	5 mg tablets, 5 mg/5 mL, 15 mg/5 mL		
Prednisone	1, 2.5, 5, 10, 20, 50 mg tablets; 5 mg/mL, 5 mg/5 mL	Short-course "burst" to achieve control: 40–60 mg per day as single or two divided doses for 3–10 days	Short-course "burst": 1–2 mg/kg/d, maximum 60 mg/d for 3–10 days
Cromolyn and nedocromil			
Cromolyn	MDI 1 mg/puff	2–4 puffs three to four times a day	1–2 puffs three to four times a day
	Nebulizer: 20 mg/ampule	1 ampule three to four times a day	1 ampule three to four times a day
Nedocromil	MDI 1.75 mg/puff	2–4 puffs two to four times a day	1–2 puffs two to four times a day
Inhaled long-acting β_2-agonists (should not be used for symptom relief or for exacerbations; use with inhaled corticosteroids)			
Salmeterol	MDI 21 μg/puff	2 puffs every 12 h	1–2 puffs every 12 h
	DPI 50 μg/blister	1 blister every 12 h	1 blister every 12 h
Formoterol	DPI: 12 μg/single-use capsule	1 capsule every 12 h	1 capsule every 12 h
Combination medication			
Fluticasone Salmeterol combination DPI	100, 250, or 500 μg/50 μg	1 inhalation twice a day; dose depends on severity of asthma	1 inhalation twice a day; dose depends on severity of asthma
Leukotriene modifiers			
Montelukast	4 or 5 mg chewable tablet 10 mg tablet	10 mg every night	4 mg every night (2–5 years) 5 mg every night (6–14 years) 10 mg every night (> 14 years)
Zafirlukast	10 or 20 mg tablet	40 mg daily (20 mg tablet bid)	20 mg daily (7–11 years) (10 mg tablet bid)
Zileuton	300 or 600 mg tablet	2400 mg daily (give tablets qid)	
Methylxanthines [Serum monitoring is important (serum concentration of 5–15 μg/mL at steady state)]			
Theophylline	Liquids, sustained-release tablets, and capsules	Starting dose 10 mg/kg/d up to 300 mg max; usual max 800 mg/d	Starting dose 10 mg/kg/d: usual max: < 1 year of age: 0.2 (age in weeks) + 5 = mg/kg/d ≥ 1 year of age: 16 mg/kg/d

From NAEPP. Guidelines for the diagnosis and management of asthma—update on selected topics 2002: NIH-NHLBI. NIH Publication No. 02-5075, 2002. www.nhlbi.nih.gov. DPI, dry powder inhaler; MDI, metered dose inhaler.

C. INHALED BRONCHODILATORS

Bronchodilators, which are used to relieve symptoms by relaxing airway smooth muscle, also come in various forms. The short-acting β-agonists are the most important bronchodilators and are used to treat acute symptoms. Short-acting β-agonists should be used only on an as-needed basis, not regularly. Their onset of action is rapid and sustained for 4–6 h, usually long enough to allow patients to participate in sports and activities.

Levalbuterol, a new single isomer (R-isomer) of albuterol, is now available, and is thought to have advantages over the racemic mixture.

Two long-acting β-agonists are available in the United States, salmeterol and formoterol (Table 6–3). Both have a 12 h duration of action, but formoterol begins working within 5 min, whereas salmeterol's onset of action is approximately 20–30 min. In addition to acting as bronchodilators, inhaled β-agonists have also been shown to have antiinflammatory properties, and

Table 6–4. Estimate comparative daily dosages for inhaled corticosteroids.

Drug	Low daily dose		Medium daily dose		High daily dose	
	Adult	Child	Adult	Child	Adult	Child
Beclomethasone CFC 42 or 84 µg/puff	168–504 µg	84–336 µg	504–840 µg	336–672 µg	> 840 µg	> 672 µg
Beclomethasone HFA 40 or 80 µg/puff	80–240 µg	80–160 µg	240–640 µg	160–320 µg	> 640 µg	> 320 µg
Budesonide DPI 200 µg/inhalation	200–600 µg	200–400 µg	600–1200 µg	400–800 µg	> 1200 µg	> 800 µg
Inhalation suspension for nebulization (child dose)	0.5 mg		1.0 mg		2.0 mg	
Flunisolide 250 µg/puff	500–1000 µg	500–750 µg	1000–2000 µg	1000–1250 µg	> 2000 µg	> 1250 µg
Fluticasone MDI: 44, 110, or 220 µg/puff DPI: 50, 100, or 250 µg/inhalation	88–264 µg	88–176 µg	264–660 µg	176–440 µg	> 660 µg	> 440 µg
Triamcinolone acetonide 100 µg/puff	400–1000 µg	400–800 µg	1000–2000 µg	800–1200 µg	> 2000 µg	> 1200 µg

From NAEPP. Guidelines for the diagnosis and management of asthma—update on selected topics 2002: NIH-NHLBI. NIH Publication No. 02-5075, 2002. www.nhlbi.nih.gov. CFC, chlorofluorocarbon propellant; DPI, dry powder inhaler; HFA, hydrofluoroalkane propellant; MDI, metered dose inhaler.

specifically appear to enhance the effectiveness of inhaled steroids.

Other bronchodilators include inhaled ipratropium, an anticholinergic agent. This is a weaker bronchodilator than the β-agonists, but does provide an additional benefit when used together with these agents. Patients with asthma respond less well to ipratropium than do patients with chronic obstructive pulmonary disease (COPD). The antileukotriene agents also have bronchodilating effects, but these are mild and these drugs are considered more important in chronic treatment and control of underlying inflammation. Finally, theophylline is also a bronchodilator, but doses that produce bronchodilation are often associated with side effects, such as gastrointestinal upset or headache. Theophylline, like ipratropium, does add benefit to the β-agonists, and may be used in emergency room or intensive care unit settings. However, it is considered to be more important as a chronic treatment, perhaps by modifying inflammation.

D. NIH–WHO GUIDELINES TO TREATMENT

Deciding which agents to use and how to use them is a primary goal of the NIH–WHO guidelines (Table 6–5). The key principle is categorizing the clinical nature and severity for each individual, and then modifying therapy according to that category. A general rule is to start at high doses of medication to gain control of the symptoms, and then reduce dosing to find the lowest possible doses that maintain control. End points in determining successful treatment include reduced frequency and intensity of symptoms, ability to perform normal daily activities including sports and exercise,

ability to sleep through the night without exacerbations, limited use of an as-needed β-agonist for acute relief of bronchoconstriction, and maximum improvement in pulmonary function. Some studies have also shown the benefit of attempting to normalize airway hyperresponsiveness. Judging these end points requires inquiry not only of patients' symptoms and well-being, but also periodic measurement of pulmonary function. A useful index of symptom control is the Juniper asthma control questionnaire.

The guidelines begin by first differentiating intermittent from persistent symptoms of asthma. Persistent symptoms are then further differentiated into mild, moderate, and severe. In those with only intermittent symptoms, such as in response to exercise or other known, discreet stimuli, an as-needed use of bronchodilator may be appropriate, as long as such use is not excessive. Once such use occurs daily, then a classification of mild, persistent asthma should be considered. With the onset of mild, persistent symptoms, one crosses the threshold into use of chronic antiinflammatory therapy. This may consist of cromolyn or nedocromil in children, or inhaled corticosteroids in any patient. If daily symptoms still persist, a long-acting bronchodilator such as salmeterol or formoterol should be added. As symptoms become moderate, and then severe, increasing doses of inhaled steroid, if not the addition of a short course of oral steroids, is indicated. In addition, if mild-to-moderate persistent asthma is not controlled well on inhaled steroids and long-acting bronchodilators, adjuvant treatment with oral antileukotriene agents or theophylline may be helpful.

Table 6–5. Stepwise approach for managing asthma in adults and children older than 5 years of age: treatment.

Classify Severity: Clinical Features before Treatment or Adequate Control			Medications Required to Maintain Long-Term Control
	Symptoms/day *Symptoms/night*	*PEF or FEV₁* *PEF variability*	*Daily medications*
Step 4 Severe persistent	Continual Frequent	≤ 60% > 30%	• Preferred treatment: —High-dose inhaled corticosteroids AND —Long-acting inhaled β₂-agonists AND, if needed, —Corticosteroid tablets or syrup long term (2 mg/kg/d, generally do not exceed 60 mg/d) (make repeat attempts to reduce systemic corticosteroids and maintain control with high-dose inhaled corticosteroids)
Step 3 Moderate persistent	Daily > 1 night/week	> 60%–< 80% > 30%	• Preferred treatment: —Low to medium-dose inhaled corticosteroids and long-acting inhaled β₂-agonists • Alternative treatment (listed alphabetically): —Increase inhaled corticosteroids within medium-dose range OR —Low to medium-dose inhaled corticosteroids and either leukotriene modifier or theophylline
			If needed (particularly in patients with recurring severe exacerbations). • Preferred treatment: —Increase inhaled corticosteroids within medium-dose range, and add long-acting inhaled β₂-agonists • Alternative treatment (listed alphabetically): —Increase inhaled corticosteroids in medium-dose range, and add either leukotriene modifier or theophylline
Step 2 Mild persistent	> 2/week but < 1 time day > 2 nights/month	≥ 80% 20–30%	• Preferred treatment: —Low-dose inhaled corticosteroids • Alternative treatment (listed alphabetically): cromolyn, leukotriene modifier, nedocromil, OR sustained release theophylline to serum concentration of 5–15 µg/mL
Step 1 Mild intermittent	≤ 2 days/week ≤ 2 nights/month	≥ 80% < 20%	• No daily medication needed • Severe exacerbations may occur, separated by long periods of normal lung function and no symptoms; a course of systemic corticosteroids is recommended
All patients	• Short-acting bronchodilator: 2–4 puffs short-acting inhaled β₂-agonists as needed for symptoms • Intensity of treatment will depend on severity of exacerbation; up to three treatments at 20-min intervals or a single nebulizer treatment as needed; course of systemic corticosteroids may be needed • Use of short-acting inhaled β₂-agonists on a daily basis, or increasing use, indicates the need to initiate or increase long-term control therapy		

(continued)

Table 6–5. Stepwise approach for managing asthma in adults and children older than 5 years of age: treatment. (continued)

Step down
Review treatment every 1 to 6 months; a gradual stepwise reduction in treatment may be possible

Step up
If control is not maintained, consider step up; first, review patient medication technique, adherence, and environmental control

Note
• The stepwise approach is meant to assist, not replace, the clinical decision making required to meet individual patient needs
• Classify severity; assign patient to most severe step in which any feature occurs (PEF is % of personal best; FEV_1 is % predicted)
• Gain control as quickly as possible (consider a short course of systemic corticosteroids): then step down to the least medication necessary to maintain control
• Provide education on self-management and controlling environmental factors that make asthma worse (eg, allergens and irritants)
• Refer to an asthma specialist if there are difficulties controlling asthma or if step 4 care is required; referral may be considered if step 3 care is required

• Minimal or no chronic symptoms day or night
• Minimal or no exacerbations
• No limitations on activities; no school/work missed

• PEF > 80% of personal best
• Minimal use of inhaled short-acting β_2-agonist (< 1 time per day, < 1 canister/month)
• Minimal or no adverse effects from medications

From NAEPP. Guidelines for the diagnosis and management of asthma—update on selected topics 2002: NIH-NHLBI. NIH Publication No. 02-5075, 2002. www.nhlbi.nih.gov.

Certain principles of combined therapy have recently been identified. First, many studies have now shown that adding a long-acting bronchodilator is more effective at improving symptoms and pulmonary function than increasing the dose of inhaled steroid alone. The use of a fixed combination of fluticasone and salmeterol has been more efficacious than use of identical doses of each component taken separately, perhaps because of improved adherence to therapy. Second, the addition of a long-acting bronchodilator may allow for a reduced dose of inhaled steroid, in order to avoid unnecessary adrenal suppression and possible side effects. However, switching to monotherapy with a long-acting β-agonist alone may result in a significant loss of asthma control, due to masking of underlying inflammation or tolerance to the bronchoprotective and bronchodilating properties of long-acting β-agonists. This tolerance is attenuated with concomitant use of inhaled steroids, which may work by upregulating β-receptors. Interestingly, however, different polymorphisms of the β-receptor appear to have different sensitivities to such tolerance. Third, the addition of salmeterol to inhaled steroids appears superior to the addition of the antileukotriene agent montelukast, although adding montelukast continues to improve symptoms beyond using inhaled steroids alone.

E. FUTURE DIRECTIONS IN PHARMACOLOGICAL TREATMENT OF ASTHMA

Although inflammation plays a key role in asthma pathogenesis, our current antiinflammatory therapies are far from perfect at treating asthma. Other drugs with antiinflammatory effects, such as methotrexate, cyclosporine, and gold, have been shown to have moderate clinical effects in asthma, but are associated with potential serious side effects. Intravenous immunoglobulin, with its broad effects on the immune response, has also been shown to improve asthma control and result in the ability to lower steroid usage, but treatment is very expensive.

One reason for the failure of general antiinflammatory therapy in asthma is that there is a tremendous amount of heterogeneity in the clinical manifestations of the syndrome, including the response to treatment (eg, with inhaled steroids or antileukotrienes). This heterogeneity likely arises because of the unique association of environmental factors acting on specific genetic backgrounds in each individual. Many different mechanisms are likely involved in producing asthma.

A new approach in asthma research is to target specific mechanisms. This has been successful in developing the antileukotriene agents and monoclonal antibodies to immunoglobulin E (IgE). The antileukotriene agents appear to be most useful as add-on controller therapy in patients with persistent asthma, or perhaps as monotherapy in patients with mild, persistent asthma who cannot tolerate inhaled corticosteroids. The use of monoclonal anti-IgE antibody has just been approved for use in adolescents and adults with allergies and moderate to severe persistent asthma that are poorly controlled on inhaled corticosteroids. Clinical trials have shown the drug to reduce the incidence of asthma exacerbations. This targeted approach is also being tried in a variety of different areas. These areas include agents to deviate TH2 to TH1 immune responses (eg, IL-12, interferon-γ, and antigen-linked CpG nucleotides), anticytokines (eg, anti-IL-13), agents to inhibit mast cell and epithelial cell function, and novel antioxidants and bronchodilators. A future goal is to identify the genetic basis for the specific clinical forms of asthma, so that appropriate prophylactic measures and targeted treatment can be used.

F. NONPHARMACOLOGICAL TREATMENT OF ASTHMA

Other treatment principles that do not involve drug therapy are also important in asthma therapy. One of these is environmental control. Inquires should be made into known triggers of asthma exacerbation, including allergens, dust, smoke, fumes, foods, and other stimuli. If a patient with asthma is known to be sensitive to certain allergens, for example, then control measures should include reducing allergen exposure and allergen avoidance. Immunotherapy is indicated for allergic patients, who, despite optimal therapy, have poorly controlled asthma and have documented sensitivity to specific well-defined allergens, such as dust mites, cat dander, and pollens.

Education about asthma is another important aspect of asthma treatment. Like diabetes, asthma cannot be cured, but patients can learn to control the syndrome and lead normal lives. To do this, they must thoroughly understand the importance of inflammation, and the difference between medications that control ongoing inflammation and bronchoconstriction and those that treat acute bronchoconstriction. They must learn to recognize when asthma symptoms and control are worse, thereby prompting increased intensity of treatment. For some patients, symptom recognition is sufficient, but for others, symptoms may not be as evident as early changes in lung function. For these patients, learning to measure and record lung function by home peak flow monitoring is critical to the early recognition of a worsening condition. Home peak flow monitoring seems to provide the most benefit for those patients with moderate to severe persistent asthma. Likewise, the use of a written action plan has proven useful in these patients and in patients with a history of severe exacerbations.

These include concrete instructions on what to do if asthma becomes worse. In this way, patients can act on symptoms quickly and, by learning to control symptoms without the immediate involvement of their physician, they gain a sense of autonomy in their lives.

As anxiety and stress can clearly play a role in asthma control, psychiatrists, psychologists, and social workers may provide care in areas such as fear of disease, dealing with school, jobs, and peers, and paying for costly medications.

To facilitate the educational and multidisciplinary nature of asthma care, comprehensive outpatient care programs have been designed. These improve asthma control and reduce unscheduled doctor visits, emergency room visits, and costs of care.

Despite international guidelines and a better understanding of the pathophysiology of asthma, the goals of the guidelines are not met in the medical community at large. Studies have shown that general practitioners are less likely to prescribe controller medications, measure pulmonary function, and carefully evaluate patient triggers than are specialists. The large 1998 survey "Asthma in America" has documented that less than desired targets are being met in the areas of improving pulmonary function, optimal pharmacotherapy, improving daily activities, and reducing exacerbations. Overall compliance with asthma treatment is only 50%. Clearly, better education of both health care professionals and patients is strongly needed.

Asthma in America Landmark Survey: www.asthmainamerica.com. (This was a large U.S. survey of over 700 health care workers and over 2500 current asthma patients that found that asthma management in the United States is falling far short of the goals established by the NIH guidelines.)

Barnes PJ: Current issues for establishing inhaled corticosteroids as the antiinflammatory agents of choice in asthma. J Allergy Clin Immunol 1998;101:S427. [PMID: 9563367]. (A comprehensive review of the data supporting use of corticosteroids as first-line therapy in chronic asthma.)

CAMP Research Group: Long-term effects of budesonide or nedocromil in children with asthma. N Engl J Med 2000;343:1054. [PMID: 11027739]. (The longest-term study to date in children documenting the beneficial effects and safety of use of inhaled corticosteroids.)

Donohue JF, Ohar JA: New combination therapies for asthma. Curr Opin Pulm Med 2001;7:62. [PMID: 11224725]. (A comprehensive review of data supporting combined therapy in asthma.)

George MR et al: A comprehensive educational program improves clinical outcome measures in inner-city patients with asthma. Arch Intern Med 1999;159:1710. [PMID: 10448773]. (An example of the benefit provided by a comprehensive educational program in the treatment of asthma.)

Haahtela T: The disease management approach to controlling asthma. Respir Med 2002;96(Suppl A):S1. [PMID: 11858560]. (A concise overview of asthma diagnosis and management.)

Lazarus SC et al: Long-acting β-agonist monotherapy vs. continued therapy with inhaled corticosteroids in patients with persistent asthma. A randomized controlled trial. JAMA 2001; 285:2583. [PMID: 11368732].

Lemanske RF et al: Inhaled corticosteroid reduction and elimination in patients with persistent asthma receiving salmeterol. A randomized controlled trial. JAMA 2001;285:2594. [PMID: 11368733]. (This pair of articles highlights the principle of improved asthma symptoms and control using a combination of inhaled steroid and long-acting β-agonist.)

Milgrom H, et al for the RhuMAb-E25 Study Group: Treatment of allergic asthma with monoclonal anti-IgE antibody. N Engl J Med 1999;341:1966. [PMID 106078013]. (A randomized trial of two doses of this anti-IgE antibody versus placebo in patients with moderate to severe asthma shows improved symptoms at 12 weeks in both treatment groups.)

National Asthma Education and Prevention Program, Expert Panel Report 2. Guidelines for the diagnosis and management of asthma: NIH-NHLBI. NIH Publication No. 97-4051, 1997. www.nhlbi.nih.gov. (The most comprehensive national guidelines on asthma.)

National Asthma Education and Prevention Program. Guidelines for the diagnosis and management of asthma—update on selected topics 2002: NIH-NHLBI. NIH Publication No. 02-5075, 2002. (An update on selected topics from the 1997 report.)

Szefler SJ et al: Significant variability in response to inhaled corticosteroids for persistent asthma. J Allergy Clin Immunol 2002;109:410. [PMID: 11897984]. (This article reports the important observation that there is extreme variability in the response of patients to inhaled steroids).

Special Considerations

A. DIFFICULT TO CONTROL ASTHMA

Some patients have severe asthma that is not controlled despite apparent use of optimal therapy. In these patients, a systematic approach to reassessment and treatment may be indicated. First, it is necessary to reassess the diagnosis of asthma. Are patients not responding to treatment because they actually have congestive heart failure, vocal cord dysfunction (VCD), or other lung disease? Pulmonary function studies, including methacholine challenge testing, allergy evaluation, and chest x-ray should be performed if the diagnosis is uncertain.

If asthma diagnosis is certain, then reconsider asthma classification and ensure that treatment guidelines are being met. This includes use of a peak flow meter and a written action plan. Then question the correct use of inhalers and dosing regimens. Asking the patient to demonstrate use of an MDI, for examination-ple, is the best way to ensure correct usage. Asthma control should be pursued quickly with a short oral course of steroids, with subsequent resumption of inhaled corticosteroids.

It is important to determine whether environmental factors and concomitant disorders might be exacerbating asthma. These factors include allergen exposure, infection, rhinosinusitis, gastroesophageal reflux disease (GERD), and psychosocial issues. Aggressive treatment of sinus disease with inhaled nasal steroids and nasal saline washes, or of GERD with proton pump inhibitors and nonmedical means of reducing acid reflux, may be crucial to regaining asthma control. If the patient has significant allergies, treatment with the new intravenous anti-IgE has been shown to work well when more conventional therapies have proved suboptimal. Obesity has recently been recognized as an important factor that exacerbates asthma symptoms. Patients should be counseled in proper nutrition and exercise to facilitate weight loss. Finally, consider enrolling a patient with severe asthma into a pulmonary rehabilitation program, which can provide valuable additional education, psychosocial counseling, and specific exercises to improve aerobic conditioning. Improved conditioning usually results in reduced levels of dyspnea and increased exercise tolerance, both of which can substantially improve a patient's well-being.

Proceedings of the ATS workshop on refractory asthma: Am J Respir Crit Care Med 2000;162:2341. [PMID: 11112161]. (An official ATS workshop report on diagnosing and managing patients with difficult to control asthma.)

B. STATUS ASTHMATICUS

The patient with acute, severe asthma must be treated aggressively to avoid respiratory failure. As mentioned, patients with severe asthma may present with signs that indicate severe airflow limitation and increased work of breathing, along with variable degrees of hypoxia. These patients should be admitted to the intensive care unit for close observation and aggressive treatment. Such treatment begins with supplemental oxygen and involves use of intravenous steroids and high doses of inhaled β-agonists, usually initially by nebulization. Helium–oxygen mixtures (heliox) in an 80:20 to 60:40 mix are used to reduce turbulent flow in the proximal airways and thereby reduce the work of breathing, affording relief and time for steroids to take effect to reduce inflammation. Heliox may also improve peripheral deposition of medication, although it is unknown whether this has clinical benefit. Noninvasive ventilation may also reduce the work of breathing and buy time if the patient can tolerate the face mask. Intravenous aminophylline and oral antileukotriene agents have also been used in the management of severe bronchospasm. Intravenous magnesium sulfate may also be tried, but results from many trials fail to demonstrate consistent benefit. There is no evidence that outcome is improved by adding antibiotics to standard care unless clear evidence of infection is present.

It is important to avoid intubation and mechanical ventilation in status asthmaticus because of the substantial risk of barotrauma, but many times this is necessary. In these situations, oxygenation is rarely a problem, but providing adequate ventilation without increasing static airway pressures or excessive autoPEEP (positive end-expiratory pressure) is challenging. An overall strategy is to provide adequate ventilation to maintain an arterial pH of at least 7.20, without concern for the $PaCO_2$ level per se, unless contraindications to hypercapnia exist. Such contraindications include extreme hemodynamic instability and elevated intracranial pressure. Otherwise, in most circumstances, this strategy of so-called permissive hypercapnia is well tolerated. Intravenous bicarbonate may be used to maintain pH > 7.2.

Barotrauma and hemodynamic compromise from dynamic hyperinflation and the generation of high autoPEEP are serious concerns in the mechanically ventilated asthmatic. To reduce these complications, try to maximize expiratory time on the ventilator using low respiratory rates, low tidal volumes, and relatively high flow rates, and to keep plateau pressure below 35 cm H_2O. The use of PEEP is contraindicated in asthma, because PEEP presents further hinderance to expiration and could worsen dynamic hyperinflation. Reducing the work of breathing and controlling the pattern of respiration may require heavy sedation and possibly paralytic agents. Rarely is bronchoscopy indicated to remove excessive airway secretions or mucous plugs, but this should be considered in situations with segmental or subsegmental atelectasis that fail to respond to conventional chest physiotherapy.

C. NOCTURNAL ASTHMA

Although many patients with asthma experience nighttime symptoms, some appear to have pronounced difficulties with their asthma at night. These symptoms typically are worse at around 4 AM, which corresponds to the normal circadian variation in lung function that has its peak at 4 PM and nadir at 4 AM. Whether nocturnal asthma represents a distinct entity or is just a marker of asthma severity is controversial, but there are data to suggest that patients with nocturnal asthma have more airway inflammation and distinct physiological abnormalities compared to patients with asthma without nocturnal worsening of symptoms. Important treatment strategies include optimizing therapy for persistent asthma and assessing whether sinus disease, GERD, or bedroom exposure to allergens and other irritants are involved. Clinical trials have demonstrated improvement in nocturnal symptoms with the use of evening doses of salmeterol or long-acting theophylline, as well as the use of oral or inhaled steroids at 3 PM, rather than at 8 AM or 8 PM.

D. EXERCISE-INDUCED ASTHMA

Exercise-induced asthma is thought to occur because of airway cooling and drying that takes place during the high minute ventilation of exercise. These physical stimuli likely activate mast cells or other pathways that constrict in airway smooth muscle and increase airway narrowing. The majority of patients with exercise-induced asthma are easily treated with regular use of prophylactic bronchodilators, in addition to control of underlying persistent asthma, if present. A dose of albuterol, two to four puffs 20 min before exercise abolishes most symptoms of exercise-induced asthma. The addition of two to four puffs of cromolyn may also help. The longer-acting salmeterol and formoterol may also prevent exercise-induced symptoms, and are especially useful in school children who are then protected throughout the day as they spend time in sports and activities. Remember, though, that long-acting β-agonists should not be used alone in the treatment of any degree of persistent asthma. The antileukotriene agents have also been shown to attenuate exercise-induced asthma, and may be especially useful in select patients.

Many patients also have a so-called refractory period of up to 6 h following exercise, representing a time when bronchospasm is less likely to occur. To take advantage of this phenomenon, these patients should warm up prior to their main exercise to induce mild bronchospasm, and then should be able to engage in their main exercise with minimal symptoms following a period of approximately 30 min rest. Many patients also recognize that exercise involving high minute ventilation in cold, dry air (eg, cross country skiing) causes more bronchospasm than exercise involving lower minute ventilation in warm, humid environments (eg, swimming). Patients who fail to respond to bronchodilators should be reevaluated for the diagnosis of asthma, with special attention to the diagnosis of VCD.

E. OCCUPATIONAL ASTHMA

Many patients develop asthma symptoms in response to inhaled irritants in the workplace. Such irritants can be broadly classified as organic dusts, inorganic dusts, and toxic gases. Documenting bronchospasm in a temporal relation with exposure to these agents is the key to diagnosing occupational asthma. The use of a symptom diary and peak flow recording over periods of time encompassing the in- and out-of-work environment can be very useful. Avoidance of exposure is the best solution, but minimizing exposure by personal protective gear and environmental control measures in the workplace may also help. In some cases, a one-time substantial exposure to an inhaled irritant may elicit new-onset asthma, a syndrome known as reactive airways dysfunction syndrome.

F. DIVING AND HIGH-ALTITUDE EXPOSURE

Many asthmatics engage in scuba diving. As a diver descends, gas is forced into solution in the blood, only to reappear as a gas upon ascent. If the rate of ascent is excessive, nitrogen bubbles emerge in the blood and result

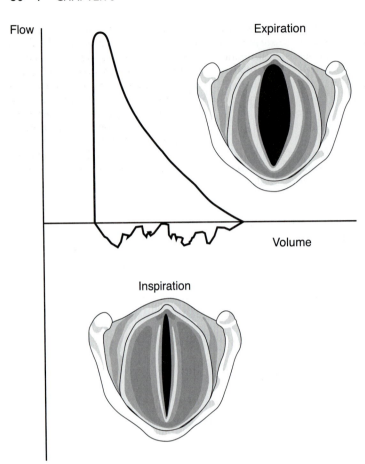

Figure 6–2. Vocal cord dysfunction. VCD is characterized by paradoxical closure of the vocal cords during inspiration, as seen here in conjunction with a flow-volume loop. During expiration, the cords are open, and expiratory airflow is unimpeded, but during inspiration, the cords have partially closed, resulting in an uneven truncation of inspiratory airflow.

in the painful and dangerous condition known as the bends. In addition to gas in solution, all thoracic gas is compressed during descent from the surrounding increased ambient pressure, and upon ascent, such gas reexpands. If the diver cannot exhale the reexpanded gas in a proper fashion, barotrauma may result. This is especially a concern in patients with areas of lung in poor communication with the airways, such as bullous lesions. This concern also applies to patients with asthma, in whom gas expansion within narrowed airways may result in barotrauma from pneumothorax, pneumomediastinum, or air embolism. In addition, the physical activity of swimming and breathing cold, dry tank air may elicit exercise-induced bronchospasm. For these reasons, patients with asthma should use extreme caution in diving, and dive only if their asthma is under excellent control. This may be documented by performing an exercise challenge under premedication. The addition of inhalation of cold, dry air during the exercise challenge and the measurement of lung vol-

umes to document hyperinflation are also useful to screen for safe diving. Limited, retrospective studies have shown that asthmatics with persistent decrements in expiratory flow at low lung volumes are at increased risk of barotrauma from diving.

At high altitude, air is also cold and dry, so asthmatics may experience bronchospasm during exercise. On the other hand, air is less dense at altitude, and airflow is usually increased under such circumstances. In addition, high-altitude air is usually cleaner and freer of allergens, so the net effect of high-altitude exposure on asthma is unpredictable. As with all forms of physical activity and exercise, patients with asthma should be prepared by carrying an inhaled β-agonist to use for short-term relief of bronchospasm.

G. Vocal Cord Dysfunction (VCD)

Paradoxical closure of the vocal cords during inspiration is a common condition that mimics asthma. The etiology of VCD is unknown. As many as 40% of patients carrying a diagnosis of asthma may have concomitant VCD, and many patients thought to have asthma may only have VCD. The best way to distinguish the two is to take a careful history, with special attention to symptoms. VCD occurs abruptly and may be accompanied by difficulty speaking, hoarse voice, or discomfort, including pain, in the throat region. These symptoms typically abate as quickly as they come on, unlike true asthma. The most telling point is that the patient is refractory to conventional asthma therapy. Indeed, many patients with VCD are incorrectly treated for asthma for many years. Proper diagnosis includes documentation of abnormal inspiratory flow on a flow-volume loop, and confirmation of paradoxical closure of the vocal cords during inspiration by direct visualization by laryngoscopy (Figure 6–2). Direct fiberoptic laryngoscopy can be performed quickly and comfortably in the office setting, and is especially important to do during times of symptoms. Because methacholine or exercise challenge commonly bring on symptoms, performing laryngoscopy at the time of these tests may be most useful. Treatment of VCD is primarily through speech therapy, although some patients benefit from the addition of psychotherapy as well.

Chronic Obstructive Pulmonary Disease

7

Thomas L. Petty, MD

Chronic obstructive pulmonary disease (COPD) is our nation's most rapidly growing health problem. It is now the fourth most common cause of death and the only disease in the top 10 that continues to rise in prevalence and mortality. Approximately 16 million adult Americans now have symptomatic stages of COPD. It is estimated that an equal number may have undiagnosed disease. Recent calculations indicate that COPD results in $30.4 billion in direct and indirect costs, presenting a huge economic impact on our society. The purpose of this chapter is to characterize COPD as a major healthcare problem in the United States and present a systematic approach to diagnosis and treatment of various stages of disease, using a case-based approach.

Definition

COPD is an all-inclusive and relatively nonspecific term that is applied to a spectrum of disease that includes chronic bronchitis, emphysema, and asthmatic bronchitis. Cardinal symptoms are chronic cough, mucus hypersecretion, dyspnea on exertion, and occasional wheeze. Characteristically, there is progressive reduction in expiratory airflow. Lung hyperinflation occurs in the majority of patients.

Historical Perspective

Laennec, who invented the stethoscope in 1819, was the first to characterize emphysema. His *Treatise of Diseases of the Chest* contains the following profound statement, "In emphysema the air makes its escape from the air cells much slower than in the healthy state of the organ. This seems to indicate either more difficult communication between air contained in the air cells or that of the bronchi, or else diminished elasticity of the air cells themselves. Perhaps both of these causes conspire to produce the effect in question." Other astute observers recognized the importance of loss of elastic recoil, as COPD began to be characterized physiologically in the early twentieth century. Elastic recoil is a result of stretching the lungs and thorax during a full inspiration. Both lungs and thorax contain elastic fibers. Expiratory airflow is due to the deflation of the system, very much like an inflated balloon empties when released.

The first clear definitions of COPD were developed by the American Thoracic Society and published in 1962. Concepts about COPD have since evolved based on improved understandings of the pathogenesis and the course and prognosis of disease.

Pathogenesis

COPD is a product of inflammatory damage to the conducting airways, both small and large, and loss of elastic recoil due to damage of alveolar structures. Loss of elasticity and premature loss of alveolar walls are parallel processes, but are not related by cause and effect. Together loss of elastic recoil and increased airways resistance reduce expiratory airflow, which is the major indicator of disease severity and prognosis.

The inflammatory mechanisms resulting in COPD are different from asthma. In COPD the CD8 T-lymphocyte is involved, along with macrophages that produce chemotactic factors that stimulate neutrophils to release elastases and toxic oxygen species. Interleukin 8 and tumor necrosis factor α also appear to be involved. In contrast, with asthma the CD4 T-lymphocyte, activated mast cells, eosinophils, and interleukins 4, 5, and 13 are involved.

Whatever the biochemical and cellular events are that damage the alveoli and small airways, physiological alterations begin very early in the natural course of disease. Once the elastic recoil begins to decrease, the total lung capacity (TLC) and the forced vital capacity (FVC) increase. This is why the normal ratio of forced expiratory volume (FEV_1) to FVC of > 70% begins to drop. Said another way, the denominator increases (FVC) before the numerator (FEV_1) becomes reduced.

Epidemiology

COPD has been considered "a smoker's disease that clusters in families and worsens with age." Familial clustering is well established in the α_1-antitrypsin deficiency state (ZZ, SZ, and Null phenotypes). MZ heterozygotes have a mildly increased risk. Family clustering also occurs in patients with normal α_1-antitrypsin phenotypes and serum levels of this protective glycoprotein. Roughly 85% of patients with COPD have

Table 7–1. Classification of COPD by severity (GOLD).

Stage	Characteristics
0: At risk	Normal spirometry Chronic symptoms (cough, sputum production)
I: Mild	$FEV_1/FVC < 70\%$ $FEV_1 \geq 80\%$ predicted With or without chronic symptoms (cough, sputum production)
II: Moderate	$FEV_1/FVC < 70\%$ $30\% \leq FEV_1 < 80\%$ predicted (11A: $50\% \leq FEV_1 < 80\%$ predicted) (11B: $30\% \leq FEV_1 < 50\%$ predicted) With or without chronic symptoms (cough, sputum production, dyspnea)
III: Severe	$FEV_1/FVC < 70\%$ $FEV_1 < 30\%$ predicted or $FEV_1 < 50\%$ predicted plus respiratory failure[1] or clinical signs of right heart failure

[1]Respiratory failure = arterial partial pressure of oxygen (Pao_2) < 8.0 kPa (60 mm Hg) with or without arterial partial pressure of CO_2 ($Paco_2$) > 6.7 kPa (50 mm Hg).

been smokers, often beginning at a young age and with heavy tobacco consumption. Up to 15% of patients with established COPD have not been direct consumers of tobacco. Some of these patients may have been exposed to environmental tobacco smoke in their daily lives, however. The physician must look beyond smoking for identification of COPD.

Assessments

COPD is characterized by chronic cough, mucus hypersecretion, and dyspnea on exertion in smokers as well as some nonsmokers.

Patients with advanced stages of disease usually present with hyperinflation, decreased breath sounds, and sometimes signs of pulmonary hypertension with or without congestive right heart failure. These individuals are easy to diagnose on clinical grounds alone. By contrast, patients with asymptomatic stages have neither signs or symptoms of disease nor x-ray or EKG manifestations. Thus, spirometry must be done on all patients to make a diagnosis. Spirometry is to the assessment of COPD as the sphygmomanometer is to the diagnosis of hypertension.

Other physiological tests that help characterize COPD are the lung compartments, ie, TLC and residual volume (RV), which measure air trapping and hyperinflation. Measurement of gas transfer across the air–blood interface, known as the diffusion test, is also a good physiological indicator of emphysema when alveolar walls are lost.

High-resolution computed tomography (CT) scans are also highly indicative of the lesions of emphysema, ie, loss of alveolar tissue on a large region of destruction known as bullae. With increased resolution, airways lesions can also be evaluated by CT scanning.

Staging

A new classification proposed by the Global Initiation of Lung Disease (GOLD) is presented in Table 7–1. Other classifications have been offered by the American Thoracic Society (ATS), the European Respiratory Society, and the British Thoracic Society (BTS), but it is probably best to adhere to one system. Because the GOLD is a new international initiative, the classification should be embraced, in the opinion of the author. The British Thoracic Society also proposed a symptomatic scoring system (Table 7–2).

The National Lung Health Education Program

Another new healthcare initiative that focuses on COPD is the National Lung Health Education Program (NLHEP). The consensus statement of the

Table 7–2. British Thoracic Society scoring system for symptoms.

Stable COPD	Mild	Moderate	Severe
Cough	"Smoker's cough"	Cough with or without sputum	Prominent cough
Dyspnea	Minimal	On exertion	On exertion or at rest
Lung examination	Normal	With or without wheeze	Hyperinflation, wheeze
Other examination	Normal	Normal	Cyanosis, edema

Source: British Thoracic Society. The COPD Guidelines Group of the Standards of Care Committee of the British Thoracic Society: BTS guidelines for the management of chronic obstructive pulmonary disease. Thorax 1997;52:S1.

NLHEP recommends spirometric testing in all smokers age 45 or older and anyone with chronic cough, dyspnea on exertion, mucus hypersecretion, or wheeze. Spirometric testing finds abnormalities in both asymptomatic and symptomatic patients. Of course, some asthmatics will be found in the screening of symptomatic patients. Asthma is also a COPD, sometimes confused with emphysema; overlaps are common. The course and prognosis of bronchial asthma under treatment are quite different from emphysema. Reversibility of airway obstruction and complete stabilization of disease should be the goal in asthma management. In COPD, management is aimed at providing maximum reversibility of airflow obstruction, achieving clinical and functional stability, and preventing premature declines in FEV_1. These are key therapeutic goals, along with control of symptoms and improving or maintaining quality of life.

Course & Prognosis

The natural history of COPD covers 30 or more years. The course is insidious and the patient is usually without symptoms for 20 or more years before finally being diagnosed on the basis of symptoms, or, hopefully earlier, by spirometry as recommended by the NLHEP. In fact, up to 75% of lung function may be lost before patients are limited by dyspnea on exertion or troubled by chronic cough and expectoration. This is the reason why spirometry is so important in assessing asymptomatic patients as well as patients with established disease. The course varies and is a function of the age at which the ventilatory measurements reach the symptomatic threshold, which is usually $FEV_1 < 1.5$ L/s in an average-sized, middle-aged individual. The course and prognosis are also a function of the rate of decline in FEV_1, the age of the patient, and the type of COPD, ie, asthmatic bronchitis, chronic bronchitis, or emphysema. Overlaps and combinations of these clinical types of COPD are common.

Treatment

A. SMOKING CESSATION

Smoking cessation is necessary to prevent or forestall progression of disease. All patients with COPD absolutely must stop smoking. Details of the strategies in stopping smoking are lengthy and complex, and go beyond the scope of this presentation. The reader is referred to the reference by Dale et al. for a succinct review on this topic.

Approximately 3% of patients will stop smoking on the advice of a physician. It is important for patients to modify their behavioral patterns associated with their cues to light a cigarette. Deciding to quit and choosing a quit date are fundamental principles. A growing number of nicotine replacement products are available both over-the-counter and by prescription to deal with symptoms of nicotine withdrawal (Table 7–3). Bupropion is a nonnicotine antidepressant drug that is effective in mitigating nicotine withdrawal. Together, the physician's advice, the decision on the part of the patient to quit, the selection of a quit date, and the use of pharmacological strategies during the initial 2 weeks of nicotine withdrawal may lead to successful cessation in up to 30% of patients.

B. VACCINES

All patients with any stage of COPD should receive influenza virus vaccine each fall. Because of antigenic shift and waning immunity, a newly constituted vaccine given before the influenza season, usually in October or November, is required annually. A pneumococcal vaccine should be given at least once in a lifetime. Both influenza and pneumococcal vaccines can be given at the same time, which is more cost effective than giving each vaccine alone.

Table 7–3. Drugs used for smoking cessation.

Drug and Method of Administration	Unit Dose	Dose Interval
Nicotine polacrilex (oral)	2 to 4 mg	Every 1 to 2 h[1]
Transdermal nicotine patch	21, 14, and 7 mg	Over 24 h
	15, 10, and 5 mg	Over 16 h
	22 and 11 mg	Over 24 h
Nasal nicotine spray	0.5 mg/inhalation/nostril	8 to 40 mg/d in hourly or as needed dosing
Nicotine inhaler	10 mg/inhaler	Continuous puffing for 20 min 6 to 16 times/day
Nicotine lozenge	2 mg	Every 1 to 2 h
Bupropion sustained-release tablets	150 mg	150 mg for 3 days, then 300 mg/d
Buspirone tablets	15, 10, and 5 mg	7.5 mg twice a day, starting dose; 60 mg/d, maximum dose

[1]Fifteen to 30 pieces may be chewed over 24 h.

C. The Growing Therapeutic Armamentarium for COPD

A growing number of bronchodilators, including inhaled anticholinergics and β-agonists, used alone or in combination, are available to deal with symptomatic stages of COPD. Most patients with COPD have some degree of airflow improvement with the use of inhaled bronchodilators. A combination of ipratropium with albuterol in the same metered-dose inhaler (MDI) is most convenient and economical. Long-acting β-agonists can be used in conjunction with anticholinergics in maintenance management. A stepped care approach is suggested in Table 7–4. In addition, both inhaled and oral corticosteroids are valuable for acute exacerbations. Antibiotics are used for episodes of purulent bronchitis (Table 7–5). Oxygen is useful in maintenance management in both chronic stable hypoxemia and in exacerbations of disease.

Long-term oxygen therapy improves the length of life in selected patients with advanced COPD and chronic stable hypoxemia. This is the only therapy proven to alter the natural course of COPD in later stages. Pulmonary rehabilitation, which involves patient education, breathing training, breathing exercise, and systemic exercise on a regular basis, has become the standard of care for ambulatory patients and is effective in increasing exercise tolerance and in improving quality of life (see below).

Both noninvasive and invasive mechanical ventilation can be lifesaving. Surgical approaches, including lung volume reduction surgery and lung transplantation, may be palliative in selected patients.

COPD begins as an asymptomatic reduction in airflow that often persists for 30 or more years before the combined symptoms of dyspnea on exertion, chronic cough, and expectoration and wheeze occur. The various therapies appropriate for COPD are best discussed in a case management approach. The following three case examples give practical advice on the management of various stages of COPD. The possible strategies of therapy suggested are evidence based, whenever possible.

Case-Based Approaches to Management

A. Patient 1

You see a 59-year-old man previously diagnosed as having COPD in the clinic 3 months following discharge from the Intensive Care Unit (ICU) for a severe exacerbation of COPD. The patient was advised to stop smoking, but failed on several attempts. He had received influenza virus vaccine in the past fall. Following an outing for Christmas shopping, the patient developed a cold, which "settled in his chest." Increased sputum with purulence and fever was followed by worsening dyspnea. He suddenly became extremely dyspneic and was admitted to the ICU via the emergency room. Following treatment with oxygen, antibiotics, and systemic corticosteroids, the patient improved slowly and was discharged on home oxygen delivered by a concentrator. Corticosteroids were not continued after discharge.

Table 7–4. Stepped care for COPD.

	Agent and Purpose	**Indication**
Step 1	For episodic symptoms, eg, dyspnea, cough, wheeze	Short acting β-agonist, eg, albuterol, metered-dose inhaler (MDI)—two puffs every 3–4 h or ipratropium MDI—4–6 h, reduce on control of symptoms
Step 2	For persistent symptoms due to reversible bronchospasm	Ipratropium MDI—two puffs two to four times a day or ipratropium/albuterol combination—two puffs two to three times a day
Step 3	For above symptoms with exercise dyspnea	Add long-acting theophylline 400–800 mg/d
Step 4	For persistent symptoms and nocturnal worsening	Consider a long-acting β-agonist, salmeterol MDI—two puffs twice daily or salmeterol disc inhalers, twice daily, or formeterol, dry powder inhaler twice daily
Step 5	For persistent symptoms and FEV_1 < 50% predicted and frequent exacerbations	Add fluticasone, budesonide, or triamcinolone inhalers
Step 6	For acute exacerbations of COPD with worsening dyspnea and sputum	Prednisone 60–80 mg daily
Step 7	For acute exacerbations with purulent sputum	Add antibiotics to prednisone—see Table 7–5

Table 7–5. Choice of empirical antibiotic therapy for COPD exacerbation with purulent sputum.

Treatment	Dosage[1]
First line	
Amoxicillin (Amoxil, Trimox, Wymox)	500 mg three times a day
Trimethoprim-sulfamethoxazole (Bactrim, Cotrim, Septra)	1 tablet (80/400 mg) twice a day
Doxycycline	100 mg twice a day
Second line[2]	
Amoxicillin and clavulanate (Augmentin)	500–875 mg twice a day
Second- or third-generation cephalosporin [eg, cefuroxime (Ceftin)]	250–500 mg twice a day
Macrolides	
Clarithromycin (Biaxin)	250–500 mg twice a day
Azithromycin (Zithromax)	500 mg on Day 1, then 250 mg a day for 4 days
Quinolones	
Ciprofloxacin (Cipro)	500–750 mg twice a day
Levofloxacin (Levaquin)[3]	500 mg a day
Moxifloxacin (Avelox)	400 mg a day

[1]May need adjustment in patients with renal or hepatic insufficiency.
[2]For patients in whom first-line therapy has failed and those with moderate to severe disease or resistant or gram-negative pathogens.
[3]Although the newer quinolones have better activity against *Streptococcus pneumoniae*, ciprofloxacin may be preferable in patients with gram-negative organisms.

When seen in your clinic 1 month later, the patient was accompanied by his daughter, who is wheeling the oxygen E-cylinder that was prescribed for portability. Your patient reported that he remained severely short of breath and could not regain the 10 pounds of weight that he had lost during the acute exacerbation. He commented on being "depressed" over the fact that he needed to "wear oxygen." His appetite was poor and he had difficulty sleeping. He had rarely gone outside of his home since discharge. The patient was receiving albuterol by MDI three times daily, ipratropium by MDI three times daily, and sustained release theophylline, 600 mg at bedtime. Your patient is moderately short of breath. He is alert and cooperative. Physical examination reveals decreased breath sounds. Cardiac and extremity examination are normal. Edema is absent. The patient's FEV_1 is 1.10 L/s (29% of predicted), FVC is 3.42 (75% of predicted), and FEV_1/FVC ratio is 46%.

(No previous spirometric tests had ever been done before!) The patient's oxygen saturation, measured by a pulse oximeter, is 97%, while receiving oxygen by a nasal cannula at 2 L/min. You consider the following treatment options (choose the one most appropriate for this patient):

1. Add a selective serotonin reuptake inhibitor (SSRI) antidepressant
2. Add oral corticosteroids
3. Measure theophylline blood level
4. Add a salmeterol MDI
5. Stop oxygen and do oximetry after 20 min
6. Continue the present treatment and see the patient again in 3 months

Comment: Of course, any patient's problem may suggest more than one therapeutic option. This patient, with severe COPD, who has just recovered from his first bout of acute respiratory failure and is now depressed and receiving oxygen, is in need of aggressive systematic therapy to prevent relapse and readmission. But of greater importance is the challenge of improving the patient to a state of general health and quality of life.

Probably the choice least likely to help would be to add an antidepressant. Depression, anxiety, and somatic preoccupation are common in patients with advanced COPD. In most cases, the depression is reversible through methods of pulmonary rehabilitation and adjustments in therapy. More recent studies of patients who receive home oxygen have shown a high prevalence of depression, often a result of reduced mobility and opportunities for social interaction.

You might be tempted to add corticosteroids once again, as they have been shown to be helpful in acute exacerbations of disease. In fact, there is some suggestion from uncontrolled clinical trials that long-term administration of corticosteroids may slow the rate of decline in ventilatory function, but no randomized controlled clinical trials have shown an improvement in survival.

Theophylline often has a beneficial effect on respiratory muscle function, and usually does not lead to insomnia in patients with COPD. The effect on respiratory muscle function is not directly related to blood theophylline levels. These measurements are also expensive. Thus, in the absence of gastrointestinal upset or cardiac arrhythmias, measurement of theophylline blood levels is not commonly done to guide theophylline therapy.

Salmeterol, a long-acting β-agonist, may be useful in the maintenance management of COPD. Salmeterol provides equal clinical benefit when compared with ipratropium. However, salmeterol cannot be used for breakthrough attacks because of its prolonged duration of action. Either albuterol or ipratropium is required for this purpose. Using the combination of albuterol with ipratropium in a single MDI would be a reasonable and useful strategy in either exacerbations or in maintenance management.

Stopping oxygen for 20 min and repeating pulse oximetry would be the most important option. Because this patient has a 97% saturation on 2 L, it could be that room air hypoxemia is not present. Too many patients are encumbered by oxygen, often inappropriately delivered via a stationary system, which may, in fact, result in reduced activities of daily living and depression. Today, ambulatory oxygen is the standard of care for patients who can and will increase their activities and exercise both inside and outside of the home.

Continuing with the same treatment and seeing the patient again 3 months later might be the treatment option selected by some physicians. However, this would probably promote a further period of unnecessary self-exile, because of the patient's preoccupation with the need for oxygen therapy. The continued use of an inappropriate home oxygen system would not be desirable. A more active treatment strategy would be more appropriate.

What happened? Oxygen was stopped at the time of the physical examination and counseling. After 20 min patients with hyperinflation and air trapping, as a result of increased RV and temporary "storage" of oxygen, reach a steady state. Following the discontinuation of oxygen, pulse oximetry was repeated on room air and oxygen saturation was 92%. On walking around the clinic while breathing air, the patient's oxygen saturation was 90% with an accompanying pulse of 88.

Stopping the oxygen 3 months after discharge is important because it helps both the physician and the patient understand that oxygen is no longer necessary, at least at the present time. By learning this fact, the patient can be encouraged to gradually increase walking to 20–30 min or more each day. This can be accomplished by walking outside on good weather days or walking in shopping malls or within other covered structures to improve exercise tolerance during periods of poor weather. Regular daily exercise is the key ingredient of pulmonary rehabilitation.

Pulmonary rehabilitation, the details of which go beyond the scope of this chapter, can briefly be described as focusing on patient education, breathing retraining, physical reconditioning, and the adjustment of pharmacological agents. Oxygen is useful only in those patients with chronic stable hypoxemia. The Nocturnal Oxygen Therapy Trial (NOTT) demonstrated a survival benefit from long-term ambulatory oxygen, compared with shorter periods of oxygen administration via a stationary system. Whether the improved survival with ambulatory oxygen in the NOTT study (Figure 7–1) was due to the duration of oxygen or the method of delivery has never been adequately studied. A reevaluation of the NOTT study strongly suggests that patients who had better walk tolerance during exercise training prior to receiving oxygen, compared with those with poorer walk tolerance, had a much better survival with ambulatory oxygen than with stationary oxygen alone. Even patients with poor exercise tolerance did better with ambulatory oxygen than with stationary oxygen.

The prognosis for patients with advanced COPD has been improving in recent years. This is probably

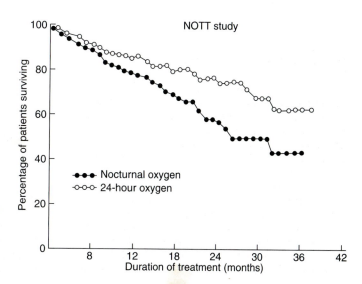

Figure 7–1. Comparison of survival in nocturnal oxygen (NOT) patients compared with continuous oxygen therapy (COT) patients. Survival is significantly better at each year of observation (Nocturnal Oxygen Therapy Trial).

due to the fact that today more aggressive therapy is given to prevent exacerbations of COPD, which helps to prevent acute respiratory failure. More effective strategies to achieve smoking cessation, advances in the treatment of acute respiratory failure, and the use of oxygen and pulmonary rehabilitation have together improved the length and quality of life for many patients with advanced COPD.

B. PATIENT 2

You see a 41-year-old woman in the clinic because of her concerns about emphysema and lung cancer. Her worry is over the fact that her mother, who has severe emphysema, has recently been found to have lung cancer, which is inoperable because of its location near the carina. The patient had started smoking at age 13, and had consumed, on average, 1.5 packs of cigarettes per day (42 pack-years). She reports a "cigarette cough" and poor pep and energy. She is still able to work as a secretary in a large law firm. Because smoking in the office is prohibited, she takes numerous "coffee breaks" and smokes outside of the building to deal with her nicotine craving. Her mother is receiving radiation therapy for lung cancer in an attempt to improve the staging, with the possibility of a lung resection later.

Physical examination is normal. Which one of the following diagnostic procedures would be appropriate at this time?

1. Chest x-ray
2. Arterial blood gases
3. Spirometry
4. α_1-Antitrypsin deficiency
5. Sputum cytology
6. CT scan of chest

Because her mother has lung cancer, and lung cancer has a familial component, you might be tempted to do a chest x-ray, even at the patient's young age. In fact, most physicians are now beginning to realize that women are more susceptible to developing lung cancer than men at a given age and level of smoking. In fact, women tend to have lung cancer at a younger age than men. A chest x-ray, however, is not nearly as sensitive as CT scanning in diagnosing early-stage lung cancer. Low-radiation dose spiral CT scanning would be appropriate if airflow obstruction were present. The risk of lung cancer is four- to sixfold greater in patients with airflow obstruction, compared with normal airflow, with all other background factors being equal (ie, smoking, occupational risk, and family history).

Accordingly, spirometry is the most practical and necessary option in this patient. It is the most important method of diagnosing COPD and assessing responses to therapy.

α_1-Antitrypsin could be considered in view of the family history of emphysema, but only about 3% of COPD is due to α_1-antitrypsin deficiency. It is much more important to identify airflow obstruction by spirometry in assessing patients with a family history of emphysema. Sputum cytology could also be considered and, because of heavy smoking and airflow obstruction, could reveal dysplastic premalignant lesions or even roentgenographically occult lung cancer.

Her spirometry results are as follows: FEV_1 is 2.05 (67% of predicted), FVC is 4.10 (110% of predicted), and FEV_1/FVC ratio is 51%. Thus, this patient clearly has airflow obstruction with an FEV_1 of less than 70% of predicted and the interesting fact that the FVC is 110% of predicted. By the GOLD criteria, the stage of this woman's COPD would be classified as moderate. Other ATS and BTS criteria would classify her as mild. Of greater importance, in view of her young age and significant loss of airflow, most experienced clinicians would consider her severity as moderate and in need of treatment immediately.

Of course, the most important therapy for this patient is smoking cessation. The Lung Health Study has clearly shown that patients between the ages of 35 and 60 have a significant improvement in FEV_1 following smoking cessation, compared with accelerated losses during continued smoking, over a 5-year period (see Figure 7–2). Today, there are improved strategies in smoking cessation, with a growing number of pharmacological agents available to use before or on the quit date. These products are listed in Table 7–3. Assuming this patient had normal ventilatory function at age 20, which may not be true since she started smoking as a teenager, she has lost a total of 1500 mL in 21 years, or a loss of over 71 mL per year. Normal losses for a person this age and height (5 foot 5 inches) are approximately 25 mL per year. Thus, with a similar decline over the next 20 years with continued smoking, at 61 years (her mother's age) she will have lost another 1420 mL. By age 61 her FEV_1 will have declined to 0.73 L, which is in the range of far advanced and disabling emphysema (see Figure 7–3). By contrast, if she stops smoking and only loses FEV_1 at the rate of 25 mL per year, she will lose 500 mL and her FEV_1 will be 1.55 at age 61, which is compatible with a state of reasonably good health (see Figure 7–3). Thus, a key to success in this patient is smoking cessation to prevent a disastrous outcome.

This patient succeeds in stopping smoking and you see her again on follow-up 1 year later. On this occasion, her FEV_1 is 2.20 L/s. She is now concerned about a 12-pound weight gain and has further concerns about the future, because her mother has died of a massive hemorrhage. She again asks about her risk of lung cancer. The following should be considered now:

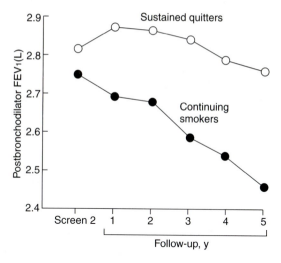

Figure 7–2. Mean postbronchodilator forced expiratory volume at 1 s (FEV$_1$) for participating in the smoking intervention and placebo groups who were sustained quitters and continuing smokers. The two curves diverge sharply after baseline. (Adopted from Anthonisen NR et al: Effects of smoking intervention and the use of an inhaled anticholinergic bronchodilator on the rate of decline of FEV$_1$. The Lung Health Study. JAMA 1994;272:1502.)

1. Sputum cytology
2. CT scan
3. Reassurance that her smoking cessation at a young age will be sufficient
4. Chest x-ray
5. Appetite suppressants

This patient is certainly at high risk for lung cancer, even though she has stopped smoking. Today more lung cancer is found in former smokers than in current smokers. Although still controversial, it would be appropriate, based upon recent studies, to order a low-radiation dose spiral CT scan looking for an occult peripheral nodule, and sputum cytology to find indications of dysplastic preneoplastic or neoplastic lesions. Today, the combination of sputum cytology and CT scanning offers the greatest promise in early identification of lung cancer. Both sputum cytology and CT scans identify patients in early stages, where the likelihood of cure is 60% to 80%. When lung cancer is diagnosed by accident by chest x-rays that are done for other reasons, or on the basis of symptoms, the 5-year survival is a dismal 14%. Chest x-rays are not as sensitive as CT scans in the diagnosis of early lung cancer.

Many smokers gain some weight on stopping, but this occurs mostly in the initial stage of quitting and often does not progress. Dietary counseling would be appropriate because of the weight gain, but the use of anorectic agents should be avoided.

C. PATIENT 3

A 45-year-old man sees you for a "routine physical." He prides himself on a state of good physical fitness. He plays golf each weekend, and jogs at least 30 min per day. This program was begun after an earlier diagnosis of hypertension, hypercholesterolemia, and insulin resistance. Following the exercise and weight loss program, the patient's blood pressure returned to normal. Serum lipids became high-density lipoprotein (HDL) 60, low-density lipoprotein (LDL) 105, triglycerides 200, and fasting blood sugar 90. He had smoked a pack per day for 21 years, but stopped 2 years ago when he began his physical reconditioning program.

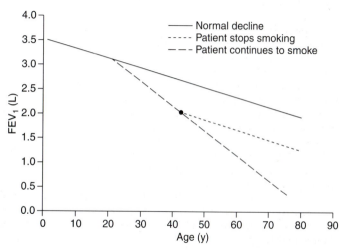

Figure 7–3. Patient 2 case example: FEV$_1$ projections. This illustrates the accelerated losses of FEV$_1$ that have occurred at age 41, assuming that the patient's lung function was normal at age 20. The two projections portray a slower decline in FEV$_1$ due to stopping smoking, compared with a more rapid decline if she continues to smoke.

You review the patient's records and find that a chest x-ray, EKG, and SMA-22 done in the past year as a part of an insurance evaluation were normal. Spirometric tests have never been done on this patient. His height is 5 foot 11 inches. Spirometry reveals FEV_1 is 3.43 L/s (80%), FVC is 5.28 (100%), and FEV_1/FVC ratio is 65%. You recognize that this patient has early stage COPD because the FEV_1/FVC ratio is less than 70%, even though his FEV_1 is only borderline low. The patient's FEV_1 elevates by 350 mL to 3.84 L/s, an increase of 12%, in response to albuterol. This patient asks you if there is any therapy that will prevent the decline of his FEV_1 over his lifetime. You consider one of the following options:

1. Reassurance that stopping smoking is sufficient to ensure good health
2. Ipratropium, two puffs, three times daily
3. Salmeterol, two puffs, twice daily
4. Inhaled corticosteroids
5. Oral theophylline

Although this patient meets the criterion of a significant bronchodilator response, ie, a 12% improvement of FEV_1 in response to an inhaled agent, there is no evidence that the long-term use of either a β-agonist or an anticholinergic will alter the rate of decline in ventilatory function. During the Lung Health Study, ipratropium remained effective during the 5 years that it was used, but it did not change the rate of decline of baseline FEV_1. Another study, however, showed that ipratropium had the effect of elevating baseline lung function. Thus, if a bronchodilator were to be used, ipratropium would probably be superior to a β-agonist. It would also have fewer side effects of tremor, tachycardia, or palpitations.

Recently there has been great interest in determining whether corticosteroids can slow the rate of decline in FEV_1 in COPD. Five studies have failed to show a sustained benefit in baseline FEV_1. One study showed a slight improvement in a subset of patients, but an overall rate of decline equal to that of placebo. At least two studies have shown an improvement in symptoms and quality of life, whereas one study has shown a statistically significant reduction in bone density.

In this patient, who has previously demonstrated insulin resistance, steroid systemic effects might worsen insulin resistance and ultimately result in diabetes. Thus, inhaled corticosteroids should not be used. Judged by his FEV_1 and state of physical fitness, this patient does not face premature morbidity and mortality from COPD. He does not require any medications for his lungs as long as he remains asymptomatic and maintains a near normal FEV_1. New drugs are under study that may slow the rate of decline in FEV_1 by opposing the inflammatory and other damaging mechanisms that result in airway inflammation and loss of alveolar walls.

Summary

COPD is a result of genetically determined susceptibility factors and environmental exposures, most commonly tobacco smoking. Treatment strategies vary, depending on the stage of disease, the age of the patient, and the success or failure of smoking cessation. The early identification and management of COPD and related disorders remain a major challenge for medicine.

American Thoracic Society: Statement on definitions and classifications of chronic bronchitis, asthma, and pulmonary emphysema. Am Rev Respir Dis 1962;85:762. (Original definitions of COPD.)

Anthonisen NR et al: Effects of smoking intervention and the use of an inhaled anticholinergic bronchodilator on the rate of decline of FEV_1. The Lung Health Study. JAMA 1994;272:1497. [PMID: 7966841]. (Stopping smoking improved lung function in COPD. The most common cause of death was lung cancer.)

Barnes PJ: Chronic obstructive pulmonary disease. N Engl J Med 2000;343:269. [PMID: 10911010]. (A review of the mechanisms of COPD pathogenesis and established and newer therapies.)

Burrows B et al: The emphysematous and bronchial types of chronic airways obstruction. A clinicopathological study of patients in London and Chicago. Lancet 1966;1(7442):830. [PMID: 4159957]. (A comparison of COPD phenotypes in the UK and North America. The presentations in both countries are similar.)

Burrows B et al: The course and prognosis of different forms of chronic airways obstruction in a sample from the general population. N Engl J Med 1987;317:1309. [PMID: 3683459]. (Different survival results in different types of COPD.)

Dahl M et al: Change in lung function and morbidity from chronic obstructive pulmonary disease in alpha 1-antitrypsin MZ heterozygotes: a longitudinal study in the general population. Ann Intern Med 2002;136:270. [PMID: 11848724]. (Evidence that $α_1$ heterozygotes have an increased prevalence of COPD.)

Dale LC et al: Treatment of nicotine dependence. Mayo Clin Proc 2000;75:1311. [PMID: 11126841]. (A summary of treatment strategies for nicotine dependence.)

Ferguson GT et al: Office spirometry for lung health assessment in adults. A consensus statement from the National Lung Health Education Program. Chest 2000;117:1146. [PMID: 10767253]. (Recommendations for spirometric testing in all smokers age 45 and older in anyone with dyspnea on exertion, cough, mucus hypersecretion, or wheeze.)

Henschke CI et al: Early lung Cancer Action Project: overall design and findings from baseline screening. Lancet 1999;354:99. [PMID: 10408484]. (Results of baseline screening for lung cancer with CT.)

Klein JS et al: High resolution CT diagnosis of emphysema in symptomatic patients with normal chest radiographs and isolated low diffusing capacity. Radiology 1992;182:817. [PMID: 1535900]. (CT evidence of emphysema.)

Lacasse Y, Rousseau L, Maltais F: Prevalence of depressive symptoms and depression in patients with severe oxygen-dependent chronic obstructive pulmonary disease. J Cardiopulm Rehabi 2001;20:80. [PMID: 11314288]. (Evidence of a high prevalence of depression in COPD patients who receive oxygen.)

Lung Health Study Research Group: Effect of inhaled triamcinolone on the decline in pulmonary function in chronic obstructive lung disease. N Engl J Med 2000;343:1902. [PMID: 11136260]. (Inhaled corticosteroids did not slow the rate of decline in FEV$_1$ but reduced disease exacerbations.)

Mahler DA et al: Efficacy of salmeterol xinafoate in the treatment of COPD. Chest 1999;115:957. [PMID: 10208192]. (A comparison of salmeterol with ipratropium. Responses were similar.)

Mannino DM et al: Obstructive lung disease and low lung function in adults in the United States. Arch Intern Med 2000;160:1685. [PMID: 10847262]. (A large population study documenting a huge underdiagnosis of COPD.)

Nocturnal Oxygen Therapy Trial Group: Continuous or nocturnal oxygen therapy in hypoxemic chronic obstructive lung disease. A clinical trial. Ann Intern Med 1980;93:391. [PMID: 6776858]. (The original report showing the superiority of ambulatory oxygen over stationary oxygen.)

Pauwels RA et al: Long-term treatment with inhaled budesonide in persons with mild chronic obstructive pulmonary disease who continue smoking. European Respiratory Society Study on Chronic Obstructive Pulmonary Disease. N Engl J Med 1999;340:1940. [PMID: 10379018]. (A controlled clinical trial of inhaled corticosteroids showed no change in rate of decline in FEV$_1$.)

Pauwels RA et al: Global strategy for the diagnosis, management and prevention of chronic obstructive pulmonary disease. Am J Respir Crit Care Med 2001;163:1256. [PMID: 11316667]. (The Global Initiative for COPD.)

Petty TL: Home oxygen—a revolution in the care of advanced COPD. Med Clin North Am 1990;74:715. [PMID: 2335990]. (A review of methods for home oxygen therapy and outcomes.)

Petty TL (Chairman, Combivent Inhalation Aerosol Study Group): In chronic obstructive pulmonary disease, a combination of ipratropium and albuterol is more effective than either agent alone. An 85-day multicenter trial. Chest 1994;105:1411. [PMID: 8181328]. (Results of a multicenter trial of Combivent.)

Petty TL (ed): Strategies in preserving lung health and preventing COPD and associated diseases. The National Lung Health Education Program (NLHEP). Chest 1998(Suppl);113:123s. [PMID: 9484245]. (The resource document of the NLHEP provides background for the NLHEP.)

Petty TL: Screening strategies for early detection of lung cancer, the time is now. JAMA 2000;284:1977. [PMID: 11035898]. (The case for lung cancer screening in high risk persons.)

Petty TL, Bliss PL: Ambulatory oxygen therapy, exercise, and survival with advanced chronic obstructive pulmonary disease (The Nocturnal Oxygen Therapy Trial revisited). Respir Care 2000;45:204. [PMID: 10771792]. (A retrospective review of the NOTT Study. Ability to exercise with ambulatory oxygen resulted in better outcomes compared with stationary oxygen.)

Petty TL, Silvers GW, Stanford RE: Mild emphysema is associated with reduced elastic recoil and increased lung size but not with airflow limitation. Am Rev Respir Dis 1987;136:867. [PMID: 3662240]. (Evidence of increased lung volumes and FVC before FEV$_1$ declines.)

Petty TL, Weinmann GG: Building a national strategy for the prevention and management of and research in chronic obstructive pulmonary disease. National Heart, Lung, and Blood Institute Workshop Summary. JAMA 1997;277:246. [PMID: 9005275]. (Initiative of the NLHEP.)

Prescott E et al: Gender and smoking-related risk of lung cancer. The Copenhagen Center for Prospective Population Studies. Epidemiology 1998;9:77. [PMID: 9430273]. (Suggests that women are more susceptible to lung cancer than men.)

Rennard SI et al: Extended therapy with ipratropium is associated with improved lung function in patients with COPD. A retrospective analysis of data from seven clinical trials. Chest 1996;110:62. [PMID: 8681667]. (Evidence that ipratropium improved baseline lung function.)

Ries AL et al: Effects of pulmonary rehabilitation on physiologic and psychosocial outcomes in patients with chronic obstructive pulmonary disease. Ann Intern Med 1995;122:823. [PMID: 7741366]. (A controlled clinical trial showing improved outcomes with pulmonary rehabilitation.)

Sandford AJ, Weir JD, Pare PD: Genetic risk factors for chronic obstructive pulmonary disease. Eur J Respir Dis 1997;10:1380. [PMID: 9192947]. (A review of genetic background factors in COPD.)

Silverman EK et al: Genetic epidemiology of severe, early onset chronic obstructive pulmonary disease. Am J Respir Crit Care Med 1998;157:1770. [PMID: 9620904]. (Family clusters of COPD with normal α_1-antitrypsin.)

Chronic Bronchiectasis & Cystic Fibrosis

Milene T. Saavedra, MD, & Jerry A. Nick, MD

8

ESSENTIALS OF DIAGNOSIS

- *Bronchiectasis is characterized by chronic cough productive of purulent sputum.*
- *Chest radiography demonstrates abnormally dilated airways and mucous plugging, characterized by "ring" shadows, "gloved finger" shadows, or air-filled cystic spaces that may include fluid levels.*
- *Spirometry reveals a pattern of airflow obstruction.*
- *Cystic fibrosis is one of the most common causes of bronchiectasis. The classic CF phenotype includes chronic sinopulmonary disease, pancreatic exocrine insufficiency, and abnormal sweat chloride levels.*

General Considerations

Bronchiectasis is a pathological description of abnormally dilated, distorted thick-walled medium-sized bronchi that are chronically inflamed and infected by bacteria. The essential clinical feature is chronic production of purulent sputum. Bronchiectasis is not a single disease, but a pathological entity now recognized to be associated with many different conditions. The process occurs in airways that have sustained inflammatory injury with subsequent loss of structural integrity of muscle, elastic tissue, and bronchial cartilage. These abnormal dilated airways are susceptible to bacterial colonization, which leads to neutrophil influx. Proteolytic neutrophil products further damage lung tissue and disrupt ciliary function, and this continued bronchial wall damage predisposes to further colonization with bacteria.

Cystic fibrosis (CF) is the most common inherited disorder among whites in the United States, affecting one in 3200. One in 25 is a carrier of the disease. The disease is caused by mutations in a single gene, called the cystic fibrosis transmembrane conductance regulator (CFTR), and is inherited in an autosomal recessive fashion. Defective chloride transport across epithelial cells leads to dehydrated secretions and exocrine gland dysfunction. Although multiple organs are affected, the progression of bronchiectasis is the most common cause of death and disability. Over 800 mutations in the gene that encodes CFTR have been described, with the most common mutation, δF508, seen in 66% of CF chromosomes.

Barker AF: Bronchiectasis. N Engl J Med 2002;346:1383. [PMID: 11986413]. (A recent review of bronchiectasis that provides an excellent overview of the subject.)

Pathogenesis

Bronchiectasis is caused by a variety of insults to the airways. A number of congenital and/or hereditary factors predispose certain individuals to develop it, but bronchiectasis is not present at birth. Primary or secondary infections are the most frequently identified initiating factor in patients predisposed to bronchiectasis. Other proinflammatory insults such as inhalation of toxins, aspiration of gastric contents, abnormal immune responses (such as autoimmune diseases), or environments exposures (tobacco smoke) can accelerate the lung disease. Damage to the bronchial mucosa and accompanying impairment of host defense eventually lead to chronic infection of the airways regardless of the initial insult. A persistent inflammatory response is established resulting in chronic sputum production and perpetuation of airway injury. The most clearly defined mechanism resulting in bronchiectasis is mutation of CFTR in CF.

CFTR functions as a cyclic adenosine monophosphate (cAMP)-regulated chloride channel located in the apical membranes of epithelia affected by CF. This defect leads to excess absorption of salt and water at airway surfaces, dehydrating secretions and contributing to the development of thick tenacious mucus. Bacteria, particularly *Pseudomonas aeruginosa*, colonize these mucus plugs. The plugs are difficult to clear from the airways, leading to persistent excessive airway recruitment of inflammatory cells whose proteases injure the structural integrity of airways. This chronic bacterial presence in sinuses leads to tissue inflammation and mucosal thickening in a cycle that results in ostial obstruction and unhindered bacterial growth in what becomes an undrainable cavity. Dehydration of ductal fluid results in pancreatic duct obstruction from intraductal precipitation of secreted protein. Progressive degradation and atrophy of pancreatic acini ultimately occur and the pancreas becomes fibrotic. This destructive process also affects pancreatic islet β cells. CF-related diabetes affects 24% of patients by age 24; this number climbs to 76% by age 30. Mucus and feces containing inspissated intestinal contents may lead to impaction in the terminal ileum, cecum, and right-sided colon. Mild to severe hepatobiliary disease may result from localized stasis and obstruction of biliary ducts. Retention of hepatotoxic bile acids initiates a cascade of inflammatory cytokine release, free radical production, and lipid peroxidation, all of which may contribute to the progression of necrosis and cirrhosis. The male reproductive tract ductal structures are affected with impairment of vas deferens and epididymis development with subsequent infertility.

Prevention

Bronchiectasis could clearly be avoided in some individuals. Childhood immunization against pertussis and measles for the general population as well as influenza and pneumococcal vaccination in high-risk groups reduce the prevalence and morbidity of the disease. In cases due to untreated childhood infections or airway obstruction by a foreign body, appropriate early medical intervention could prevent the chronic sequelae. However, patients with bronchiectasis typically present as adults with irreversible damage and the primary focus becomes reducing progression of lung disease.

Singleton R et al: Bronchiectasis in Alaska Native children: causes and clinical courses. Pediatr Pulmonol 2000;29:182. [PMID: 10686038]. (This report provides insights as to how bronchiectasis can be prevented by examining the causes of bronchiectasis in this remote population.)

Clinical Findings

A. Symptoms and Signs

Patients with bronchiectasis typically complain of chronic mucopurulent sputum production. Airways involvement results in wheezing and dyspnea. Chronic inflammation in the airways leads to enlargement and tortuosity of bronchial arteries, which may subsequently bleed. Health care providers should be aware that small amounts of hemoptysis frequently herald respiratory infections and need for antibiotic therapy. Massive hemoptysis (greater than 240–300 mL of

blood in 24 h) may occur and carries a high mortality rate.

Clinical manifestations of CF disease are highly variable due to both the plethora of mutations and widespread organ involvement. The principal organs involved are discussed below and are listed in Table 8–1.

1. Sinopulmonary disease—Symptoms are related to progressive compromise of the airway lumen secondary to a mucus biofilm and massive quantities of inflammatory exudate. Patients manifest productive cough with purulent sputum that may be accompanied by hemoptysis during acute exacerbations of airways disease. Persistently brown-tinged sputum with airways reactivity should prompt consideration of allergic bronchopulmonary aspergillosis (ABPA). Airways reactivity is exceedingly common, occurring in approximately 40% of patients. Patients with severe disease or acute exacerbations may be hypoxemic and/or hypercapnic. Cor pulmonale is frequently present in end-stage disease. Patients who are newly diagnosed as adults frequently harbor a history of chronic respiratory ailments, but as a group have milder lung disease and less infection by *P aeruginosa*.

Sinus disease may present with headache, nasal obstruction, mouth breathing, facial pain, halitosis, and purulent nasal discharge. A mucopyocele may lead to erosion of sinus walls with ophthalmological findings such as proptosis and double vision. The most frequent complaint is postnasal drip, detectable by a "cobblestoned" appearance of the posterior oropharynx. This feature of sinus disease may contribute to worsening of pulmonary disease. Rhinorrhea with purulent nasal discharge and obstruction of nasal airflow, as well as distortion of facial features, suggests the presence of nasal polyposis.

2. Pancreatic disease—Pancreatic exocrine insufficiency is generally a feature of patients diagnosed from childhood. Eighty-five to 90% of patients with CF have pancreatic exocrine insufficiency, defined by elevated fecal fat excretion. Pancreatic insufficiency is less common in the small subset of patients diagnosed with CF as adults; those with milder mutations of CFTR may possess sufficient pancreatic function to preclude pancreatic enzyme supplementation. However, these patients are at increased risk for acute or chronic pancreatitis.

The presence of pancreatic insufficiency is often associated with fat-soluble vitamin deficiencies. Deficiencies of vitamins A, D, E, and K are often diagnosed biochemically through screening programs before becoming clinically apparent. Nevertheless, occurrence of hemoptysis should prompt evaluation of prothrombin time. Deficiencies of vitamins E and A tend to occur as later sequelae of malabsorption. Vitamin E deficiency

Table 8–1. Extrapulmonary manifestations of cystic fibrosis.

Organ System	Useful Diagnostic Test	Therapeutic Approach
Pancreas (exocrine)		
Pancreatitis	Elevated amylase and lipase, exclusion of other causes	Bowel rest, pain management
Pancreatic insufficiency	Steatorrhea, elevated fecal fat	Enteric-coated microencapsulated enzymes containing proteases and lipases
Nutritional deficiencies	Albumin, prealbumin; levels for vitamins A, E, and D, Protime (vitamin K)	Aggressive caloric intake, including a high fat diet, replacement of vitamin A, E, D, and K
Pancreas (endocrine)		
CF-related diabetes (CFRD)	Random glucose ≥ 200 mg/dL on two or more occasions or a fasting blood glucose (FBG) ≥ 126 mg/dL on two or more occasions or a FBG ≥ 126 mg/dL in association with a casual glucose > 200 mg/dL; an oral glucose tolerance test (OGTT) in ambiguous cases	Insulin with continued high calorie diet
Hepatobiliary		
Multilobular biliary cirrhosis	Work-up includes liver function tests, ultrasound, ERCP, and exclusion of other causes of liver disease; liver biopsy often not needed	Ursodeoxycholic acid (UDCA)
Gallstones		
Microgallbladder		
Hepatic steatosis		
Hepatic congestion from cor pulmonale		
Gastrointestinal		
Neonatal meconium ileus	History, examination and abdominal radiographs	Systemic hydration polyethylene glycol electrolyte (PEG) solutions by mouth or enemas, laparotomy and bowel resection (very rarely)
Distal intestinal obstruction syndrome (DIOS)		
Clostridium difficile associated colitis	Stool cultures and toxin, colonoscopy or abdominal CT scan	Antibiotic treatment
Fibrosing colonopathy	Contrast enema	Reduced enzyme dose, occasionally colonic resection
Appendicitis	Examination, ultrasound, abdominal CF scan	Appendectomy
Bone and joint disease		
Osteoporosis	Dual energy x-ray absorptiometry (DEXA)	Calcium and vitamin D supplements, consider bisphosphonates
Arthritis	Serological analysis to exclude other causes of arthritis	Short courses of nonsteroidal and steroidal anti-inflammatory medications
Hypertrophic pulmonary osteoarthropathy	Radiographs of long bones	Short courses of nonsteroidal and steroidal anti-inflammatory medications
Reproductive disease		
CBAVD resulting in azoospermia	Semen analysis	Reproduction possible through sperm retrieval and assisted reproductive techniques
Cervical mucus abnormalities	Fertility may be normal	Counseling on contraception options, reproductive issues, and family planning

presents clinically with ophthalmoplegia, absent deep tendon reflexes, tremors in the hands, and ataxia. Spinocerebellar degeneration or hemolytic anemia may also occur. Night blindness suggests vitamin A deficiency. Evaluation for metabolic bone disease due to vitamin D deficiency should be performed if osteopenia is present on dual-energy x-ray absorptiometry (DEXA) screening or bony fractures develop.

Progressive destruction and fibrosis of the pancreas causes development of cystic fibrosis-related diabetes mellitus (CFRD). This complication increases in frequency as patients live longer into adulthood. Using the oral glucose tolerance test, one CF center reported CFRD in 43% of patients over age 30. CFRD is associated with deterioration in body mass and pulmonary function. Microvascular complications of CFRD, including retinopathy, neuropathy, and nephropathy, are all relatively common; however, the macrovascular complications of stroke and coronary artery disease are rare. The Cystic Fibrosis Foundation recommends aggressive screening and treatment of CFRD. Management of this form of diabetes requires special considerations and should be done in conjunction with a CF specialist or an endocrinologist.

3. Hepatobiliary disease—Mild elevations of hepatic transaminases or alkaline phosphatase are relatively common on yearly liver function evaluations. One retrospective review of 233 adults over 15 years of age found hepatomegaly or persistently abnormal liver blood tests in 24%. The fibrosis and cirrhosis that occur secondary to impaired bile secretion and localized stasis leads to multilobular biliary cirrhosis in 2–5% of patients, gallstones in 4–12%, other gallbladder abnormalities including microgallbladder in 24–45%, and fatty liver in 15–30%. Obstructive jaundice in adults may be secondary to cholelithiasis, sclerosing cholangitis, or common bile duct stenosis. Use of endoscopic retrograde cholangiopancreatography (ERCP) to reveal strictures should be considered carefully, as seeding of the endoscope with *P aeruginosa* and subsequent bacterial cholangitis have been reported.

4. Gastrointestinal disease—Chloride transport abnormalities in the gut and relative dehydration of intestinal contents contribute to development of meconium ileus in neonates and distal intestinal obstruction syndrome (DIOS) in older children and adults. Intestinal motility also appears to be altered in patients with CF, although the mechanism is not known. Periumbilical and hypogastric pain in adults with CF is most commonly caused by DIOS, with recurrent episodes seen in up to 3.5% of the population. Clinicians not accustomed to caring for patients with CF frequently misdiagnose DIOS as appendicitis, Crohn's disease, or intussusception. Exploratory laparotomy for these misdiagnoses is commonly associated with considerable worsening of DIOS and should be avoided. Abdominal bloating and hypogastric complaints are common in patients with CF and are usually due to malabsorption that allows ingested nutrients to reach the colon where bacteria metabolize them to gaseous products. Malabsorption as a cause of abdominal pain is commonly accompanied by steatorrhea. Less common causes of abdominal pain in adult patients with CF include *Clostridium difficile*-associated colitis. Fibrosing colonopathy, secondary to ingestion of very high doses of pancreatic enzymes, is manifested by inflammation and

strictures in the right colon. It occurs primarily in the pediatric age group.

5. Bone and joint disease—Multiple factors contribute to metabolic bone disease in patients with CF, including accelerated bone resorption, diminished bone formation, low vitamin D levels, and reduced calcium absorption. Low bone mineral density has been widely reported in children and adults with CF and is linked with low body mass index and low lung function. The prevalence of osteoporosis in adults with CF varies from 38% to 77%, which is higher than rates reported in children (19% to 67%).

Arthropathy occurs in up to 12% of the adult CF population. Pathogenesis appears to be immunological but is not well understood. Hypertrophic pulmonary osteoarthropathy, with a prevalence of 8%, presents with clubbing and chronic symmetrical bony pain or swelling at the knee, wrist, or ankle and frequently accompanies pulmonary exacerbations. An episodic arthropathy, characterized by high sedimentation rates, incapacitating asymmetric joint pain and swelling, fever, and occasionally rash due to leukocytoclastic vasculitis may occur. Rheumatoid arthritis, amyloidosis, drug-induced arthritis secondary to fluoroquinolones, and granulomatous arthritis with features of sarcoidosis have all been described in patients with CF.

6. Reproductive disease—Nearly all males with CF have abnormal reproductive tract anatomy, particularly involving the vas deferens, with subsequent azoospermia. Approximately 1–2% of men with less severe mutations and mild lung disease are fertile. Female patients with CF have normal reproductive anatomy. Although cervical mucus has lower water content in females with CF compared to nonaffected woman, more than 100 females with CF become pregnant every year. Maternal issues to consider include prepregnancy pulmonary function, frequency of need for antibiotics, and nutritional status, all of which have bearing on fetal health and maternal postpregnancy outcomes. Pregnancy, per se, has not been shown to have an independent negative effect on the mother in clinical studies. Infant outcomes are significantly better if the mother's disease remains stable during pregnancy, but there are considerably higher rates of preterm delivery in mothers with CF.

Yankaskas JR et al: Cystic fibrosis adult care consensus conference report. Concepts in CF care. CF Foundation 1999;IX, Section 3:1. (A comprehensive review of present recommendations for the care of adults with CF; this is the most complete, current document on the subject to date.)

B. LABORATORY FINDINGS

Patients with bronchiectasis often have normal laboratory profiles. White blood count can be normal or only mildly elevated despite chronic pulmonary infections.

Liver function test may be abnormal in patients with CF or α_1-antitrypsin deficiency. A number of specific tests are available that help support or exclude rare causes of bronchiectasis. These are discussed below and are listed in Table 8–2.

A quantitative pilocarpine iontophoresis sweat test should be the initial test performed in a case of suspected CF. The sweat chloride concentration will be abnormal (>60 mmol/L) in more than 90% of diagnosed patients. However, a normal sweat chloride value cannot be used as the sole criterion for excluding the diagnosis of CF. CFTR mutation analysis should be performed in suspect cases with normal or borderline sweat chloride values. The sensitivity of genetic testing is limited because current commercial panels screen for only a minority of the more than 1000 identified CF mutations and patients diagnosed after the age of 18 years are more likely to carry infrequent or unidentified mutations. Nasal potential difference may be measured to confirm the diagnosis in cases in which a diagnosis cannot be made on the basis of identification of two CFTR mutations. However, this technique is not available at all medical centers.

Sputum cultures are useful in both supporting a diagnosis and planning therapy. Sputum may be mucoid, mucopurulent, or purulent, depending on the clinical state. In advanced cases the sputum, on standing, separates into a frothy top layer, a mucoid middle layer, and a yellow-to-green layer of pus and debris at the bottom. Cultures should be analyzed for bacteria, fungus, and acid-fast bacteria (AFB). Special media are required to facilitate growth of organisms such as *Burkholderia cepacia*. Growth of *Staphylococcus aureus* or a mucoid strain of *P aeruginosa* is suggestive of CF. Cultures with multiple organisms should not be interpreted as nondiagnostic. In older patients with CF, many pathogenic bacteria can be present in a single specimen. Multiply-resistant gram-negative organisms such as *B cepacia*, *Stenotrophomonas maltophilia,* and *Alcaligenes xylosoxidans* are found in up to one-third of adults with CF. This has significant implications for management and infection control. The microbiology laboratory must be capable of distinguishing these organisms and performing extended antimicrobial susceptibility panels. Antibiotic synergy testing may be helpful in some situations and is available at the Cystic Fibrosis Foundation-sponsored reference laboratory at Columbia University for patients followed at accredited CF Care Centers. Confirmed or suspected *B cepacia* isolates should be sent to the Cystic Fibrosis Foundation-sponsored reference laboratory at the University of Michigan for confirmation of identity and further characterization.

C. IMAGING STUDIES

Evidence of bronchiectasis on chest radiograph or computed tomography (CT) includes dilated, nontapering, thick-walled bronchi appearing as thin radiodense lines ("tram tracks") when seen longitudinally. The dilated bronchi are accompanied by a smaller round pulmonary artery ("ring shadow" or "signet ring") when viewed on end. These dilated airways may be filled with secretions and appear as thick linear densities ("mucous plugs") or as branching Y- or V-shaped densities ("gloved-finger sign"). Cysts may be quite large (up to 3 cm), have a course honeycombed pattern, and be filled or partially filled with fluid. Three types of bronchiectasis have been described. Cylindrical bronchiectasis is associated with bronchi that are uniformly dilated and terminate abruptly in mucous plugs. Varicose bronchiectasis has varicose vein-shaped bronchi on longitudinal section. Cystic or saccular bronchiectasis is the most severe form and has dilated bronchi that end in cystic pus-filled cavities with reduced bronchial subdivisions (Figure 8–1).

Posterior/anterior and lateral chest radiographs should be obtained every 2–4 years in patients with stable clinical status. Imaging also should be considered for patients with signs or symptoms consistent with a significant acute pulmonary exacerbation, pneumothorax, lobar atelectasis, or hemoptysis. High-resolution computed tomography (HRCT) is superior to plain radiographs in establishing the diagnosis of bronchiectasis, but cannot be recommended on a routine basis. CT scans are utilized in patients being considered for lung transplant.

D. SPECIAL TESTS

Abnormalities of pulmonary function tests are nearly always present in bronchiectasis. A pattern of airflow obstruction is typically present as a result of bronchospasm, mucosal edema, mucous plugging, and increased dynamic compression. Lung volumes are usually normal or reduced. The carbon monoxide diffusion capacity may be reduced and the $P(A–a)O_2$ gradient increased. Bronchodilator-induced reversibility of airway obstruction may be present.

Kumar NA et al: Bronchiectasis: current clinical and imaging concepts. Semin Roentgenol 2001;36:41. [PMID: 11204758]. (A concise review of the radiographic features of bronchiectasis.)

Differential Diagnosis

The typical history that suggests bronchiectasis is chronic cough with mucopurulent secretions. Bronchiectasis can be confirmed with chest radiographs and HRCT. The differential diagnosis of bronchiectasis is one of the most challenging in pulmonary medicine. Bronchiectasis occurs in several suppurative lung diseases. One useful distinction is that of focal versus diffuse disease. Bronchiectasis involving a single lobe or segment of the lung

Table 8–2. Diseases associated with development of bronchiectasis.

Associated Condition	Appropriate Tests and Typical Findings
Diffuse Infection (primary)	Sputum cultures and serological assays
Bacteria: Klebsiella pneumonia, S aureus, H influenzae, B pertussis	
Mycobacteria: M tuberculosis, NTM Mycoplasma	
Viruses: Influenza, adenovirus, measles, HIV	
Fungus	
Allergic bronchopulmonary aspergillosis (ABPA)	Elevated serum IgE, specific *Aspergillus fumigatus* IgE levels, eosinophilia, immediate skin hypersensitivity to aspergillin, (+) fungal serum IgG precipitins, central bronchiectasis, refractory asthma, transient infiltrates, mucous plugs
Mucoid impaction	Radiographic findings
Bronchocentric granulomatosis	Work-up of primary disorder, biopsy
Cystic fibrosis (CF)	Sweat chloride, CFTR mutation analysis
Primary ciliary dyskinesia	Ultrastructural examination of cilia from nasal biopsy by electron
Kartagener's syndrome	microscopy; sperm transport studies
Young's syndrome	Obstructive azoospermia from intraluminal epididymal obstruction with normal spermatogenesis, normal sweat chloride
Immunodeficiency states	
IgG deficiency	Quantitative serum total IgM, IgA, IgG, and IgG subclass levels (IgG_1,
IgG subclass deficiency	IgG_2, IgG_3, IgG_4)
IgA deficiency	
Leukocyte dysfunction	Neutrophilia, neutrophil respiratory burst or chemotaxis studies
Lymphocyte dysfunction	
Complement deficiencies	Total hemolytic complement (CH_{50}) and C_3 level reduced
α_1-Antitrypsin deficiency	Serum α_1-antitrypsin level, P_i typing
Autoimmune or hyperimmune disorders	Work-up of primary disorder
Rheumatoid arthritis	
Ulcerative colitis	
Cutaneous vasculitis	
Hashimoto's thyroiditis	
Pernicious anemia	
Primary biliary cirrhosis	
Relapsing polychondritis	
Celiac disease	
Yellow nail syndrome	Yellow nails, lymphedema of lower extremities, recurrent pneumonia
Diseases of tracheal or bronchial cartilage	
Williams–Campbell syndrome	CT and bronchoscopy, expiratory collapse of proximal bronchi
Tracheobronchomegaly (Mounier–Kuhn)	CT and bronchoscopy
Inhalation of noxious fumes and dust, anhydrous ammonia, silica, sulfur dioxide, talc, cork, bakelite	History of exposure
Heroin	History of exposure
Chronic fibrosing diseases	Work-up of primary disorder, lung biopsy
Chronic gastric aspiration	Functional studies documenting aspiration
Marfan's syndrome	Work-up of primary disorder
Heart–lung transplant	CT scan in appropriate clinical setting
Idiopathic	Exclusion of other plausible diagnosis

(continued)

Table 8–2. Diseases associated with development of bronchiectasis. (continued)

	Associated Condition	Appropriate Tests and Typical Findings

Focal	Infection (primary)
	  Klebsiella pneumonia, S aureus, H influenzae,
	    M tuberculosis, NTM
		Sputum cultures

	Luminal bronchial obstruction
	  Foreign body
	  Broncholith
	  Endobronchial tumor
	  Mucoid impaction
	  Bronchial stenosis
		CT scan, bronchoscopy

	Extrinsic bronchus obstruction Lymph node, aneurysm, tumor, granuloma	CT scan, bronchoscopy
	Pulmonary sequestration	CT scan, angiogram
	Unilateral hyperlucent lung (Swyer–James syndrome)	Fluoroscopy, angiography, CT scan

typically results from focal bronchial obstruction or severe lobar pneumonia. Patients present with a history of recurrent or persistent lobar pneumonia. Bronchial obstruction proximal to the region of bronchiectasis may be secondary to a foreign body, carcinoma, broncholith, or lymph nodes (as occurs in middle lobe syndrome). Multilobar disease is usually secondary to diffuse infections such as influenza, *S aureus, P aeruginosa,* or *Klebsiella* species, to toxic inhalation, or to defects in host defense. The latter occurs in chronic granulomatous infections, immunodeficiency disorders, autoimmune diseases, and congenital diseases (Table 8–2).

A careful medical history and physical examination can significantly narrow the differential diagnosis in many patients with bronchiectasis. Chronic sinusitis or extrapulmonary infections strongly suggest impaired host defense. A family history of lung disease suggests CF, α_1-antitrypsin deficiency, or primary ciliary dyskinesia (PCD). Infertility in males is associated with several causes of bronchiectasis, including immotile sperm with PCD and obstructive azoopermia in patients with CF and Young's syndrome. Specific tests are available to help establish or exclude specific causes of bronchiectasis (Table 8–2). Radiographic distribution of disease may be helpful. Both cystic fibrosis and ABPA are characterized by predominantly upper lobe disease. Disease localized to the right middle lobe or lingula should raise suspicion of *Mycobacterium avium* complex infection. Bronchiectasis secondary to other causes generally is localized to the lower lobes.

Patients are frequently afflicted with multiple conditions that are all associated with bronchiectasis. For example, a patient can present with bronchiectasis, infection with nontuberculous mycobacteria (NTM), and ABPA. Further work-up may reveal that the patient has CF. Although CF, NTM, and ABPA are all primary

causes of bronchiectasis, it is likely in this patient that bronchiectasis occurred as a result of CF. ABPA and infection with NTM occurred as secondary events in airways already damaged by CF. In addition, bronchiectasis is often misdiagnosed as asthma, chronic bronchitis, or emphysema. However, in rare incidents, each of these common diseases can develop into bronchiectasis. For example, asthma associated with ABPA or emphysema due to α_1-antitrypsin deficiency can ultimately result in bronchiectasis.

Estimates of the relative prevalence of various causes of bronchiectasis are difficult to determine as the identified etiologies of bronchiectasis have changed over time with improved treatments and diagnostic techniques. Older studies report a preponderance of postinfectious or undiagnosed (idiopathic) cases. However, patients with bronchiectasis from many causes can relate a history of multiple pulmonary infections in childhood; thus in the absence of other evidence, postinfectious bronchiectasis is a diagnosis of exclusion. With modern childhood immunizations and antibiotics, postinfectious bronchiectasis is probably quite rare, except for isolated populations or in developing nations with poor access to health care. Even after exhaustive evaluation, no specific etiology is identified in up to 50% of bronchiectasis cases. CF is the most common cause of bronchiectasis when an etiology is identified. As the ability to sequence the entire CFTR gene becomes widely available, many idiopathic cases will likely be identified as atypical forms of CF. Other causes of bronchiectasis are likely quite rare, each comprising less then 1% of the total.

Establishing a conclusive diagnosis of CF can be challenging, given the differences in severity of the phenotype and the high frequency of CF carriers among individuals of Northern European descent. The Cystic

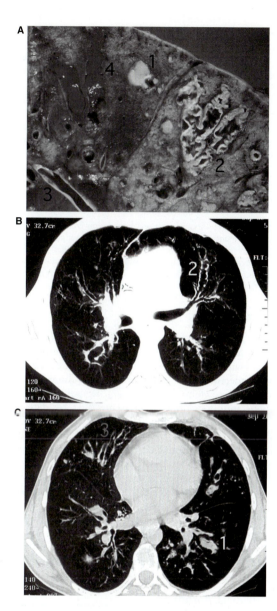

Figure 8–1: Pathological and radiographic features of cystic fibrosis. ***A:*** Gross lung pathology. Typical features of cystic fibrosis lung disease include (1) cystic bronchiectasis with plugging of the segment with mucous, pus, and cellular debris; (2) varicose bronchiectasis; (3) cylindrical bronchiectasis; and (4) localized hemorrhage associated with cylindrical bronchiectasis plugging of airways. ***B:*** High-resolution CT scan demonstrating segments of (2) varicose bronchiectasis. ***C:*** High-resolution CT scan demonstrating (1) plugging of cystic bronchiectasis and (3) cylindrical bronchiectasis. (**A:** Courtesy of Joseph R. Siebert and Joel E. Haas, used with permission.)

Fibrosis Foundation consensus statement requires the presence of at least one clinical feature consistent with CF, along with a demonstration of dysfunction of CFTR. Bronchiectasis fulfills the clinical criteria for CF. Bronchiectasis may be negligible in some individuals, but single-organ manifestations such as chronic sinusitis, idiopathic pancreatitis, or congenital bilateral absence of the vas deferens (CBAVD) may also be the clinical manifestation of CF. Other accepted manifestations include a history of CF in a sibling or a positive newborn screen, but these are rarely applicable to the adult patient. Evaluation for CFTR dysfunction should begin with a sweat chloride test. CFTR mutation analysis should be performed in individuals with elevated sweat chloride values that fail to reach the diagnostic threshold (40–60 mol/L). Identification of two known CFTR mutations also satisfies the criteria for demonstrating CFTR dysfunction. However, nearly all mutation analyses to date have been restricted to the most common CFTR mutations and individuals with normal sweat chloride values often possess rare CFTR mutations. Recently, a CFTR analysis (Ambry Genetics, Costa Mesa, CA) that relies on sequencing the gene has become commercially available and will likely identify a number of patients with rare CFTR mutations who did not meet criteria for CF using conventional testing. A positive nasal potential difference (NPD) can also provide sufficient evidence for CFTR dysfunction. Approximately 10% of patients with CF have a negative sweat chloride test; these atypical presentations are more likely to remain undiagnosed early in life. A diagnosis of CF should be assigned to patients only if there is documentation of elevated sweat chloride values, two CF mutations, or an abnormal NPD measurement, in addition to the necessary clinical features.

Immune-mediated diseases may also be associated with bronchiectasis. Deficiencies of immunoglobulin (Ig) G (IgG), and more rarely IgM and IgA, lead to recurrent sinopulmonary infections and bronchiectasis. Humoral immunity can be assessed through quantitative measurement of serum total IgM, IgA, IgG, and IgG subclass levels (IgG_1, IgG_2, IgG_3, and IgG_4). Autoimmune conditions associated with bronchiectasis include rheumatoid arthritis, systemic lupus erythematosus, Sjögren's syndrome, and relapsing polychondritis. Inflammatory bowel disease, especially ulcerative colitis, has also been associated with bronchiectasis. Unfortunately bowel resection does not palliate the airways disease. Tests for neutrophil respiratory burst or chemotaxis can be diagnostic in selected patients. A positive test, however, supports the diagnosis only in the proper clinical setting. For example, evidence of *P aeruginosa* in sputum cultures does not represent the cause of bronchiectasis, but rather an infectious complication of damaged airways.

Mycobacterium avium complex (MAC) infection and ABPA are two infectious etiologies that require special consideration. MAC infection has been increasingly recognized in middle-aged women. These patients are immunocompetent, nonsmokers without a history of structural lung disease, and with disease primarily in the right middle lobe and lingula. Thoracic wall abnormalities, such as pectus excavatum and kyphoscoliosis, have also been associated with NTM infection in these women. Treatment of MAC is complicated, involving three drug regimens for approximately 2 years, or 12 months past the last negative sputum culture. ABPA requires the four major findings of asthma, anatomic central bronchiectasis by CT, blood or sputum eosinophilia (with an elevated serum immunoglobulin E level), and immediate and late dermal hypersensitivity to *Aspergillus* antigens. The mainstay of treatment is bronchodilators and corticosteroids as the disease is an immune response to *Aspergillus*. Itraconazole therapy has recently been shown to reduce corticosteroid requirements.

Pasteur MC et al: An investigation into causative factors in patients with bronchiectasis. Am J Respir Crit Care Med 2000;162:1277. [PMID: 11029331]. (This report describes a comprehensive evaluation of 150 adults with idiopathic bronchiectasis. Specific causes or plausible conditions associated with bronchiectasis were found in 47% of this highly selected group.)

Complications

Acute pulmonary exacerbations are common in adults with bronchiectasis. Exacerbations in the adult CF population can occur several times a year, often preceded by a viral upper respiratory infection (URI). The presentation is usually a subacute worsening of respiratory status over several days or weeks. Antibiotic therapy in patients with bronchiectasis should be considered if four of the following nine symptoms have occurred: worsening of dyspnea, cough, wheezing, fatigue, or pulmonary function, change in sputum production, chest examination, or baseline chest radiograph, or fever. Sputum will typically become darker, more copious, and blood streaked. Decreased appetite, weight loss, pulmonary congestion, and/or chest pain are often reported. Adult patients with CF can usually predict with a high degree of certainty the onset of a pulmonary exacerbation. Examination is most significant for increased respiratory rate and rhonchi, especially in the upper lobes. A reduction in forced expiratory volume (FEV_1) compared to baseline values is typical and decreased arterial oxygen saturation (SaO_2) can occur depending on the severity of the patient's lung disease. Laboratory studies can demonstrate mild leukocytosis. Radiographic changes such as increased opacities in

areas of preexisting bronchiectasis can be seen, but true pneumonias are uncommon.

Treatment centers on aggressive correction of existing coagulopathies and supportive care when hemoptysis occurs. Arterial embolization or local pulmonary resection may be required for patients with massive hemoptysis.

Patients with bronchiectasis commonly exhibit progressive airflow obstruction. Up to 90% of patients with CF die of complications arising from respiratory failure. Supplemental oxygenation and assisted ventilation in patients with advanced lung disease are discussed below.

Schidlow DV et al: Cystic Fibrosis Foundation consensus conference report on pulmonary complications of cystic fibrosis. Pediatr Pulmonol 1993;15:187. [PMID: 8327283]. (Specific recommendations on the treatment of pneumothorax, hemoptysis, and respiratory failure in bronchiectasis from cystic fibrosis.)

Treatment

Specific treatment guidelines have been developed for only a few causes of bronchiectasis. For example, patients with immunoglobulin deficiency experience fewer infections and less progression of lung disease with immune globulin replacement. Response to intravenous immunoglobulin can be assessed by demonstrating inadequate antibody responses to *Haemophilus influenzae* or pneumococcal vaccine. Specific recommendations for patients homozygous for α_1-antitrypsin deficiency include antiprotease replacement therapy. Individuals with ABPA are treated with corticosteroids with close monitoring of serum IgE levels. Itraconazole may be used as a corticosteroid-sparing agent in patients poorly responsive to corticosteroids or intolerant of corticosteroid side effects. Recurrent sinusitis should be treated aggressively with a combination of medical and surgical therapies. Gastroesophageal reflux should be treated if present.

A. SURGICAL APPROACH

Bronchiectasis from an obstructing foreign body or associated with deeply damaged segments that are sources of ongoing infection is occasionally treated surgically. Lobectomy has a role in removing damaged localized regions of lung containing *M tuberculosis* or *M avium* complex when applied in a selective manner by an experienced thoracic surgeon. However, lobectomy is very rarely indicated in the setting of diffuse bronchiectasis such as CF and should be considered carefully in patients who may eventually be candidates for lung transplant. In very rare cases lobectomy can be successful in controlling massive hemoptysis unresponsive to conservative treatment or arterial embolization.

Development of therapeutic guidelines for many forms of bronchiectasis has been hindered by the relatively small numbers of patients. However, treatment of bronchiectasis from CF has been studied systematically and evidence-based recommendations exist. Current treatment options for CF lung disease are described below. In the absence of specific recommendations, physicians may consider using the therapeutic approaches proven to be of benefit in patients with CF as a basis for developing treatment strategies for individuals with bronchiectasis of unknown etiology.

B. MAINTENANCE CARE FOR PATIENTS WITH CF

The cornerstones of treatment for patients with CF are antibiotics, airway clearance, and nutritional support. A standard treatment regimen includes antibiotics for pulmonary exacerbations and chronic suppressive therapy, airway clearance and exercise, mucolytic agents, bronchodilators, antiinflammatory agents, supplemental oxygen, and nutritional support. Patients with CF should be cared for at a comprehensive CF Care Center by a multidisciplinary health care team that includes a physician, nurse, respiratory therapist, dietician, and social worker. The pulmonary status of patients should be regularly monitored through assessment of symptoms, physical examination, and spirometry. Percent predicted FEV_1 is accepted as the single most useful objective measure of pulmonary status. Oxygen saturation at rest, during exercise, and/or sleep should be measured routinely in patients with moderate-to-severe pulmonary disease to assess need for supplemental oxygen. A complete microbiological assessment of expectorated sputum including antibiotic susceptibility testing should be performed on at least an annual basis. Microbiology laboratories should follow published guidelines for processing CF sputum in order to isolate the wide range of organisms found in these specimens.

1. Chronic suppressive antibiotic therapy—Treatment of pulmonary exacerbations rarely eradicates lung infections in adults with preexisting bronchiectasis. Antibiotics serve to significantly reduce the quantity of bacteria in the airways, resulting in decreased inflammation and sputum production. Aerosolized tobramycin (TOBI) has been shown over a 24-week period to produce significant improvement in pulmonary function, to decrease the density of P $aeruginosa$ in sputum, and to decrease the number of days that patients with CF with moderate to severe pulmonary disease are hospitalized. Twenty-four-month open-label follow-up of these trials has demonstrated sustained improvement in FEV_1 as compared to control groups.

A significant long-term concern in using chronic suppressive therapy is emergence of antimicrobial resistance. The TOBI trials showed no increase in the prevalence of B $cepacia$ or other resistant organisms.

There was a modest but detectable shift in the minimum inhibitory concentrations of P $aeruginosa$ strains infecting the TOBI-treated subjects. Sustained improvement in pulmonary function appears to outweigh the theoretical risk of tobramycin resistance that may develop over time, but this must be carefully considered for each individual.

Chronic suppressive antibiotic therapy with a number of other antimicrobials has been attempted. Various dosage and formulations of inhaled tobramycin (other then TOBI), gentamicin, and colistin (Colimycin) have been reported in smaller, less rigorous clinical trials. Scheduled parenteral antipseudomonal therapy administered in 2-week courses of therapy four times per year is an alternative suppressive strategy popularized in Denmark. Oral antibiotics are also frequently used for chronic suppression. However, for each of these agents, either a lack of studies, failure to show efficacy, or significant methodological concerns with trials prevent recommendation of these treatments at this time.

Several recent studies have shown benefit from longterm administration of azithromycin in patients with CF. Patients receiving azithromycin demonstrated improved pulmonary function and decreased hospitalizations. Azithromycin has little effect against P $aeruginosa$ but may suppress anaerobic bacteria. In addition, azithromycin has potent intrinsic antiinflammatory effects that may contribute to its observed efficacy in CF and diffuse panbronchiolitis.

2. Sputum clearance—Mobilization of sputum and airway clearance is an essential component of the treatment of bronchiectasis. Sputum in CF contains numerous cytotoxic compounds that are by-products of neutrophil recruitment, activation, and necrosis in response to chronic infection. There are a variety of airway clearance techniques available, each of which can be beneficial when applied correctly. Conventional chest physiotherapy, which utilizes percussion and postural drainage, is commonly used in pediatric patients, but is often impractical in adults. Alternative modalities have been developed, including active cycle breathing, forced expiratory technique, positive expiratory pressure (PEP) devices, autogenic drainage, the high-frequency chest wall oscillation system (the Vest), the Flutter device, and the intrapulmonary percussive device. A detailed description of each of these methods can be found in Hardy and Anderson (1996). Meta-analysis suggests that several of these modalities are equivalent in efficacy to conventional chest physiotherapy. The most popular airway clearance mechanisms utilized by adult patients include the Vest, exercise, and PEP devices.

Physical activity augments airway clearance and is an important adjunct to airway clearance techniques, provided adequate oxygenation can be maintained during exercise. Airway clearance regimens can be tailored to patients' life-styles and severity of disease. The frequency and duration of each treatment should be individualized. Patients with minimal to mild symptoms may require only one session a day whereas those with a greater volume of thick secretions may need three or more sessions per day. Poor patient adherence is common, especially during clinically stable periods.

Chronic production of purulent sputum is the central clinical feature of bronchiectasis, thus mucolytic agents are of considerable interest in treatment. Recombinant human DNase (Pulmozyme) decreases the viscosity of CF sputum by degrading extracellular DNA into smaller pieces. Patients receiving DNase demonstrate modest improvements in pulmonary function, decreased rates of respiratory tract infections, and improvement in CF-related symptoms. Fewer respiratory tract infections results in less days in the hospital and fewer days on parenteral antibiotics. Over longer time periods, the benefits of DNase appear relatively small, but the treatment is safe and well tolerated. All patients with CF should be considered for a several month therapeutic trial of once per day DNase. The drug can be started safely during acute pulmonary exacerbations as well as stable periods. DNase is not presently recommended for the treatment of idiopathic bronchiectasis.

No well-validated alternative mucolytics are available at this time. N-Acetylcysteine reduces viscosity of sputum in vitro, presumably by breaking disulfide bonds. The nebulized form of the drug has been used in CF but has not been carefully studied. N-Acetylcysteine can be irritating to the upper airway and cause bronchoconstriction. Some, but not all, European studies have suggested a modest benefit from oral N-acetylcysteine, particularly in patients with moderate to severe disease. However, it is not clear that adequate amounts of orally administered drug penetrate into the airways to produce a mucolytic effect. For these reasons, N-acetylcysteine cannot be recommended.

There has been renewed interest in using nebulized hypertonic saline to facilitate airway clearance. Improved mucociliary clearance is likely due to its effects on sputum viscoelasticity. A short-term (2-week) clinical trial demonstrated that 6% saline nebulized twice a day resulted in improvement in pulmonary function tests compared to a control group that used isotonic saline. Hypertonic saline may cause bronchospasm in patients with CF, but this can be prevented by pretreatment with bronchodilators. Less concentrated solutions (starting at 3%) may be better tolerated.

A component of reactive airways disease overlaps with bronchiectasis in nearly all adults with CF. Nebulized β-adrenergic agonists provide symptomatic relief and facilitate clearance of the airways prior to chest physiotherapy. They may also help preserve lung function in patients with CF. Although most patients demonstrate improved pulmonary function with bronchodilators, some patients may worsen with this therapy. Airflow may decrease paradoxically or hyperinflation may worsen because of smooth muscle relaxation and decreased airway elasticity. Oral β-agonist preparations have no advantage over the inhaled medications in reversing bronchospasm. Long-acting aerosolized β-adrenergic agonists may also have a role in treatment, particularly in maintaining pulmonary function through the night.

Anticholinergic bronchodilators are well tolerated and may be more effective than β-adrenergic agonists in adults with CF. The adult CF airway may more closely mimic that of patients with chronic bronchitis, with less bronchospasm and more secretions, than children with CF. For this reason some individuals are more responsive to parasympathomimetic agents or combination therapy with a β-adrenergic agonist and an anticholinergic agent. Theophylline increases mucociliary clearance, diaphragmatic contractility, and central nervous system respiratory drive, but is not widely used in CF due to a narrow therapeutic range and significant adverse effects.

Antiinflammatory agents have a role in managing CF lung disease. Patients with asthma-like symptoms may require treatment with short courses of oral glucocorticoids or chronic administration of inhaled corticosteroids. Significant side effects prevent recommendation of long-term oral corticosteroids, despite demonstrated benefit in pulmonary function. Higher doses of inhaled corticosteroids have shown some promising preliminary results, but larger studies with longer-term data are needed before this therapy can be globally recommended. High-dose ibuprofen, with monitoring of blood levels, slowed progression of pulmonary disease in mildly affected patients (FEV_1 >60%), particularly in children 5–12 years of age. Adverse events, primarily gastrointestinal and renal, combined with a lack of data in patients with moderate to severe obstructive airways disease (FEV_1 <60% predicted) have limited widespread use of this treatment. Studies are underway examining the use of leukotriene modifiers in the CF population, but sufficient evidence is not yet available to recommend their use.

3. Oxygen—Clinically apparent cor pulmonale is a poor prognostic indicator. Subclinical pulmonary hypertension develops in a significant proportion of patients with CF and strongly correlates with hypoxemia, independent of pulmonary function. Subclinical pulmonary hypertension is associated with increased mortality as compared to patients with a similar degree of spirometric impairment without pulmonary hypertension. Supplemental oxygen improves exercise tolerance and survival in hypoxic patients with chronic obstructive pulmonary disease. The criteria for supplemental oxygen includes PaO_2 less than 55 mm Hg during the daytime on room air or less than 59 mm Hg in the presence of pedal edema, polycythemia, or electrocardiographic evidence of impairment of the right side of the heart. Oxygen is also indicated during exercise if exercise oxygen saturation falls below 88–90%. Nocturnal oxygen is indicated if oxygen saturation is less than 88–90% for 10% or more of total sleep time.

C. Pulmonary Exacerbations

Management of pulmonary exacerbations relies heavily on aggressive antibiotic treatment, typically intravenous antibiotics for a duration of 2 weeks. The best response is achieved by administering two antipseudomonal antibiotics in combination, preferably an antipseudomonal β-lactam (cefepime or ceftazidime) and an aminoglycoside (tobramycin). Fluoroquinolones are often used for mild exacerbations, but older patients are frequently infected with strains of *P aeruginosa* that are resistant to these agents. Antibiotics should be selected on the basis of recent sputum cultures. *P aeruginosa* is the most common and clinically significant pathogen in adults with CF. Intravenous access is usually achieved through temporary peripherally inserted central catheters (PICC lines) or permanent port-a-caths. Abnormalities in antibiotic pharmacokinetics associated with CF may necessitate higher doses and shorter dosing intervals. Other treatments including sputum clearance, bronchodilators, and nutritional support should be intensified during periods of pulmonary exacerbation. Patients with reactive airway disease may require oral corticosteroids. Depending on the severity of the exacerbation and the patient's support system, many adults can be treated at home, although others require admission to the hospital.

Treatment for one or more multidrug-resistant organisms (MROs) such as *B cepacia* or selected strains of *P aeruginosa* usually requires specific antibiotic combinations chosen on the basis of antimicrobial susceptibility testing. MROs that are resistant *in vitro* to all acceptable antibiotics may respond to combinations of antibiotics *in vivo*, either selected empirically or through synergy testing. The optimal approach has not been validated in clinical trials.

Concurrent diagnoses such as asthma, NTM infection, sinus disease, and gastroesophageal reflux should be considered in patients whose symptoms, clinical course, or response to treatment are atypical for CF. ABPA mimics many of the clinical signs and symptoms of exacerbations of bronchiectasis, especially in patients with CF, and often complicates these conditions. The presence of NTM in the sputum also represents a difficult clinical scenario. NTM can cause bronchiectasis, but may also represent a later infection with variable

clinical significance. NTMs classified as rapid growers, such as *Mycobacterium abscessus, M chelonae,* or *M fortuitum,* usually represent an aggressive infection that must be treated with a combination of antibiotics over months to years. MAC may be less significant as patients often do not demonstrate clinical improvement following aggressive treatment. However, in the setting of clinical decline MAC in the sputum should probably be treated.

D. Lung Transplantation

Lung transplantation became a viable option for patients with CF more than 10 years ago, but there is substantial morbidity and mortality associated with the procedure. Five-year posttransplant survival is approximately 50%. Patients with limited survival who have exhausted conventional therapies should be considered for transplantation. Patients with CF considered to be candidates for transplant should be referred for initial evaluation when their percent predicted FEV_1 falls below 30%. Although FEV_1 alone is inadequate in identifying appropriate candidates for transplantation, the relative shortage of available organs necessitates listing patients up to a year prior to the anticipated need for transplant. Patients with severe but relatively stable pulmonary disease can postpone transplantation for years, but close communication between the patient, CF care team, and transplant center is essential in determining the optimal time for the procedure. A subset of patients with CF who are more likely to gain survival advantage from the procedure can be identified with a validated survival model that incorporates parameters including FEV_1, gender, nutritional status, diabetic status, and sputum microbiology.

E. Extrapulmonary Manifestations of CF

CF is a multisystem disease. A comprehensive review of management of these issues exceeds the scope of this chapter, but has been reviewed by Yankaskas et al. (1999). Management of these multiple issues is best coordinated at specialized CF centers. The most important aspects of extrapulmonary CF treatment are outlined in Table 8–1.

F. End-of-Life Options

Despite substantial therapeutic advances, CF remains uniformly fatal. End-of-life care eventually becomes important for all patients. Predicting mortality in patients with advanced lung disease is difficult, as some individuals can enter long, relatively stable periods despite remarkably poor lung function. Discussions of dying are frequently avoided in patients awaiting lung transplantation. Headaches and chest pain sharply increase in the last 6–12 months prior to death in adults. Palliative care is important in managing symptoms such as pain and dyspnea, and addressing issues such as anxiety, depression, and fatigue is critical. Advance care planning, including designation of a medical proxy, is essential and should occur early in the course of illness to ensure that patients' wishes are respected. Most adults with CF have considered their end-of-life options, are aware of decisions made by others with CF, and are likely to be relieved when physicians discuss these issues with honesty and sensitivity. Finally, the physician and CF team should be flexible and offer choices regarding the location of terminal care, including a critical care unit, private hospital room, hospice, or home with requisite support.

Aggressive care for respiratory failure was historically viewed as futile in the context of CF. However, many patients with respiratory failure may benefit from noninvasive ventilatory support. This therapy should be considered in all patients with CF with advanced lung disease, particularly in patients awaiting lung transplantation. ICU care, including tracheal intubation and mechanical ventilation, is appropriate in the setting of potentially reversible events, such as massive hemoptysis or an acute pulmonary exacerbation. ICU care for patients with respiratory failure as a consequence of progressive disease may also be appropriate, especially if lung transplant is imminent. However, end-of-life care may be more difficult in a critical care setting. Although offering some hope, the care team must also be realistic in presenting options to patients and their families. At most centers only a minority of patients survive an episode of respiratory failure long enough to undergo lung transplantation.

Hardy KA, Anderson BD: Noninvasive clearance of airway secretions. Respir Care Clin North Am 1996;2:323. [PMID: 9390886]. (A useful review of airway clearance techniques.)

Liou TG et al: Survival effect of lung transplantation among patients with cystic fibrosis. JAMA 2001;286:2683. [PMID: 11730443]. (Survival benefit following transplantation occurred only in patients with CF with a predicted 5-year survival of less than 30%.)

Sood N et al: Outcomes of intensive care unit care in adults with cystic fibrosis. Am J Respir Crit Care Med 2001;163:335. [PMID: 11179102]. (A large series of patients with CF admitted to the ICU demonstrated a much greater rate of survival than previously assumed.)

Yankaskas JR et al: Cystic fibrosis adult care consensus conference report. Concepts in CF care. CF Foundation 1999;IX, Section 3:1. (A comprehensive review of present recommendations for care of adults with CF; the most complete and current document on the subject to date.)

Prognosis

Prognosis for patients with bronchiectasis varies according to the underlying cause of their condition and the severity of their disease. Median survival for patients with CF in the United States has increased dramatically in the past 30 years, from 16 years in 1970 to 32 years in 2000. Patients born in the 1990s can expect survival to more than 40 years. There will be more than 10,000 adult patients with CF in the United States by the year 2005. However, many patients with CF continue to die of respiratory failure in early adulthood. A study of the Finland National Hospital Discharge Register of patients diagnosed later in life with bronchiectasis (typically not due to CF) reported a mean age at presentation of 56 years. Twenty-five percent of these patients had died after an average of 9 years of follow-up. This survival rate was somewhat better than patients presenting with chronic obstructive pulmonary disease, but worse than those presenting with asthma.

Keistinen T et al: Bronchiectasis: an orphan disease with a poorly-understood prognosis. Eur Respir J 1997;10:2784. [PMID: 9493661]. (Interesting report of the long-term survival of older patients with bronchiectasis.)

Obstruction of Large Airways

Ron Balkissoon, MD, FRCP (C)

ESSENTIALS OF DIAGNOSIS

- *Obstruction may be caused by structural/anatomic abnormalities (tumors, foreign bodies, infections) or functional abnormalities (vocal cord dysfunction, muscle tension dysphonia).*
- *Symptoms include cough, stridor, shortness of breath, globus sensation, hoarseness.*
- *Pulmonary function testing including flow volume loops showing truncation.*
- *Laryngoscopy reveals cause of mechanical or anatomical obstruction.*
- *Bronchoscopy may be necessary if obstruction occurs in the subglottic large airway including trachea and main bronchi.*

General Considerations

In this chapter the large airways will be considered to include the pharynx, larynx, trachea, and main bronchi. Obstruction of the large airways should be considered when patients present with symptoms and signs of obstructive airways disease but do not have findings consistent with asthma or chronic obstructive lung disease or have these conditions but demonstrate a pronounced worsening of symptoms not controlled with standard medication. In the young age groups, foreign bodies and congenital webs are the most common abnormalities; whereas in the elderly population, tumors both benign and malignant and laryngeal manifestations of systemic diseases such as sarcoidosis or collagen vascular diseases are of greatest concern.

Pathogenesis

There are both acute and chronic causes of upper airway obstruction. Acute causes include aspiration of a foreign body as well as causes associated with direct blunt trauma such as fractures of the laryngeal cartilages, arytenoid cartilage dislocation, hematoma formation, and bilateral vocal cord paralysis. These injuries may be overlooked if the patient is intubated following massive trauma (eg, trauma resulting from motor vehicle accidents or falls). Only after the patient is extubated may such injuries be appreciated. The physician should be alert to evaluating these patients by laryngoscopy during intubation and soon after extubation. Intubation and various invasive surgical and medical procedures of the head and neck area lead to vocal cord paralysis and/or obstruction due to hematoma or formation of infectious abscess. There are a variety of drugs that lead to upper airway obstruction including the sedative hypnotics such as benzodiazepines that produce somnolence, respiratory depression, reduction in upper airway muscle tone, reduced cough response, and a blunted respiratory drive to hypoxia and hypercarbia. Use of the anticoagulants warfarin and heparin may put patients at risk for formation of hematoma secondary to relatively minor trauma.

Large airway obstruction caused by bacterial infection is seen in children and is less common in adults. Noniatrogenic infections including tracheitis and supraglottitis are commonly due to *Staphylococcus aureus* and *Streptococcus* species. Adult croup may be due to viral rather than bacterial sources. Retropharyngeal abscesses and dental, sublingual, submandibular, and other oral cavity infections are commonly due to *Streptococcus* or oral anaerobic species. Miscellaneous causes for acute upper airway obstruction include thermal injuries, systemic anaphylaxis, and rapid thyroid enlargement such as during pregnancy or postradiation therapy edema.

Chronic or slowly progressive causes of airflow obstruction include vocal cord polyps or granulomas and tumors of the aerodigestive tract, particularly invasive malignancies such as squamous cell carcinomas, lymphomas, or thyroid cancers. Children, in particular, may have tonsillar or lingual enlargement due to chronic infections. Other etiologies include papilloma formation leading to internal narrowing in the larynx and trachea or benign thyroid tumors causing extrinsic compression. Tracheal stenosis can occur after traumatic or prolonged intubation where the endotracheal cuff tube has been overinflated leading to local ischemia and consequent formation of granuloma. A significant number of chronic diseases can have laryngeal manifestations including rheumatoid arthritis, lupus, progressive systemic sclerosis, Wegener's granulomatosis, and relapsing polychondritis (Table 9–1).

Table 9–1. Causes of upper airway obstruction.

Extra thoracic lesions (pharynx, larynx, upper trachea)
  Malignant or benign tumors (eg, papillomas, polyps)
  Infection (eg, croup, epiglottitis, tonsillar abscess)
  Vocal cord paralysis or dysfunction
  Cricoarytenoid (eg, rheumatoid arthritis)
  Edema or hypertrophy (eg, angioneurotic edema, obstruc-
    tive sleep apnea)
  Trauma (eg, cricoid fracture, cervical subluxation, precervi-
    cal hematoma)
  Burn injury
  Tracheal stenosis
  Extrinsic compression (eg, goiter)
  Foreign body
  Amyloid
  Congenital abnormalities
Intrathoracic lesions (lower trachea)
  Tracheal tumors
  Tracheal stenosis (eg, after intubation or tracheostomy)
  Inflammatory diseases (eg, Wegener's granulomatosis,
    relapsing polychondritis, herpes)
  Tracheomalacia
  Trauma
  Extrinsic compression (eg, mediastinal tumors)
  Foreign bodies
  Amyloid
  Congenital (eg, vascular rings)

In contrast to self-explanatory mechanisms for upper airway obstruction related to a mass effect or neurological impairment of the upper airway, vocal cord dysfunction (VCD) has gained recognition as a cause of episodic recurrent upper airway obstruction that is often misdiagnosed as asthma or chronic airflow limitation both in children and adults. The pathogenesis of this problem appears to be the development of reflex closure of the vocal cords upon exposure to a wide variety of triggers not unlike those reported by asthmatics. This often leads to the erroneous diagnosis of asthma and resultant severe iatrogenic disease related to indiscriminate use of steroids often without any clear benefit. Vocal cord dysfunction has a high degree of association with gastroesophageal reflux and postnasal drip, suggesting that chronic irritation to the larynx by refluxate, postnasal drip, or occupational/environmental irritant exposures can lead to a chronic habituated hyperresponsiveness with reflex vocal cord closure to protect the lower airways.

Prevention

With the list of etiologies noted above, prevention strategies for the iatrogenic causes include judicious use of sedative hypnotic medications and optimum surgical and procedural techniques to minimize complications such as nerve paralysis, hematoma, or infection. Avoidance or cessation of smoking will obviously reduce the risk of oropharyngeal cancers as well as cerebral vascular accidents. Parents can prevent foreign body aspiration by keeping small objects out of the reach of toddlers.

Clinical Findings

A. SYMPTOMS AND SIGNS

Aside from patients being obviously dyspneic, the signs and symptoms of upper airway obstruction vary according to the cause of the obstruction. Acute upper airway obstruction due to foreign bodies, trauma, or allergic anaphylactic reactions is associated with abrupt onset of throat constriction, panic, and inability to phonate. Cough may be muted or weak if a foreign body is firmly lodged in the trachea such that passage of air is virtually impossible. Salivation may occur. Patients may grab at their throat as a sign of the point of blockage; vital signs may show tachycardia and elevated blood pressure or the converse depending on the degree of hypoxia or carbon dioxide retention. Similarly, level of consciousness will be affected by the same factors. If the obstruction is almost complete there may be almost no audible breath sounds, whereas if the obstruction is partial, laryngeal wheezes that may refer to the chest will be best appreciated directly over the trachea. Causes of slow onset upper airway obstruction may be associated with progressive dyspnea starting with symptoms just with exertion. Complaints may include a dry chronic cough, hemoptysis (rare), sore throat, and/or voice changes. In certain circumstances with mass lesions, patients may also report orthopnea, or shortness of breath related to positional changes of the neck and consequent compression of the upper airway. There may be visible evidence of a neck mass such as an obvious goiter or more subtle signs such as an asymmetry, bulge, or displacement of the trachea. Individuals with cerebral vascular accidents or central nervous system (CNS) neoplasms may demonstrate facial asymmetry or cranial nerve deficits.

Individuals with VCD will report the above symptoms, particularly shortness of breath, triggered by exercise, irritants including temperature extremes, and sometimes emotional distress. They may also report symptoms of gastroesophageal reflux disease (GERD) and/or paroxysmal nocturnal dyspnea.

B. LABORATORY FINDINGS

Routine complete blood count (CBC) could identify a hematological malignancy. Thyroid function tests may suggest a cause as may serology for collagen vascular diseases [erythrocyte] sedimentation rate (ESR), antinuclear antibodies (ANA), antineutrophilic cytoplasmic antibodies (ANCA), or rheumatoid factor]. Arterial blood gases are helpful to assess severity and judge the urgency for invasive intervention.

C. IMAGING STUDIES

Chest radiographs are generally not helpful in identifying tracheal narrowing or other pathology of the upper airway. To visualize the upper airway, high-resolution scans of the high thorax and neck are useful and three-dimensional computed tomography (3-D CT) reconstruction of the airways can demonstrate anatomical sites of narrowing and characterize the nature of the obstruction. Dynamic imaging with ultrafast CT can provide additional information.

D. SPECIAL TESTS

Spirometric studies demonstrate characteristic features that help to identify the nature of the obstruction. Fixed obstructive lesions of the extrathoracic trachea will demonstrate a plateau of the inspiratory loop, whereas fixed obstructive lesions in the intrathoracic trachea will cause a plateau of the inspiratory and expiratory limb of the flow volume loop. Lesions that are mobile can demonstrate variable effects on the expiratory loop with primarily an expiratory truncation with a ball valve-like action. Individuals with VCD may demonstrate variable truncation of inspiratory or expiratory loops and may only be intermittent based on exposure to a trigger. To distinguish VCD from asthma, methacholine testing, irritant provocation, cold air challenge, or exercise testing can be chosen to elicit a VCD episode.

E. SPECIAL EXAMINATIONS

Direct visualization of the upper airway is the gold standard for making a definitive diagnosis and assessing the nature and severity of the upper airway obstruction. Flexible fiberoptic rhinolaryngoscopy or bronchoscopy will most often be sufficient to perform the evaluation, however, if it is an emergent problem, rigid bronchoscopy may be needed to secure a patent airway. This technique requires general anesthesia and performance by experienced personnel, generally an ear, nose, and throat (ENT) or thoracic surgeon or pulmonologist.

Differential Diagnosis

The myriad causes of clinically significant upper airway obstruction are listed in Table 9–1. Occasionally, obstructive sleep apnea or even snoring is confused with other upper airway obstruction. Although this is technically correct, these conditions do not merit the approach to diagnosis or treatment outlined in this chapter. For further discussion of sleep apnea, which often is caused by collapse of the airway at the base of the tongue during sleep, see Chapter 29.

Treatment (Table 9–2)

In cases of emergent airway compromise, establishing adequate oxygenation and gas exchange are of primary importance. Ideally patients should be mildly sedated and kept awake if at all possible. Paralytic agents may be hazardous in upper airway obstruction, particularly if it is difficult to intubate the patient. When possible, paralytic agents should be avoided. In cases in which there is severe tracheal obstruction, an open ventilating rigid bronchoscope may be used, which allows for a secure airway during visualization and ensures adequate oxygenation. Insertion of a rigid bronchoscope also dilates an emergent narrowing airway. Once the airway is secured, a detailed examination of the upper airway and the tracheobronchial tree can be performed.

Depending on the nature of the lesion in the upper airway, several options can be used as therapeutic strategies. For many cancers, external beam radiation alone is the treatment of choice if there is time for this to work since the radiation effect reaches layers of tissue outside the airway lumen. For space-occupying lesions where removal is indicated, a rigid bronchoscope has the advantage that it can be used for laser interventions. Where airway compromise is not a major concern, a flexible bronchoscope can be used. For stenotic lesions, balloon dilation is a temporizing measure but will often require subsequent reevaluation and repeat dilatation. The use of rigid endoscopy may also be advantageous if there are concerns about significant bleeding or airway instability. Dilation is immediately effective for stenotic lesions but at best is generally a temporizing measure ideally followed by laser therapy and/or stenting. Mechanical dilation procedures run the risk of generating granulation tissue that generally requires laser therapy anyway.

Laser therapy with an Nd:YAG laser can be used with a rigid bronchoscope by most, but can also be

Table 9–2. Management options for mechanical obstructive lesions.

Initial stabilizing measures
   Endotracheal intubation
   Open ventilating rigid bronchoscope
Rigid or balloon dilation
Laser therapy
Electrocautery
Argon plasma coagulation
Photodynamic therapy
Cryotherapy
External beam radiation
Brachytherapy
Airway stents

used with a flexible bronchoscope by experienced endoscopists. Laser energy is used to create thermal tissue damage and is indicated for treating short endobronchial central airway lesions such as malignant intrinsic airway obstruction or postintubation tracheal stenosis. Other options include electrocautery and argon plasma coagulation therapies, which also use thermal energy to destroy malignant or scar tissue. Argon plasma coagulation specifically utilizes a gas that is ionized when exposed to high-frequency current in an electrical arc, which leads to immediate desiccation and tissue destruction without direct contact. It generally operates at a depth reliably of 2–3 mm.

In the case of space-occupying lesions such as malignancies with intrinsic obstruction of the lumen that do not respond to laser therapy, photodynamic therapy should be considered. This technique involves the injection of a photosensitizing agent that, after a suitable interval of time, followed by intraluminal exposure to laser light of 630 nm causes delayed cell death by a nonthermal phototoxic reaction. Cryotherapy and external beam radiation with brachytherapy (direct placement of a hollow catheter with a radioactive source within the airway) are other options.

Airway stents using silicone or metal devices are generally well tolerated but require periodic follow-up. Stents are particularly useful for external compressive lesions and for proximal bronchopleural and tracheoesophageal fistulas. Silicone stents require insertion with a rigid bronchoscope, whereas metal stents can be inserted with a flexible bronchoscope. Recognized complications include reobstruction, stent migration, and/or stent occlusion.

Upper airway obstruction due to functional problems such as vocal cord paralysis or VCD requires identification of contributing factors (medications, underlying medical problems) and optimal treatment. Treatment of acute VCD attacks can involve use of throat relaxation techniques, heliox, nebulized lidocaine, sedatives, or continuous positive airway pressure (CPAP). Long-term management of VCD requires a multidisciplinary approach that optimizes treatment for contributing problems such as GERD and postnasal drip with voice rehabilitation therapy that emphasizes laryngeal musculature relaxation techniques and psychological counseling where indicated. Vocal cord paralysis may benefit from surgical fixation of the vocal cords.

Hoppe H et al: Multidetector CT virtual bronchoscopy to grade tracheal bronchial stenosis. AJR Am J Roentgenol 2002;178:1195. [PMID: 11959731]. [This study compares the efficacy of noninvasive multidetector CT (virtual bronchoscopic images, axial CT slices, coronal reformatted images, and sagittal reformatted images) in depicting and allowing accurate grading of tracheobronchial stenosis with that of flexible bronchoscopy. It concludes that multidetector CT virtual bronchoscopy is a reliable noninvasive method that allows accurate grading of tracheobronchial stenosis. However, it should be combined with the interpretation of axial CT images and multiplanar reformatted images for evaluation of surrounding structures and optimal spatial orientation.]

Newman KB et al: Clinical features of vocal cord dysfunction. Am J Respir Crit Care Med 1995;152:1382. [PMID: 7551399]. (Case series of patients with classic vocal cord dysfunction seen at one institution in the early 1990s. Largest cohort series to date of VCD patients.)

Perkner JJ et al: Irritant associated vocal cord dysfunction. J Occup Environ Med 1998;40:136. [PMID:9503289]. (Report on 11 cases of VCD in which there was a temporal association between VCD onset and occupational or environmental exposure. Chart review of 11 cases that met IVCD case criteria compared to 33 control VCD subjects. Noted statistical differences between the groups for ethnicity and chest discomfort but not for gender, tobacco smoking habits, symptoms, or pulmonary function parameters. First description of IVCD published.)

Ryu HJ et al: Obstructive lung diseases: COPD, asthma, and many imitators. Mayo Clin Proc 2001;76:1144. [PMID: 11702903]. [Review of chronic obstructive pulmonary disease (COPD) including less common causes such as bronchiectasis, upper airway lesions, bronchiolar diseases, and some interstitial lung diseases that are associated with airflow obstruction. These less common forms of obstructive lung diseases are often misdiagnosed because of infrequent occurrence and poor recognition. A heterogeneous spectrum of disorders that can present with evidence of airflow obstruction is described and a diagnostic approach to obstructive lung disease is outlined.]

Seijo LM et al: Interventional pulmonology. N Engl J Med 2001;344:740. [PMID: 11236779]. (Review of interventional techniques to deal with benign and malignant causes of airway obstruction including laser, cryotherapy, brachytherapy, stenting, and photodynamic therapy.)

Stephens KE et al: Bronchoscopic management of central airway obstruction. J Thorac Cardiovasc Surg 2000;119:289. [PMID: 10649204]. (Case series of 97 patients with central airway obstruction who were critically ill, with impending suffocation, and underwent bronchoscopic procedures for the management of central airway obstruction. Concluded that endobronchial surgical techniques can be used safely and systematically for the relief of benign and malignant central airway obstructions; diverse approaches and interventions were required to produce and maintain palliation of airway symptoms.)

SECTION III

Interstitial Lung Disease

Idiopathic Interstitial Pneumonia | 10

Harold R. Collard, MD, & Talmadge E. King, Jr., MD

The idiopathic interstitial pneumonias (IIPs) are a group of interstitial lung diseases (ILDs) of unknown etiology. There are over 100 known causes of ILD, including certain inherited conditions, collagen vascular diseases, drugs, and dozens of occupational and environmental exposures. Historically, conditions that remained idiopathic have been collectively called by various names including "diffuse interstitial fibrosis," "diffuse fibrosing alveolitis," "Hamman-Rich syndrome," "idiopathic pulmonary fibrosis," and IIP. The currently preferred term for these conditions is IIP, and it will be used for the remainder of the chapter.

CLASSIFICATION SCHEMA

The definition and classification of the IIPs have been a source of confusion for many years. It is now quite clear that classification of the IIPs based on the histopathological appearance of surgical lung biopsy specimens helps guide therapy and aids in prognostication. In 1969, Liebow and Carrington described five histopathological subgroups of IIP: undifferentiated or "usual" interstitial pneumonia (UIP), diffuse lesions similar to UIP with superimposed bronchiolitis obliterans termed bronchiolitis interstitial pneumonia (BIP), desquamative interstitial pneumonia (DIP), lymphoid interstitial pneumonia (LIP), and giant cell interstitial pneumonia (GIP). This classification was revised by Katzenstein and Myers in 1998, and updated by the American Thoracic Society/European Respiratory Society (ATS/ERS) in 2002.

The current ATS/ERS classification schema for the IIPs includes seven distinct conditions based largely on histopathological appearance (Table 10–1): idiopathic pulmonary fibrosis (IPF) defined by the presence of a UIP pattern, nonspecific interstitial pneumonia (NSIP) defined by the presence of an NSIP pattern, cryptogenic organizing pneumonia (COP) defined by the presence of an organizing pneumonia pattern, acute interstitial pneumonia (AIP) defined by the presence of a diffuse alveolar damage (DAD) pattern, DIP defined by the presence of a DIP pattern, a closely related pattern termed respiratory bronchiolitis associated ILD (RBILD) defined by the presence of a respiratory bronchiolitis (RB) pattern, and lymphocytic interstitial pneumonia (LIP) defined by the presence of an LIP pattern. An integrated approach is critical to achieving an accurate diagnosis in patients with suspected IIP. Clinical, radiographic, and pathological data should be equally considered, with careful attention given to identifying known causes of ILD.

American Thoracic Society/European Respiratory Society: International multidisciplinary consensus classification of the idiopathic interstitial pneumonias. Am J Respir Crit Care Med 2002;165(2):277. [PMID: 11790668]. (A thorough review of the current classification schema for the idiopathic interstitial pneumonias and descriptions of the individual conditions.)

Katzenstein AA, Myers JL: Idiopathic pulmonary fibrosis: clinical relevance of pathologic classification. Am J Respir Crit Care Med 1998;157(4, Pt 1):1301. [PMID: 9563754]. (The seminal article describing the new histopathological classification schema for idiopathic interstitial pneumonia and its clinical relevance.)

Nicholson AG et al: The prognostic significance of the histologic pattern of interstitial pneumonia in patients presenting with the clinical entity of cryptogenic fibrosing alveolitis. Am J Respir Crit Care Med 2000;162(6):2213. [PMID: 11112140]. (This article demonstrates the prognostic importance of histopathology in the idiopathic interstitial pneumonias.)

Table 10–1. Idiopathic interstitial pneumonia: clinical diagnosis and histopathologic correlation.

Clinical Diagnosis	Histopathological Pattern
Idiopathic pulmonary fibrosis	Usual interstitial pneumonia
Nonspecific interstitial pneumonia	Nonspecific interstitial pneumonia
Cryptogenic organizing pneumonia	Organizing pneumonia
Acute interstitial pneumonia	Diffuse alveolar damage
Respiratory bronchiolitis-associated interstitial lung disease	Respiratory bronchiolitis
Desquamative interstitial pneumonia	Desquamative interstitial pneumonia
Lymphocytic interstitial pneumonia	Lymphocytic interstitial pneumonia

IDIOPATHIC PULMONARY FIBROSIS

 ESSENTIALS OF DIAGNOSIS

- *Chronic, progressive dyspnea and cough.*
- *No identifiable cause of interstitial lung disease.*
- *Predominantly basilar, subpleural, reticular abnormalities, honeycombing, and minimal ground-glass abnormality on high-resolution computed tomography (CT) scan.*
- *Temporal heterogeneity, minimal inflammation, and fibroblastic foci on surgical lung biopsy.*
- *Poor response to medical therapy and poor survival.*

General Considerations

Idiopathic pulmonary fibrosis (also called cryptogenic fibrosing alveolitis) is the most common form of IIP and is defined by the presence of UIP on surgical lung biopsy. Separating patients with IPF from those with other forms of IIP is important, as IPF has a distinctly poor response to therapy and prognosis. Recent insight into the mechanisms of progressive fibrosis in IPF has led to potential new therapeutic approaches.

Clinical Findings

The most common presentation for patients with IPF is progressive dyspnea over months to years and chronic nonproductive cough. The typical patient is 50 to 70 years old with a slight male predominance. Physical examination may reveal digital clubbing and the presence of bibasilar fine inspiratory crackles (so called "dry" or "Velcro" crackles). Pulmonary function testing commonly reveals restrictive lung disease [reduced total lung capacity (TLC), functional residual capacity (FRC), and residual volume (RV) with decreased forced expiratory volume in 1 s (FEV_1) and forced vital capacity (FVC) but usually normal or increased FEV_1/FVC ratio] and abnormal gas exchange [decreased diffusing capacity of the lung for CO (DL_{CO}) and resting or exercise hypoxemia].

High-resolution CT (HRCT) scanning is the most useful imaging technique in ILD and should be performed routinely on patients suspected of having IIP. The characteristic findings in patients with IPF include patchy, predominantly basilar, subpleural reticular abnormalities, absent or limited ground-glass abnormalities, traction bronchiectasis, and honeycombing. Atypical findings include extensive ground-glass abnormality, nodularity, upper or mid-zone predominance, and prominent hilar or mediastinal lymphadenopathy.

Histopathological Findings

The histopathological pattern seen in patients with IPF is UIP. UIP pattern is characterized by a heterogeneous, predominantly subpleural distribution of involvement. Importantly, there is temporal heterogeneity, with areas of end-stage fibrosis and "honeycombing" (thickened collagenous septae surrounding airspaces lined by bronchial epithelium) abutting areas of active proliferation of fibroblasts and myofibroblasts. These discrete areas of acute fibroblastic proliferation have been termed "fibroblastic foci," and are essential to the histopathological diagnosis of a UIP pattern. There is generally minimal interstitial inflammation, suggesting a primarily fibroproliferative process.

The histopathological observations of temporal heterogeneity and fibroblastic foci have led to the hypothesis that IPF is a result of ongoing diffuse microscopic alveolar epithelial injury. The predominant pathophysiological paradigm for the IIPs has held that chronic inflammation eventually leads to widespread fibrosis. IPF appears to be pathophysiologically distinct from this model, characterized by minimal inflammation and chronic fibroproliferation likely due to abnormal parenchymal wound healing. The lack of a significant inflammatory component in IPF may explain its poor response to antiinflammatory therapies such as corticosteroids, discussed below.

Differential Diagnosis

The clinical presentation of IPF is similar to many forms of ILD, and a careful history and physical examination must be performed to identify any known causes of ILD. Importantly, a UIP pattern on surgical lung biopsy is not specific for IPF. It can be seen in collagen-vascular diseases (eg, scleroderma, rheumatoid arthritis), asbestosis, and hypersensitivity pneumonitis. However, recent studies show that an NSIP pattern is most often found in these settings.

Treatment

Corticosteroids have been the mainstay of therapy for IPF for over 50 years. Unfortunately, the response of IPF to corticosteroid therapy is minimal. The best data on corticosteroid responsiveness in IPF were published in 1978 by Carrington et al: They retrospectively reviewed patients with a UIP pattern and found that 11% improved as measured by a combination of clinical, physiological, and radiographic indices. Recent studies have found similarly poor response rates (8–17%). All of these studies likely contained patients with histopathology that would now be classified as NSIP, a more steroid-responsive pattern. How many of the responders in these studies were actually patients with NSIP is unknown, but the actual response rate of IPF to corticosteroids is surely lower than published data suggest. Some argue that IPF is uniformly unresponsive to corticosteroids, and that patients who show clinical improvement have been misdiagnosed.

The immunomodulatory agents azathioprine and cyclophosphamide have failed to show a statistically significant benefit over steroids alone in patients with IIP. Antifibrotic agents have been tried alone or in combination with corticosteroids in patients with IPF. Colchicine has shown no significant benefit. However, two other antifibrotic agents, perfenidone and interferon-γ, have shown promising preliminary results and are currently being studied in large clinical trials.

The current recommendation for the treatment of IPF is high-dose steroids (0.5–1.0 mg/kg/day initially, then tapered) in combination with immunomodulator therapy (cyclophosphamide or azathioprine) for at least 3 months, following clinical, radiographic, and physiological parameters to assess response to therapy. If there is no improvement, therapy should be stopped and consideration given to enrollment in clinical trials of antifibrotic agents. Lung transplantation should be considered in all patients with progressive disease who are unresponsive to medical treatment. Referral for transplantation should be made in patients with a vital capacity below 60% predicted, and a diffusing capacity corrected for alveolar volume below 50%. Lung transplantation has been shown to improve survival in patients with IPF. Unfortunately, patients with IPF are often referred for transplantation too late, with 30% or more of patients dying while on the waiting list.

Prognosis

Survival in IPF is poor, with mean survival of 2–3 years from time of diagnosis and 5-year survival of around 20%. Prognostic indicators have been difficult to identify, but recent data suggest that a combination of factors including age, smoking history, level of dyspnea, severity of changes in lung function or gas exchange, the presence or absence of clubbing, the degree of radiographic abnormality, and the extent of young connective tissue present within the fibroblastic foci on surgical lung biopsy are predictive of survival.

American Thoracic Society: Idiopathic pulmonary fibrosis: diagnosis and treatment. International consensus statement. American Thoracic Society (ATS), and the European Respiratory Society (ERS). Am J Respir Crit Care Med 2000;161(2, Pt 1):646. [PMID: 10673212]. (This is a thorough review of the current management of IPF.)

King TE Jr et al: Predicting survival in idiopathic pulmonary fibrosis: scoring system and survival model. Am J Respir Crit Care Med 2001;164(7):1171. [PMID: 11673205]. (This article describes a clinical/radiographic/physiological predictor model of survival in patients with IPF.)

King TE Jr et al: Idiopathic pulmonary fibrosis: relationship between histopathologic features and mortality. Am J Respir Crit Care Med 2001;164(6):1025. [PMID: 11587991]. (This paper demonstrates the prognostic significance of fibroblastic foci on surgical lung biopsy in patients with IPF.)

Mapel DW et al: Corticosteroids and the treatment of idiopathic pulmonary fibrosis. Past, present, and future. Chest 1996;110(4):1058. [PMID: 8874268]. (A review of the data evaluating corticosteroids in IPF.)

Raghu G et al: Azathioprine combined with prednisone in the treatment of idiopathic pulmonary fibrosis: a prospective double-blind, randomized, placebo-controlled clinical trial. Am Rev Respir Dis 1991;144(2):291. [PMID: 1859050]. (This study showed no statistically significant benefit to the addition of azathioprine to prednisone in patients with IPF.)

Ziesche R et al: A preliminary study of long-term treatment with interferon gamma-1b and low-dose prednisolone in patients with idiopathic pulmonary fibrosis. N Engl J Med 1999;341(17):1264. [PMID: 10528036]. (A small study showing significant benefit to interferon-γ in patients with IPF.)

Zisman DA et al: Cyclophosphamide in the treatment of idiopathic pulmonary fibrosis: a prospective study in patients who failed to respond to corticosteroids. Chest 2000;117(6):1619. [PMID: 10858393]. (This study shows no benefit to adding cyclophosphamide in patients with IPF who failed corticosteroid therapy.)

NONSPECIFIC INTERSTITIAL PNEUMONIA

 ESSENTIALS OF DIAGNOSIS

- Subacute or chronic, progressive dyspnea and cough.
- No identifiable cause of interstitial lung disease, with special attention to the presence of collagen vascular disease and environmental exposures.
- Temporal uniformity and varying degrees of inflammatory and fibrotic abnormalities on surgical lung biopsy.
- Variable responsiveness to medical therapy, better survival that IPF.

General Considerations

Nonspecific interstitial pneumonia originated as a histopathological categorization reserved for surgical lung biopsies that did not demonstrate a clearly identifiable pattern (eg, UIP). An NSIP pattern is seen with a number of known causes of ILD including drugs, collagen-vascular disease, and hypersensitivity pneumonitis; therefore the identification of an NSIP pattern should prompt a careful search for these conditions. The current definition of NSIP as a clinical form of IIP is troublesome, as it has no distinctive clinical, radiographic, or histopathological description. Until further definition is available, however, the diagnosis of NSIP will remain provisional.

Clinical Findings

Like IPF, NSIP typically presents with chronic dyspnea and cough, although the duration of symptoms is generally shorter. Patients typically present between age 40 and 50. Fever and finger clubbing may occur and bibasilar fine inspiratory crackles are common. Pulmonary function testing shows a restrictive pattern, similar to that seen in IPF.

High-resolution CT scanning reveals a predominance of ground-glass abnormality, most commonly bilateral and subpleural in distribution, and is associated with lower lobe volume loss. Patchy areas of airspace consolidation and reticular abnormalities may be present, but honeycombing is unusual. Importantly there is

a continuum of findings in NSIP, with some cases radiographically indistinguishable from IPF.

Histopathological Findings

The surgical lung biopsy in NSIP is characterized by varying degrees of inflammation and fibrosis, with some biopsies showing a predominance of inflammatory changes ("cellular" pattern) and others a predominance of fibrotic reaction ("fibrotic" pattern). Although an NSIP pattern may have significant fibrosis, it is usually temporally uniform, and fibroblastic foci and honeycombing, if present, are rare. The temporal uniformity is distinctly different from the temporal heterogeneity seen in a UIP pattern. Nonetheless, a fibrotic NSIP pattern can be difficult to reliably distinguish from a UIP pattern, and there is significant variability in interpretation even among expert pathologists.

Differential Diagnosis

Clinically, the most common diagnosis confused with NSIP is IPF. A nonspecific interstitial pneumonia pattern is seen with a number of known causes of ILD including drugs, collagen-vascular disease, and hypersensitivity pneumonitis. The diagnosis of an NSIP pattern on surgical lung biopsy should prompt the clinician to revisit the clinical data carefully looking for these conditions.

Treatment

There are no prospective data on treatment for NSIP. Two retrospective reviews have suggested generally favorable responsiveness to corticosteroids. Patients with a primarily cellular NSIP pattern respond better than patients with a fibrotic NSIP pattern. High dose corticosteroids (0.5–1.0 mg/kg/day initially, then tapered) are usually given for at least 3 months, following clinical, radiographic, and physiological parameters to assess response to therapy. If there is no improvement, therapy should be stopped. If hypersensitivity pneumonitis is suspected, removal from exposure to potential causative agents should be attempted.

Prognosis

There are several excellent retrospective studies suggesting upward of 70% 5-year survival in NSIP (Figure 10–1). Patients with a fibrotic NSIP pattern on surgical lung biopsy appear to have worse 10-year survival than those with a cellular NSIP pattern: 35–90% vs. 100%, respectively.

Bouros D et al: Histopathological subsets of fibrosing alveolitis in patients with systemic sclerosis and their relationship to outcome. Am J Respir Crit Care Med 2002;165:1581. [PMID: 12070056]. (This report describes the pathological features

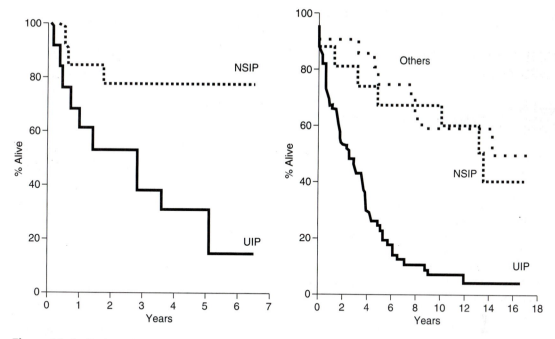

Figure 10–1: Kaplan–Meier survival curves in patients with IIP based on histopathological classification. **Left:** Survival from presentation was significantly greater in patients with an NSIP pattern compared with those with a UIP pattern (*p* = 0.005). (Reprinted with permission from Daniil et al: A histologic pattern of nonspecific interstitial pneumonia is associated with a better prognosis than usual interstitial pneumonia in patients with cryptogenic fibrosing alveolitis. Am J Respir Crit Care Med 1999;160(3):899. [PMID: 10471616].) **Right:** Data from 104 patients with histopatologically confirmed IIP. The survival difference between patients with a UIP pattern and all others was statistically significant (*p* < 0.001) with a mean survival of 2.8 years. (Reprinted with permission from Bjoraker et al: Prognostic significance of histopathological subsets in idiopathic pulmonary fibrosis. Am J Respir Crit Care Med 1998;157:199.) PMID: 9445300

found in systemic sclerosis and found that NSIP is by far the most common pattern.)

Daniil ZD et al: A histologic pattern of nonspecific interstitial pneumonia is associated with a better prognosis than usual interstitial pneumonia in patients with cryptogenic fibrosing alveolitis. Am J Respir Crit Care Med 1999;160(3):899. [PMID: 10471616]. (This article demonstrates the prognostic significance of NSIP when compared to IPF.)

Katzenstein AA, Fiorelli RF: Nonspecific interstitial pneumonia/-fibrosis. Histologic features and clinical significance. Am J Surg Pathol 1994;18(2):136. [PMID: 8291652]. (The seminal article describing NSIP.)

Travis WD et al: Idiopathic nonspecific interstitial pneumonia: prognostic significance of cellular and fibrosing patterns: survival comparison with usual interstitial pneumonia and desquamative interstitial pneumonia. Am J Surg Pathol 2000;24(1):19. [PMID: 10632484]. (This paper demonstrates the improved survival of a cellular vs. a fibrotic NSIP pattern on surgical lung biopsy in patients with NSIP.)

Vourlekis JS et al: Nonspecific interstitial pneumonitis as the sole histologic expression of hypersensitivity pneumonitis. Am J Med 2002;112(6):490. [PMID: 11959061]. (This article demonstrates the importance of revisiting the clinical evaluation when the histological pattern is NSIP.)

CRYPTOGENIC ORGANIZING PNEUMONIA

 ESSENTIALS OF DIAGNOSIS

- Acute to subacute dyspnea, cough, and fever.
- No identifiable associated condition.
- Patchy terminal/respiratory bronchiolar and alveolar inflammation with proliferation of connective tissue filling the alveolar space.
- Excellent clinical response to corticosteroids with improved survival compared with IPF.

General Considerations

Cryptogenic organizing pneumonia (COP) is an idiopathic lung disease characterized by proliferation of granulation tissue (ie, organizing pneumonia) in the alveolar airspaces, alveolar ducts, and small airways, with relative sparing of the interstitium. Organizing pneumonia can be found on surgical lung biopsy in association with a number of diseases (eg, postinfectious, drug related, connective tissue disease related, posttransplant). It is also commonly seen accompanying other histopathological patterns (eg, UIP). The diagnosis of COP is reserved for isolated organizing pneumonia in patients without an identifiable associated disease. The term bronchiolitis obliterans organizing pneumonia (BOOP) historically encompassed COP but is no longer recommended for this idiopathic condition.

Clinical Findings

Cryptogenic organizing pneumonia typically presents with dyspnea and cough developing over a few days to a few months. Fever is relatively common, and COP is often misdiagnosed as community-acquired pneumonia. Patients with COP present over a wide range of ages, with the mean age around 50 years. Bibasilar inspiratory crackles are common. Finger clubbing is rare. Pulmonary function testing shows a mild to moderate restrictive pattern similar to that seen in the other IIPs.

High-resolution CT scanning reveals a predominance of bilateral, patchy consolidation, most commonly with a subpleural or peribronchial distribution. Peribronchovascular nodules (occasionally quite large) and irregular linear, subpleural opacities are also seen. Ground-glass opacities may occasionally be prominent findings. Honeycombing is rarely, if ever, present.

Histopathological Findings

The histopathological appearance of organizing pneumonia is a uniform temporal appearance of mild interstitial chronic inflammation associated with an intraluminal organizing fibrosis in distal airspaces (bronchioles, alveolar ducts, and alveoli). The lung architecture is generally well preserved, and honeycombing is not described.

Differential Diagnosis

The clinical presentation of COP can be mistaken for community-acquired pneumonia or ILD, depending on the duration and constellation of presenting symptoms. The histopathological appearance of organizing pneumonia should prompt a careful search for other histopathological patterns that may be present, such as UIP, NSIP, DAD, DIP, and RBILD. When found in association with another histopathological pattern, it is usually considered a secondary phenomenon and is not consistent with the diagnosis of COP. Organizing pneumonia on surgical lung biopsy should also suggest the associated clinical conditions mentioned above.

Treatment

Although a small percentage of patients with COP improve spontaneously, corticosteroids are the mainstay of therapy. Treatment is usually given at high doses (0.5–1.0 mg/kg/day initially, then tapered) for at least 6 months. Shorter courses of therapy are associated with a high rate of recurrent disease. The vast majority (>80%) of patients will respond to corticosteroid treatment. A small percentage of patients will have progressive disease despite therapy. Alternative agents such as cyclophosphamide have been used but few data support any benefit. Although patients usually show signs of improvement within days of starting treatment, it is recommended that treatment with tapering doses of corticosteroids be given for 6 months or longer.

Prognosis

Survival in patients with COP is excellent, with 5-year survival estimated at close to 100%. An occasional case of COP may progress to respiratory failure and death. This usually occurs when the diagnosis and subsequent treatment are delayed.

Alasaly K et al: Cryptogenic organizing pneumonia. A report of 25 cases and a review of the literature. Medicine (Baltimore) 1995;74(4):201. [PMID: 7623655]. (A review of the literature describing COP.)

Epler GR: Bronchiolitis obliterans organizing pneumonia. Arch Intern Med 2001;161(2):158. [PMID: 11176728]. (A review of organizing pneumonia with a thorough description of associated conditions.)

Izumi T: Proceedings of the international congress on bronchiolitis obliterans organizing pneumonia. Chest 1992;102;1S.

ACUTE INTERSTITIAL PNEUMONIA

 ESSENTIALS OF DIAGNOSIS

- *Acute to subacute dyspnea, cough, with rapid progression to respiratory failure.*
- *No identifiable cause of acute lung injury.*
- *Evidence of diffuse alveolar damage on surgical lung biopsy.*
- *Unclear response to medical therapy, poor prognosis, may be recurrent.*

General Considerations

Acute interstitial pneumonia (AIP, also called Hamman-Rich disease) is an acute form of IIP generally characterized by rapid progression to respiratory failure over days to weeks. Histopathology reveals diffuse alveolar damage (DAD). Diffuse alveolar damage is a common histopathological pattern of acute lung injury, and is the typical finding in patients with acute respiratory distress syndrome (ARDS). The diagnosis of AIP is given to patients with DAD in the absence of known risk factors for ARDS (so called "idiopathic ARDS").

Clinical Findings

Acute interstitial pneumonia presents with dyspnea and cough developing over a few days to weeks. Fever is occasionally present. Many patients report a viral prodrome consisting of myalgias and upper respiratory symptoms. The mean age at presentation is 50 years. Diffuse inspiratory crackles are common. Pulmonary function testing shows a restrictive pattern. Rapidly progressive hypoxemia and respiratory failure develop in most patients.

High-resolution CT scanning reveals ground-glass abnormality and consolidation, predominantly basilar but often located throughout all lung fields. Early stages of AIP may have patchy involvement whereas more advanced cases show diffuse abnormality. Honeycombing is rarely seen, but may be present in advanced cases.

Histopathological Findings

There are two histopathological stages to DAD. In the acute stage, edema, epithelial necrosis and sloughing, fibrinous exudates in airspaces, and hyaline membrane formation are characteristic findings. The process is usually widespread and temporally uniform. In the second, or organizing stage, proliferation of type II pneumocytes, resolution of hyaline membranes and alveolar exudates, and fibroblastic proliferation occur. Thrombi are commonly seen in small to medium sized vessels. This organizing stage is the most common pattern seen at the time of surgical lung biopsy in patients with AIP, but either stage is consistent with the diagnosis. With time, end-stage fibrosis develops and large cystic airspaces form resembling honeycombing. These cystic spaces, however, are lined with alveolar epithelium, in contrast to the bronchial epithelium seen in the honeycomb spaces associated with a UIP pattern.

Differential Diagnosis

The differential diagnosis of AIP includes community-acquired pneumonia, *Pneumocystis carinii* pneumonia, congestive heart failure, ARDS, and other causes of rapidly progressive respiratory failure. Patients with AIP are commonly misdiagnosed. As they progress to respiratory failure in the absence of any identifiable diagnosis, surgical lung biopsy often reveals DAD.

Treatment

There is no proven treatment for AIP. The majority of reported cases received coticosteroids and antibiotic therapy without any clear benefit. Although data from patients with DAD of known cause (ARDS) would suggest no benefit from early corticosteroid treatment, extrapolation of these data to patients with AIP is questionable.

Prognosis

Survival in AIP is worse than in ARDS, with a greater than 50% mortality reported in the literature. Whether lung protective ventilatory strategies proven to work in ARDS are beneficial in AIP is unknown.

Olson J et al: Hamman-Rich syndrome revisited. Mayo Clin Proc 1990;65(12):1538. [PMID: 2255216]. (A review of AIP describing its clinical presentation, histopathological appearance, and clinical course.)

Vourlekis JS et al: Acute interstitial pneumonitis. Case series and review of the literature. Medicine 2000;79(6):369. [PMID: 11144035]. (A thorough review of the literature on AIP.)

RESPIRATORY BRONCHIOLITIS-ASSOCIATED INTERSTITIAL LUNG DISEASE & DESQUAMATIVE INTERSTITIAL PNEUMONIA

 ESSENTIALS OF DIAGNOSIS

- *Chronic, progressive dyspnea and cough.*
- *Almost always associated with current or former cigarette smoking.*
- *Pigment-laden macrophages in and surrounding respiratory bronchioles (RBILD) and diffusely throughout alveoli (DIP).*
- *Good response to smoking cessation and corticosteroids, good prognosis.*

General Considerations

Respiratory bronchiolitis-associated interstitial lung disease (RBILD) and desquamative interstitial pneumonia (DIP) are arguably different clinical manifestations of the same histopathological condition, with RBILD progressing to DIP over time. Although they are discussed together in this chapter, RBILD and DIP are still generally considered distinct clinical diagnoses.

Clinical Findings

Both RBILD and DIP present with chronic, progressive dyspnea and cough. The mean age at diagnosis is in the third to fourth decade of life. The vast majority of patients with either condition are current or former smokers, or have had environmental exposure to passive cigarette smoke. Physical examination usually reveals bibasilar inspiratory crackles, and clubbing is occasionally present in DIP. Pulmonary function testing is usually normal or mildly obstructive in RBILD, likely due to concomitant chronic obstructive pulmonary disease. A restrictive pattern is generally seen in DIP.

In patients with RBILD, HRCT often reveals central and peripheral bronchial wall thickening (proximal to subsegmental bronchi), centrilobular nodules, ground-glass opacity, and air trapping. None of these findings has a zonal predominance. DIP demonstrates more diffuse ground-glass abnormality, often peripheral in distribution. Honeycombing can be seen but is usually limited.

Histopathological Findings

The most striking histopathological feature of both RBILD and DIP is the presence of pigment-laden macrophages (macrophages containing dusty brown cytoplasm, often positive on iron stains). These macrophages were originally, and incorrectly, thought to be "desquamated" epithelial cells, thus the name "desquamative" interstitial pneumonia. Accumulation of pigmented macrophages in the respiratory bronchioles, called respiratory bronchiolitis, is a common histopathological pattern seen in smokers. In patients with suspected IIP and a predominantly bronchiolar and peribronchiolar distribution on histopathology (ie, respiratory bronchiolitis), the term RBILD pattern is used. If there is more widespread alveolar involvement, the term DIP pattern is used. The alveolar septae are mildly thickened by inflammatory infiltrates in both conditions.

Differential Diagnosis

RBILD and DIP must be distinguished from each other. They are also easily confused with other forms of ILD. The histopathological findings of an RBILD pattern are often patchy and subtle, so careful review of surgical lung biopsy specimens is critically important in patients with suspected RBILD.

Treatment

Many cases of RBILD and DIP have resolved with smoking cessation alone. Corticosteroids are the mainstay of therapy, but there are no prospective treatment studies in either condition. Almost all patients with RBILD reported in the literature to date have improved with smoking cessation and corticosteroids (0.5–1.0 mg/kg/day initially, then tapered). The best data on steroid responsiveness of DIP suggest around 60% of patients improve. Corticosteroids are generally continued for at least 3 months, as in the other IIPs.

Prognosis

The prognosis for both RBILD and DIP is good, with greater than 70% survival at 5 years. No patient with RBILD has been reported to progress to pulmonary fibrosis, although the number of cases to date is small. DIP will occasionally progress to end-stage fibrosis and respiratory failure despite therapy. Once thought to possibly represent early IPF, a progressive DIP pattern is histopathologically distinct from a UIP pattern.

Carrington CB et al: Natural history and treated course of usual and desquamative interstitial pneumonia. N Engl J Med 1978;298(15):801. [PMID: 634315]. (This article is still the best review to date of DIP.)

Myers JL et al: Respiratory bronchiolitis causing interstitial lung disease. A clinicopathologic study of six cases. Am Rev Respir Dis 1987;135(4):880. [PMID: 3565934]. (The initial description of RBILD.)

Park JS et al: Respiratory bronchiolitis associated interstitial lung disease: radiologic features with clinical and pathologic correlation. J Comput Assist Tomogr 2002;26:13. [PMID: 11801899]. (This article reviews the radiographic manifestations of RBILD.)

Yousem SA et al: Respiratory bronchiolitis-associated interstitial lung disease and its relationship to desquamative interstitial pneumonia. Mayo Clin Proc 1989;64(11):1373. [PMID: 2593722]. (A comparative review of 18 cases of RBILD and 36 cases of DIP.)

LYMPHOCYTIC INTERSTITIAL PNEUMONIA

 ESSENTIALS OF DIAGNOSIS

- *Chronic, progressive dyspnea and cough.*
- *No evidence for autoimmune disorder or immunodeficiency.*
- *Evidence of dense interstitial lymphoid infiltrate on surgical lung biopsy.*
- *Unclear response to medical therapy, generally good prognosis.*
- *Progression to lymphoma is a major concern.*

General Considerations

Initially described as a form of IIP by Liebow and Carrington, LIP was subsequently considered a preneoplastic condition. Although the clinical and histopathological findings of LIP are often the presenting signs of underlying malignancy, autoimmunity (eg, rheumatoid arthritis and Sjögren's syndrome), or congenital immunodeficiency, there remains a minority of cases that appears to be idiopathic.

Clinical Findings

The clinical presentation of LIP is often indistinguishable from that of the other forms of IIP. Patients with LIP tend to be young (30 to 50 years old) and predominantly female. Symptoms are generally slowly progressive, with dyspnea and cough most prominent. Bibasilar crackles are common and lymphadenopathy is occasionally present. Pulmonary function generally reveals restriction. High-resolution CT scanning commonly shows diffuse ground-glass abnormality, poorly defined centrilobular nodules, thickened bronchovascular bundles, lymph node enlargement, and cysts.

Histopathological Findings

Surgical lung biopsy in LIP reveals a dense interstitial lymphoid infiltrate with variable and usually minor peribronchial involvement. The infiltrates are mostly comprised of T-lymphocytes, plasma cells, and macrophages. There is often associated type II cell hyperplasia. Lymphoid follicles are often present. Granuloma formation and mild fibrosis may rarely be seen.

Differential Diagnosis

There are many conditions associated with the histological finding of a cellular, primarily lymphoid, parenchymal infiltrate: follicular bronchiolitis, nodular lymphoid hyperplasia, and Castleman's disease being the most common. Follicular bronchiolitis and LIP may well represent a spectrum of the same process. The two together are sometimes referred to as "diffuse pulmonary lymphoid hyperplasia." Further, LIP can be histopathologically indistinguishable from hypersensitivity pneumonitis or cellular nonspecific interstitial pneumonia, so careful clinicopathological diagnosis is essential.

Treatment

LIP is generally treated with corticosteroids with or without immunomodulator therapy. Although there are no good data to support their use, corticosteroids are anecdotally thought to improve outcomes.

Prognosis

The clinical course is quite variable. Most patients with LIP stabilize or improve, with 5-year survival estimated at around 60%. The minority of patients progress to diffuse pulmonary fibrosis and death.

Koss MN et al: Lymphoid interstitial pneumonia: clinicopathological and immunopathological findings in 18 cases. Pathology 1987;19(2):178. [PMID: 3453998]. (A review of LIP supporting the hypothesis that it is a distinct, nonpreneoplastic condition.)

Nicholson AG et al: Reactive pulmonary lymphoid disorders. Histopathology 1995;26(5):405. [PMID: 7544761]. (A review of LIP and the closely related condition, follicular bronchiolitis.)

APPROACH TO DIAGNOSIS

A full description of the diagnostic approach to the IIPs would require a discussion of the general diagnostic approach to ILD, which is beyond the scope of this chapter. Once the diagnosis of IIP is suspected, the most important clinical distinction to make is whether the patient has IPF, as IPF has a distinctly poor response to therapy and prognosis. The discussion below will focus primarily on the ability of different diagnostic modalities to distinguish IPF from the other IIPs (Table 10–2).

History, Physical Examination, Pulmonary Function Testing

The history, physical examination, and pulmonary function evaluation have little diagnostic accuracy in IIP. Dyspnea and cough are common to all forms of IIP. A shorter duration of symptoms and the presence of fever suggest AIP or COP. In IPF, NSIP, RBILD, DIP, and LIP, patients usually present with slowly progressive symptoms, and fever is uncommon. Fine inspiratory crackles are common to all the IIPs. Digital clubbing is most common in IPF, occasionally present in NSIP and DIP, and rarely present in the other IIPs. Pulmonary function testing commonly reveals restrictive lung disease and abnormal gas exchange.

Chest Radiography

The chest radiograph lacks diagnostic specificity in IIP, with the exception of honeycombing, which is suggestive of IPF. It correlates poorly with the histopathological pattern, anatomic distribution of disease, and severity of involvement. Although the conventional chest radiograph still serves an important screening purpose, patients suspected of having IIP should undergo HRCT, which is much more diagnostically useful.

Table 10–2. IIP: summary of clinical presentation, histopathology, response to therapy, and survival.[1]

	IPF	NSIP	COP	AIP	RBILD	DIP	LIP
Demographic	50–70s, slight male predominance	40–50s, equal male:female	All ages (mean 50), equal male:female	All ages (mean 50), equal male:female	30–50s, predominantly smokers	40–50s, predominantly smokers	30–50s, female predominance
Clinical	Chronic dyspnea and cough, crackles, clubbing	Chronic dyspnea and cough, crackles, occasional clubbing	Acute to subacute (days to weeks) dyspnea, cough, fever, crackles, no clubbing	Acute to subacute (days to weeks) rapidly progressive dyspnea, cough, occasional fever, crackles, no clubbing	Chronic dyspnea and cough, crackles, no clubbing	Chronic dyspnea and cough, crackles, occasional clubbing	Chronic dyspnea and cough, crackles no clubbing, occasional lymphadenopathy
Radiographic (HRCT)	Bilateral lower lobe, subpleural, reticular abnormality; minimal ground glass; honeycombing	Bilateral lower lobe, subpleural ground glass; occasional reticular abnormality	Bilateral lower lobe, subpleural ground glass and consolidation; nodules; no reticular abnormality or honeycombing	Bilateral diffuse ground glass; rare reticular abnormality and honeycombing	Patchy ground glass; centrilobular nodules; thickened airway walls; no honeycombing	Bilateral lower lobe, subpleural ground glass; rare reticular abnormality and no honeycombing	Patchy ground glass; centrilobular nodules; thickened bronchovascular bundles; cysts
Histopathological	UIP pattern	NSIP pattern	OP pattern	DAD pattern	RB pattern	DIP pattern	LIP pattern
Response to corticosteroids	Poor (10% or less)	Good (50–90%)	Excellent (> 80%)	Unclear, likely poor	Excellent (> 90%)	Good (60%)	Unclear, likely good
Prognosis	Poor (20% 5-year survival)	Good (70% 5-year survival)	Excellent (> 90% 5-year survival)	Poor (< 50% short-term survival)	Excellent (> 90% 5-year survival)	Good (70% 5-year survival)	Good (60% 5-year survival)

[1]HRCT, high-resolution computed tomography; IPF, idiopathic pulmonary fibrosis; NSIP, nonspecific interstitial pneumonia; COP, cryptogenic organizing pneumonia; AIP, acute interstitial pneumonia; RBILD, respiratory bronchiolitis-associated interstitial lung disease; DIP, desquamative interstitial pneumonia; LIP, lymphocytic interstitial pneumonia; UIP, usual interstitial pneumonia; OP, organizing pneumonia; DAD, diffuse alveolar damage; RB, respiratory bronchiolitis.

High-Resolution Computed Tomography

The characteristic radiographic features of the various IIPs on HRCT have been described above. The ability of HRCT scanning to confidently diagnose IPF has been widely investigated, with reported sensitivities of 43–78% and specificities of 90–97%. Based on these data, HRCT can make a confident, highly specific diagnosis of IPF in half to two-thirds of patients with IIP. Its specificity for other forms of IIP is poor. Ground-glass abnormality is present in all cases of NSIP, COP, AIP, RBILD, DIP, and LIP, and there are no reliably diagnostic patterns.

Bronchoscopy

There are, unfortunately, no bronchoalveolar lavage (BAL) findings specific to the IIPs. Patients with IPF demonstrate a nonspecific increase in BAL neutrophils, eosinophils, and, less commonly, lymphocytes. Several studies have suggested that a predominance of BAL lymphocytes predicts both steroid responsiveness and improved survival. This has led to the recommendation that isolated BAL lymphocytosis should suggest an alternative diagnosis to IPF. This finding is, however, neither sensitive nor specific. Transbronchial biopsy is of limited utility due to the small size of the biopsy obtained and the lack of histological preservation due to mechanical crushing of the tissue. Its main purpose is to rule out alternative diagnoses such as sarcoidosis, occult infection, and malignancy.

Surgical Lung Biopsy

The decision whether to pursue surgical lung biopsy (either via open thoracotomy or, more commonly, thoracoscopy) is one of the most important in the care of patients with suspected IIP. The utility of an accurate histopathological diagnosis is clear; choice of therapy, responsiveness to treatment, and prognosis are all affected. It is our opinion that surgical lung biopsy should be pursued in all patients who cannot be confidently diagnosed on clinical and radiographic grounds, unless too frail or ill to tolerate it. With the widespread use of thoracoscopic biopsy, the number of patients unable to tolerate surgical biopsy is increasingly small.

The ATS/ERS have recently published a consensus statement describing criteria for the clinical diagnosis of IPF (Table 10–3). The presence of all four major criteria and at least three of four minor criteria increases the likelihood of a correct clinical diagnosis. A recent study using these criteria showed the clinical diagnosis of IPF to have a sensitivity of 62% and a specificity of 97%, when compared to the histopathological diagnosis. Ultimately, it is up to individual clinicians and patients to decide with what degree of diagnostic specificity they are comfortable.

Table 10–3. ATS/ERS criteria for the clinical diagnosis of IPF.[1]

Major criteria (must have all four):
1. Exclusion of other known causes of ILD, such as certain drug toxicities, environmental exposures, and connective tissue diseases.
2. Abnormal pulmonary function studies that include evidence of restriction (reduced VC often with an increased FEV_1/FVC ratio) and impaired gas exchange (increased alveolar–arterial oxygen gradient with rest or exercise, or decreased DL_{CO}).
3. Bibasilar reticular abnormalities with minimal ground glass opacities on HRCT scans.
4. Transbronchial lung biopsy or bronchoalveolar lavage showing no features to support an alternative diagnosis.

Minor criteria (must have at least three of four):
1. Age greater than 50 years.
2. Insidious onset of otherwise unexplained dyspnea on exertion.
3. Duration of illness of 3 or more months.
4. Bibasilar, inspiratory dry crackles (Velcro type).

[1]The presence of all four major and three of four minor criteria establishes a presumptive clinical diagnosis of IPF. IPF, idiopathic pulmonary fibrosis; ILD, interstitial lung disease; VC, vital capacity; FEV_1, forced expiratory volume in 1 s; FVC, forced vital capacity; DL_{CO}, diffusing capacity for the lung for carbon monoxide; HRCT, high-resolution computed tomography
Reprinted with permission from American Thoracic Society: Idiopathic pulmonary fibrosis: diagnosis and treatment. International consensus statement. American Thoracic Society (ATS), and the European Respiratory Society (ERS). Am J Respir Crit Care Med 2000;161(2, Pt 1):646.

American Thoracic Society/European Respiratory Society International multidisciplinary consensus classification of the idiopathic interstitial pneumonias. Am J Respir Crit Care Med 2002;165(2):277. [PMID: 11790668]. (A thorough review of the idiopathic interstitial pneumonias including a discussion of the approach to diagnosis and the role of surgical lung biopsy.)

Ferson PF, Landreneau RJ: Thoracoscopic lung biopsy or open lung biopsy for interstitial lung disease. Chest Surg Clin North Am 1998;8(4):749. [PMID: 9917923]. (A thorough review and comparison of both open surgical and thoracoscopic lung biopsy for interstitial lung disease.)

Hunninghake G et al: Utility of lung biopsy for the diagnosis of idiopathic pulmonary fibrosis. Am J Respir Crit Care Med 2001;164:193. [PMID: 11463586]. (This article examines the value of surgical lung biopsy or HRCT in making the diagnosis of IPF.)

Raghu G et al: The accuracy of the clinical diagnosis of new-onset idiopathic pulmonary fibrosis and other interstitial lung disease: A prospective study. Chest 1999;116(5):1168. [PMID: 10559072]. (This article suggests a confident diagnosis of IPF can be made in approximately half of patients without surgical lung biopsy.)

Pulmonary Manifestations of Collagen Vascular Diseases

11

Gregory P. Cosgrove, MD

The collagen vascular diseases (Table 11–1) are a heterogeneous group of idiopathic, inflammatory, systemic diseases. Common to these diseases is an aberrant immunological response resulting in end-organ damage. Pulmonary involvement results in significantly increased morbidity and mortality independent of that associated with the underlying connective tissue disease. Therefore, physicians must be aware of the pulmonary manifestations of the connective tissue diseases. In doing so, appropriate therapy and surveillance may be instituted to limit or ameliorate progressive dysfunction.

Pulmonary abnormalities occur in the airways, lung parenchyma, pulmonary vasculature, or pleura. Dysfunction may be either a direct effect of the underlying disease process or a secondary complication due to treatment toxicities and opportunistic infection. Although infectious complications are numerous, this chapter will focus solely on the noninfectious aspects of lung involvement of the connective tissue diseases. Specifically, the focus will be on the common pulmonary manifestations of rheumatoid arthritis (RA), systemic lupus erythematosus (SLE), systemic sclerosis (SSc), and polymyositis/dermatomyositis (PM/DM). Pulmonary manifestations of less common diseases such as Sjögren's syndrome and mixed connective tissue disease will be highlighted briefly. The pulmonary vasculitides are discussed in Chapter 20.

RHEUMATOID ARTHRITIS

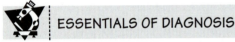

ESSENTIALS OF DIAGNOSIS

- *Elevated rheumatoid factor.*
- *Symmetric, small joint arthralgias with stiffness that may progress to joint deformities.*
- *Dyspnea with or without a productive cough.*

General Considerations

Rheumatoid arthritis is a systemic inflammatory disease predominantly affecting the synovial membranes of the diarthrodial joints. The disease affects all ethnicities, with an increasing prevalence between the fourth and sixth decades. In North America, the annual incidence is estimated to be 0.3–1.5%. The prevalence in women is 2.5 times higher than in men. However, pulmonary manifestations (Table 11–2) are more common in men, with a 3:1 ratio, and in those who develop disease later in life.

Pathogenesis

Rheumatoid arthritis appears to be a disease in which there is an aberrant immunological response in genetically susceptible individuals. Infectious agents, both bacterial and viral, have been implicated in the development of RA, but the association remains tenuous despite intense investigation. The immune response in RA is primarily centered within the synovial membrane with an antigen-specific T lymphocyte infiltration to a yet unidentified autoantigen. The resultant T lymphocyte-mediated inflammatory response initiates a cytokine cascade with subsequent immune complex deposition. Tumor necrosis factor-α (TNF-α) appears to have a major role in the persistent inflammatory response seen in RA, which leads to progressive articular destruction through a variety of mechanisms. Whether TNF-α has a prominent role in the pulmonary manifestations of the disease, is currently being investigated. Experimental animal models do suggest that immune complex-mediated lung injury is also responsible for the pulmonary manifestations of RA. To date, an antigen has not been identified.

Clinical Findings

A. SYMPTOMS AND SIGNS

Symptomatic pulmonary disease most often occurs in individuals with late-onset RA with the majority of pa-

Table 11–1. Collagen vascular diseases.

Rheumatoid arthritis (RA)
Systemic lupus erythematosus (SLE)
Systemic sclerosis (SSc)
Polymyositis/dermatomyositis (PM/DM)
Mixed connective tissue disease (MCTD)
Sjögren's syndrome
Relapsing polychondritis
Ankylosing spondylitis
Behcet's disease
Systemic vasculitides (Wegener's granulomatosis, Churg-
    Strauss syndrome)

tients presenting between the ages of 50 and 60 years. Lung disease usually follows the articular manifestations of RA, but does not necessarily correlate with the extent of articular disease. Pulmonary involvement may also antedate overt joint disease, as is the case in up to 20% of patients who develop interstitial lung disease (ILD) complicating RA.

Table 11–2. Pulmonary manifestations in rheumatoid arthritis.

Airways disease
    Cricoarytenoid arthritis
    Airflow limitation (obstruction)
    Follicular bronchiolitis
    Bronchiolitis obliterans (constrictive)
    Bronchiectasis
Pleural disease
    Pleuritis
    Empyema (aseptic or septic)
    Pneumothorax secondary to a ruptured necrobiotic nodule
    Bronchopleural fistula
Rheumatoid nodules (necrobiotic nodules)
Interstitial lung disease
    Interstitial pulmonary fibrosis
    Bronchiolitis obliterans organizing pneumonia
    Caplan's syndrome
    Apical fibrobullous disease
    Amyloidosis
Drug-induced lung disease
    Methotrexate pneumonitis
    D-Penicillamine
    Gold
Thoracic cage immobility
Pulmonary vascular disease
    Pulmonary artery hypertension
    Vasculitis
Infections
    Reactivation of tuberculosis

Dyspnea, a productive or nonproductive cough, and pleurisy are the most common initial symptoms patients experience. However, incidental radiographic abnormalities are commonly detected as necrobiotic nodules, early interstitial lung disease, or small to moderate-sized pleural effusions in otherwise asymptomatic patients.

Pleural disease is one of the more common pulmonary manifestations of RA, with approximately 20% of RA patients reporting a history of pleurisy. Autopsy studies document that 38–72% of patients with RA have demonstrable pleural involvement at the time of death. These findings range from pleural thickening, or small to moderate-sized pleural effusions, to pyogenic or nonpyogenic empyema. Spontaneous pneumothoraces complicating RA are rare but have been reported. Pneumothoraces are thought to result from necrosis and cavitation of subpleural necrobiotic nodules. Pleural effusions may be seen concomitantly with necrobiotic nodules and/or interstitial lung disease. Effusions are characteristically exudative, with glucose concentrations < 30 mg/dL in up to 80% of patients. Additionally, the pleural fluid rheumatoid factor is typically elevated and is higher than that detected in the serum.

Airflow obstruction is another common pulmonary manifestation of RA. Of all the connective tissue diseases, RA most commonly affects the airways. Isolated airflow obstruction in the absence of prior tobacco use, bronchiolitis obliterans (constrictive bronchiolitis), follicular bronchiolitis with or without an underlying Sjögren's syndrome, bronchiectasis, bronchiolitis obliterans with obstructing pneumonia (BOOP), and cricoarytenoid arthritis have all been reported in RA. Cricoarytenoid arthritis is of particular concern as it occurs in up to 25% of patients and predisposes patients to possibly life-threatening acute laryngeal obstruction. Bronchiolitis obliterans (BO) presents with an abrupt onset of dyspnea, nonproductive cough, inspiratory crackles, and a mid-inspiratory squeak. Both D-penicillamine and secondary Sjögren's syndrome have been associated with bronchiolitis obliterans in RA. In contrast to RA-associated ILD, which typically affects men more often than women, BO is most often reported in middle-aged women.

Interstitial lung disease in RA is frequently insidious in onset and is associated with progressive dyspnea on exertion and a chronic, nonproductive cough. Bibasilar crackles, tachypnea, and exertional hypoxia are frequently observed. Clubbing is present in up to 75% of patients. Signs of pleural disease are commonly noted with concomitant pleural-interstitial lung disease occurring in 20% of patients. In the absence of overt articular disease, the clinical presentation of RA-associated ILD is similar to that of idiopathic pulmonary fibrosis

(IPF). The notable difference between the two diseases is the frequent pattern of clinical stability in the absence of therapy in RA-associated ILD in distinct contrast to the progressive course commonly characterizing IPF.

Bronchiolitis obliterans organizing pneumonia may also occur in RA and presents with fever, cough, and patchy alveolar infiltrates. BOOP differs from BO by the presence of infiltrates and alveolar involvement. The course of BOOP in RA may be more recalcitrant and less responsive to steroids than typically noted in other forms of the disease in which prognosis is excellent.

Drug-induced lung disease secondary to methotrexate, D-penicillamine, or gold must be considered in patients with pre-existing exposure to these medications. D-Penicillamine and gold have been associated with BO whereas methotrexate has been reported to result in diffuse pneumonitis, pleuritis, and noncardiogenic pulmonary edema. Drug-induced lung diseases are discussed in further detail in Chapter 33.

Pulmonary vascular disease in the absence of overt fibrotic lung disease is manifest less frequently in RA than in other connective tissue diseases. Secondary pulmonary hypertension with cor pulmonale may, however, complicate chronic fibrotic ILD from RA. Pulmonary capillaritis causing diffuse alveolar hemorrhage, either isolated or in association with systemic rheumatoid vasculitis, has been reported.

B. Laboratory Findings

The presence of rheumatoid factor (RF), which is autoantibody to the Fc portion of immunoglobulin G, is the most common laboratory abnormality in RA. The presence of RF, however, is not necessary for the diagnosis of RA as only 85% of RA patients are RF seropositive. RF can be detected in healthy volunteers as well as others with chronic inflammatory diseases or viral or chronic bacterial infections, and in organ transplant recipients. The presence of RF, especially in high titers, is associated with the development of extraarticular disease. Hypergammaglobulinemia, thrombocytosis, eosinophilia, and hypocomplementemia may be observed. An elevated erythrocyte sedimentation rate (ESR) or C-reactive protein (CRP) is noted during periods of active inflammation and occurs more frequently with extraarticular involvement.

C. Imaging Studies

Pleural effusions are the most common radiographic abnormalities in patients with RA. In up to 20% of patients, dense reticular or reticulonodular opacities suggestive of ILD are present. Radiographic honeycombing is usually a basilar, peripheral predominant process. Upper lobe fibrosis or fibrobullous disease may occur but is less common. Necrobiotic nodules, which fre-

quently cavitate, are seen in the lung periphery and may be several centimeters in diameter. Airways disease may be evident with signs of basilar bronchiectasis or air trapping from BO or follicular bronchiolitis. Patchy alveolar opacities may represent RA-associated BOOP, however, infection must always be considered.

Differential Diagnosis

The pulmonary manifestations of RA must be distinguished from medication-related side effects, infectious complications, or other connective tissue disease that presents in a similar manner. Interstitial lung disease secondary to RA mimics that seen in IPF. These diseases must be distinguished from one another, as the rate of progression in IPF is significantly faster without the variable course characterizing RA.

Complications

Infectious complications are common in RA and respiratory infections result in approximately 20% of patient deaths. Common bacterial and viral pathogens as well as opportunistic agents should be considered in all patients with new pulmonary disease, especially in those who are receiving immunosuppressive therapy. An increased risk of reactivation of latent tuberculosis has recently been reported in patients receiving anti-TNF-α therapy. Gold, methotrexate, cyclophosphamide, and D-penicillamine all have pulmonary toxicities. Therefore, drug-related side effects should be considered in all patients who develop pulmonary disease while on therapy.

Treatment

Disease-modifying antirheumatic drugs (DMARDs) such as corticosteroids are commonly used to treat the pulmonary manifestations of RA. Both objective physiological and radiographic improvements as well as a subjective improvement in dyspnea have been reported with corticosteroid therapy. There is less evidence to support the use of other agents such as methotrexate, cyclophosphamide, azathioprine, or anti-TNF-α therapies. In those who do respond to immunosuppressive therapy, either subjectively or objectively, the addition of a cytolytic agent such as cyclophosphamide or azothioprine may allow chronic immunosuppression with low-dose prednisone and decreased corticosteroid-related side effects.

Prognosis

Pulmonary involvement, especially the presence of ILD, portends a significantly reduced survival. In RA, the 5-year mortality in patients with extraarticular involvement is twice that of patients without extraarticular disease. However, a significant degree of variation exists in disease progression. Some patients have a rapidly progressive course whereas others progress slowly with long periods of stability. Therefore, serial monitoring is essential to assess disease progression for each patient.

Akira M, Sakatani M, Hara H: Thin-section CT findings in rheumatoid arthritis-associated lung disease: CT patterns and their courses. J Comput Assist Tomogr 1999;23(6):941. [PMID: 10589572]. (Useful diagnostic and prognostic information may be provided by thin section CT scanning.)

Anaya JM et al: Pulmonary involvement in rheumatoid arthritis. Semin Arthritis Rheum 1995;24(4):242. [PMID: 7740304]. (Detailed review of pathological findings.)

Gochuico BR: Potential pathogenesis and clinical aspects of pulmonary fibrosis associated with rheumatoid arthritis. Am J Med Sci 2001;321(1):83. [PMID: 11202484]. (Interesting update on the pathophysiology of rheumatoid arthritis and the lung.)

Rajasekaran BA et al: Interstitial lung disease in patients with rheumatoid arthritis: a comparison with cryptogenic fibrosing alveolitis. Rheumatology (Oxford) 2001;40(9):1022. [PMID: 11561113]. (A comparison of clinical features and prognosis in rheumatoid ILD and idiopathic pulmonary fibrosis.)

Rovere Querini P et al: Miliary tuberculosis after biological therapy for rheumatoid arthritis. Rheumatology (Oxford) 2002;41 (2):231.

Schwarz MI et al: Isolated pulmonary capillaritis and diffuse alveolar hemorrhage in rheumatoid arthritis and mixed connective tissue disease. Chest 1998;113(6):1609. [PMID: 9631801]. (Unusual cause of capillaritis.)

SYSTEMIC LUPUS ERYTHEMATOSUS

 ESSENTIALS OF DIAGNOSIS

- *Young female.*
- *Elevated ANA titer.*
- *Serositis.*
- *Hematological abnormalities.*

General Considerations

Systemic lupus erythematosus (SLE) is the classical autoimmune disease characterized by antibodies to nuclear and cytoplasmic antigens and multiorgan involvement affecting the skin, kidneys, central nervous system (CNS), musculoskeletal system, and lungs. Lung involvement occurs more commonly in SLE than in any other connective tissue disease with more than 50% of patients experiencing pulmonary manifestations (Table

11–3) at some point during the course of their illness. As with RA, all compartments of the lung may be affected.

SLE is primarily a disease of young women. The peak incidence occurs between the ages of 15 and 40 years. The female:male ratio is 6–10:1. Most cases are sporadic in origin. A genetic predisposition may exist, as SLE is more common in family members of affected patients. The current hypothesis is that disease occurs in genetically predisposed individuals in whom either endogenous or exogenous factors trigger an aberrant immune response with subsequent autoimmunity resulting in clinical disease.

Pathogenesis

Autoantibodies and B cell hyperactivity are the most prominent immunological features associated with SLE. Although antinuclear antibodies (ANAs) are not specific to SLE, they occur in > 95% of patients with this disease and are directed against different nuclear and cytoplasmic epitopes (antigenic molecules). End-organ dysfunction is thought to be secondary to autoantibody-induced immune complex deposition. The pathogenic mechanisms have been extensively studied in patients with lupus nephritis in whom anti-double-stranded (ds) DNA antibodies can be detected by immunofluorescence within glomeruli and mesangium as

Table 11–3. Pulmonary manifestations in systemic lupus erythematosus.

Airways disease
  Bronchiectasis
  Bronchiolitis obliterans (constrictive)
  Bronchiolitis obliterans organizing pneumonia
  Epiglottitis, laryngitis, cricoarytenoid arthritis
Pleural disease
  Pleuritis
  Pleural effusions
  Pleural thickening
Interstitial lung disease
  Acute lupus pneumonitis
  Chronic interstitial pneumonitis
  Bronchiolitis obliterans organizing pneumonia
  Diffuse alveolar hemorrhage
Cardiogenic pulmonary edema
Acute reversible hypoxemia syndrome
Pulmonary vascular disease
  Pulmonary artery hypertension
  Vasculitis
  Thromboembolism
Atelectasis
Diaphragmatic dysfunction/shrinking lung syndrome

---

well as in serum in high titers during active episodes of glomerulonephritis.

Clinical Findings

A. SYMPTOMS AND SIGNS

Symptoms attributable to the pulmonary manifestations of SLE vary significantly depending on the lung compartment involved. Infections are the most common manifestations of pulmonary involvement in SLE. Humoral and cellular immunological dysfunction underlying SLE in addition to those risks associated with aggressive immunosuppressive therapy predisposes patients to infection. Because of this, patients are infected with usual pathogens as well as opportunistic pathogens. Of particular note, mycobacterial and nocardial infections are increased in SLE. As for other immunosuppressed patients, infectious symptoms may be attenuated, atypical, and difficult to distinguish from the disease itself.

Pleural disease is common in patients with SLE and may occur in up to 93% of patients at the time of autopsy. Clinically significant disease may manifest as pleurisy, which occurs in 50% of patients at some point during the course of their disease. Pleural effusions, often bilateral, frequently accompany episodes of pleurisy and are associated with fever and dyspnea. Effusions are mild to moderate in size, and exudative in nature. Glucose concentrations are normal in contrast to RA, in which pleural glucose is low. Autoantibodies (ANA, anti-dsDNA) may be present in the pleural fluid in titers >1:320. Although autoantibody testing is not sensitive for the disease, it is specific for lupus pleuritis.

Pulmonary vascular disease occurs in up to 25% of patients with SLE. In contrast to systemic sclerosis, pulmonary hypertension in the absence of parenchymal lung disease is uncommon. Thromboembolic disease occurs in up to 25% of patients and is associated with significantly increased mortality. Antiphospholipid antibodies, which occur in approximately 30% of patients with SLE, are associated with pulmonary emboli and infarction, capillaritis, diffuse pulmonary hemorrhage, postpartum idiopathic pneumonia syndrome, and pulmonary hypertension. Of SLE patients who develop pulmonary hypertension, approximately 60% have antiphospholipid antibodies.

SLE-associated ILD may be acute or chronic in nature. Severe, acute-onset dyspnea may be secondary to two life-threatening disorders: acute lupus pneumonitis or diffuse alveolar hemorrhage. Acute lupus pneumonitis usually occurs in patients with established disease, but may be the initial manifestation of SLE in young women. The risk of acute lupus pneumonitis is increased in postpartum SLE patients. Alveolar hemorrhage is a life-threatening complication of SLE, with

fulminant respiratory failure secondary to either pulmonary involvement from a systemic infection, an isolated pulmonary capillaritis, or diffuse alveolar damage. Acute lupus nephritis occurs concurrently with alveolar hemorrhage in 60–90% of patients. Hemoptysis is evident in < 40% of patients on presentation, but in up to 80% of patients at some point in their illness. The mortality associated with either acute lupus pneumonitis or alveolar damage is significant, approaching 50% in recent studies. Therefore, prompt recognition is essential for aggressive and appropriate treatment.

Chronic ILD occurs in SLE but not to the same extent as seen in RA, SSC, or PM/DM. Insidious onset dyspnea similarly occurs, but is commonly associated with pleuritic chest discomfort and mildly productive cough. The physical examination is similar to other chronic ILDs. Clubbing is less common than for RA.

Dyspnea, in the absence of overt parenchymal or vascular disease, may occur in patients with SLE due to diaphragmatic weakness or dysfunction. This is termed shrinking lung syndrome or acute reversible hypoxemia syndrome. Shrinking lung, or vanishing lung syndrome is associated with restrictive physiology and abnormalities of ventilation. The restriction, often difficult to distinguish from ILD by pulmonary function testing, is due to weakness of muscles of respiration including the diaphragm. On examination, systemic weakness may not be identified; there is selective involvement of the diaphragm and respiratory muscles. Acute reversible hypoxemia syndrome is seen in acutely ill patients with fever and a widened alveolar–arterial (A–a) oxygen difference. It is thought that excessive complement activation induces a transient leukoocclusive vasculopathy with diffusion abnormalities. The syndrome is transient and usually responds to antiinflammatory therapy with corticosteroids and aspirin.

Airways disease, especially of the upper airways, is uncommon in SLE. Acute epiglottitis, laryngitis, vocal cord edema or paralysis, and ulcerative tracheitis have been reported. Bronchiectasis and BO, constrictive BO, or BOOP are less frequent than in RA. BOOP is difficult to diagnose. It may resemble infectious pneumonia in presentation and therefore may be more common than reported given the increased incidence of respiratory infections in SLE and the tendency to empirically treat patients rather than pursue pathological clarification.

B. LABORATORY FINDINGS

Positive ANAs occur in > 90% of patients with lupus. Low titer ANAs are also present in 2% of normal healthy females. The anti-dsDNA may reflect disease activity in some patients with nephritis. Other specific ANAs fail to correlate with disease activity. Anemia, leukopenia, and thrombocytopenia are common in

SLE, reflecting the multisystem involvement of the disease. Progressive anemia in a patient with alveolar infiltrates should raise a strong concern for alveolar hemorrhage as hemoptysis is present in only 40% of patients during the initial presentation.

C. IMAGING STUDIES

Small lung volumes with atelectasis are commonly present on chest radiographs. The low lung volumes may be secondary to diaphragmatic dysfunction or restrictive lung disease. Parenchymal abnormalities in SLE are frequent but nonspecific with patchy airspace disease being present in BOOP, lupus pneumonitis, alveolar hemorrhage, pulmonary emboli, or infections. Reticular (linear) opacities, most prominently in the bases, are common in chronic diffuse ILD. Pleural disease, either pleural thickening or bilateral effusions, may occur with or without chest pain. Effusions in the absence of chest pain are more often related to renal failure rather than active pleuritis.

Differential Diagnosis

The pulmonary manifestations of lupus are nonspecific. Infectious processes must always be considered given the marked immunological dysfunction and high incidence of respiratory infections in SLE.

Treatment

Corticosteroids are the primary therapy for SLE-related noninfectious pulmonary disease. Azathioprine and cyclophosphamide are adjuncts for refractory disease and serve as steroid-sparing agents in those who need chronic immunosuppression. Pulse dose cyclophophamide therapy is used for diffuse alveolar hemorrhage and lupus pneumonitis in those who do not respond to high-dose corticosteroids. As is the case with other connective tissue diseases, the efficacy of such therapy remains unclear.

Prognosis

Pulmonary involvement in SLE is associated with significant morbidity and increased mortality. The risk of death has been estimated to be more than twofold higher in SLE patients with clinically evident pulmonary disease. Diffuse alveolar hemorrhage and lupus pneumonitis portend a significantly increased acute mortality approaching 50% in most series.

Cheema GS, Quismorio FP Jr: Interstitial lung disease in systemic lupus erythematosus. Curr Opin Pulmon Med 2000;6(5): 424. [PMID: 10958234]. (Details of acute and chronic onset ILD are discussed.)

Fishback N, Koss MN: Pulmonary involvement in systemic lupus erythematosus. Curr Opin Pulm Med 1995;1(5):368. [PMID: 936098]. (A broad perspective on pulmonary symptoms in this disorder.)

Karim MY et al: Presentation and prognosis of the shrinking lung syndrome in systemic lupus erythematosus. Semin Arthritis Rheum 2002;31(5):289. [PMID: 11965593]. (The rare manifestations of shrinking lung in 7 of 2650 lupus patients.)

Murin S, Wiedemann HP, Matthay RA: Pulmonary manifestations of systemic lupus erythematosus. Clin Chest Med 1998;19 (4):641. [PMID: 9917958]. (Pulmonary findings in SLE and drug-induced SLE.)

Wu CY et al: Severe pulmonary hemorrhage as the initial manifestation in systemic lupus erythematosus with active nephritis. Lupus 2001;10(12):879. [PMID: 11787879]. (Case report of capillaritis.)

SCLERODERMA

 ESSENTIALS OF DIAGNOSIS

- *Proximal scleroderma (proximal to the metacarpophalangeal or metatarsophalangeal joints) with two or more of the following:*
  - *Sclerodactyly.*
  - *Digital pitting scars or loss of substance from the finger pads.*
  - *Bibasilar pulmonary fibrosis.*

General Considerations

Systemic sclerosis (SSc) is an acquired, autoimmune disease of unknown etiology associated with excessive deposition of extracellular matrix and a small vessel vasculopathy involving the skin, gastrointestinal tract, lungs, kidneys, and heart. The lungs are the fourth most commonly affected organ. However, lung disease is the leading cause of death in patients with SSc. The incidence of SSc is approximately 19 cases per million per year with women being 7–12 times as likely to develop the disease as men. Most patients present between the ages of 35–65 years. Children are rarely affected. Pulmonary manifestations are listed in Table 11–4.

Pathogenesis

The current paradigm to conceptualize SSc pathogenesis suggests that in a susceptible host, exposure to certain environmental agents leads to immune system activation with resultant endothelial cell damage and

Table 11–4. Pulmonary manifestations in progressive systemic sclerosis.

Airways disease
   Airflow limitation
   Follicular bronchiolitis
Pleural disease
   Pleuritis
   Pleural effusions
   Spontaneous pneumothorax
Interstitial lung disease
   Interstitial pulmonary fibrosis
   Aspiration pneumonitis
   Diffuse alveolar hemorrhage
   Diffuse alveolar damage
Pulmonary vascular disease
   Pulmonary artery hypertension
Pulmonary scar carcinoma
Infections

fibroblast activation. The subsequent, perpetuating cascade results in an obliterative vasculopathy and fibrosis with end-organ damage. In contrast to other connective tissue diseases, complement activation and immune complex deposition do not appear to be involved in the pathogenesis of SSc.

Clinical Findings

A. SYMPTOMS AND SIGNS

SSc is classified into two forms: limited and diffuse. In the limited form, cutaneous thickening is found in the distal limbs without truncal involvement. The *CREST* (*C*alcinosis, *R*aynaud's phenomenon, *E*sophageal dysmotility, *S*clerodactyly, and *T*elangiectasias) variant of SSc is a form of limited scleroderma. In limited SSc, Raynaud's phenomenon may antedate other organ involvement by years. Diffuse SSc is classified by both distal and proximal limb skin thickening or truncal involvement, signs of digital ischemia, or pulmonary fibrosis. In contrast to limited SSc, the interval between Raynaud's phenomenon and multiorgan involvement is months in duration. Severe, diffuse interstitial pulmonary fibrosis is more common with the diffuse form of SSc, whereas isolated pulmonary hypertension is more common with the CREST variant of SSc. Diffuse interstitial fibrosis or pulmonary hypertension may occur in either limited or diffuse SSc.

   ILD is the classic pulmonary manifestation in SSc. Physiological abnormalities have been documented in 30–60% of patients, whereas at autopsy 60–100% of patients have signs of diffuse ILD. Dyspnea, initially with exertion and later at rest, is a common presenting symptom. Cough, usually nonproductive or productive of only scant mucoid sputum, occurs in up to 20% of patients. The cough may be from interstitial fibrosis or secondary to recurrent aspiration/reflux in those with esophageal dysfunction. Up to 50% of patients will have fine, mid-to-late inspiratory crackles on examination. Signs of pulmonary hypertension may be evident, although these are difficult to appreciate. In severe pulmonary hypertension, an accentuated fixed, split S_2 or a right-side heave may be the first examination finding. In advanced disease, overt signs of right heart failure such as an S_3 gallop, jugular venous distention, tricuspid regurgitation, or pedal edema may be present.

   Pleural disease is evident in 50–80% of patients at the time of autopsy. In contrast, pleuritic chest pain is reported in only 20% of patients. Spontaneous pneumothoraces secondary to ruptured subpleural cysts in the lung bases are rare. Clubbing is uncommon, especially in patients with obliterative vasculopathy. The cutaneous manifestations of SSc are usually the most apparent manifestation of the disease. However, the extent of cutaneous involvement does not correlate with the severity of pulmonary disease.

B. LABORATORY FINDINGS

Antinuclear antibodies are found in approximately 90% of patients with SSc. An elevated anticentromere antibody occurs more frequently with limited SSc, whereas the anti-Scl-70 (antitopoisomerase I antibody) and antihistone antibodies are detected more commonly in the diffuse form of SSc.

C. IMAGING STUDIES

Basilar reticular or reticulonodular opacities suggesting pulmonary fibrosis are present in 25–45% of patients with SSc on plain chest radiographs. Radiographic honeycombing may become evident as the disease progresses, in a pattern similar to that seen in IPF, RA, or asbestosis. Esophageal dilation is present in approximately 80% of patients with diffuse interstitial fibrosis. Dilation of the main pulmonary artery in conjunction with either diffuse interstitial fibrosis or esophageal dilation is suggestive of SSc or mixed connective tissue disease. Typically, the degree of pulmonary artery dilation is out of proportion to the degree of pulmonary fibrosis in SSc.

Differential Diagnosis

Features of SSc may be present in patients with an overlap syndrome such as mixed connective tissue disease (MCTD) in whom different aspects of SLE, Sjögren's syndrome, and PM/DM are also present. In those patients, cutaneous involvement may be accompanied by alopecia, photosensitivity, an inflammatory myopathy, arthralgias, and myalgias. Anti-U1RNP antibodies are commonly present in high titers. However, anti-U1RNP antibodies are not characteristic of MCTD as they occur in approximately 30% of patients with SLE.

Complications

Aspiration, due to hypopharyngeal or esophageal dysfunction, is a significant problem in a large number of patients with SSc and should be assessed in all patients. Medication-related side effects should also be considered in patients receiving cyclophosphamide or D-penicillamine as diffuse alveolar damage and constrictive bronchiolitis have been reported as complications of therapy.

Treatment

Given the variable course of disease in SSc, therapy is dependent upon demonstration of progressive disease, whether it be diffuse interstitial fibrosis or pulmonary hypertension. Retrospective and uncontrolled trials suggest that immunosuppressive regimens using oral cyclophosphamide and low-dose prednisone result in significant lung function improvement that is durable for 12 months. The use of D-penicillamine in early SSc demonstrated an improvement in skin thickness, gas exchange abnormalities as measured by diffusing capacity of the lung for CO (DL_{co}), improved 5-year survival, and a decreased rate of new visceral involvement compared with untreated controls. Supplemental oxygen therapy, diuretic therapy for right heart failure, and anticoagulation are the mainstay of therapy for mild to moderate pulmonary hypertension. In patients who develop moderate to severe pulmonary hypertension, continuous infusion of epoprostenol or oral bosentan may be used as both have been demonstrated to improved exercise capacity and decrease dyspnea. Lung or heart–lung transplantation is a therapeutic option for those with severe, advanced disease.

Prognosis

The course of disease in SSc is variable and relapses may occur. The prognosis for the diffuse form of the disease, a 10-year survival of 40–60%, is significantly worse than that of the limited form or CREST, which has a 70% 10-year survival rate.

Prognosis is linked to the extent of visceral involvement in SSc. The 5-year survival in patients who develop SSc-associated lung involvement is approximately 40%.

Co HT, Block JA, Sequeira W: Scleroderma lung: pathogenesis, evaluation, and current therapy. Am J Ther 2000;7(5):321. [PMID: 11317180]. (Review of pathogenesis and treatment.)

Rubin LJ et al: Bosentan therapy for pulmonary arterial hypertension. N Engl J Med 2002;346(12):896. [PMID: 110-7289]. (Results for the first effective oral therapy for pulmonary hypertension. The study includes patients with scleroderma.)

White B: Evaluation and management of pulmonary fibrosis in scleroderma. Curr Rheumatol Rep 2002;4(2):108. [PMID 11890875]. (Another perspective on diagnosis and treatment options.)

White B et al: Cyclophosphamide is associated with pulmonary function and survival benefit in patients with scleroderma and alveolitis. Ann Intern Med 2000;132(12):947. [PMID: 10858177]. (Cellularity on biopsy is characteristic of those who respond well to treatment.)

POLYMYOSITIS/DERMATOMYOSITIS

 ESSENTIALS OF DIAGNOSIS

- Symmetric, proximal muscle weakness.
- Characteristic muscle biopsy with nonsuppurative inflammation.
- Elevation of serum muscle enzymes (creatine phosphokinase, aldolase).
- Characteristic electromyelogram (EMG) abnormalities.
- Heliotropic rash or erythematous dermatitis on the dorsum of the hands, face, knees, elbows, or neck is necessary for the diagnosis of dermatomyositis.

General Considerations

Polymyositis/dermatomyositis (PM/DM) is an inflammatory myopathy of unknown etiology. The disease may be idiopathic, associated with other connective tissue diseases, or concomitant with an underlying neoplasia. The annual incidence is estimated at approximately 0.5 to 8 cases per million, several thousandfold less common that RA. In contrast to most other connective tissue diseases, PM/DM has a bimodal age distribution with peaks in childhood (ages 10–15 years) and adulthood (ages 45–60 years). Women are affected twice as frequently as men, with the highest incidence in African-American females.

Polymyositis and dermatomyositis are distinguished by the presence of a prominent skin rash often antedating muscle disease by a year or more. Malignancy-associated PM/DM has been reported in patients with lung, colon, breast, prostate, and uterine carcinomas. A diagnosis of PM/DM may antedate, occur simultaneously, or follow the diagnosis of an associated malignancy. Pulmonary manifestations are given in Table 11–5.

Pathogenesis

Aberrant cell-mediated immunity is thought to be an important mechanism underlying the inflammatory myopathy and dermatitis associated with PM/DM. Viral infections have been implicated as potential triggering events, especially in light of seasonal variability in the incidence of PM/DM. Genetic factors may also have an important role as individuals with HLA-DR subtypes are at increased risk for developing inflammatory myopathies.

Clinical Findings

A. Symptoms and Signs

Insidious onset proximal muscle weakness in the upper or lower extremities is commonly the initial manifestation of PM/DM. Overt myalgias may or may not be present. Progressive weakness typically occurs over a period of 3–6 months. However, an acute fulminant course has been documented, especially in those who present with alveolar hemorrhage secondary to pulmonary capillaritis or diffuse alveolar damage. Fever, in the absence of infection, may accompany other systemic symptoms. In DM, a characteristic rash may antedate, coincide, or follow weakness. The rash varies, manifesting as a pink or violaceous, macular or papular,

Table 11–5. Pulmonary manifestations in polymyositis/dermatomyositis.

Aspiration pneumonia
Respiratory muscle dysfunction
   Ventilatory failure
   Hypostatic pneumonia
   Restrictive lung disease
   Diaphragmatic dysfunction
   Atelectasis
Interstitial lung disease
   Interstitial pulmonary fibrosis
   Aspiration pneumonitis
   Bronchiolitis obliterans organizing pneumonia
   Diffuse alveolar hemorrhage
   Pulmonary alveolar proteinosis
Pulmonary vascular disease
   Pulmonary artery hypertension
   Necrotizing pulmonary capillaritis
Malignancy
Drug-induced lung disease
Infections

symmetric, nonpruritic rash on the dorsal aspect of the interphalangeal joints, elbows, patellae, or medial malleoli. The rash may also present with heliotropic discoloration of the eyelids, posterior shoulders, anterior neck, face, or forehead. The muscle disease is typically a less prominent feature in DM than in PM. Raynaud's phenomenon occurs in up to 20% of patients. Involvement of the striated skeletal muscles of the hypopharynx and esophagus produces dysphonia and dysphagia. This predisposes patients to aspiration, which is the most common form of pulmonary disease associated with PM/DM. Respiratory muscle involvement may be subtle, but often parallels the course seen with the peripheral musculature. Hypostatic pneumonia in dependent regions of the lung with pulmonary edema may occur. Progressive ventilatory failure with hypercarbia is rare. This involves diaphragmatic weakness leading to hypoventilation and occasionally requiring ventilatory support.

PM/DM-associated parenchymal lung disease includes diffuse interstitial fibrosis or patchy alveolar opacities. As with other collagen vascular diseases, ILD may antedate, coincide, or follow the extrapulmonary manifestations of the disease. ILD occurs in more than 30% of patients with PM/DM and appears to be associated with arthralgias and myalgias. Dyspnea, with or without cough, is accompanied by diffuse basilar crackles on examination. Pathologically, usual interstitial pneumonitis, nonspecific interstitial pneumonitis, diffuse alveolar damage, or BOOP may be present. Alveolar proteinosis has been reported to occur in PM/DM. Pleural disease, which is common in SLE, MCTD, and RA, is uncommon in PM/DM. Pulmonary vascular disease may complicate chronic fibrotic lung disease in PM/DM. Isolated pulmonary hypertension is less common but has been reported. Capillaritis, a form of vasculitis, has been reported in PM/DM. Cardiac involvement, with inflammatory myositis or fibrosis, may also present with conduction abnormalities or ventricular dysfunction.

B. Laboratory Findings

Elevations of serum muscle enzymes (creatine phosphokinase, aldolase, lactate dehydrogenase, aspartate aminotransferase), up to tenfold that of normal, occur at some point during the course of disease in PM/DM. However, in early disease or after severe chronic disease with significant muscle atrophy, muscle enzymes may be normal. This sometimes leads to confusion of this disease with IPF. In the absence of any other associated connective tissue disease, antinuclear antibodies are negative in PM/DM. Muscle-specific autoantibodies, such as anti-Jo-1, are present in up to 20% of patients. In those who develop ILD, 50–60% have positive anti-Jo-1 serologies.

C. IMAGING STUDIES

Radiographs are nonspecific in PM/DM as they are in many other connective tissue diseases and may demonstrate diffuse, basilar predominant, reticular, or nodular abnormalities. Severe, chronic disease may result in honeycomb changes at the bases. Radiographic evidence of airspace consolidation usually represents a manifestation of either BOOP or diffuse alveolar damage in the absence of infection. Ground glass abnormalities and linear opacities are the most common abnormalities seen in high-resolution CT imaging of patients with PM/DM.

Differential Diagnosis

Primary metabolic diseases such as McArdle's glycogen storage disease, hyperthyroidism, mitochondrial disorders of lipid transport, and atypical presentations of neurological disorders should be considered when evaluating patients for PM/DM. Medications such as gemfibrazole, zidovudine (AZT), and hydroxymethylglutaryl coenzyme A (HMG-CoA) reductase inhibitors as well as opportunistic infections such as toxoplasmosis, trichinellosis, cryptococcosis, cytomegalovirus, and *Mycobacterium avium intracellulare* infections should also be considered in those with signs of myositis and systemic illnesses.

Complications

Opportunistic or secondary infections commonly complicate the course of pulmonary disease secondary to PM/DM due to the significant risk of aspiration.

Treatment

Corticosteroids are the treatment of choice for most patients. The response to therapy is often dependent upon the extent of disease and type of lung involvement at the time of therapy. If treatment is initiated early, > 90% of patients will experience subjective and objective improvement in weakness and approximately 50% will achieve remission. In 40% of patients, corticosteroid therapy may result in remission or symptomatic, radiographic, and physiologic improvement. The response to therapy in lung disease is dependent upon the degree of cellularity present on biopsy. A fibrotic usual interstitial pneumonitis pattern suggests a less favorable response to corticosteroids than either the more cellular nonspecific pneumonitis or BOOP. In corticosteroid-resistant patients, the addition of azathioprine or cyclophosphamide may afford better control and disease stabilization. Other agents such as methotrexate, cyclosporine, and plasmapheresis have been used with variable success.

Cancer screening should be considered, especially in males over age 40 with dermatomyositis. In up to one-third of patients, myositis will coincide with an underlying malignancy.

Prognosis

ILD, dysphagia, concomitant Raynaud's phenomenon, cardiac involvement, the presence of aspiration, and older age are poor prognostic factors.

Akira M, Hara H, Sakatani M: Interstitial lung disease in association with polymyositis-dermatomyositis: long-term follow-up CT evaluation in seven patients. Radiology 1999;210(2):333. [PMID: 10207411]. (Sequential patterns are shown radiographically.)

Douglas WW et al: Polymyositis-dermatomyositis-associated interstitial lung disease. Am J Respir Crit Care Med 2001;164(7):1182. [PMID: 11673206]. (The relatively good prognosis of the ILD is discussed.)

Grau JM et al: Interstitial lung disease related to dermatomyositis. Comparative study with patients without lung involvement. J Rheumatol 1996;23(11):1921. [PMID: 8923367]. (ILD does not worsen overall disease prognosis in dermatomyositis.)

Hirakata M, Nagai S: Interstitial lung disease in polymyositis and dermatomyositis. Curr Opin Rheumatol 2000;12(6):501. [PMID: 11092199]. (Good overall review.)

Marie I et al: Pulmonary involvement in polymyositis and in dermatomyositis. J Rheumatol 1998;25(7):1336. [PMID: 9676766]. (Pulmonary physiology and lab studies are reviewed.)

Schwarz MI: The lung in polymyositis. Clin Chest Med 1998;19 (4):701. [PMID: 9917961]. (Comprehensive review.)

MISCELLANEOUS CONNECTIVE TISSUE DISEASES

Mixed Connective Tissue Disease

Patients with mixed connective tissue disease (MCTD) present with features from various different connective tissue diseases such as SLE, SSc, polymyositis, and Sjögren's syndrome. MCTD presents with a constellation of symptoms including an inflammatory myopathy, cutaneous disease with Raynaud's syndrome, alopecia, sclerodactyly, or photosensitivity, and moderate to severe deforming arthritis of the proximal interphalangeal, distal interphalangeal, and metacarpophalangeal joints. Pulmonary manifestations include pleural disease with pleurisy with or without effusions, marked pulmonary hypertension, chronic aspiration for the approximately 80% of patients who develop esophageal dysmotility, and ILD marked by diffuse interstitial fibrosis with BOOP or nonspecific interstitial pneumonitis. Pulmonary vasculitis and diffuse alveolar hemorrhage have been reported.

Therapy in MCTD is focused on preventing aspiration in those with esophageal dysfunction, immunosuppressive regimens for the cellular pneumonias such as BOOP and nonspecific interstitial pneumonia (NSIP), and aggressive therapy for pulmonary hypertension, which may be pronounced.

Kozuka T et al: Pulmonary involvement in mixed connective tissue disease: high-resolution CT findings in 41 patients. J Thorac Imaging 2001;16(2):94. [PMID: 11292211]. (The frequent CT findings are discussed for an unselected sample of 41 patients.)

Saito Y et al: Pulmonary involvement in mixed connective tissue disease: comparison with other collagen vascular diseases using high resolution CT. J Comput Assist Tomogr 2002;26(3):349. [PMID: 12016361]. (There is less ground glass pattern in the lungs of patients with MCTD compared to other connective tissue diseases.)

Schwarz MI et al: Isolated pulmonary capillaritis and diffuse alveolar hemorrhage in rheumatoid arthritis and mixed connective tissue disease. Chest 1998;113(6):1609. [PMID: 9631801]. (Unusual cause of capillaritis.)

Sjögren's Syndrome

Sjögren's syndrome is an autoimmune disease with lymphocytic infiltration of glandular organs producing a complex of keratoconjuctivitis, xerostomia, and an underlying connective tissue disease such as SLE, RA, MCTD, or PM/DM. Primary Sjögren's syndrome occurs in the absence of an underlying connective tissue disease, which accounts for approximately 40% of cases.

Pulmonary involvement in Sjögren's syndrome primarily manifests in the form of ILD and small airway disease. Lymphocytic infiltration, similar to that within exocrine glands, may occur in the form of lymphocytic interstitial pneumonia (LIP). Treatment consists of immunosuppression and serial monitoring, especially in those with LIP, as the potential exists for malignant conversion of LIP to lymphoma.

Deheinzelin D et al: Interstitial lung disease in primary Sjögren's syndrome. Clinical-pathological evaluation and response to treatment. Am J Respir Crit Care Med 1996;154(3, Pt 1): 794. [PMID: 8810621]. (The frequent finding of ILD and treatment responses are discussed.)

O'Donnell PG, Tung KT: Lymphomas in the lung associated with Sjögren's syndrome. AJR Am J Roentgenol 1998;171(3):895. [PMID: 9725353]. Relationship of Sjögren's with pneumonia is discussed.)

Sarcoidosis

Yasmine S. Wasfi, MD, & Andrew P. Fontenot, MD

ESSENTIALS OF DIAGNOSIS

- Sarcoidosis is a systemic granulomatous disorder of unknown etiology, primarily affecting the lung.
- Diagnostic criteria:
- Compatible clinical and radiographic presentation (see specifics below).
- Histopathological demonstration of noncaseating granulomatous inflammation.
- Exclusion of other diseases capable of producing a similar clinical/radiographic/histopathological picture.

General Considerations

In 1899, Boeck used the term "multiple benign sarkoid of the skin" to describe a disorder characterized by multiple raised skin lesions. Subsequently, similar pathological findings were seen in other organ systems, including the lung and lymph nodes, and the term "sarcoidosis" was derived from these descriptions. Sarcoidosis occurs worldwide, affecting individuals of all races, all ages, and both sexes, although with a slight female predominance. Most patients are diagnosed between the ages of 20 and 40 years, with a peak incidence in the 20–29 year age group. Estimates of disease prevalence in the United States range from <1 to 40 per 100,000 with certain ethnic and racial groups having an increased incidence of disease. For example, age-adjusted incidence rates in the United States are 35.5 per 100,000 for African-Americans and 10.9 per 100,000 for whites. African-Americans also tend to present with more severe disease.

Newman LS, Rose CS, Maier LA: Sarcoidosis. N Engl J Med 1997;336:1224. [PMID: 9110911]. (Good general review of clinical manifestations, diagnosis, and treatment of sarcoidosis.)

Pathogenesis

Although the cause(s) of sarcoidosis is unknown, evidence suggests that the immune response occurs follow-ing a specific environmental exposure in genetically susceptible individuals. Whether an infectious or noninfectious environmental agent is responsible for initiation of the inflammatory response remains unknown. Several epidemiological studies of disease clusters support the existence of shared environmental exposures. These include a case–control study of a sarcoidosis cluster on the Isle of Man, which revealed that a significantly greater percentage of cases as compared to control subjects had previous contact with a sarcoidosis patient. In addition, clusters of disease have been found among nurses, firefighters, and individuals exposed to pine pollen.

Large numbers of activated macrophages and T-lymphocytes accumulate at sites of ongoing inflammation. The T cells express a CD4$^+$ phenotype and secrete Th1-type cytokines such as interleukin-2 and interferon-γ. CD4$^+$ T cell alveolitis likely represents the earliest event in generation of the noncaseating granuloma. The CD4$^+$ T cells result from oligoclonal expansion, suggesting development of a conventional antigen-stimulated immune response.

The variation in incidence, severity, and manifestations of disease among different racial and ethnic groups suggests a genetic predisposition to disease development. Another observation that supports genetic susceptibility is familial clustering of disease. For example, sarcoidosis occurs two to four times more frequently in monozygotic than in dizygotic twins. Similarly, up to 19% of affected African-American families and 5% of white families have more than one affected family member. Results from a case–control etiological study of sarcoidosis (ACCESS) further support these observations. This study enrolled over 700 case–control pairs in the United States matched for age, gender, race, and ethnicity. Analysis of nearly 11,000 first-degree and over 17,000 second-degree relatives of these groups demonstrated an overall adjusted familial relative risk of developing sarcoidosis of 4.7 (95% CI = 2.3–9.7). In this study whites had a much higher familial relative risk compared to African-Americans (18.0 versus 2.8; $p = 0.098$). It is likely given these observations that multiple genes, rather than a single gene, are involved in the genetic predisposition to sarcoidosis.

Studies of polymorphisms in the HLA family of genes have yielded inconsistent results. Associations between specific HLA-DR, -DQ, and -DP alleles and the presence of sarcoidosis or specific characteristics of the disease have been identified, and the associated alleles have differed based on race and ethnicity. In contrast, the ACCESS study results demonstrate a significant association between sarcoidosis and HLA-DRB1*1101 across the entire patient cohort, including African-Americans and whites. Despite these and other associations of genetic polymorphisms with disease, the exact nature of the genetic predisposition to sarcoidosis remains unclear.

Rossman M et al: Association with human leukocyte antigen class II amino acid epitopes and interaction with environmental exposures. Chest 2002;121:1S4. [PMID: 11893656]. (Review of data that supports the theory that sarcoidosis results from environmental exposures in genetically susceptible populations.)

Rybicki BA et al: Familial aggregation of sarcoidosis. A case–control etiologic study of sarcoidosis (ACCESS). Am J Respir Crit Care Med 2001;164:2085. [PMID: 11739139]. (Epidemiological study that identifies increased risk of sarcoidosis in close relatives of sarcoidosis patients.)

Vourlekis JS, Sawyer RT, Newman LS: Sarcoidosis: developments in etiology, immunology, and therapeutics. Adv Intern Med 2000;45:209. [PMID: 10635050]. (General review of the pathogenesis and therapy of sarcoidosis.)

Clinical Findings

The clinical presentation of sarcoidosis varies widely based on the organs involved and the extent of their involvement. Some patients are asymptomatic at presentation and are brought to medical attention due to abnormalities identified on a screening chest radiograph. Others present with nonspecific constitutional symptoms such as fatigue, malaise, weight loss, and fever. Most commonly, individuals present with symptoms referable to the involved organ(s). These are discussed below.

A. Lungs

The majority of patients with sarcoidosis (>90%) present with pulmonary involvement. Common symptoms include dyspnea on exertion, a dry nonproductive cough, and vague chest discomfort. Physical examination may reveal crackles and/or wheezing, but may also be normal. The most common abnormalities seen on pulmonary function tests are reductions in the diffusing capacity for carbon monoxide (DL_{CO}), lung volumes, and vital capacity. Obstructive defects may also be seen and are thought to result from endobronchial involvement or airway distortion due to parenchymal disease. Endobronchial involvement may result in significant airway stenosis. The resulting obstructive defects show little or no reversibility after the inhalation of bron-

chodilators. The physiological abnormalities seen in sarcoidosis may not correlate with the severity of changes present on chest radiographs.

The chest radiograph is abnormal in >90% of sarcoidosis patients. Table 12–1 describes a staging classification based on radiographic abnormalities. Normal chest radiographs occur in 5–10% of patients at presentation. Stage I radiographs are seen in 40–50% of cases and 20–30% of subjects present with stage II radiographic changes. Ten to 20% of subjects present with stage III radiographic abnormalities. Despite increased sensitivity of chest computed tomography (CT) compared to plain chest radiography, CT is usually not indicated unless there is an atypical clinical or radiographic presentation or suspicion of a pulmonary complication. However, chest CT when performed confirms the radiographic abnormalities, typically demonstrating reticulonodular infiltrates that follow a bronchovascular distribution, thickened interlobular septae, and hilar and/or mediastinal lymphadenopathy.

B. Lymphatic System

Lymphadenopathy is a common feature of sarcoidosis and is most often observed in hilar lymph nodes (up to 90% of patients). Five to 30% of patients have peripheral lymphadenopathy, most commonly in cervical, axillary, epitrochlear, and inguinal nodes. These nodes are typically nontender and mobile and may cause some deformity, but rarely have clinically important sequelae. Lymph node biopsy can be used to make the diagnosis of sarcoidosis with two important caveats. First, if granulomatous inflammation is seen in one section the entire lymph node must be examined as lymphoma or carcinoma can also cause a granulomatous reaction. Second, extrathoracic lymph node biopsy demonstrating noncaseating granulomatous inflammation (without evidence of infection or malignancy) is not sufficient to make a diagnosis of sarcoidosis in the absence of other organ involvement. Such isolated granuloma-

Table 12–1. Radiographic stages of sarcoidosis.

Stage	Radiographic Abnormalities
0	None
I	Bilateral hilar and/or mediastinal adenopathy without pulmonary parenchymal abnormalities
II	Hilar and/or mediastinal adenopathy with pulmonary parenchymal abnormalities (generally a diffuse interstitial pattern)
III	Diffuse pulmonary parenchymal disease without nodal enlargement
IV	Pulmonary fibrosis with evidence of honeycomb change (end-stage lung disease)

tous inflammation of nonthoracic lymph nodes or the liver is designated as "granulomatous lesions of unknown significance (GLUS)."

C. HEART

Prevalence estimates for cardiac sarcoidosis range from <1% to as high as 58% depending on the population screened and case definitions. The range of clinical manifestations is equally broad. Sudden death due to ventricular arrhythmias or complete heart block is a common presentation of cardiac sarcoidosis. It may be the first sign of cardiovascular involvement. Other manifestations of cardiac sarcoidosis include supraventricular tachycardias, ventricular aneurysms, other conduction defects (first- or second-degree atrioventricular block, intraventricular conduction delay), and cardiomyopathy/congestive heart failure. Myocarditis and pericardial involvement occur rarely.

D. SKIN

Approximately 25% of patients with sarcoidosis have skin involvement. The classic skin lesions are erythema nodosum and lupus pernio. Erythema nodosum is a vasculitic lesion that presents as raised, tender, erythematous nodules, 1–2 cm in diameter. Lesions typically occur on anterior surfaces of the lower legs and may be accompanied by knee and ankle arthralgias or arthritis. The combination of erythema nodosum, arthralgias, fever, and bilateral hilar adenopathy is known as Löfgren's syndrome. Both erythema nodosum and Löfgren's syndrome resolve spontaneously and usually do not recur. Lupus pernio is usually associated with chronic sarcoidosis. The skin lesions of lupus pernio appear as purplish plaques found over the nose, cheeks, lips, and ears. Lupus pernio is rare, occurring more commonly in African-American women. It typically is associated with lung fibrosis, upper respiratory tract disease, bone cysts, and/or lacrimal gland involvement.

Although erythema nodosum and lupus pernio are the most characteristic skin changes seen in sarcoidosis, other dermatological abnormalities occur. These include macular and papular red-brown to orange lesions, nodules, keloids, and areas of hyper- or hypopigmentation. These less characteristic lesions are usually presumed to be due to sarcoidosis when they occur in patients with a prior biopsy-proven diagnosis of the disease. Skin biopsy demonstrating noncaseating granulomas provides definitive evidence of skin involvement.

E. OCULAR

Estimates of the prevalence of ocular involvement range from 15 to 54%. The most common manifestation of ocular sarcoidosis is uveitis. Anterior uveitis is more common in African-American patients. It may present acutely with pain, photophobia, lacrimation, and redness or with a more chronic course. Posterior uveitis is more common in whites, gradual in onset, and likely to result in visual impairment. The second most common ocular manifestation is conjunctival nodules. These are usually asymptomatic unless extensive, in which case diplopia or keratoconjunctivitis sicca may occur. Lacrimal gland enlargement is another characteristic finding but is rare. Disease of the posterior segment of the eye may also occur. It is associated with a higher prevalence of central nervous system involvement. Examples of posterior segment disease include posterior uveitis, vitreous hemorrhage, cataracts, glaucoma, cystoid macular edema, and retinal ischemia with neovascularization. The most severe visual morbidity from ocular sarcoidosis is usually due to vitreous hemorrhage, retinal ischemia, and rare cases of retinal detachment. Evaluation for ocular involvement includes routine ophthalmological evaluation including slit-lamp examination. Fluorescein angiography is also useful, particularly for detection of microvascular involvement. Finally, conjunctival biopsy is useful in diagnosing sarcoidosis, even in the absence of ocular symptoms or other evidence of ocular disease.

F. NERVOUS SYSTEM

Neurosarcoidosis occurs in both the central and peripheral nervous systems. Clinically apparent nervous system involvement occurs in less than 10% of patients. The most easily recognizable manifestations are cranial nerve abnormalities. Unilateral seventh nerve palsies are most common. Space-occupying brain lesions may occur. These commonly present with symptoms of hypothalamic or pituitary disease, such as diabetes insipidus and high prolactin secretion. Leptomeningeal involvement and peripheral neuropathy have also been observed. Magnetic resonance imaging (MRI) is helpful in the evaluation of neurosarcoidosis through demonstration of brain lesions and/or a typical pattern that occurs with leptomeningeal involvement. Evaluation of cerebrospinal fluid may also support the diagnosis. Typical findings include lymphocytic pleocytosis and elevated protein levels. Electrodiagnostic studies and biopsy can sometimes be useful in the diagnosis of peripheral neuropathy.

G. PAROTID GLANDS

Parotid enlargement is a rare feature of sarcoidosis. Unilateral or bilateral parotitis occurs in less than 5% of patients. Parotid enlargement in the context of fever, facial palsy, and anterior uveitis is known as Heerfordt's syndrome or uveoparotid fever.

H. ENDOCRINE AND RENAL

Disordered calcium metabolism is the most common endocrine abnormality in sarcoidosis. Increased production of 1,25-dihydroxyvitamin D by activated macrophages in sarcoid granuloma leads to hypercalcemia and hypercalciuria. Hypercalcemia occurs in 2–10% of patients with sarcoidosis. Persistent hypercalcemia and hypercalciuria may result in nephrolithiasis, nephrocalcinosis and rarely renal failure. Other renal manifestations are rare, but include interstitial nephritis and mass lesions. The latter are usually granulomas. Hypothalamic or pituitary involvement may result in diabetes insipidus or the syndrome of inappropriate antidiuretic hormone (SIADH).

I. Liver

Liver involvement by sarcoidosis has been demonstrated in 50–80% of patients who have undergone liver biopsy. Many of these patients, however, do not demonstrate clinical evidence of liver disease. Clinically apparent liver disease most commonly manifests as palpable hepatomegaly and cholestatic liver function abnormalities. Radiographic abnormalities include multiple low-density lesions on CT or MRI.

J. Musculoskeletal System

Muscles, bones, and joints may be involved by sarcoidosis. Joint symptoms are most common, with pain reported in 25–39% of patients with sarcoidosis. Deforming arthritis is rare. When it occurs, the knees, ankles, and small joints of the hands and feet are most commonly affected. Bony involvement is also rare, observed in about 5% of patients. Typical bone lesions consist of cysts that are most easily seen in the phalanges. Bone cysts commonly occur in association with chronic disease and cutaneous involvement. Muscle involvement is also a rare complication of sarcoidosis and includes muscle nodules, acute myositis, and chronic myopathy. Symptoms of muscle weakness should be carefully distinguished from steroid-induced myopathy.

K. Hematological

Anemia, leukopenia, and thrombocytopenia have all been observed in sarcoidosis. Leukopenia, and specifically lymphopenia, occurs in one-third of patients. It is sometimes due to granulomatous inflammation in the bone marrow but more commonly results from redistribution of lymphocytes from peripheral blood to areas of active inflammation. Prevalence estimates of anemia are approximately 20%. Half of these cases are due to granulomas in the bone marrow, whereas the remainder result from nonspecific bone marrow suppression from chronic disease. Thrombocytopenia is rarely seen. Splenomegaly in sarcoidosis usually is not clinically relevant; however, it contributes to decreased cell counts

in some patients, particularly white blood cells and platelets.

L. Other

The sections above summarize the most common abnormalities seen in sarcoidosis, although virtually any organ system can be affected. Other sites of documented disease include the upper respiratory tract, gastrointestinal tract, and reproductive organs.

Judson MA et al: Defining organ involvement in sarcoidosis: the ACCESS proposed instrument. ACCESS Research Group. A Case Control Etiologic Study of Sarcoidosis. Sarcoidosis Vasc Diffuse Lung Dis 1999;16:75. [PMID: 10207945]. (Discussion of a proposed longitudinal mechanism to monitor the spectrum of organ involvement in patients with established, biopsy-proven diagnosis of sarcoidosis.)

Statement on sarcoidosis: Joint Statement of the American Thoracic Society (ATS), the European Respiratory Society (ERS) and the World Association of Sarcoidosis and Other Granulomatous Disorders (WASOG). Am J Respir Crit Care Med 1999;160:736. [PMID: 10430755]. (Comprehensive review of clinical presentation, diagnosis, and treatment of sarcoidosis.)

Diagnosis

The diagnosis of sarcoidosis requires a compatible clinical presentation and evidence of granulomatous inflammation in an involved organ. In the appropriate clinical setting, bilateral hilar adenopathy in asymptomatic patients may be adequate to establish a presumptive diagnosis of sarcoidosis. The major differential diagnosis in such patients is lymphoma. Most patients with lymphoma, however, have constitutional symptoms. Nonetheless, we recommend confirming the diagnosis by biopsy to exclude infection or malignancy.

The diagnosis of sarcoidosis is most commonly made by fiberoptic bronchoscopy with transbronchial biopsy. The yield of this approach is 40–90%, varying with operator experience and the number of biopsies obtained. Endobronchial biopsies can also be diagnostic but have a lower yield (40–60%). Other bronchoscopic findings that are suggestive but not diagnostic of sarcoidosis are bronchoalveolar lavage (BAL) lymphocytosis and an elevated BAL $CD4^+/CD8^+$ T cell ratio. If bronchoscopic biopsies are nondiagnostic, other diagnostic approaches include biopsy of mediastinal nodes by mediastinoscopy, video-assisted thoracoscopic lung biopsy, or open lung biopsy. Mediastinoscopy is the preferred procedure if mediastinal adenopathy is present on chest CT scan. Presence of an elevated serum angiotension-converting enzyme (ACE) level, anergy, and an abnormal gallium scan are supportive but not diagnostic of sarcoidosis. Alterations in the serum ACE levels do not predict clinical course, nor do measures of BAL inflammatory activity such as $CD4^+/CD8^+$ T cell ratios. Table 12–2 highlights the recommended initial evaluation of patients with presumed sarcoidosis.

The diagnostic feature on lung histopathology is the sarcoid granuloma. This is a well-formed noncaseating epithelioid cell granuloma surrounded by a rim of lymphocytes and fibroblasts. Other characteristic features include a perilymphatic interstitial distribution of granulomas in the lung and giant cell cytoplasmic inclusions known as asteroid or Schaumann bodies.

Diagnosis of cardiac sarcoidosis can be difficult. Electrocardiograms are abnormal in as many as 50% of patients with sarcoidosis but are nonspecific. Echocardiographic abnormalities are also nonspecific. Radionuclide imaging using thallium-201, gallium-67, or technetium-99 has been used to identify abnormalities in patients with cardiac sarcoidosis. Unfortunately, the sensitivity and specificity of these techniques are not well documented. Endomyocardial biopsy is a highly specific test. The presence of noncaseating granulomas is diagnostic. Unfortunately, the sensitivity of this approach is only 25–50%.

Differential Diagnosis

The differential diagnosis of sarcoidosis depends in part on the primary organ(s) involved at initial presentation. The differential diagnosis of pulmonary sarcoidosis includes any disorder characterized by granulomatous inflammation. This includes infections by Mycobacterium tuberculosis, nontuberculous mycobacteria, and fungi. Hypersensitivity pneumonitis and some pneumoconioses are also associated with granulomatous in-

Table 12–2. Recommended initial evaluation of patients with sarcoidosis.

Baseline
  Thorough history, including environmental and occupational exposures
  Complete physical examination with emphasis on potential involved organs (eg, heart, liver, eye)
  Chest radiograph (PA and lateral)
  Pulmonary function testing with at minimum spirometry and a diffusing capacity
  Electrocardiogram
  Ophthalmological evaluation with slit-lamp examination
  Laboratory evaluation including assessment of renal function, hepatic function, serum calcium, complete blood count, and 24-h urine calcium
Follow-up
  Periodic monitoring for disease progression or new organ involvement, with referral to specialists as appropriate
  Use of most sensitive, least invasive tests for assessment of organs of interest

flammation. Of particular interest is chronic beryllium disease, which is clinically, pathologically, and radiographically identical to sarcoidosis. Other metals such as titanium and aluminum also induce granulomatous reactions. Less likely considerations include Wegener's granulomatosis and chronic interstitial pneumonias such as lymphocytic interstitial pneumonia.

Lymph node involvement by noncaseating granulomas also suggests a broad differential diagnosis. In addition to mycobacterial pathogens, brucellosis, toxoplasmosis, and cat-scratch disease also cause granulomatous lymphadenopathy. Malignancies such as Hodgkin's disease, non-Hodgkin's lymphoma, and metastatic carcinoma may also be associated with granulomatous lymphadenopathy. Each of these diseases can cause a sarcoid-like reaction and can be confused with sarcoidosis if the entire lymph node is not examined histopathologically. As mentioned previously, isolated nonthoracic lymph node granulomas without an identified etiology are insufficient evidence to establish a diagnosis of sarcoidosis.

The differential diagnosis of noncaseating granulomas in other organs is similar. Notable considerations include foreign body reactions in skin lesions, schistosomiasis, and primary biliary cirrhosis in liver disease and Crohn's disease for liver or gut lesions.

Newman LS: Metals that cause sarcoidosis. Semin Respir Infect 1998;13:212. [PMID: 9764952]. (Review of granulomatous lung disease following inhalation of various metals.)

Complications

Complications of sarcoidosis vary by organ involvement. More extensive granulomatous inflammation and eventual replacement of granulomatous inflammation with fibrosis characterize disease progression. End-stage lung disease with extensive honeycombing of the lung parenchyma may develop. In fibrocystic sarcoidosis (stage IV), colonization of the cystic spaces with fungus balls (mycetoma) can result in life-threatening hemoptysis. Fibrosis may also contribute to cardiac and neurological dysfunction as well as loss of vision. Finally, untreated hypercalcemia and/or hypercalciuria can lead to development of renal calculi and renal failure.

Prognosis

The natural history of sarcoidosis is quite variable and has been difficult to evaluate due to the common practice of early treatment with corticosteroids. However, as many as two-thirds of patients undergo spontaneous remissions. Despite this, half of all patients have at least mild long-term dysfunction of affected organs. Several clinical features predict a good prognosis with a high likelihood of spontaneous remission. Radiographic stage I disease resolves in 55–90% of cases. Individuals who present with erythema nodosum, fever, arthritis, or Löfgren's syndrome have an excellent prognosis. More than 80% of these patients undergo spontaneous remission without recurrence of disease.

Several clinical features are strongly associated with more chronic or progressive illness. Increasing radiographic stage is linked to decreasing likelihood of spontaneous remission. Forty to 70% of stage II patients remit, whereas only 10–20% of those with stage III disease spontaneously resolve. Individuals with stage IV disease have fibrosis and do not undergo spontaneous remission. More than 85% of remissions occur within 2 years of diagnosis. Failure to resolve within that time period predicts a more chronic or progressive course. Other characteristics associated with a worse prognosis include African-American race, older age at disease onset, and specific forms of nonpulmonary disease, in particular neurological involvement, cardiac involvement, chronic uveitis, lupus pernio, and chronic hypercalcemia with or without nephrocalcinosis. Overall mortality is low; only 1–5% of deaths in patients with sarcoidosis are attributed to the underlying disease. Most deaths in this subset are due to cardiac involvement, progressive respiratory failure, or neurological disease.

Treatment

There are no strict guidelines regarding indications for treatment of sarcoidosis. Most experts agree that certain extrapulmonary manifestations of disease require systemic therapy. These include cardiac sarcoidosis, neurosarcoidosis, hypercalcemia, and ocular sarcoidosis unresponsive to topical therapy. In addition, progressive pulmonary disease and other progressive extrapulmonary manifestations are usually treated with systemic therapy.

The first-line agent for all of the above forms of sarcoidosis is systemic corticosteroids. Numerous randomized and nonrandomized studies have examined the impact of systemic corticosteroids on pulmonary sarcoidosis. Although short-term relief of symptoms has been observed, most studies fail to demonstrate significant long-term benefit to steroid therapy in patients with radiographic stage II or III disease. There are numerous criticisms of these studies, including the heterogeneity of patient populations, lack of standardized therapeutic intervention and outcome evaluation, and difficulty in distinguishing between corticosteroid effect and natural course of disease. However, two recent studies support a beneficial role for steroids.

The British Thoracic Society study enrolled patients with stage II or III pulmonary sarcoidosis who did not have extrathoracic disease that required therapy. Patients were observed for 6 months. Those who did not require corticosteroid intervention during that time were then randomized to receive either long-term corticosteroid therapy or corticosteroids in response to symptom progression or functional decline. After 2 years, patients in the long-term treatment arm had slight but statistically significant improved lung function compared to the symptomatic therapy group. A more recent study evaluated whether early treatment with corticosteroids in patients with stage I and II disease was beneficial. Patients were randomized within 3 months of diagnosis to receive either corticosteroids (3 months of oral corticosteroids followed by 15 months of inhaled steroids) or placebo. This was done independent of lung function or symptoms. The majority of patients had normal lung function at the time of enrollment. Radiographic, physiological, and laboratory evaluations were performed at baseline, 18 months, and annually for 5 years. At the 5-year follow-up, several findings suggested a benefit of early therapy for patients with stage II disease. First, significantly more placebo-treated subjects had persistent radiographic changes. Second, placebo-treated subjects required more frequent corticosteroid treatment. Finally, corticosteroid-treated subjects had significantly greater improvement in forced vital capacity and DL_{CO} compared to the placebo group.

A meta-analysis of corticosteroid therapy in pulmonary sarcoidosis analyzed eight randomized controlled trials with data suitable for analysis. The combined results demonstrated that therapy of patients with stage II and III disease with oral corticosteroids for 6–24 months improved chest radiographic appearance, vital capacity, and diffusing capacity.

Although there is evidence to support benefit from corticosteroid therapy, the issues of patient selection, timing of initiation, and duration of therapy remain unresolved. There is also no consensus regarding the ideal dose. Suggestions range from 40 mg of prednisone every other day to 1 mg/kg daily. Most clinicians evaluate the response to a daily dose of 30–40 mg of prednisone for 4–12 weeks. Patients who do not improve within this time period are unlikely to respond and prednisone should be slowly tapered. Patients who do respond begin a gradual taper after 3 months to a minimum effective dose as low as 10 mg every other day by 6–12 months. It is recommended that steroid responders continue therapy for a total of 12–18 months before discontinuing steroids.

There are alternatives to therapy with corticosteroids. These are typically used in individuals who have had continued deterioration despite use of corticosteroids or who cannot tolerate corticosteroid side effects. Methotrexate is frequently the first alternative therapy used. It was initially reported to be effective in the treatment of cases of dermatological sarcoidosis. It has subsequently been used in patients with pulmonary disease as well as other organ involvement. The largest case series described outcomes in 50 patients primarily with pulmonary disease treated with methotrexate for at least 2 years. Approximately two-thirds of these patients experienced a positive clinical response. In addition, 25 of 30 patients who were on corticosteroids at the time of initiation of methotrexate were able to decrease their dose or discontinue corticosteroids altogether. It was subsequently reported that approximately two-thirds of 209 methotrexate-treated patients experienced either disease stabilization or remission.

Other agents that have been used to treat sarcoidosis include azathioprine, chloroquine/hydroxychloroquine, cyclophosphamide, chlorambucil, pentoxifylline, thalidomide, and cyclosporin. Supporting evidence for most of these agents is limited to case reports and case series, typically in patients refractory to corticosteroid therapy. The most rigorous investigation of the utility of cyclosporin enrolled 20 patients for 6 months of therapy and demonstrated no clinical improvement. Despite early encouraging case reports, cyclosporin is therefore not recommended as an alternative treatment for sarcoidosis. Chloroquine is no longer used secondary to ocular toxicity; however, hydroxychloroquine appears to be particularly effective in the treatment of hypercalcemia, hypercalciuria, and skin manifestations. Use of cyclophosphamide is usually limited by its toxicities, however, in one series it was effective in management of neurosarcoidosis in patients refractory to corticosteroids. Anti-tumor necrosis factor therapy may represent another promising alternative, however, only case reports support its use. A randomized, blinded, placebo-controlled trial of an anti-tumor necrosis factor agent is currently underway. General guidelines for instituting systemic therapy and recommended doses of

Table 12–3. Guidelines for the initiation of therapy.

Clinical Status	Recommendation
Asymptomatic pulmonary disease	Observation; may consider oral followed by inhaled steroids if recently diagnosed stage II disease
Stage II or III pulmonary disease with symptoms and/or abnormal function	Systemic therapy
Severe extrapulmonary disease, including heart, central nervous system, eyes, kidneys	Systemic therapy

the agents discussed above are provided in Tables 12–3 and 12–4.

Transplantation is an option for patients who fail medical therapy. Successful lung, heart–lung, heart, liver, and kidney transplants have been performed in patients with sarcoidosis. Available data suggest that survival for lung and liver transplants is similar in sarcoid and nonsarcoid patients. This is true in lung transplants despite the frequent recurrence of granulomas in lung allografts (reported at 17–67%). In general, disease recurrence does not appear to impact significantly on patient or graft survival.

Baughman RP: Methotrexate for sarcoidosis. Sarcoidosis Vasc Diffuse Lung Dis 1998;15:147. [PMID: 9789892]. (General review of treatment of sarcoidosis with methotrexate.)

Baughman RP, Sharma OP, Lynch JP 3rd: Sarcoidosis: is therapy effective? Semin Respir Infect 1998;13:255. [PMID: 9764955]. (Review of appropriate use and monitoring of various drugs used to treat sarcoidosis, including their toxicities.)

Table 12–4. Therapeutic options for sarcoidosis.

Agent	Dose	Side Effects
Prednisone	30–60 mg/day	Weight gain, hypertension, glucose intolerance, depression, osteoporosis
Methotrexate	7.5–25 mg/week	Liver toxicity, pulmonary toxicity, stomatitis, bone marrow suppression
Azathioprine	100–200 mg/day	Nausea, anorexia, pancreatitis, bone marrow suppression
Hydroxychloroquine	200–400 mg/day	Nausea, headache, skin hyperpigmentation, ocular toxicity
Cyclophosphamide	Oral: 75–150 mg/day; intravenous pulse: 0.5–0.75 g/m^2/month	Bone marrow suppression, nausea, hemorrhagic cystitis, oncogenesis, ovarian failure/impaired spermatogenesis
Chlorambucil	2–8 mg/day	Bone marrow suppression, oncogenesis, azospermia/anovulation, oral ulcers, rashes, gastrointestinal toxicity
Pentoxifylline	25 mg/kg/day	Nausea, headache, dizziness
Thalidomide	100–200 mg/day	Muscle weakness; extremity pain, numbness, tingling, burning; rash

Gibson GJ et al: British Thoracic Society Sarcoidosis study: effects of long term corticosteroid treatment. Thorax 1996;51:238. [PMID: 8779124]. (Five-year longitudinal study evaluating long-term corticosteroid therapy for asymptomatic patients with sarcoidosis and persistent radiographic abnormalities.)

Lower EE, Baughman RP: Prolonged use of methotrexate for sarcoidosis. Arch Intern Med 1995;155:846. [PMID: 7717793]. (Review of safety and efficacy of methotrexate in 50 patients treated for at least 2 years for sarcoidosis.)

Paramothayan S, Jones PW: Corticosteroid therapy in pulmonary sarcoidosis: a systematic review. JAMA 2002;287:1301. [PMID: 11886322]. (Comprehensive review of efficacy of corticosteroids in pulmonary sarcoidosis.)

Pietinalho A et al: Early treatment of stage II sarcoidosis improves 5-year pulmonary function. Chest 2002;121:24. [PMID: 11796428]. (Five-year longitudinal study of efficacy of early corticosteroid therapy for stage I and II sarcoidosis.)

Sulica R, Teirstein A, Padilla ML: Lung transplantation in interstitial lung disease. Curr Opin Pulmon Med 2001;7:314. [PMID: 11584182]. (General review of lung transplantation in the management of various types of interstitial lung disease.)

Relevant Web Site

http://www.nlm.nih.gov/medlineplus/druginformation.html

Pulmonary Alveolar Proteinosis

13

James H. Ellis, Jr., MD

 ESSENTIALS OF DIAGNOSIS

- Symptoms are nonspecific and include dyspnea, cough, fatigue, and malaise.
- Chest radiograph demonstrates diffuse alveolar infiltrates.
- Computed tomography of the chest demonstrates an alveolar filling process with a characteristic "crazy paving" pattern.
- Diagnosis confirmed by detection of periodic acid–Schiff-positive material in bronchoalveolar lavage or lung biopsy.

General Considerations

Pulmonary alveolar proteinosis (PAP) was identified in 1958, based on experience with 27 patients in whom the major histological finding was filling of alveolar spaces by a lipid-rich, insoluble, periodic acid–Schiff-positive lipoproteinaceous material. The first case dated to 1953; the pathology was sufficiently distinctive that it was unlikely to have escaped previous notice. Subsequent studies of the abnormal alveolar contents revealed that the major biochemical components of this substance were phospholipids with small amounts of protein. Prakash suggested that the term "pulmonary alveolar phospholipoproteinosis" more appropriately characterized the disorder. However, this term is rarely used today.

The amorphous, insoluble, proteinaceous material is deposited in alveoli and can exude into bronchioles. This material is unique in that it does not appear to stimulate an inflammatory response, although fibrosis is noted in some biopsies, particularly in late stages of disease.

PAP is an uncommon, idiopathic disease. It is difficult to determine its exact frequency because of the absence of a national registry. The disease has been reported throughout the United States and in virtually all industrialized countries. In 1969, only 139 cases of PAP had been reported worldwide; by 1980, approximately 260 cases were recognized. Even now fewer that 500 cases have been reported. The ratio of male to female patients in most series is about 4 to 1, with most being 30 to 50 years of age. Many of the patients in published reports had been exposed to various dusts and chemicals such as silica and aluminum dust, but existence of the disease in unexposed siblings also suggests a genetic predisposition. Superimposed infections by unusual pathogens may occur. Infection by *Nocardia asteroides* is most commonly reported, followed by fungal and atypical mycobacterial infections. Amiodarone lung toxicity in humans has some features of a lung phospholipidosis. Experimental animals exposed to a variety of chemicals demonstrate pathological features identical to those in human PAP, and reports describe morphological findings identical to those in PAP following exposure to silica, fiberglass, volcanic ash, and aluminum dust. PAP is also associated with malignant diseases, especially acute or chronic myeloid leukemias. These forms are termed secondary PAP. Initial reports were in patients with chronic myeloid leukemias, but the disease also occurs in acute leukemia, multiple myeloma, Waldenstrom's disease, and lymphoma. Primary and secondary PAP are indistinguishable from a morphological perspective as they share the same microscopic and ultrastructural pattern. However, their clinical response to lavage therapy is different. Secondary PAP is a rare cause of respiratory failure in patients with cancer and probably results from concomitant events, including exposure to pulmonary irritants as well as functional defects of alveolar macrophages. Recent data suggest that granulocyte–macrophage colony-stimulating factor (GM-CSF) may be important in the pathogenesis of PAP, and that alveolar macrophages are likely key factors contributing to the development of secondary PAP.

Prakash U et al: Pulmonary alveolar phospholipoproteinosis: experience with 34 cases and a review. Mayo Clin Proc 1987; 62:499. [PMID: 3553760]. (Review of 34 cases, describing clinical presentation and efficacy of lung lavage.)

Rosen SH, Castleman B, Liebow AA: Pulmonary alveolar proteinosis. N Engl J Med 1958;258:1123. (Original case series describing PAP.)

Pathology

The lungs of patients with PAP are heavy, containing insoluble yellow material that exudes from cut lung surfaces. This material is muddy in texture and beige in color. Blood-tinged discoloration may be seen in very active cases. It resists degradation by trypsin, acetylcysteine, and heparin. The material affects the lungs in patches, taking on an acinar distribution in appearance. Honeycombing is absent and the pleural surfaces appear regular and smooth. Periodic acid–Schiff (PAS)-positive, amorphous, granular material, rich in lipids, is deposited in the alveolar spaces, rising up into the bronchioles in severe cases. The alveolar lining cells are cuboidal and contain PAS-positive cytoplasm. Some lung sections show an increase in type II alveolar pneumocytes. This cell's principal functions are synthesis, storage, and secretion of surfactant. Large macrophages are commonly found as single cells in the midst of the insoluble alveolar material. The macrophages appear to incorporate the alveolar material, but are unable to digest it, subsequently becoming large and relatively immobile. They eventually die and become "ghost cells." Less typically, thickened septa and interstitial fibrosis may be present, although this is probably due to repeated or chronic infection as opposed to the underlying PAP.

Pathogenesis

PAP is a disorder of surfactant homeostasis. In most respects, the material in the alveoli is qualitatively similar to normal surfactant except for an increase in serum proteins and specific immunoglobulins. Surfactant, a complex mixture of phospholipids, neutral lipids, and proteins, is responsible for the variable and low surface tension within lungs. Following secretion as lamellar bodies from type II pneumocytes, surfactant passes through a series of aggregate forms of various sizes during its cycle within the alveolus. Surfactant components are in a dynamic cycle of secretion and reuptake by type II secretory cells. Precise concentrations of surfactant proteins and lipids are maintained in the alveolar space by a careful balance among synthesis, recycling, and catabolism. PAP is associated with accumulation of surfactant lipids and proteins in alveolar spaces. Critical factors that may contribute to its pathogenesis include a synthesis stimulus, increased replication of type II pneumocytes, increased surfactant production, and impaired removal of surfactant and dying cells.

GM-CSF activates alveolar macrophages and increases their rate of surfactant clearance. GM-CSF deficiency or dysfunction has been implicated in the pathogenesis of alveolar proteinosis. Disruption of production of GM-CSF or the common β-subunit of the GM-CSF receptor in mice causes alveolar proteinosis that is histologically similar to that seen in human patients. The defect in surfactant homeostasis in this model is caused by decreased surfactant clearance, mediated in part by dysfunction of alveolar macrophages.

Local production of GM-CSF corrects the alveolar proteinosis in GM-CSF-deficient mice, and transplantation of bone marrow cells expressing the common β-subunit of the GM-CSF receptor restores surfactant homeostasis.

Evidence in humans also implicates GM-CSF in the development of PAP. GM-CSF production by alveolar macrophages is decreased in some patients with PAP, despite normal GM-CSF gene expression of GM-CSF-specific mRNA. However, circulating monocytes and alveolar macrophages from PAP patients synthesize and respond to GM-CSF normally, suggesting no intrinsic abnormalities in GM-CSF signaling. In contrast, the cytokine interleukin-10 (IL-10), a potent inhibitor of macrophage GM-CSF production, is increased in the bronchoalveolar lavage (BAL) of patients with PAP. These studies suggest that in some patients PAP may result from decreased availability of GM-CSF due to GM-CSF blocking activity and reduced GM-CSF production by either GM-CSF-neutralizing antibodies or IL-10.

Tchou-Wong KM et al: GM-CSF gene expression is normal but protein release is absent in a patient with pulmonary alveolar proteinosis. Am J Respir Crit Care Med 1997;156:1999. [PMID: 9412586]. (Study of GM-CSF production and GM-CSF gene expression by alveolar macrophages in a patient with PAP.)

Thomassen MJ et al: Pulmonary alveolar proteinosis is a disease of decreased availability to GM-CSF rather than an intrinsic cellular defect. Clin Immunol 2000;95:85. [PMID: 10779401]. (Study of response of alveolar macrophages and circulating monocytes to GM-CSF.)

Clinical Findings

A. Signs and Symptoms

The major symptoms of PAP are shortness of breath and dyspnea on exertion. Some patients have a mild cough with occasional sputum production. Chest pain and hemoptysis are extremely unusual, but fatigue and malaise are common. Fever suggests a superinfection. There are few physical signs of disease, and chest examination reveals surprisingly little. Breath sounds are usually normal, although fine rales may be present. Digital clubbing is rare.

B. Chest Imaging

The disease process usually affects both lungs relatively uniformly. Infiltrates are generally more pronounced in perihilar regions and less dense peripherally. Infiltrates are alveolar in nature, with loss of the vascular pattern and presence of air bronchograms. Lymphadenopathy and pleural disease are rare. High-resolution computed tomography (CT) may demonstrate the extent and pattern of regional lung involvement better than chest roentgenograms. High-resolution CT findings of PAP include ground glass opacities with superimposed interlobular septal thickening and intralobular interstitial thickening. When this pattern is most pronounced it appears as white, branching linear opacities that have been termed the "crazy-paving" appearance (Figure 13–1). Although the crazy-paving pattern is highly suggestive of PAP, it is not specific and has also been described in *Pneumocystis carinii* pneumonia, usual interstitial pneumonia, pulmonary hemorrhage, acute radiation pneumonitis, acute respiratory distress syndrome (ARDS), drug-induced pneumonitis, alveolar cell carcinoma, and exogenous lipoid pneumonia.

C. LABORATORY TESTS

Routine complete blood count (CBC) and comprehensive laboratory screens are usually normal with the exception of lactate dehydrogenase, which is characteristically increased. Pulmonary function studies generally show a reduction in vital capacity, total lung capacity,

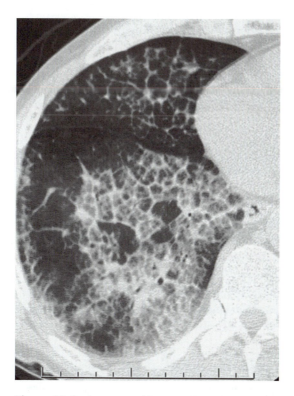

Figure 13-1. A 54-year-old man with mild dyspnea on exertion. CT shows a typical crazy paving pattern of alveolar proteinosis. [Reproduced, with permission, from Lynch, Newell, Lee (eds): *Imaging of Diffuse Lung Disease.* Decker, 2000.]

and diffusing capacity. Arterial oxygen tension and saturation are reduced. Carbon dioxide tension is also reduced, but pH is normal, reflecting a chronic compensated respiratory alkalosis. Arterial oxygen desaturation worsens with progressive increase in work rate. These abnormalities may reverse completely following whole lung lavage.

Murayama S et al: "Crazy paving appearance" on high resolution CT in various diseases. J Comput Assist Tomogr 1999;5:749. [PMID: 10524860]. (Differential diagnosis of "crazy paving" pattern on high resolution CT.)

Diagnosis

The diagnosis of PAP can be made from BAL, transbronchial lung biopsy during bronchoscopy, or open lung biopsy. In patients with a productive cough it is occasionally possible to identify the alveolar phospholipid material or lipid-laden macrophages in expectorated sputum, or to identify the material in a segmental bronchial lavage at the time of fiberoptic bronchoscopy. However, this technique does not distinguish PAP from other disorders such as *Pneumocystis carinii* pneumonia. Lung biopsy is still the most reliable way to establish the diagnosis and to diagnose infection through cultures and special stains. Biopsy is preferred before proceeding to therapy with whole lung lavage. Recent data, however, suggest that detection of serum anti-GM-CSF antibodies may be a sensitive and specific marker for PAP. Future research is required to determine whether this laboratory test will replace lung biopsy in the diagnosis of PAP.

Bonfield TL et al: Autoantibodies against granulocyte macrophage colony-stimulating factor are diagnostic for pulmonary alveolar proteinosis. Am J Respir Cell Mol Biol 2002;27:481. [PMID: 12356582]. (Report of sensitivity and specificity of serum anti-GM-CSF antibodies for PAP.)

Natural History & Prognosis

Untreated patients with PAP may have a variable course. Without definitive therapy, about one-third of patients progressively deteriorate and die, one-third remain stable but symptomatic, and one-third spontaneously improve. Most deaths are due to progressive hypoxemia. About 10 times more adult than pediatric cases have been reported, and the severity of PAP increases with earlier onset of symptoms. Mortality is >80% among infants less than 1 year old and 100% in infants with neonatal onset of disease. Use of whole lung lavage (see below) has dramatically improved prognosis in adult patients. Deaths directly related to PAP are rare in patients treated with whole lung lavage and usually result from fibrosis, infection, or, in secondary PAP, the underlying illness. Unfortunately, the procedure is difficult to perform in infants because the airways are too small for introduction of double lumen tubes.

My personal experience has involved 25 patients over 32 years with biopsy-proven PAP (19 males and 6 females; average age at onset 38 years; range 23–46 years). A total of 394 lavages have been performed, ranging from 2 to 134 on the same patient over the course of active disease. The longest period of remission has been 25 years. PAP became inactive on average 4 years following the initial diagnosis, after an average of 12 whole lung lavages. Chronic active disease has been seen in two patients ranging from 16 to 20 years. *Nocardia asteroides* was diagnosed in five patients, mycobacteria were cultured in five patients during the course of their lavages, and two had both *Nocardia* and *Mycobacterium avium-intracellulare.* Two patients had chronic myelocytic leukemia, one of whom had *Aspergillus fumigatus* cultured from the lavage effluent. There was one successful pregnancy during which lavage was not required, but PAP remained active for the next 6 years after childbirth.

Larson RK, Gordinier R: Pulmonary alveolar proteinosis: report of six cases, review of the literature and formulation of a new theory. Ann Intern Med 1965;62:292. (First article suggesting PAP resulted from abnormal surfactant homeostasis.)

Seymour JF, Presneill JJ: Pulmonary alveolar proteinosis: progress in the first 44 years. Am J Respir Crit Care Med 2002;166:215. [PMID: 12119235]. (Excellent state of the art review of clinical presentation, pathogenesis, natural history, and treatment of PAP.)

Treatment

Once the diagnosis of PAP has been established, the physician is faced with the dilemma of observing the patient in hope of a spontaneous remission or intervening early therapeutically. Pivotal to this decision is the degree of dyspnea and exercise limitation due to respiratory compromise produced by the disease and presence of infection.

The therapeutic alternatives that have been tried to treat PAP include inhalation of enzymatic (trypsin) or mucolytic (acetylcysteine) agents, limited BAL through a flexible fiberoptic bronchoscope, and whole lung lavage. Inhalation treatments have been abandoned due to complications and ineffectiveness. Similarly, lavage through a flexible fiberoptic bronchoscope had serious limitations due to time constraints and limited ability to instill adequate volumes of lavage fluid. The preferred treatment subsequently became whole lung lavage using a double-lumen endotracheal–endobronchial tube under general anesthesia.

A. WHOLE LUNG LAVAGE

Ramirez took the bold step of using a Carlens endotracheal tube to separate both lungs, degassing one lung, and then flooding it with saline containing heparin and acetylcysteine, while providing gas exchange with the other lung. The patient was given only local anesthesia and allowed to take deep breaths to mix the saline with the proteinaceous alveolar contents. The saline was then drained, suctioned, and coughed out. Wasserman modified the technique to perform whole lung lavage in anesthetized patients in whom the lung remained degassed for 2–3 h while it was lavaged with fresh saline solutions. Lavage was continued until the effluent was almost clear (20 L or more). Chest percussion during the procedure considerably enhanced the yield, and lavage was performed with warmed isotonic saline without additives. Some reports suggested additional clinical improvement if trypsin was added to the lavage fluid, at least in patients treated with BAL via a fiberoptic bronchoscope. A number of techniques have been described for whole lung lavage including the lavage of each lung on two separate days, one lung at a time on the same day, and in children, both lungs while on partial cardiopulmonary bypass. A hyperbaric chamber has also been used to maintain adequate oxygen saturation during whole lung lavage. My practice is to lavage the second lung on the next day. The indications for whole lung lavage are listed in Table 13–1. Many patients recognize by their symptoms when repeat lavage is necessary.

The technique of whole lung lavage requires a trained staff that includes a physician knowledgeable in the procedure and its potential complications, an anesthesiologist with double-lumen tube skills, and support personnel. A respiratory therapist provides mechanical chest percussion throughout the procedure. General anesthesia and muscle paralysis are induced and then the patient is intubated with a left-sided double-lumen tube (sizes 35 to 41) allowing lung separation and independent lung ventilation. Correct positioning is confirmed by fiberoptic bronchoscopy. A pediatric fiberoptic bronchoscope that can be passed through both lumen of a #35 double-lumen tube is used. Spillage of lavage fluid into the contralateral ventilated lung can be detected by auscultation with an esophageal stetho-

Table 13–1. Indications for whole lung lavage.

Arterial hypoxemia
Increasing oxygen requirements
Progressive dyspnea and impairment of daily activities
Severe cough
Deteriorating pulmonary function

scope as well as by rapid appearance of lavage fluid in the endotracheal tube lumen ventilating the nonlavaged lung. If spillage is detected, the procedure is halted, the lavaged lung is drained, and the tube is repositioned using the fiberoptic bronchoscope. Isotonic saline warmed to 37°C prevents hypothermia, as does a warming blanket. The container holding the sterile, warmed, isotonic saline is positioned above the patient's chest to provide hydrostatic filling pressure and connected to the appropriate endotracheal tube lumen. Using a Y-connector and tubing, the lung is filled with the isotonic saline while the draining arm is clamped. When the fluid flow decreases or a predetermined volume is instilled, the filling arm is clamped and the draining arm is unclamped. The patient is placed and kept in an oblique position with the lavaged lung dependent, and the head is lowered into the Trendelenburg position to facilitate drainage. During the filling and drainage cycles, chest percussion is performed over the lavaged lung. Increments of isotonic saline from 500 to 1500 mL are instilled depending on the patient's size and response to the protein removed. Fluid volumes are monitored and effluent is collected in large-volume containers that allow observation of clearing of the effluent. The procedure continues until the effluent is nearly clear; a total of 12–40+ L of lavage fluid may be required. Following lavage, the lung is ventilated and in most cases patients are extubated in the operating room before transfer to the recovery area. Prolonged ventilatory support is rarely required. The initial effluent is sent for appropriate cultures.

The first lavage is usually the most difficult to perform because appropriate tube size has to be determined and respiratory compromise from underlying lung disease is at its worst. Positive end-expiratory pressure on the ventilated lung may assist in management of hypoxemia. Continuous oxygen saturation monitoring is mandatory, however, extracorporeal membrane oxygenation or cardiopulmonary bypass is rarely needed (in my experience only once in nearly 500 lavages). Use of a pulmonary artery catheter is rarely necessary, but the invasive hemodynamic monitoring data associated with whole lung lavage are well described. Transesophageal echocardiographic changes during whole lung lavage may provide useful measurements in a difficult case. Complications of whole lung lavage include worsening hypoxemia, hydropneumothorax, fever, hoarseness, and pneumonia.

Loubser PG: Validity of pulmonary artery catheter-derived hemodynamic information during bronchopulmonary lavage. J Cardiothor Vascul Anesth 1997;7:885. [PMID: 9412892]. (Report of changes in central hemodynamic parameters that occur during whole lung lavage.)

Ramirez J, Kieffer RF, Ball WC: Bronchopulmonary lavage in man. Ann Intern Med 1965;63:819. [PMID: 5848630]. (Early report of use of lung lavage to manage PAP.)

Wasserman K, Blank N, Fletcher G: Lung lavage (alveolar washing) in alveolar proteinosis. Am J Med 1968;44:611. [PMID: 564277]. (Early report of whole lung lavage performed under general anesthesia.)

B. GM-CSF

Studies implicating GM-CSF in the pathogenesis of PAP suggest repletion of this cytokine may be valuable in management of the disorder. An early report described clinical, physiological, and radiographic changes in response to the initiation, withdrawal, and reintroduction of GM-CSF therapy in a patient with PAP. Kavuru reported preliminary results in four patients with PAP treated with GM-CSF. Three of the four patients improved. Similarly, Seymour reported a GM-CSF response rate of 43% in 14 patients. These preliminary studies are promising, suggesting that GM-CSF may eventually become an alternative or adjunctive therapy to whole lung lavage, however, additional studies are still required to evaluate its efficacy.

Kavuru MS et al: Exogenous granulocyte-macrophage colony-stimulating factor administration for pulmonary alveolar proteinosis. Am J Respir Crit Care Med 2000;161:1143. [PMID: 10764303]. (Clinical response of four PAP patients treated with GM-CSF.)

Seymour JF et al: Therapeutic efficacy of granulocyte-macrophage colony-stimulating factor in patients with idiopathic acquired alveolar proteinosis. Am J Respir Crit Care Med 2001;163:524. [PMID: 11179134]. (Case series of 14 PAP patients treated with GM-CSF.)

Seymour JF et al: Efficacy of granulocyte-macrophage colony-stimulating factor in acquired alveolar proteinosis. N Engl J Med 1996;335:1924. [PMID: 8965913]. (Case report documenting clinical, physiological and radiographic response following treatment with GM-CSF in a patient with PAP.)

Summary

PAP is a rare, fascinating, and relatively recently identified disease actively being altered by time, improved techniques, and knowledge. It currently is managed by a combination of whole lung lavage and GM-CSF, but the best sequence of therapy has to be determined. Additionally, the coexistence of infection(s) is being increasingly recognized. Management of infections may also alter the disease course and outcome.

Pulmonary Langerhans'-Cell Histiocytosis, Lymphangioleiomyomatosis, & Bronchiolitis Obliterans with Organizing Pneumonia

14

James M. O'Brien, Jr., MD

PULMONARY LANGERHANS'-CELL HISTIOCYTOSIS

 ESSENTIALS OF DIAGNOSIS

- *Nonproductive cough and dyspnea with or without systemic symptoms.*
- *Extrathoracic involvement (5–15%) of bones, skin, hypothalamus, liver, spleen, and lymph nodes.*
- *Nodular or cystic pattern on high-resolution computed tomography with basal sparing.*
- *Demonstration of Langerhans' cells and bronchiolocentric granuloma on lung biopsy or increased (>5%) CD1a-positive cells on bronchoalveolar lavage.*

General Considerations

Pulmonary Langerhans'-cell histiocytosis (PLH) is part of a spectrum of diseases characterized by proliferation of and infiltration by Langerhans' cells into various organs. Several organ systems may be involved in Langerhans'-cell histiocytosis (LCH), including the lungs, bone, skin, pituitary gland, liver, lymph nodes, and thyroid (Figure 14–1). Lung involvement may occur either in isolation or as part of a multisystem syndrome. When lung disease is part of the clinical presentation in adult patients, the term pulmonary Langerhans'-cell histiocytosis is used.

The nomenclature of these syndromes is diverse. Older classification schemes used designations such as systemic histiocytosis X, eosinophilic granuloma, Letterer–Siwe disease, Hand–Schuller–Christian syndrome, Hashimoto–Pritzker syndrome, and Langerhans cell granulomatosis. To avoid confusion due to eponymous conflicts, the Histiocyte Society established a simplified classification scheme based on a spectrum of presentations that varies from those involving single organs to more aggressive, disseminated disease. These diseases should be referred to as Langerhans'-cell histiocytosis and the presence of specific organ involvement should be described. In patients with pulmonary manifestations, the lung is the only organ system affected in approximately 85%, whereas multisystem disease is seen in 5–15%.

The exact prevalence and incidence of PLH are unknown. However, it appears that this is a rare disease. In one study of those undergoing open-lung biopsy for interstitial lung disease, only 15 cases of PLH were detected among 501 patients over 6 years, whereas 274 cases of sarcoidosis were found. Another study of biopsy specimens from patients with interstitial lung disease found PLH in 5%. However, it has been suggested that PLH may be underdiagnosed as some patients have a paucity of symptoms or undergo a spontaneous remission and never undergo a confirmatory biopsy.

There does not seem to be a familial basis to PLH. The specific genetic factors involved are not known. It appears to be a disease largely of white individuals with no specific geographic predilection. Likely, there is no gender predominance. Early series suggested a male bias, but more recent series have called this into question. Changing patterns in tobacco consumption, with more women now smoking, may have caused this ap-

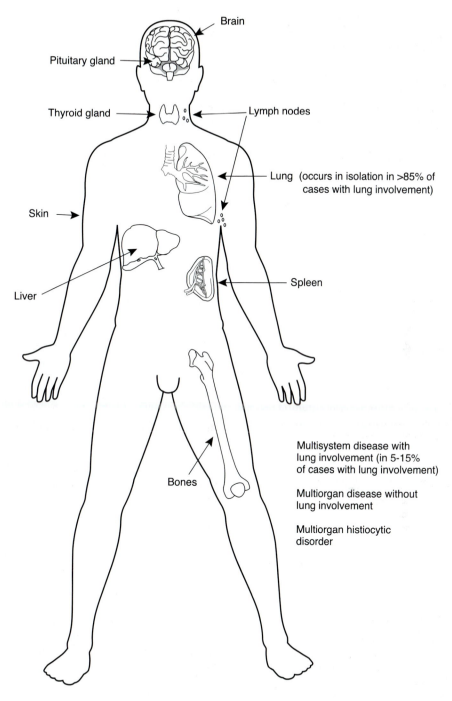

Figure 14–1. Organ involvement in Langerhans'-cell hystiocytosis in adults.

parent shift. Most patients are between 20 and 40 years of age, but pulmonary involvement has been described in individuals from 3 months to 69 years of age.

The one identifiable and consistent risk factor for PLH is cigarette smoking. In series after series, over 90% of affected individuals are current smokers and almost all have some history of exposure. Often daily cigarette consumption exceeds one pack, although lifetime smoke exposure may be modest. This finding has led to the investigation of cigarette smoke as a causative agent in PLH. Two major lines of inquiry involve the recognition that smoking causes an accumulation of Langerhans' cells in lungs unaffected by PLH and that tobacco exposure causes a proliferation of neuroendocrine cells that may increase inflammation and influx of Langerhans' cells via secretion of bombesin. In Langerhans'-cell histiocytosis syndromes in children, X-linked polymorphic DNA probes have indicated a monoclonal origin. However, this is not well established in adults with PLH.

Clinical Findings

A. Symptoms and Signs

Clinical manifestations of PLH are varied and up to 25% of patients are asymptomatic at presentation. The most common presenting symptoms are a nonproductive cough and dyspnea. Approximately one-third of patients will have constitutional symptoms (weight loss, fever, night sweats, anorexia, etc). Hemoptysis is an uncommon occurrence and, even in the presence of an established diagnosis of PLH, should lead to an investigation for other pathology, including bronchogenic carcinoma.

Chest pain is an uncommon finding and may be due to a variety of mechanisms. Pneumothorax complicates PLH in 10–20% of cases and may be recurrent or bilateral. Also, bone lesions may occur in the ribs, leading to thoracic pain. Extrapulmonary involvement may be responsible for the initial diagnostic evaluation in 5–15% of patients. Symptoms include pain due to bone involvement, polyuria and polydipsia due to diabetes insipidus from hypothalamic involvement, rash due to cutaneous LCH, adenopathy from lymph node disease, and abdominal discomfort and early satiety due to infiltration of the liver and spleen.

B. Laboratory Findings

Routine laboratory investigation is rarely helpful. Leukocytosis is uncommon and the cellular differential is usually normal. The erythrocyte sedimentation rate (ESR) can be moderately elevated and low titers of autoantibodies and immune complexes have been described. The angiotensin-converting enzyme level is usually normal.

C. Pulmonary Function Testing

Physiological testing is variable and may depend on the stage of disease. A frequent finding is a disparity between relatively marked radiographic abnormalities and minimal changes in pulmonary function testing. In 10–15% of patients, pulmonary function testing is normal. The most commonly described abnormality is a decrease in the diffusing capacity of carbon monoxide, seen in 60–90% of patients in different series. Other common findings are a decreased vital capacity and an elevated residual volume–total lung capacity ratio. However, restrictive, obstructed, and mixed patterns have been seen. It has been argued that as the disease progresses, obstructive patterns predominate. Cardiopulmonary testing often discloses decreased exercise tolerance with exertional widening of the alveolar–arterial oxygen gradient. Findings suggestive of pulmonary vascular disease have also been described.

D. Imaging Studies

1. Chest radiography—The majority of patients with PLH have an abnormal chest radiograph and the abnormalities appear to evolve as the disease progresses. However, up to 10% will have a normal chest radiograph at presentation. The early radiographic findings of PLH are described as poorly demarcated micronodules and reticular shadows. These abnormalities are more widespread in the upper and middle lung zones and a sparing of the bases and costophrenic angles has been highlighted as a clue to the diagnosis of PLH (Figure 14–2A). As the disease progresses, cystic lesions (up to 2 cm in diameter) become more common (Figure 14–2B). This appearance can mimic emphysema and lymphangioleiomyomatosis. Ultimately, lung honeycombing may be seen, representing severe lung fibrosis. Lung volumes are normal to increased. Less common findings include alveolar infiltrates, hilar adenopathy, and prominent pulmonary arteries. Pleural effusions are rare, having been seen in only 8% of cases in one series.

2. High-resolution computed tomography—High-resolution computed tomography (HRCT) has proved to be an important diagnostic tool in patients with PLH. Characteristically, abnormalities are seen interspersed on a background of normal lung parenchyma. Again, sparing of basal lung regions is seen. Early disease is characterized by centrilobular nodules. Subsequently, there is a transition toward more cystic abnormalities. These cysts are variable in size, but are usually less than 20 mm with a thin wall and an irregular shape. In fact, the combination of diffuse, irregularly shaped cystic spaces with small peribronchiolar nodular opacities is highly suggestive of PLH (Figure 14–2C). Often, a presumptive diagnosis may be made on the HRCT appearance alone. In one study, HRCT was

A

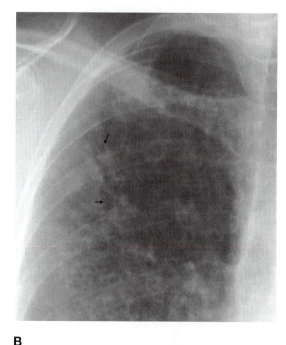

B

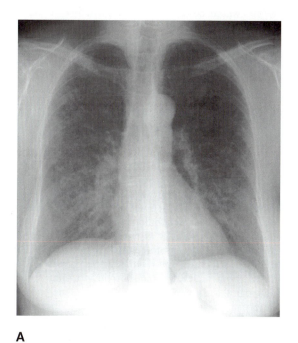

C

Figure 14–2. A 59-year-old female with mild dyspnea and Langerhans'-cell hystiocytosis. **A:** Chest radiograph shows profuse nodules predominating in the mid- and upper zones with sparing of the lower lungs, and particularly the costophrenic sulci. Lung volumes are preserved. **B:** Detail view of the right upper lobe shows nodules and cysts. **C:** HRCT shows the characteristic combination of poorly defined nodules and cysts of varying sizes.

used to correctly diagnose PLH in 88–94% of cases. In the same series, chest radiography was diagnostic in only 53–65% of patients. Other abnormalities include pulmonary artery enlargement, ground glass densities, adenopathy, and lower lobe cystic changes without nodules.

3. Bronchoalveolar lavage and lung biopsy—Bronchoscopy with bronchoalveolar lavage can be of help in the diagnosis of PLH. Bronchoscopic examination is generally normal, although changes associated with smoking may be seen. Most commonly, the total cell count retrieved in the bronchoalveolar lavage is increased, with a large number of pigment-laden macrophages. Moderate increases in the percentage of neutrophils and eosinophils have been described. Lymphocyte percentages are normal or decreased and the CD4/CD8 ratio is decreased, as in most smokers. Langerhans' cells may be identified in the bronchoalveolar lavage, most commonly by staining for the presence of CD1a, a transmembrane protein related to MHC-I that may play a role in antigen presentation. A finding of more than 5% of CD1a-positive cells is highly suggestive of PLH. Unfortunately, intermediate numbers of Langerhans' cells (2–5%) are most common and carry a sensitivity of < 25%. Transbronchial biopsy results are variable, but have been cited to have a diagnostic yield of 10–40% in PLH. Transbronchial biopsy may carry an increased risk of pneumothorax in those with PLH, an argument against its routine use.

A definitive diagnosis of PLH requires the demonstration of the characteristic lesion on histopathological specimens. Because of the patchy nature of the disease, this most commonly requires a surgical biopsy and video-assisted thoracoscopy is most often used. Directing the biopsy to sites involved with nodules on HRCT can increase the diagnostic yield. In patients who smoke and have characteristic changes of PLH on HRCT, biopsy can often be avoided. However, diagnosis by pathology should be pursued in those requiring surgical treatment of pneumothorax, in women with cystic lung disease (to differentiate PLH from lymphangioleiomyomatosis), in symptomatic patients with nodules for whom corticosteroid treatment is considered, and in patients with atypical presentations.

The characteristic lesion of PLH is the presence of activated Langerhans' cells organized in loose granulomas with associated lymphocytes and inflammatory cells (especially macrophages and eosinophils). The earliest lesion is thought to be a proliferation of Langerhans' cells along the small airways. These cellular lesions expand into bronchiolocentric nodules that include a mixed population of cells with variable numbers of Langerhans' cells, eosinophils, lymphocytes, plasma cells, fibroblasts, and pigmented alveolar macrophages. Ultimately, the granulomatous lesions become fibrotic and destroy the distal airways. Thus, PLH is truly a bronchiolitis. The fibrotic nodules become more stellate and connect to other nodules to form a honeycombed lung with enlargement of distal air spaces and hyperinflation (Figure 14–3). Pathologically, cystic lesions represent encasement of the residual dilated lumen of destroyed bronchioles by the fibrotic reaction. Other pathological lesions are not uncommon and include respiratory bronchiolitis and desquamative interstitial pneumonitis. In experienced hands, Langerhans' cells can be identified without special histological stains. However, S-100, anti-CD1a, and HLA-DR stains have been employed to highlight Langerhans' cells. The pathognomonic sign of Langerhans' cells is the presence of Birbeck granules (pentalaminar, rod-shaped intracellular structures) seen on electron microscopy. However, this technique is rarely employed in clinical practice.

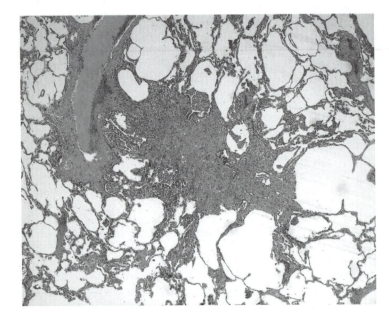

Figure 14–3. Langerhans'-cell histiocytosis. A stellate scar is centered on a bronchiole.

Treatment

Because the natural history of PLH is not well known, it is difficult to determine the impact of various treatment strategies. In fact, no treatment or intervention has been shown to be efficacious in a controlled manner. Spontaneous remissions and exacerbations have been described. Due to the epidemiological association with cigarette smoking, tobacco abstinence is considered imperative. Although the influence of smoking cessation has not been systematically studied, clinical and radiographic improvements have been described and the majority of patients experience a stabilization of symptoms with abstinence. At the very least, the patient will be spared other adverse effects of tobaccoism. Avoidance of environmental smoke must also be stressed.

Corticosteroids are the most commonly employed pharmacological therapy. Several series have reported improved symptoms and chest radiographs in association with this therapy (almost always in concert with smoking cessation). Commonly used doses of prednisone are from 0.5 to 1.0 mg/kg/day. Generally, this is tapered over 6–12 months, but recurrences have been described with discontinuation. Because of the uncertainty of its efficacy, deciding about corticosteroid administration is difficult. A reasonable approach is to use corticosteroids in those with progressive disease or persistent symptoms following smoking cessation. It has been suggested that patients with nodular disease are more likely to respond to therapy. In those with steroid-unresponsive disease or multisystem involvement, vinblastine, methotrexate, cyclophosphamide, etoposide, and cladaribine have been tried with variable results.

Lung transplantation should be considered for those with advanced PLH associated with severe respiratory insufficiency. There are no established disease-specific guidelines for lung transplantation or poor prognosis. Therefore, rapidly declining lung function or severe limitation unresponsive to smoking cessation and immunosuppressives should prompt evaluation for transplantation. Recurrences of PLH have been described in the transplanted lung. This has occurred in those who resume tobacco use, as well as in those who continue to abstain. For those in whom transplantation is considered, aggressive pleurodesis should be avoided, if possible, to reduce posttransplant pleural complications.

Prognosis

Because of a lack of long-term studies, little is known about the natural history of PLH. However, a number of retrospective studies suggest that most patients have a good prognosis. Approximately 50% have a favorable course, either with no treatment or with corticosteroid therapy. However, another 10–20% have a rapid downhill course. Others have slowly progressive disease that proceeds insidiously over decades. Radiological series suggest that nodular lesions regress in 13–55% and progress in 7–21% of patients. Confounding this is the finding that nodular lesions may appear to regress but are, in fact, becoming cystic lesions. Poor prognostic signs have included disease onset at the extremes of age, persistence of systemic symptoms, recurrent pneumothorax, nonbony extrathoracic disease, the presence of honeycombing on chest radiograph, major pulmonary function test abnormalities [especially a decreased forced expiratory volume/forced vital capacity (FEV_1/FVC) ratio], and a failure to stop smoking. Mortality ranges from 2 to 25%. Recently, the Mayo Clinic reviewed its experience with 102 adults with PLH. With a median follow-up of 4 years, these patients had an overall median survival of 12 years with an estimated rate of survival 5 years after diagnosis of 74% and an estimated 10-year survival of 64%. This was significantly shorter than for age- and gender-matched healthy persons. In this series, shorter survival was associated with older age, a lower carbon monoxide diffusing capacity, a lower FEV_1, a higher residual volume, and a lower ratio of FEV_1 to FVC.

In addition to extrathoracic disease, other disease processes can complicate PLH. Most notably, patients with Langerhans'-cell histiocytosis appear to be at a higher risk for neoplastic disease. This association has been best established in pediatric patients with multisystem PLH and is less clear in adults. It has been suggested that lymphoma and bronchogenic carcinoma may occur at a greater frequency in patients with PLH than in the unaffected population. In the most recent reported series in adults, there were 628 person-years of follow-up for hematological cancers, with 2 observed and 0.172 expected cases, producing a risk ratio of 11.6. As with other cystic and cavitary lung disease, PLH may be complicated by fungal infections that can be devastating in the face of immunosuppression. Pulmonary hypertension is being recognized as a more common complication of PLH and may occur even in the absence of severe impairment in ventilatory function or hypoxemia.

Murin S et al: Other smoking-affected pulmonary diseases. Clin Chest Med 2000;21:121. [PMID: 10763094]. (Review covers less common lung diseases associated with smoking, including PLH, respiratory bronchiolitis-associated interstitial lung disease, idiopathic pulmonary fibrosis, and asbestosis.)

Tazi A et al: Adult pulmonary Langerhans'-cell histiocytosis. Thorax 2000;55:405. [PMID: 10770823]. (Review covers clinical aspects of PLH as well as theories and investigation into the pathogenesis of PLH.)

Vassallo R et al: Clinical outcomes of pulmonary Langerhans'-cell histiocytosis in adults. N Engl J Med 2002:346:484. [PMID: 11844849]. (A recent clinical review of the Mayo Clinic experience with PLH.)

Vassallo R et al: Pulmonary Langerhans'-cell histiocytosis. N Engl J Med 2000;342:1969. [PMID: 10877650]. (Comprehensive clinical review that briefly touches on pathogenesis.)

LYMPHANGIOLEIOMYOMATOSIS

 ESSENTIALS OF DIAGNOSIS

- *Nonspecific pulmonary symptoms in a woman of reproductive age.*
- *Pleural involvement, including recurrent and bilateral pneumothoraces and chylous effusions, is common.*
- *Renal angiomyolipomas are seen in 50% of patients.*
- *Presence of multiple thin-walled cysts seen diffusely throughout the lungs on HRCT.*
- *Demonstration of proliferation of smooth muscle cells that occlude bronchioles, lymphatics, and venules.*
- *Identification of lymphangioleiomyomatosis cells by staining with HMB-45.*

General Considerations

Lymphangioleiomyomatosis (LAM) is a rare disease that affects women almost exclusively, often during their reproductive years. Pathologically, it is characterized by nonneoplastic proliferation of atypical smooth muscle cells around airways, blood vessels, and lymphatics. Although the disease is most commonly centered in the thorax, lymph nodes in the abdomen and pelvis may also be involved, and renal angiomyolipomas are seen in up to 50% of patients. This latter finding has led to the investigation of LAM as a part of the tuberous sclerosis complex (TSC). The genetic defects in TSC are known and have opened an avenue of research into the pathogenesis of LAM.

Because of the rarity of LAM, much of the knowledge of the disease comes from case reports and series collected at referral centers. Recently, registries have been started in the United States, the United Kingdom, and France. The hope is that by compiling the information gleaned from these individual patients, more can be learned about the disease. Prevalence is estimated at approximately one per one million persons in the United States and Western Europe. However, the true prevalence is likely greater due to misdiagnosis and subclinical disease. Typically, LAM is a disease of women of childbearing age. One case–control series found that women with LAM were less likely than a control population to have been pregnant or have had children and

tended to have had more spontaneous abortions and a greater incidence of fibroids. The average age of disease onset was 34 years in one large series, with onset after menopause uncommon. Of 186 patients in one report, only eight (4%) were postmenopausal at presentation. Of these eight patients, six were receiving estrogen-replacement therapy. This has led to the hypothesis that LAM is mediated or affected by hormonal influences. However, a few cases of LAM have been reported in men, as well as in a male bottle-nosed dolphin, and in children, suggesting the response to hormonal manipulation is not complete. Therefore, other mechanisms of disease are being sought.

Recently, a potential relationship between LAM and the TSC has been investigated. TSC is an autosomal dominant disease with an equal gender distribution characterized by hamartomas in multiple organs. The pathological lesions found in LAM are identical to those seen in patients with pulmonary involvement by TSC. In fact, LAM is considered sufficient for a presumptive diagnosis of TSC when it presents alone and constitutes a definitive diagnosis when in combination with at least one other secondary diagnostic criterion (such as renal angiomyolipoma) (Table 14–1). Furthermore, the incidence of pulmonary involvement in TSC is <0.1–2.3%; however, those with pulmonary involvement are almost exclusively female. Because of these similarities, a search has begun for a common pathogenesis. In TSC, germ line mutations are found in one of two genes, TSC-1 or TSC-2. A second somatic mutation in the same gene results in a loss of heterozygosity and a loss of production of the gene product in a cell. The TSC genes appear to function as tumor suppressor genes and their loss results in the growth of the hamartomas characteristic of the disease. Interestingly, a loss of heterozygosity was found for TSC-2 in renal angiomyolipomas of 7 of 13 patients with LAM but no other evidence of TSC. These findings have led to the proposal that LAM is an atypical form (*forme fruste*) of TSC. Further research is needed to define the relationship between these disorders.

Clinical Findings

A. SYMPTOMS AND SIGNS

As mentioned previously, LAM is seen almost exclusively in women. However, the presenting profile of these patients is otherwise often unremarkable. Symptoms may occur before radiological or physiological abnormalities, and there is often a delay between the onset of symptoms and accurate diagnosis. In several of the reported series, the diagnosis of LAM was established a mean of 3 years after initial symptoms appeared.

Table 14–1. Revised diagnostic criteria for tuberous sclerosis complex.

Major features

1. Facial angiofibromas or forehead plaque
2. Nontraumatic ungual or periungual fibroma
3. Hypomelanotic macules (more than three)
4. Shagreen patch (connective tissue nevus)
5. Multiple retinal nodular hamartomas
6. Cortical tuber[1]
7. Subependymal nodule
8. Subependymal giant cell astrocytoma
9. Cardiac rhabdomyoma, single or multiple
10. Lymphangiomyomatosis[2]
11. Renal angiomyolipoma[2]

Minor features

1. Multiple randomly distributed pits in dental enamel
2. Hamartomatous rectal polyps[3]
3. Bone cysts[4]
4. Cerebral white matter migration lines[1,4]
5. Gingival fibromas
6. Nonrenal hamartoma[3]
7. Retinal achromic patch
8. "Confetti" skin lesions
9. Multiple renal cysts[3]

Definite TSC: Either two major features or one major feature with two minor features
Probable TSC: One major feature and one minor feature
Possible TSC: Either one major feature or two or more minor features

---

From www.tsalliance.org/whatisTSC/table1.asp.
[1]When cerebral cortical dysplasia and cerebral white matter migration tracts occur together, they should be counted as one rather than two features of TSC.
[2]When both lymphangiomyomatosis and renal angiomyolipomas are present, other features of TSC should be present before a definitive diagnosis is assigned.
[3]Histological confirmation is suggested.
[4]Radiographic confirmation is sufficient.

The most common presenting symptoms are dyspnea and pneumothorax. Each is seen in approximately 50% of patients in most series. Rarely, bilateral spontaneous pneumothoraces are the presenting feature and are suggestive of LAM. Recurrent pneumothoraces are not uncommon. Cough and chest pain are also frequent but nondescript findings. Chylous pleural effusions, chylous ascites, chyloptysis, chyluria, chylous pericardial effusion, and lower extremity lymphedema are due to interrupted lymph flow. Symptoms have been reported to develop or worsen during pregnancy. Renal angiomyolipomas are usually asymptomatic but may cause flank pain, hematuria, or a palpable mass.

The physical examination is often nonspecific. Crackles or rhonchi may be heard. The presence of a pleural effusion, ascites, or lymphedema may be more helpful. Clubbing is uncommon. LAM should be considered in women who present with dyspnea or asthma associated with pneumothorax, hemoptysis, or an abnormal chest radiograph; in women with chronic obstructive pulmonary disease in the absence of significant exposure to tobacco smoke or α_1-antitrypsin deficiency; and in women with radiographic interstitial lung disease with physiological evidence of airflow limitation.

B. LABORATORY FINDINGS

There is no specific laboratory abnormality associated with LAM. One study found elevated serum angiotensin-converting enzyme levels in two of three patients and there is a single report of a patient with LAM and an elevated CA-125. These findings are anecdotal to date and are currently of little diagnostic value.

C. PULMONARY FUNCTION TESTING

The pulmonary physiological features of patients with LAM are variable and include obstructive, restrictive, or mixed patterns. The most frequently cited abnormalities are impairment of airflow and diffusion capacity. In one study, the airflow limitation in LAM was found to be due to airway obstruction from airway narrowing rather than loss of elastic recoil. Diffusion abnormalities may result in severe gas-transfer abnormalities and hypoxia. Restrictive abnormalities are secondary to pleural effusions or changes postthoracotomy. Limitations during cardiopulmonary stress testing are usually consistent with obstructive lung disease and may also suggest pulmonary vascular abnormalities. Up to 10% of symptomatic patients have physiological measures that are within the normal range.

D. IMAGING STUDIES

1. Chest radiography—Initially, the chest radiograph may be normal. However, radiographic findings vary roughly according to disease severity and, therefore, change with the duration of disease. Subsequently, fine reticular or reticulonodular infiltrates develop (Figure 14–4A and B). Kerley B lines may be seen and are thought to represent dilation of lymphatics in the interlobular septae due to lymphatic obstruction. Lung volumes are normal or increased. The radiographic pattern may simulate those of PLH. However, the abnormalities in LAM are distributed evenly throughout the lung and do not spare the costophrenic sulci as in PLH. Ultimately, LAM progresses to honeycombing that is described as more "delicate" than that seen in idiopathic pulmonary fibrosis. In addition to the parenchymal changes seen on chest radiograph, pleural abnormalities are common. Pleural effusions are frequent and, upon

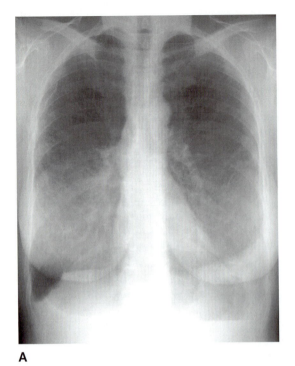

A

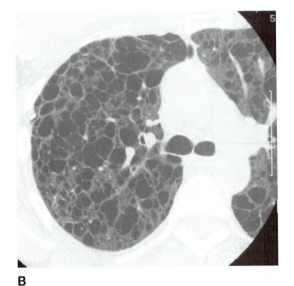

B

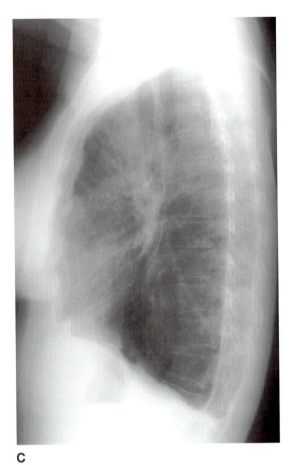

C

Figure 14–4. A 54-year-old woman with lymphangi-oleiomyomatosis. ***A, B:*** Frontal and lateral radiographs show increased lung volumes and widespread coarse reticular abnormality. There is a small left pleural effusion. ***C:*** HRCT shows profuse cysts. Each cyst has a well-defined thin wall.

sampling, are often found to be chylous. In these cases, LAM must be differentiated from other causes of chylous effusions such as traumatic or neoplastic interruption of lymphatic flow and the yellow nail syndrome. Pneumothorax is seen in almost 50% of patients at presentation and is present in up to 81% of patients at some time during the course of the disease. Pneumo-

thoraces may be bilateral. Both effusions and pneumothoraces can occur in the face of otherwise normal chest radiographs.

2. High-resolution computed tomography—Unlike the chest radiograph, HRCT is almost always abnormal at the time of diagnosis. Often the disease appears more extensive on HRCT than on radiograph. The most common finding is numerous thin-walled cysts of varying size (2–20 mm) (Figure 14–4C). The cyst walls are smooth and may be associated with reticulation (thin linear markings) at their margins that extend to the pleural surface. As the disease progresses, the cysts enlarge and become more numerous, although the intervening parenchyma is normal. There is no nodularity in contrast to PLH. As in the chest radiograph, lung volumes are normal or increased.

In addition to interstitial findings, alveolar opacities and lymphadenopathy may be seen. In one series, subtle alveolar infiltrates, thought to represent alveolar hemorrhage, were present in 60% of patients. Hilar and mediastinal adenopathy are also touted to be common abnormalities on HRCT. Furthermore, abdominal and retroperitoneal adenopathy have been described. Additionally, because renal angiomyolipomas are found in 47–60% of patients with LAM, their presence bolsters the diagnosis. Other abnormalities include pleural effusion, pneumothorax, pericardial effusion, and a dilated thoracic duct. In the setting of an appropriate history, a characteristic HRCT can be diagnostic and obviates the need for lung biopsy.

3. Bronchoalveolar lavage and lung biopsy—A surgical lung biopsy specimen is considered the gold standard for diagnosis of LAM; however, in certain circumstances transbronchial biopsies, pleural fluid cytological analysis, or lymph node pathology may be sufficient. These less invasive diagnostic modalities are more likely to yield meaningful results in the hands of experienced pathologists. Immunohistochemical staining with HMB-45, a monoclonal antibody derived from melanoma hybridomas that stains LAM cells as well as melanocytic lesions, has improved the usefulness of transbronchial biopsy in the diagnosis of LAM. Renal angiomyolipomas may also be positive for HMB-45 in LAM. Staining for this antibody may reduce the need for surgical biopsies.

On surgical biopsy or necropsy, cysts bulge from the lung surface and the cut surface shows a cystic honeycomb appearance. Cysts containing air or fluid are seen throughout the lung without regional predilection. Multiple lymph nodes may be involved and the nodes appear pale and spongy. The thoracic duct may also be enlarged and pleural adhesions and effusions may be seen.

Microscopically, LAM is characterized by proliferation of smooth muscle cells (Figure 14–5). In the lung, this proliferation tends to occur along the normal lymphatic distribution, and involves the alveolar walls and the perivascular, peribronchial, and subpleural regions. These smooth muscle cells obstruct bronchioles leading to air trapping, bullae formation, and pneumothorax. They also occlude lymphatics, cause chylothorax and chylous ascites, and block venules producing hemoptysis and hemosiderosis. As alveoli are lost in this process, cysts form. These cysts are lined with smooth muscle cells and alveolar and bronchiolar epithelium.

Further characterization of the proliferating LAM cells shows that they exhibit characteristics of smooth

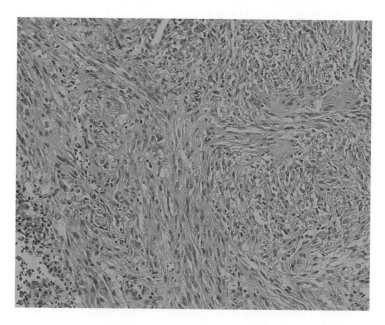

Figure 14–5. A surgical lung biopsy from a patient with lymphangioleiomyomatosis. There is a proliferation of smooth muscle in a peribronchial and perivascular distribution.

muscle cells, including the expression of smooth muscle actin and desmin. HMB-45 staining has proven to be useful in surgical specimens. The antigen that reacts with the HMB-45 antibody is a 100-kDa glycoprotein, termed gp100. Its function is not yet known but it appears to be localized within structures with morphological characteristics of immature melanosomes. HMB-45 positivity is also more common in LAM cells with a more epithelioid appearance and fewer markers of cell proliferation. The clinical significance of this marker in LAM is not yet known. Adding credence to the theory of a hormonal basis for pathogenesis, LAM cells stain for the estrogen receptor in approximately 50% of cases and may also express progesterone receptors. There is no clear evidence that patients with estrogen receptor-positive biopsies are more likely to respond to hormonal manipulation. In experienced hands, the pathological findings are relatively characteristic and the addition of HMB-45 staining has helped to exclude other diagnostic considerations such as metastatic endometrial sarcoma.

Treatment

The approach to the management of LAM is largely based on case series and retrospective analyses. The predilection of the disease for premenopausal women led to the belief that hormonal factors play an important role in the pathogenesis of LAM. Based on this observation, hormonal manipulation has become the most frequent initial treatment. The most commonly used drug is progesterone, which has had mixed results in case series. In three larger retrospective series, of a total of 32 patients who received a mean daily dose of 10 mg progesterone, 15 patients (47%) were considered to be improved or stabilized. In another review, the mean decline in FEV_1 appeared to be less in patients taking progesterone than in those receiving no treatment. In most series, response to progesterone therapy has been predicted by the presence of chylous complications. Although there have been no controlled trials, most patients receive intramuscular depot medroxyprogesterone, 400–800 mg/month, or oral progesterone, 10–20 mg/day.

Other hormonal treatments have even less evidence for efficacy. Surgical oophorectomy has been promoted by some but has most commonly been used in combination with progesterone. Mixed results have been found when tamoxifen, a partial estrogen agonist, was used alone. There are few data available on the use of gonadotropin-releasing hormone (GnRH) agonists, the newer estrogen receptor modulators (eg, raloxitene), or selective aromatase inhibitors (eg, anastrolozole). Patients should be warned that pregnancy has been associated with disease progression. Those receiving antiestrogen therapy should receive aggressive preventive therapy for osteoporosis. Occasional case reports have suggested benefit in treatments such as interferon-α or somatostatin. Corticosteroids and cytotoxic immunosuppressive agents have no role in therapy.

Because of a lack of a convincingly effective therapy, it is necessary to manage the complications that arise in patients with LAM. Because of the likelihood of recurrence of pneumothoraces in patients with LAM, most recommend early surgical intervention. Air travel should be avoided as changes in cabin pressure may increase the risk of pneumothorax. Chylous effusions can be drained to provide symptom relief but this can result in the loss of significant amounts of protein and lymphocytes. There is a temptation to attempt thoracic duct ligation in these cases, but results have been variable and unpredictable and it is rarely recommended. Medium-chain triglyceride diets can help to reduce lymph production but are unpalatable and difficult to follow. Simple low-fat diets are an alternative.

The majority of renal angiomyolipomas in LAM are small and asymptomatic. Those likely to grow and to bleed are >4 cm and multiple. The computed tomographic appearance is characteristic, and biopsy is rarely needed to confirm the diagnosis. Treatment should be considered if angiomyolipomas bleed, cause significant discomfort, grow rapidly, or if they are large at the time of detection. Because of advances in interventional radiology, selective percutaneous embolization at the site of bleeding is the treatment of choice. Some patients require partial nephrectomy.

Despite the response to hormonal therapy, most patients with LAM experience a progressive decline in respiratory function and become candidates for lung transplantation. Guidelines for transplantation include progression despite medical treatment, FEV_1/FVC <50%, total lung capacity (TLC) >130%, FEV_1 <30%, and severe cystic disease on HRCT. Most patients receive a single lung transplant and survival in these patients appears to be comparable to those receiving single lung transplants for other indications. The main problems relating to LAM in transplantation are intraoperative pleural hemorrhage and postoperative chylothorax and pneumothorax in the native lung. LAM has recurred in three cases in the allograft (all male donors). HMB-45 staining may be useful to differentiate recurrent disease from chronic allograft rejection. Continued antiestrogen therapy has been advocated because of the potential for recurrence.

As described earlier, there appears to be an unknown relationship between LAM and TSC. The diagnosis of TSC is generally made on clinical grounds and the National Tuberous Sclerosis Association (NTSA) has established diagnostic criteria (Table 14–1). Angiomyolipomas and LAM are both secondary features and hence, based on NTSA criteria, patients would be described as having TSC. However, because none of the women with isolated LAM with or without renal angiomyolipomas (but no other features of TSC) has had a child with TSC, they presumably do not have a germ line mutation in either TSC-1 or TSC-2 and do not have TSC. All women with LAM should, however, undergo a careful family history and physical examination for occult stigmata of TSC and, in cases of doubt, should be seen by a clinical geneticist.

Prognosis

The natural history of LAM is one of progressive airflow limitation leading to respiratory failure and cor pulmonale. However, there is great individual variability and it is often difficult to predict the course of each patient. In some series, a decreased FEV_1/FVC ratio, an elevated TLC, worsening grades of abnormal areas on HRCT, and cystic lesions on lung biopsy have been associated with a poor prognosis. It is believed by most that these patients have a diminished life span compared to age-matched controls, but the anticipated life expectancy is uncertain. In one series, 78% (25 of 32) of patients were alive 8.5 years after disease onset whereas in another series 38% (10 of 26) of patients were alive at the same interval. Similarly, it is difficult to know which parameters should be followed to determine disease progression. A reasonable approach for follow-up is a subjective evaluation of symptoms, pulmonary function testing, and chest radiography every 6 months, plus exercise testing and/or HRCT every year. Those with a rapid progression of disease or those on track to reach end-stage disease within 2 years should undergo evaluation for transplantation.

Obviously, there is a need for an organized approach to study these patients. To obtain more data on LAM and promote investigation into the specific pathogenesis of the disease, the National Heart, Lung, and Blood Institute sponsors a volunteer national registry for patients with LAM (http://lam.uc.edu/LAM.htm). Similar organizations have been established in Great Britain and Europe. It is hoped that by collecting clinical information on these patients under the auspices of experienced clinicians, insight will be gained into this rare disease.

Johnson S: Lymphangioleiomyomatosis: clinical features, management, and basic mechanisms. Thorax 1999:54:254. [PMID: 10332654]. (This review emphasizes the relationship between LAM and TSC, the role of hormonal factors, and the involvement of gp100.)

Kalassian KG et al: Lymphangioleiomyomatosis: new insights. Am J Respir Crit Care Med 1997:155:1183. [PMID: 9105053]. (Short perspective article focuses on investigation of the pathogenesis of LAM.)

Kelly J et al: Lymphangioleiomyomatosis. Am J Med Sci 2001: 321:17. [PMID: 11202475]. (This review provides an overview of the clinical features of LAM.)

NHLBI workshop summary: report of workshop on lymphangioleiomyomatosis. Am J Respir Crit Care Med 1999:159:679. [PMID: 9927387]. (This article outlines the scientific basis behind the NHLBI recommendations for further research in LAM.)

Sullivan EJ: Lymphangioleiomyomatosis: a review. Chest 1998: 114:1689. [PMID: 9872207]. (Another review of the clinical aspects of LAM.)

BRONCHIOLITIS OBLITERANS WITH ORGANIZING PNEUMONIA

 ESSENTIALS OF DIAGNOSIS

- *Subacute onset of flu-like symptoms with fever, nonproductive cough, and exertional dyspnea.*
- *Mild to moderate decreases in diffusion capacity and a restrictive pattern may be seen on pulmonary function testing.*
- *Poorly defined, bilateral, asymmetric consolidation is seen in the majority on chest radiography.*
- *A definitive diagnosis requires adequate tissue to demonstrate that the characteristic intraalveolar buds of granulation tissue associated with fibroblasts, myofibroblasts, and loose connective tissue are a primary pathological feature.*
- *Presumptive diagnosis may be made on classic clinical and radiographic features.*
- *Generally, this is a corticosteroid-responsive disease with an excellent prognosis.*

General Considerations

Bronchiolitis obliterans with organizing pneumonia (BOOP) is thought to be a tissue response to an unknown injury that results in the accumulation of polypoid endobronchial connective tissue masses filling the lumens of terminal and respiratory bronchioles and extending into alveolar ducts and alveoli. This response is not in itself specific, but when coupled with associated clinicoradiological and pathological patterns, it defines a distinct syndrome that has been validated in multiple clinical series. The name of this syndrome has been contested, with many preferring BOOP and others proposing cryptogenic organizing pneumonia (COP), proliferative bronchiolitis, or bronchiolitis obliterans with intraluminal polyps. Regardless of its name, this syndrome should not be confused with bronchiolitis obliterans (BO), a rare disorder of the small airways, characterized histologically by stenotic, scarred, constrictive bronchiolitis and functionally by airway obstruction. BO is most often associated with rheumatoid arthritis, bone marrow transplantation, or chronic rejection following lung transplantation.

In most cases of BOOP, there is no identifiable cause. In large series, 70–90% of cases were idiopathic. Recognized secondary causes are protean and include postinfectious, drug-related, connective tissue-associated, postradiation, environment-related, and transplantation-related factors. Table 14–2 lists some of the many conditions associated with BOOP. Men and women are affected equally, and the majority of patients are in their sixth or seventh decade. However,

cases have been described spanning 21 to 80 years of age. Smoking does not appear to be a risk factor as the majority of patients are either nonsmokers or ex-smokers at the time of diagnosis. There has been little attention paid to any ethnic predilections. In fact, no clear predisposing factors have been identified in multiple series of patients with idiopathic BOOP.

Clinical Findings

A. SYMPTOMS AND SIGNS

The majority of patients with idiopathic BOOP complain of a characteristic constellation of symptoms. Generally, there is a subacute onset of complaints over 2–10 weeks. Initially, patients suffer from a flu-like ill-

Table 14–2. Secondary causes of BOOP.

Connective tissue disease	Organ transplantation
Rheumatoid arthritis	Bone marrow transplantation
Polymyositis and dermatomyositis	Lung transplantation
Systemic lupus erythematouis	Kidney transplantation
Progressive systemic sclerosis	Environmental exposures
Sjögren's syndrome	Textile printing dyes
Mixed connective tissue disease	*Penicillium* mold dust
Polymyalgia rheumatica	House fire
Behcet's disease	Infections
Polyarteritis nodosa	Bacterial
Ankylosing spondylitis	*Streptococcus pneumoniae*
Drugs	*Chlamydia*
Antibiotics	*Legionella*
Amphotericin B	*Mycoplasma*
Cephalosporins	*Coxiella burnetti*
Minocycline	*Nocardia asteroids*
Nitrofurantoin	Viral
Sulfasalazine	Adenovirus
Sulfamethoxypyridazine	Cytomegalovirus
Bleomycin	Influenza
Gold	Parainfluenza
Methotrexate	HIV
Naproxen	Other
Sulindac	Malaria
Amiodarone	*Pneumocystis*
Acebutolol	*Cryptococcus*
Interferon	Miscellaneous disorders
L-Tryptophan	Inflammatory bowel disease
Phenytoin	Lymphoma
Carbamazepine	Myelodysplastic syndrome
Ticlopidine	T cell chronic leukemia
Cocaine	Hunner interstitial cystitis
Immunological disorders	Chronic thyroiditis
Common variable immunodeficiency	Alcoholic cirrhosis
Essential mixed cryoglobulinemia	Primary biliary cirrhosis
Radiation therapy	Seasonal syndrome with cholestasis

ness with fever and a persistent, nonproductive cough. Exertional dyspnea (generally mild), malaise, and anorexia are also common. Less common symptoms include bronchorrhea, hemoptysis, chest pain, arthralgias, and night sweats. There have been infrequent cases of a rapidly progressive course leading to respiratory failure. The true etiology in these cases has been questioned with speculation that they may have represented acute interstitial pneumonia or acute respiratory distress syndrome (ARDS) rather than BOOP.

The physical examination of patients with BOOP is rarely distinctive. In fact, the examination is normal in at least 25% of patients. The most commonly described abnormality is inspiratory crackles. These are heard sparsely across the chest, presumably over affected areas, and are of a dry character, consistent with those heard in interstitial lung diseases.

B. Laboratory Findings

No specific laboratory findings are found in BOOP. However, ESR is often elevated and is > 60 mm/h in 30% of patients. Similarly, the C-reactive protein is often elevated. A mild leukocytosis is common with an increase in the percentage of segmented neutrophils. If seen, eosinophilia is mild. Autoantibodies are rarely positive and are of a low titer when present.

C. Pulmonary Function Testing

Most symptomatic patients have abnormalities on pulmonary function testing. Almost all patients have a mild to moderate decrease in the diffusing capacity for carbon monoxide. This leads to hypoxemia that is mild and is usually seen only during exertion. In addition to the decrease in diffusion capacity, a mild to moderate restrictive pattern is frequently found. Vital capacity is reduced, but flow rates are normal, consistent with a restrictive process.

D. Imaging Studies

1. Chest radiography—Several different patterns are seen on chest radiography in patients with BOOP. The most frequent presentation is alveolar infiltration. The consolidation is characteristically patchy, bilateral, and asymmetric. Air bronchograms may be seen. The abnormalities, which are often peripheral and more profuse in the lower lobes, gradually enlarge from the original site and new lesions may appear. They also may be spontaneously migratory. These lesions can vary in size from a few centimeters to lesions that occupy an entire lobe. Their borders are hazy but, in general, individual lesions can be easily discerned. This patchy consolidative pattern is seen in 70–90% of patients with idiopathic BOOP (Figure 14–6A–C) and is the most suggestive of the diagnosis.

The next most common radiographic pattern is a diffuse, bilateral infiltrative pattern that may be reticular, nodular, or reticulonodular. Alveolar shadows may be superimposed. This pattern is found in 10–40% of patients with BOOP.

The last major radiographic category of BOOP is a solitary focal lesion that often mimics lung cancer. These are most often seen in the upper lobes and may cavitate. Air bronchograms may also be seen within the lesions. This third pattern has been associated more commonly with chest pain and hemoptysis. Pleural effusions are uncommonly appreciated on chest radiography and, when present, are small.

2. High-resolution computed tomography—The HRCT scan recapitulates the findings on chest radiography and provides greater detail of the pattern. Alveolar opacities may range from areas of true consolidation to ground glass. The peripheral lesions often take a triangular shape with the base of the triangle at the pleura. Other opacities are found in a peribronchovascular distribution. Air bronchograms are better demonstrated on HRCT than on chest radiography (Figure 14–6D and E).

The diffuse interstitial pattern may be seen as multiple radial lines following the path of bronchi to the pleura or as subpleural lines without any relation to the bronchi. These lines are more common in the lower lobes and may be associated with multifocal areas of consolidation. Nodular opacities vary from 3 to 10 mm in diameter and may be round or irregular in shape. Bronchial wall thickening and mild bronchial dilation may be present, but true bronchiectasis is not part of the presentation of idiopathic BOOP. Similar to the patchy consolidation, the solitary lesions may be more obviously an alveolar filling process with air bronchograms on HRCT than on chest radiography. Pleural effusions are more commonly seen on HRCT (5–35%) but are small and are rarely associated with pleural thickening.

3. Bronchoalveolar lavage and lung biopsy—Although diagnosis by bronchoscopy with bronchoalveolar lavage and transbronchial biopsy is frequently pursued in patients with suspected BOOP, this can provide only supportive evidence for the diagnosis. Bronchoalveolar lavage fluid usually contains increased cellularity with a mixed population of inflammatory cells. Lymphocytes are most frequently increased and may be a marker of those patients likely to respond to corticosteroids. The lymphocyte CD4/CD8 ratio is decreased. The percentage of neutrophils and eosinophils may also be increased, but not to the degree of the lymphocytosis. Foamy alveolar macrophages, mast cells, and plasma cells may also be seen. Because of the small amount of tissue obtained with transbronchial biopsy, bronchioles

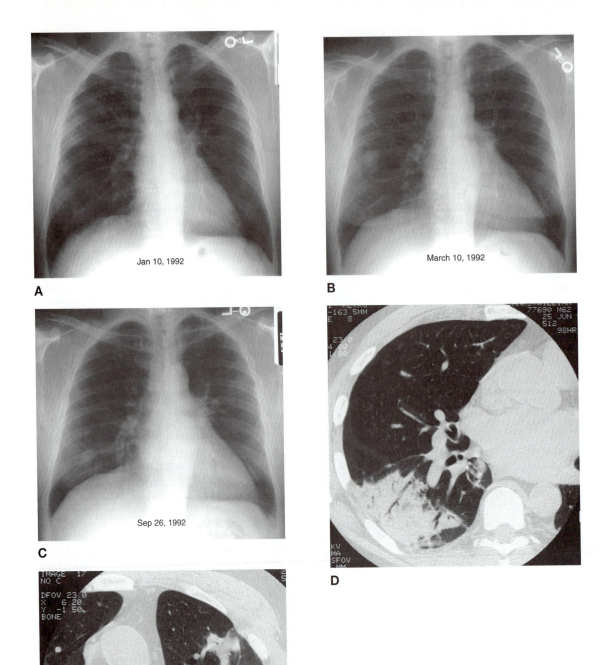

Jan 10, 1992

A

March 10, 1992

B

Sep 26, 1992

C

D

E

Figure 14–6. A 62-year-old man with recurrent migratory opacities due to BOOP. **A, B, C:** Chest radiographs show migratory poorly defined lung opacities of BOOP. **D, E:** HRCT images obtained during another exacerbation show bilateral patchy lung consolidation typical of BOOP.

may not be seen. Even in those instances in which distal airways are present, there is often not enough tissue to definitively determine whether BOOP is the dominant pathological process or simply is secondary to the primary process. In those patients with a characteristic clinical presentation and radiographic studies, a bronchoscopic biopsy may be sufficient to begin a trial of corticosteroid therapy. However, in those with an atypical presentation or lack of response to corticosteroids, a surgical lung biopsy should be considered. Because BOOP is thought to be a nonspecific reaction to lung injury, it may accompany a variety of underlying lung diseases, including vasculitis, chronic eosinophilic pneumonia, hypersensitivity pneumonitis, nonspecific interstitial pneumonitis, and usual interstitial pneumonitis (VIP). To make a definitive diagnosis of idiopathic BOOP, there must be adequate lung tissue to ensure that it is the main pathological feature and not an accessory to another lesion. For this reason, a surgical biopsy via video-assisted thoracoscopic surgery (VATS) is the preferred technique. This also allows the pathologist to provide an indication as to the severity of the process, which may guide the clinician in pursuing treatment and providing prognostic information.

Pathological examination in cases of BOOP shows intraalveolar buds of granulation tissue associated with fibroblasts, myofibroblasts, and loose connective tissue (Figure 14–7). A mixed population of inflammatory cells may be present in the granulation tissue, especially during the early stages of the process. The granulation tissue fills the lumens of terminal and respiratory bronchioles and extends in a continuous fashion into alveolar ducts and alveoli. These polypoid masses bear the eponymous name of "Masson bodies" after Masson's description of these lesions in patients with rheumatic pneumonia. The buds of connective tissue frequently extend from one alveolus to the adjacent one through the pores of Kohn, giving rise to a "butterfly" pattern. In fact, this lesion allowed for the initial description of these interalveolar conduits. Free airspaces may be filled with foamy alveolar macrophages. Chronic inflammation in the walls of surrounding alveoli may be seen in association with reactive type II pneumocytes. Despite these changes, the underlying lung architecture is preserved. This is in contrast to the findings in UIP. In UIP, intraluminal connective tissue may also be seen but the tissue appears to participate in the remodeling and destruction of the interstitium. The reason for the difference in clinical course in these two apparently related disorders is unknown. It has been suggested that this may be due to differences in angiogenesis as BOOP lesions have abundant capillaries whereas UIP lesions have minimal vascularity. A much higher apoptotic rate in BOOP lesions than in UIP suggests that apoptosis (programmed cell death) may play a role in the resolution of these abnormalities.

Treatment

Although there have been cases of spontaneous remission of BOOP lesions, the accepted treatment is corti-

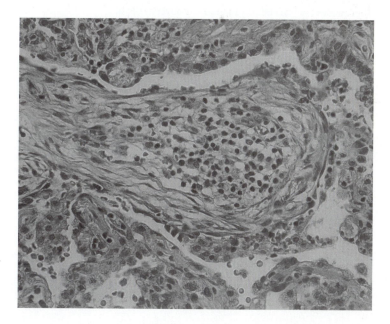

Figure 14–7. A surgical lung biopsy specimen from a patient with idiopathic BOOP. A well-formed exudate ("Masson body") composed of granulation tissue and mixed inflammatory cells is seen extending from the bronchiole and into the alveolar space.

costeroid therapy. However, the dose and duration of therapy are not well established. Most suggest initial doses of prednisone (or its equivalent dose of methylprednisolone) of between 0.75 and 1.5 mg/kg/day. This dose is maintained for 1–3 months and is then tapered over a period of 3–12 months. Because recurrences of BOOP are common as the dose of prednisone is decreased (usually at levels below 25 mg/day), most patients received corticosteroids for a minimum of 1 year in older series. However, these recurrences are easily treated with a return to higher doses and do not appear to affect the overall course or prognosis of BOOP. Therefore, attempts are now made to minimize the duration of therapy with an aggressive attempt to remove corticosteroid therapy in all patients and to provide more prolonged treatment only in those patients in whom BOOP recurs. While receiving corticosteroids, patients should receive therapy to reduce the impact of steroid-induced bone loss. Prophylaxis against *Pneumocystis* pneumonia should be strongly considered.

In patients with asymptomatic mass lesions or non-progressive disease, observation is reasonable. There are also anecdotal reports of slow improvement with prolonged erythromycin therapy and also with inhaled triamcinolone. In steroid-resistant cases, cyclophosphamide and azathioprine have been used with variable success. As most patients respond well to corticosteroids, there is little experience with lung transplantation in patients with BOOP.

Prognosis

In general, BOOP is a corticosteroid-responsive disease and carries an excellent prognosis. Between 65 and 80% of patients are cured without residua using corticosteroids alone. As mentioned, relapses are common (up to one-third of those treated for less than 1 year) but do not affect eventual cure. Some series suggest that the likelihood of recurrence is predicted by the degree of hypoxia at the time of diagnosis. A minority of patients has disease that is unresponsive to prednisone. Poor outcomes are predicted by an interstitial pattern on radiographs, a lack of bronchoalveolar lavage lymphocytosis, and histological scarring and remodeling of the lung parenchyma on biopsy. Those with secondary forms of BOOP, particularly those with connective tissue disease, have a poorer prognosis than those with the idiopathic form. Mortality in BOOP has been estimated at 3–13%. This is in stark contrast to patients with UIP, in whom survival longer than 5 years is uncommon. Epler's original series provides a good overview of the prognosis of patients with BOOP. In follow-up of 48 patients over an average of 4 years, 29 (60%) had a complete recovery, including five who did not receive any therapy. Thirteen (27%) stabilized with therapy and two (4%) suffered from progressive disease but were alive at the end of follow-up. Four patients died—two from BOOP and two from other causes. The five patients with BOOP in the presence of connective tissue disease had a worse prognosis than those with idiopathic disease.

In several small series it has been suggested that outcomes in BOOP may be more variable and worse than previously believed. Cases have been described of a rapidly progressive form of BOOP that presents following a few days of symptoms and quickly leads to respiratory failure as well as cases of BOOP that progress despite corticosteroid therapy and show significant disruption of the underlying lung architecture. Some dispute these findings and contend that these cases may not represent BOOP, but instead are cases of acute interstitial pneumonia, ARDS, or UIP. Others argue that these selected series do not represent the full spectrum of disease of BOOP and instead highlight the few instances in which the disease is unresponsive to therapy. Improved understanding of the pathogenesis of BOOP is likely to lead to a better appreciation of the course of clinical disease and more standard therapy.

Cordier JF: Organizing pneumonia. Thorax 2000:55:318. [PMID: 10722773]. (Primarily a clinical review but does include some insight into possible pathogenic mechanisms.)

Epler GR: Bronchiolitis obliterans organizing pneumonia. Arch Intern Med 2001:161:158. [PMID: 11176728]. (A concise review of the clinical, pathological, and radiological features of BOOP.)

Epler GR et al: Bronchiolitis obliterans organizing pneumonia. N Engl J Med 1985:312:152. [PMID: 3965933]. (An older paper that still provides relevant clinical information on the syndrome.)

Lynch DA: High-resolution CT of idiopathic interstitial pneumonias. Radiol Clin North Am 2001:39:1153. [PMID: 11699666]. (An excellent review of the radiological manifestations of the idiopathic lung diseases with comparisons of the various patterns of presentation. BOOP is compared to usual interstitial pneumonia, nonspecific interstitial pneumonia, desquamative interstitial pneumonia, respiratory bronchiolitis, lymphoid interstitial pneumonia, and diffuse alveolar damage.)

Acknowledgement: I would like to thank Carlyne Cool, MD for the pathological slides and David Lynch, MD for the radiologic studies.

SECTION IV

Diseases of the Alveolar Space

Acute Respiratory Distress Syndrome

15

Polly E. Parsons, MD

ESSENTIALS OF DIAGNOSIS

- *Acute onset of respiratory failure.*
- *Bilateral infiltrates consistent with pulmonary edema on chest radiograph.*
- *Hypoxemia.*
- *No evidence of left atrial hypertension.*

General Considerations

The acute respiratory distress syndrome (ARDS) was first formally described by Dr. Ashbaugh and colleagues in 1967. They reported a total of 12 cases of patients with acute respiratory failure with an overall mortality rate of 57%. The syndrome was defined in that initial description as the acute onset of severe hypoxemia that responded to initiation of mechanical ventilation with positive end-expiratory pressure (PEEP), diffuse bilateral infiltrates on chest radiograph, and decreased pulmonary compliance. Since that original description the definition of ARDS has been debated and refined. Definitions have evolved to better incorporate the clinical spectrum of disease that was recognized to occur and to try to better correlate the diagnostic definition with the pathophysiology of the syndrome. In 1994 a group of experts convened and developed the American–European Consensus Conference Committee definition that is currently utilized by most practitioners and investigators to identify ARDS. This definition has four components:

1. Acute onset of respiratory failure.
2. PaO_2/FIO_2: <300 mm Hg = acute lung injury (ALI) <200 mm Hg = acute respiratory distress syndrome (ARDS)
3. Chest radiograph: bilateral alveolar infiltrates consistent with pulmonary edema.
4. No evidence of left atrial hypertension. Pulmonary capillary wedge pressure <18 mm Hg if available.

In addition, the consensus document suggests that patients should have an identified risk factor for the development of ALI and should not have significant chronic lung disease. This definition incorporates the concept that there is a spectrum of disease. All patients with an arterial oxygen tension–pressure/fraction of inspired oxygen (PaO_2/FIO_2) ratio < 300 mm Hg have acute lung injury; only that subset with more severe hypoxemia, as reflected in a PaO_2/FIO_2 < 200 mm Hg, are now categorized as having ARDS.

The definition still has some elements that are being evaluated. The meaning of acute onset has been discussed. Studies of patients at risk for the development of ARDS have shown that the majority of patients who develop ARDS do so within 3–5 days so that is what most investigators use for the timeframe defined by acute. The chest radiograph description has also been identified as an area that needs to be more refined. Rubenfeld and colleagues had a panel of experts review a set of randomly selected radiographs from patients with PaO_2/FIO_2 < 300. They found that there was significant interobserver variability in the interpretation of these films. For example, the percentage of radiographs identified as being consistent with ALI varied from 36 to 71%. Accordingly, there is now a taskforce working to establish more rigid criteria for the interpretation of radiographs for this syndrome.

The diagnosis of left atrial hypertension may also be difficult. Recent studies suggest that as many as 25% of patients identified clinically as having ALI with no evidence of left atrial hypertension actually had pulmonary artery wedge pressures greater than 18 mm Hg when the measurements were made.

A number of clinical syndromes have been identified as risk factors for ALI (Table 15–1). The most common predisposing condition for ALI is sepsis. The incidence of ALI from sepsis ranges from approximately 30 to 50%, depending on the definition used for sepsis. Other common predisposing conditions include aspiration of gastric contents and severe trauma. Pneumonia is identified as a separate risk factor in some reviews and is incorporated under the category of sepsis in others. Risk factors can be further categorized as those associated with direct lung injury (ie, pneumonia and aspiration) and indirect lung injury (ie, nonthoracic trauma, nonpulmonary sepsis). Recent studies have found that there may be differences in some biological markers between risk factors (ie, sepsis and trauma) and in clinical response between categories of risk factors (ie, direct versus indirect injury). These observations may ultimately lead to better identification of patients who could benefit from specific therapeutic interventions.

Another recent observation that could impact development of specific therapeutic interventions is recognition that patients at risk for and with ALI are heterogeneous. These patients frequently have preexisting and comorbid conditions that have been found to impact both the incidence of ALI and mortality from the syndrome. For example, chronic alcohol abuse is associated with an increased incidence of ARDS, whereas diabetes mellitus is associated with a decreased incidence of ARDS.

The actual incidences of ALI and ARDS are still unclear. Initial estimates were made by a taskforce convened by the National Institutes of Health (NIH). That group established an incidence figure of approximately 71 patients/100,000 population in the United States.

Table 15–1. Risk factors for ARDS.

Sepsis
Aspiration of gastric contents
Trauma (thoracic or nonthoracic)
Hypertransfusion of blood products
Pancreatitis
Near drowning
Inhalation injury

Subsequent studies in the United States and other countries have yielded results ranging from 1.5 to 8 patients per 100,000 for ARDS and as high as 89 patients per 100,000 population for ALI. Studies are currently underway to better determine the incidence of this syndrome. Of note, the incidence of sepsis, the most common predisposing condition for ALI, is increasing in the United States.

Bernard GR et al: The American-European Consensus Conference on ARDS: definitions, mechanisms, relevant outcomes, and clinical trial coordination. Am J Respir Crit Care Med 1994;149:818. [PMID: 7509706]. (This is the classic article describing the current definitions of ALI and ARDS.)

Luce JM: Acute lung injury and the acute respiratory distress syndrome. Crit Care Med 1998;26:369. [PMID: 9468178]. (An excellent review of the definition and epidemiology of ARDS.)

Rubenfeld GD et al: Interobserver variability in applying a radiographic definition for ARDS. Chest 1999;116:1347. [PMID: 10559098]. (The original article that indicates the difficulty in chest radiograph interpretation.)

Ware LB, Matthay MA: The acute respiratory distress syndrome. N Engl J Med 2000;342:1334. [PMID: 10793167]. (An excellent review of all facets of ALI/ARDS.)

Pathogenesis

ALI/ARDS is characterized by injury to the alveolar epithelium and the microvascular endothelium. This injury results in an increase in permeability of the alveolar–capillary barrier and influx of fluid into the alveolar space. The original injury can be either direct or indirect, but in either case it appears that an inflammatory cascade is initiated. Inflammatory mediators and modulators are released both systemically and within the lung. Neutrophils are recruited to and retained within the lung where they release inflammatory mediators, including oxidants and proteases, that directly injure the lung and propagate the inflammatory process. The injury to the alveolar capillary barrier allows influx of protein-rich fluid that alters the integrity of the alveolar surfactant allowing further damage to occur. In many patients the process is ultimately self-limited and the alveolar capillary barrier is repaired. The mechanism by which the inflammatory cascade is shut off and the repair process is initiated is not known. In some patients the inflammatory process is not self-limited and they develop progressive fibrosis or fibrosing alveolitis.

Recent studies in animals and humans have shown that the inflammatory process can be aggravated by mechanical ventilation. In animal models, ventilation with high tidal volumes and/or low levels of PEEP can both cause and exacerbate ALI/ARDS. Lung injury in ALI/ARDS is heterogeneous with areas of dense atelectasis interspersed with areas of normal lung. The areas of normal lung are likely to be injured because they are hyperinflated when the patient is mechanically ventilated. The areas of atelectatic lung cyclically open and close with mechanical ventilation. This phenomenon is referred to as recruitment and derecruitment. Both overdistention and recruitment/derecruitment cause inflammation in animal models. Clinical trials have shown that ventilation with low tidal volumes decreases the inflammatory response as measured by decreased levels of inflammatory cytokines in both the systemic circulation and in the lung.

Ranieri VM et al: Effect of mechanical ventilation on inflammatory mediators in patients with acute respiratory distress syndrome: a randomized controlled trial. JAMA 1999;282:54. [PMID: 10404912]. (A clinical trial that showed that ventilation with low tidal volumes attenuated inflammation.)

Pathology

Histologically, the lung injury in ALI/ARDS is characterized as diffuse alveolar damage (DAD). The pattern of injury evolves through three phases, often referred to as the exudative phase, the proliferative phase, and the fibrotic phase, as the disease process progresses and then repairs. The exudative phase is characterized by development of interstitial and alveolar edema. Both the epithelium and the endothelium are injured early in the course of ALI/ARDS resulting in flooding of the alveolar space with a proteinaceous exudate. During the course of this early injury hyaline membranes, which characterize this phase of the illness, are formed. The proliferative phase can begin as early as 3 days into the course of ALI/ARDS. This phase is characterized by proliferation of type II pneumocytes with concomitant and subsequent development of fibrosis. The fibrotic phase occurs in patients with prolonged illness. During this phase total lung collagen increases and the lung becomes densely fibrotic. It is important to recognize that these three histological phases of injury and repair do not necessarily occur in all patients. Patients who recover rapidly may not progress to dense fibrosis. It is also important to recognize that although development of increased lung collagen is associated with increased mortality, patients with fibrosis do survive and may have significant resolution of their lung injury.

Tomashefski JF: Pulmonary pathology of acute respiratory distress syndrome. Clin Chest Med 2000;21:435. [PMID: 11019719]. (A detailed review of the pathology of ARDS.)

Prevention

There is no specific prevention for ALI or ARDS. Although the clinical risk factors for the syndrome have been identified there is no way to identify those patients at risk who will ultimately develop the syndrome. All preventive measures are directed at preventing the

risk factor (ie, trauma prevention, prevention of nosocomial infections, aspiration precautions, etc).

Clinical Manifestations

The clinical findings are nonspecific. Patients with ALI/ARDS present with acute onset of hypoxia and bilateral alveolar infiltrates consistent with pulmonary edema. There are no specific laboratory findings. Although ALI/ARDS are considered primary pulmonary processes, other organs are frequently involved. Development of multisystem organ failure in this patient population is generally referred to as multiple organ dysfunction syndrome (MODS). The involved organs include the central nervous system, kidneys, liver, hematological system, and cardiovascular system. Development of renal failure, hepatic dysfunction, central nervous system dysfunction, disseminated intravascular coagulation, or cardiogenic shock both individually and in aggregate increases mortality in patients with ALI/ ARDS.

Differential Diagnosis

The differential diagnosis is extensive as indicated in Table 15–2. The initial step in diagnosis is the determination that the patient has noncardiogenic pulmonary edema, thus eliminating cardiogenic pulmonary edema, a common cause of bilateral alveolar infiltrates on chest radiograph and hypoxia. Subsequent consideration of other entities in the differential diagnosis depends on clinical history [ie, high-altitude pulmonary edema (HAPE)], physical examination (ie, neurogenic pulmonary edema), laboratory assessment (ie, drug-in-

Table 15–2. Differential diagnosis.

Cardiogenic pulmonary edema
High-altitude pulmonary edema (HAPE)
Neurogenic pulmonary edema
Laryngospasm-induced pulmonary edema
Drug-induced pulmonary edema
    Heroin
    Salicylates
    Cocaine
Radiation pneumonitis
Fat embolism syndrome
Mitral stenosis with alveolar hemorrhage
Vasculitis
Hypersensitivity pneumonitis
Interstitial lung disease
(Pulmonary infections)
    Viral
    Bacterial
    Fungal

duced pulmonary edema), or other studies (ie, echocardiography for mitral stenosis).

Fat embolism syndrome (FES) may be difficult to distinguish from ALI/ARDS. History and physical examination are critical for this diagnosis. Patients who have sustained long bone fractures, particularly femur and pelvic fractures, are at risk for FES. FES usually occurs within 12–72 h of the injury and commonly presents with hypoxia and a chest radiograph consistent with pulmonary edema. Approximately 60% of patients have evidence of central nervous system (CNS) involvement manifest with symptoms ranging from agitation to coma. Many of the patients have a petechial rash across their thorax, axillae, and conjunctiva on physical examination. Neither laboratory tests, including urine, blood, and bronchoalveolar lavage for fat globules, nor chest radiograph are specific or sensitive for diagnosis of FES. Magnetic resonance imaging (MRI) may help with diagnosis in patients with CNS involvement.

The most difficult differential diagnostic category is pulmonary infection. This is listed in Table 15–2 at the bottom and in parentheses because distinguishing pure pulmonary infection from pulmonary infection with ALI may be difficult. Frequently patients with primary pulmonary infection develop ALI and frequently patients with ALI develop a nosocomial pulmonary infection. In both instances the ultimate diagnosis may be controversial. When a primary pulmonary infection actually becomes ALI may be subjective. For example, a patient with varicella pneumonia may present with bilateral alveolar infiltrates and hypoxia. Although the diagnosis may be evident if a lung biopsy was performed, these patients will be clinically indistinguishable from a patient with ALI. Therefore, they might be considered to have viral pneumonia and ALI or might be characterized as having just viral pneumonia. A potentially more straightforward example would be a patient with a left lower lobe pneumococcal pneumonia who develops bilateral alveolar infiltrates and hypoxemia. It is more likely that this patient had ARDS rather than an extension of the underlying pneumonia, although this possibility cannot be entirely ruled out. Therefore, it is not always possible to clearly distinguish pneumonia from ALI. The diagnosis of pneumonia in patients who have established ALI is discussed below.

Steinberg KP, Hudson LD: Acute lung injury and acute respiratory distress syndrome: the clinical syndrome. Clin Chest Med 2000;21:401. [PMID: 11019717]. (An excellent overview of the clinical syndrome.)

Complications

Patients with ALI/ARDS are critically ill and susceptible to all the complications associated with critical illness and intensive care unit (ICU) care. A common complication is nosocomial infection. This is a frequent cause of death in patients with ALI/ARDS so clinicians should be vigilant in monitoring for the occurrence of infection. Nosocomial pneumonia, in particular, may be difficult to diagnose in patients who already have bilateral infiltrates on chest radiographs and hypoxia. Fever, purulent sputum, increasing oxygen requirements, or increasing infiltrates on chest radiograph are signs of a possible nosocomial pulmonary infection. Initial assessment generally involves a routine gram stain and culture of expectorated or suctioned sputum. Fiberoptic bronchoscopy is performed in some patients to obtain specimens (bronchoalveolar lavage or protected brush specimens) for culture. There is some evidence that the use of quantitative cultures of bronchoscopically obtained lower respiratory tract secretions improves outcome in patients with ventilator-associated pneumonia. The best technique for obtaining material for quantitative culture continues to be debated.

Treatment

A. DRUGS

There is no specific drug treatment for ALI/ARDS. Numerous therapies directed at modulating inflammation have been tried. The list includes prostaglandin E_1, ketoconazole, N-acetylcysteine, and lisophylline. Corticosteroids have neither decreased the incidence of ARDS when administered to patients at risk nor decreased mortality from ARDS when administered early in the course. However, data from small studies suggest that the administration of corticosteroids to patients later in the course of ALI may be beneficial. This phase of the illness is referred to as late ARDS or the fibroproliferative phase of ARDS, a reflection of the pathological findings. The clinical diagnosis of late ARDS is usually made when a patient has severe, persistent hypoxemia on or about Day 7 of their illness. There is currently a large multicenter, randomized controlled trial of corticosteroids in late ARDS underway. Until the results of that study are available, most reviews do not recommend the routine use of corticosteroids in late ARDS.

Patients with ARDS have severe pulmonary hypertension and lack of resolution of this hypertension is associated with poor outcomes. This makes vasodilator therapy an attractive therapeutic option. Early studies with inhaled nitric oxide (NO) showed improvement in mortality. However, larger clinical trials did not confirm this finding, although pulmonary artery pressures were decreased and oxygenation increased in patients treated with NO. Currently inhaled NO is not recommended as routine therapy for ALI. Inhaled NO is used in some patients with refractory severe hypoxia.

Neonates with respiratory distress syndrome have a substantial improvement in mortality when treated with surfactant replacement therapy. There is a large body of evidence that suggests that adult patients with ARDS have significant surfactant dysfunction. These findings suggested that surfactant replacement therapy could benefit patients with ARDS. To date, however, no study has shown an improvement in survival with this therapy in adults. However, studies are ongoing to both improve the available surfactant preparations and the administration and delivery of the product.

Although there is no specific pharmacological therapeutic intervention for ALI/ARDS, there is now an effective intervention for the most common risk factor for ALI/ARDS, sepsis. The infusion of activated protein C substantially reduces mortality from severe sepsis. Although this agent has not been studied as a specific therapeutic agent for ALI/ARDS, a large percentage of patients in the sentinal clinical trial had multiple organ failure, required mechanical ventilation, and/or had the lungs identified as the primary source of infection.

B. MECHANICAL VENTILATION

The majority of patients with ALI require ventilatory support with endotracheal intubation and mechanical ventilation, although a small number may be treated with noninvasive ventilation alone. The appropriate way to manage the ventilator has been debated since ARDS was first described. Initial debates focused on use of PEEP. Addition of PEEP in most patients lowers FIO_2, but other potential benefits remain unproven. Initial studies failed to show that PEEP prevented the development of ARDS, but the debate on what level of PEEP is best in patients with established ALI/ARDS continues.

The concept that mechanical ventilation could cause or contribute to acute lung injury has been present for a long time. Animal models and early patient studies suggested that administration of either large volumes or extensive pressure to even a normal lung could cause damage. This has led to an intense search for the most appropriate way to manage the volumes and pressures delivered by mechanical ventilators. A group of NIH investigators recently completed a trial comparing tidal volumes of 12 mL/kg predicted body weight to 6 mL/kg predicted body weight. For this trial there was a fixed FIO_2/PEEP algorithm for all patients and plateau pressures were limited. In the study mortality was 39.8% in the 12 mL/kg group and 31.3% in the 6 mL/kg group. Although the study methods were not entirely the same, this confirmed results from an earlier smaller trial of what is now called lung protective ventilation.

C. PATIENT POSITIONING

Most critically ill patients on mechanical ventilation are kept in the supine position. However, in animal models and in patient studies, oxygenation has been shown to increase with prone positioning. This led to a large, recently completed clinical trial that found oxygenation did increase in patients with ALI/ARDS who were prone, but there was no change in mortality. Despite the lack of survival benefit, many experts recommend placing a patient in the prone position if oxygenation is difficult. The placement of a patient in the prone position is not without risk. During the change in position, equipment such as the endotracheal tube and indwelling lines can become dislodged. Care has to be taken to prevent skin ulcers in dependent areas. Currently, the optimal timing for initiation of the prone position and the optimal duration of the prone position are not known.

D. FLUID MANAGEMENT

Optimal fluid management of patients with ALI is also an area of controversy. Fluid management needs to balance the need for optimal organ perfusion with problems of fluid extravasation into the lungs and tissues that results from severe epithelial and endothelial injury. The focus is often on maintaining adequate perfusion without harming oxygenation. Achieving this goal often requires minimizing fluid resuscitation. Conversely, there was also a focus on increasing oxygen delivery to decrease the incidence of multiple organ dysfunction syndrome. Extensive studies have now shown that maximizing oxygen delivery does not offer a therapeutic benefit. Therefore, the optimal fluid management in these patients remains unknown. Also unknown are the indications for insertion of pulmonary artery catheters (PAC). In early studies of ARDS, diagnosis required measurement of the pulmonary artery capillary wedge pressure to exclude cardiogenic pulmonary edema, so many patients had PAC in place. Now that actual measurements are not needed for diagnosis and there is no evidence that maximizing oxygen delivery, which also required PAC measurements, improves outcomes, the indications for PAC insertion are not clear. There is evidence that the insertion of PAC may be associated with an increase in mortality in some patient groups, so routine insertion of PAC is not without problems.

Acute Respiratory Distress Syndrome Network. Ventilation with lower tidal volumes as compared with traditional tidal volumes for acute lung injury and the acute respiratory distress syndrome. N Engl J Med 2000;342:1301. [PMID: 10793162]. (The largest trial that has shown the benefit of protective lung ventilation.)

Bernard GR et al: Efficacy and safety of recombinant human activated protein C for severe sepsis. N Engl J Med 2001; 344:699. [PMID: 11236773]. (Description of the clinical trial of the only effective therapeutic intervention in sepsis.)

Brower RG et al: Treatment of ARDS. Chest 2001;120:1347. [PMID: 11591581]. (Review of treatments available for ARDS.)

Gattinoni L et al: Effect of prone positioning on the survival of patients with acute respiratory failure. N Engl J Med 2001; 345:568. [PMID: 11529210]. (The most recent study of prone positioning in ARDS.)

McIntyre RC et al: Thirty years of clinical trials in acute respiratory distress syndrome. Crit Care Med 2000;28:3314. [PMID: 11008997]. (Excellent review of the therapeutic interventions that have been studied in ARDS. Focuses on how to review the existing evidence to determine whether a therapy should or should not be considered.)

www.ardsnet.org (The web site for the NIH:NHLBI ARDS network, a group dedicated to the study of ARDS.)

Prognosis

In the original description of ARDS mortality was 57% and a mortality of 50–60% was frequently quoted for the syndrome. However, investigators have shown that mortality is not the same for all patients. It varies with risk factor, with extent of multiple organ dysfunction, and with some preexisting and comorbid conditions. Patients with ALI following trauma have lower mortality than patients with sepsis-related ALI. Patients with pure pulmonary involvement tend to have lower mortality than patients with multiple organ involvement. Patients who have abused alcohol have higher mortality than those who do not. Thus, there are figures for mortality for all patients in aggregate, but the actual mortality rate for each patient is variable.

Of significant interest is the observation that the mortality rate for ARDS has decreased. Currently, mortality for control groups in most clinical trials of ARDS is approximately 40%. These trials tend to exclude some of the more critically ill patients and/or those with the highest mortality, but even in epidemiological studies of ALI/ARDS the mortality rate has fallen from 50–70% to below 40%. The reason for this decline is not known. It occurred before lung protective ventilation appeared to be in widespread use and before the advent of activated protein C therapy for sepsis.

Function of patients who survive ARDS remains an area of study. The initial focus was on the pulmonary function of this group. In the absence of any large, long-term studies of pulmonary function, absolute conclusions cannot be drawn. However, review of the literature suggests that many patients who survive have essentially normal lung function by 6–12 months. Those who have the most severe ARDS quantified by degree of hypoxia and duration of mechanical ventilation are more likely to have residual pulmonary impairment.

More recently, attention has focused on the overall well-being of survivors. Using extensive health status questionnaires investigators have found that this group of patients has an overall decreased quality of life—related to both general health and pulmonary health. This impairment is recognized even when ARDS survivors are compared with patients who were similarly critically ill but who did not have ARDS. Identifying the cause of this reduction in quality of life remains the focus of extensive investigation.

Abel SJC et al: Reduced mortality in association with the acute respiratory distress syndrome (ARDS). Thorax 1998;53:292. [PMID: 9741374]. (One of several studies demonstrating the decrease in mortality in ARDS.)

Davidson TA et al: Reduced quality of life in survivors of acute respiratory distress syndrome compared with critically ill control patients. JAMA 1999;281:354. [PMID: 9929089]. (A well-designed clinical study of quality of life in survivors of ARDS. Used similarly critically ill patients as the control study group.)

Schelling G et al: Health-related quality of life and posttraumatic stress disorder in survivors of the acute respiratory distress syndrome. Crit Care Med 1998;26:651. [PMID: 9559601]. (Describes the incidence of characteristics of the decreased quality of life seen in survivors of ARDS.)

Eosinophilic Pneumonias

16

Jason S. Vourlekis, MD

ESSENTIALS OF DIAGNOSIS

- *Eosinophilic pneumonia is defined by the presence of pulmonary infiltrates and the demonstration of either peripheral blood eosinophilia, bronchoalveolar lavage fluid eosinophilia, or lung tissue eosinophilia.*
- *Eosinophilic pneumonia is classified as acute or chronic.*
- *Acute eosinophilic pneumonia presents with the rapid onset of lower respiratory tract symptoms, often culminating in acute respiratory failure.*
- *Chronic eosinophilic pneumonia has a subacute to chronic presentation associated with systemic symptoms and peripheral blood eosinophilia.*
- *Drug toxicity can cause both acute eosinophilic pneumonia and chronic eosinophilic pneumonia and should be ruled out in all cases.*

General Considerations

The eosinophilic pneumonias represent a heterogeneous group of diseases that shares the common feature of eosinophilic infiltration of lung tissue resulting in an airspace pattern on chest radiograph. Generally, the eosinophilia is defined by either: (1) pulmonary infiltrates with peripheral blood eosinophilia, (2) tissue biopsy of the lungs, or (3) bronchoalveolar lavage. Traditionally, eosinophilic pneumonia is divided into acute and chronic forms based on the clinical presentation and course. Acute eosinophilic pneumonia generally occurs in previously healthy individuals and represents a rapidly progressive disease that often culminates in acute respiratory failure. Corticosteroid therapy is very effective and relapse is extremely rare. In contrast, chronic eosinophilic pneumonia presents with a slower onset of symptoms, often in persons with a prior history of asthma or sinusitis. Corticosteroids control the disease but relapses off therapy are common. Careful attention in the history and physical examination should be given to identifying secondary causes of eosinophilic pneumonia such as medication toxicity.

ACUTE EOSINOPHILIC PNEUMONIA

Acute eosinophilic pneumonia is a rapidly progressive disease generally seen in healthy adults. There is no gender predilection. An association with the acquired immunodeficiency syndrome has been reported.

Pathogenesis

There is no known cause of acute eosinophilic pneumonia. It has been speculated that it represents an allergic response to exogenous stimuli. Bronchoalveolar lavage, which samples the alveolar air spaces, has revealed an increased number of eosinophils and an increased concentration of interleukin-5, an eosinophil chemoattractant, in patients with acute eosinophilic pneumonia. Lung biopsy reveals diffuse infiltration of alveolar spaces by eosinophils and alveolar macrophages, accompanied by a proteinaceous exudate, hyaline membranes, and interstitial expansion by eosinophils. In contrast to chronic eosinophilic pneumonia, the alveolar exudate and hyaline membranes imply an acute airspace injury and microabscesses and focal necrosis are not present.

Clinical Findings

Acute eosinophilic pneumonia is characterized initially by flu-like symptoms including fever, malaise, myalgias, and cough. Shortness of breath develops rapidly over 1 to 5 days with most patients seeking medical attention within the first week. Physical examination is notable for fever, tachycardia, hypoxia, and crackles on auscultation. Initially chest radiographs may show predominantly an interstitial pattern that rapidly progresses to diffuse, airspace disease. Small pleural effusions have been noted. Laboratory studies are notable for the absence of peripheral blood eosinophilia.

Differential Diagnosis

The diagnostic criteria for acute eosinophilic pneumonia are: (1) an acute febrile illness of less than 5 days duration; (2) hypoxic respiratory failure; (3) a mixed alveolar–interstitial or diffuse alveolar pattern on chest x-ray; (4) bronchoalveolar lavage eosinophilia (>25% eosinophils); (5) absence of other causes of eosinophilic lung disease; (6) a prompt response to corticosteroids; and (7) failure to relapse following discontinuation of therapy. At its initial presentation, acute eosinophilic pneumonia must be differentiated from all other causes of rapid-onset respiratory failure (Table 16–1). Given that peripheral eosinophilia is rarely seen in acute eosinophilic pneumonia, and if present suggests an alternative diagnosis, the confirmation of acute eosinophilic pneumonia requires the performance of either bronchoalveolar lavage or lung biopsy. Bronchoalveolar lavage, performed by instillation and subsequent aspiration of sterile normal saline within a subsegment of a lobe, can be used to obtain material for culture and to sample the inflammatory cell milieu. In acute eosinophilic pneumonia, eosinophils constitute at least 25% and often 50–60% of the total leukocytes re-

Table 16–1. Differential diagnosis of acute eosinophilic pneumonia.

Acute interstitial pneumonitis	Rapid onset of acute respiratory failure of unknown causation. The case fatality rate is 50–80%. Distinguished from acute eosinophilic pneumonia by bronchoalveolar lavage that reveals neutrophilia on biopsy.
Acute respiratory distress syndrome	Typically caused by an underlying condition, eg, pancreatitis, multiple blood transfusions, trauma, which is readily identified.
Cryptogenic organizing pneumonia	Can have a subacute to fulminant onset. The fulminant form is associated with a toxic exposure such as chemotherapy or radiation therapy involving the chest, or connective tissue disease. In the absence of an exposure history, biopsy is necessary.
Diffuse alveolar hemorrhage	Presents with shortness of breath with or without hemoptysis. Distinguished from acute eosinophilic pneumonia by bronchoalveolar lavage, which returns sanguineous fluid. Lung biopsy may be necessary for diagnosis of the underlying cause.
Drug-induced lung disease	Clinically may be differentiated from idiopathic acute eosinophilic pneumonia only by identification and removal of the causative agent.
Hypersensitivity pneumonitis	Typically, an exposure history that precedes the onset of symptoms is readily available. Eosinophilia on lavage is generally < 20% of total leukocyte count.

covered by bronchoalveolar lavage. In the absence of such eosinophilia, acute eosinophilic pneumonia is unlikely and another disease should be considered.

Acute interstitial pneumonitis is a fulminant lung disease characterized by the rapid onset of cough, shortness of breath, and diffuse airspace densities on chest x-ray. Most patients progress to acute respiratory failure and require mechanical ventilation. Acute interstitial pneumonitis is distinguished from acute eosinophilic pneumonia by the absence of bronchoalveolar lavage eosinophilia. Treatment with high-dose, parenteral corticosteroids is recommended, although its efficacy is unproven. The case fatality rate is greater than 50% and some survivors will die of either progressive pulmonary fibrosis or relapse.

Acute respiratory distress syndrome (ARDS) is an inflammatory response of the lungs to a systemic insult such as infection, pancreatitis, or trauma. Generally, the etiology of acute respiratory distress syndrome is readily identified, making it easy to differentiate from acute eosinophilic pneumonia. In ambiguous cases, bronchoalveolar lavage will reveal neutrophilia in ARDS in contradistinction to the eosinophilia seen with acute eosinophilic pneumonia.

Cryptogenic organizing pneumonia generally presents in a subacute to a chronic manner with the gradual onset of cough and shortness of breath. A more fulminant form has been reported that has a case fatality ratio of nearly 70%. In such cases, there is often an underlying history of connective tissue disease, radiation therapy, or drug therapy that helps distinguish it from acute eosinophilic pneumonia.

Diffuse alveolar hemorrhage is a clinical syndrome characterized by bleeding into airspaces. There are multiple causes of diffuse alveolar hemorrhage including Wegener's granulomatosis, antiglomerular basement membrane syndrome (Goodpasture's syndrome), systemic coagulopathy, and mitral stenosis. Diffuse alveolar hemorrhage may present with the rapid onset of fever, shortness of breath, and diffuse, airspace densities on chest x-ray. Hemoptysis often is not an initial symptom. Bronchoalveolar lavage reveals bloody or blood-tinged fluid that fails to clear with repeated lavage of the same subsegment of the lung. Surgical lung biopsy is frequently required for definitive diagnosis of the underlying disease.

Drug-induced lung disease must always be considered in the differential diagnosis of acute eosinophilic pneumonia. Table 16–2 contains a partial list of drugs and drug classes associated with eosinophilic lung disease. Withdrawal of the offending agent coupled with corticosteroid therapy often results in prompt improvement.

Hypersensitivity pneumonitis may present with acute symptoms of fever, cough, and shortness of breath,

Table 16–2. Partial list of drugs and drug classes associated with eosinophilic pneumonia.

Bicalutamide
Carbamazepine
Chlorpromazine
Crack cocaine
Dapsone
Desipramine
Ethambutol
Methotrexate
Montelukast
Nitrofurantoin
Nonsteroidal antiinflammatory drugs
Penicillin antibiotics
Phenytoin
Ranitidine
Salicylates
Sulfa drugs
Tetracycline
Trazodone
Valproic acid
Venlafaxine
Zafirlukast

typically developing within several hours of exposure to an antigen. Hypersensitivity pneumonitis is caused by an immunological response to an inhaled antigen, typically organic protein such as a microbe or microbial spore or bird dander. Farmer's lung disease, a common form of hypersensitivity pneumonitis, may present acutely following exposure to thermophilic actinomycetes within moldy hay. On bronchoalveolar lavage, eosinophilia may be present but usually with < 20% eosinophils. Withdrawal of exposure coupled with corticosteroid therapy leads to a rapid, clinical response.

Treatment

Once the diagnosis of acute eosinophilic pneumonia has been established, treatment with parenteral corticosteroids should begin. An optimal dose of corticosteroids has not been established however. Generally, 60 or 125 mg of methylprednisolone given every 6 h is rapidly effective, usually within 24–48 h. After 3 days of parenteral therapy, patients may be changed to oral prednisone at 40–60 mg/day. This dosage is continued for 2 weeks and then tapered off over the subsequent 2 weeks.

Prognosis

Acute respiratory failure requiring mechanical ventilation is the main complication of acute eosinophilic pneumonia. With early recognition and treatment of the disease, most patients do not progress to this stage. There is one reported fatality in acute eosinophilic pneumonia attributed to a complicating nosocomial pneumonia. The long-term prognosis for acute eosinophilic pneumonia is excellent. Most patients show a prompt response to corticosteroids and have complete resolution of their disease. As a rule, relapses do not occur and if suspected, an alternative diagnosis, such as chronic eosinophilic pneumonia or Churg–Strauss syndrome should be considered. Longitudinal follow-up studies suggest progressive recovery of lung function in all patients.

CHRONIC EOSINOPHILIC PNEUMONIA

Chronic eosinophilic pneumonia was first described in nine patients presenting with several months' history of productive cough, shortness of breath, fever, and persistent infiltrates on chest x-ray. The patients shared the common features of peripheral blood eosinophilia and lung tissue eosinophilia and showed a prompt therapeutic response to corticosteroid treatment.

Pathogenesis

Chronic eosinophilic pneumonia is, by definition, an idiopathic disorder. Current research has demonstrated the central role of the eosinophil in producing the lung tissue inflammation. Eosinophils are capable of releasing major basic protein, eosinophil cationic protein, and other inflammatory mediators resulting in local tissue destruction. Lung biopsy in chronic eosinophilic pneumonia reveals dense eosinophilic infiltration of alveolar spaces and septa. The interstitium is edematous and eosinophilic microabscesses may be seen. Other prominent inflammatory cells, including macrophages, lymphocytes, and plasma cells, form part of the cellular infiltrate. The roles of these latter cells in chronic eosinophilic pneumonia are not well characterized.

Clinical Findings

The onset of chronic eosinophilic pneumonia is insidious. The average patient has symptoms for several months prior to diagnosis. The disease is more common in women (male/female ratio of 2:1) with the peak prevalence of chronic eosinophilic pneumonia occurring in the third and fourth decades of life. Fever, cough, dyspnea, malaise, and sputum production are present in most patients. Night sweats, pleurisy, and myalgias have been reported. Hemoptysis occurs in 9%. Fifty percent of patients will have a preceding diagnosis of asthma.

Laboratory studies are remarkable for moderate peripheral blood eosinophilia, which is present in nearly

90% of patients. The average eosinophil count is 3000/mm^3 but counts as high as 20,000/mm^3 have been reported. Mild anemia of chronic disease and thrombocytosis also have been reported. When tested, the erythrocyte sedimentation rate is typically greater than 60 mm/h. Serum immunoglobulin E (IgE) levels are elevated in 50% of patients and may be as high as 1000 IU/mL.

The classic chest radiographic appearance of chronic eosinophilic pneumonia is the "photonegative of pulmonary edema," ie, peripheral consolidative airspace densities, located in the upper and midlung zones. This pattern is seen in approximately 33% of cases. Other radiographic patterns include central infiltrates, atelectasis, and lung nodules. Computed tomography scanning reveals adenopathy in 50% of cases.

Differential Diagnosis

The diagnosis of chronic eosinophilic pneumonia is, in part, a diagnosis of exclusion as it requires ruling out other causes of eosinophilic lung disease as discussed below (Table 16–3). In a patient without any other identifiable cause of eosinophilic lung disease and with the characteristic clinical features of chronic respiratory symptomatology, peripheral eosinophilia, and typical radiographic appearance, the diagnosis can be confidently established by demonstrating the presence of pulmonary eosinophilia by bronchoalveolar lavage fluid. A bronchoalveolar lavage fluid leukocyte composition of >20% eosinophils is consistent with chronic eosinophilic pneumonia. Surgical lung biopsy is generally not necessary to establish the diagnosis.

Allergic bronchopulmonary mycosis (ABPM) is a disorder of the airways characterized by cough, mucus production, wheezing, and fleeting, patchy airspace densities on chest radiography. Peripheral eosinophilia may be present but eosinophils rarely exceed 1000/mm^3. In most cases, the antigenic fungus is an *Aspergillus* species but other fungi including *Penicillium, Curvularia,* and *Candida* have been implicated. The mechanism of disease involves an IgE-mediated allergic response to the offending fungus. The diagnosis is established by physiological demonstration of airflow limitation [forced expiratory volume/forced vital capacity (FEV$_1$/FVC) ratio <0.7], serum IgE level >1000 IU/mL, evidence of hyperreactivity to *Aspergillus* demonstrated by both skin prick testing and *Aspergillus*-specific IgE antibodies, and a history of pulmonary infiltrates. In most cases, high-resolution computed tomography scanning demonstrates central bronchiectasis as well. Glucocorticoids provide first-line therapy for

Table 16–3. Differential diagnosis of chronic eosinophilic pneumonia.

Allergic bronchopulmonary mycosis	An allergic disorder of the airways producing asthma-type symptoms. Suspect in patients with hard to control asthma. Serum IgE level is a good initial screen but a normal level in a patient on corticosteroids does not exclude the diagnosis.
Churg–Strauss syndrome	A systemic vasculitis of the respiratory tract, with the triad of sinus disease, asthma, and peripheral eosinophilia. Biopsy demonstrating eosinophilic infiltration of blood vessels is required for definitive diagnosis.
Cryptogenic organizing pneumonia	Radiographically, the subacute and chronic forms may mimic chronic eosinophilic pneumonia. The absence of both peripheral and bronchoalveolar eosinophilia essentially rules out other chronic eosinophilic pneumonia. Lung biopsy may be necessary to establish the diagnosis.
Drug-induced lung disease	In the differential diagnosis of chronic eosinophilic pneumonia, drug-induced lung disease must always be ruled out by careful review of health products including over-the-counter, herbal, and vitamin supplements.
Helminthic infection	Typically caused by *Ascaris lumbricoides* or *Strongyloides stercoralis*, patients complain of episodic cough and wheezing. More common in residents of rural, socioeconomically depressed regions. Identification of the parasite in feces, bronchoalveolar lavage fluid, or lung tissue establishes the diagnosis.
Idiopathic hypereosinophilic syndrome	A progressive disorder characterized by peripheral blood eosinophilia and eosinophilic infiltration of tissue. It is distinguished from chronic eosinophilic pneumonia by the presence of extrapulmonary disease and the relatively poor response to corticosteroids.
Loeffler's syndrome	Characterized by migratory pulmonary infiltrates and peripheral eosinophilia. Most reported cases likely represent helminthic infections.
Tropical pulmonary eosinophilia	A chronic parasitic infection that is generally seen only in people with at least several months^2 residence in Southeast Asia.

treatment of ABPM. The antifungal drug itraconazole, which may reduce the fungal burden in ABPM, has been shown to provide a steroid-sparing effect. Clinically, ABPM may be confused with chronic eosinophilic pneumonia, but typically is distinguished by the fleeting infiltrates, the presence of bronchiectasis, and the evidence of hyperreactivity to *Aspergillus* species.

Churg–Strauss syndrome is an inflammatory disorder of the blood vessels that affects many organs but most commonly the sinuses, lungs, skin, heart, and nervous system. Churg–Strauss syndrome affects people of all ages. The disease manifests insidiously over months to years. Patients may initially present with allergic rhinitis, followed by the later development of asthma. Ultimately a systemic vasculitis develops. The disease should be considered in any patient who presents with multisystem disease and peripheral eosinophilia. The presence of any four of the following six criteria is highly suggestive of Churg–Strauss syndrome: (1) asthma, (2) peripheral blood eosinophilia (>10% eosinophils of total leukocyte count), (3) mono- or polyneuropathy, (4) migratory pulmonary infiltrates, (5) acute or chronic paranasal sinus disease, and (6) biopsy confirmation of eosinophilic infiltration of blood vessels including arteries, arterioles, or venules. It is important to distinguish Churg–Strauss syndrome from chronic eosinophilic pneumonia because the former responds best to the combination of cyclophosphamide and glucocorticoid therapy and may progress on glucocorticoid therapy alone, potentially resulting in permanent debilitation or death.

Cryptogenic organizing pneumonia, formerly known as bronchiolitis obliterans with organizing pneumonia or BOOP, radiographically mimics chronic eosinophilic pneumonia. Like chronic eosinophilic pneumonia, cryptogenic organizing pneumonia may present with multifocal, peripheral airspace consolidative infiltrates on chest x-ray. Cryptogenic organizing pneumonia often can be distinguished from chronic eosinophilic pneumonia by the absence of peripheral blood eosinophilia, although a small number of cases (fewer than 15%) of chronic eosinophilic pneumonia will also lack peripheral blood eosinophilia. In such cases, the diagnosis of chronic eosinophilic pneumonia may be established by the demonstration of bronchoalveolar lavage eosinophilia.

Drug toxicity constitutes the most common cause of chronic eosinophilic pneumonia. Table 16–2 contains a partial list of drugs and drug classes that have been associated with this disease. Important points to remember in evaluating possible drug toxicity are: (1) making a diagnosis of pulmonary drug toxicity requires a high index of suspicion, (2) drug toxicity can occur months to years after the initiation of a therapy even if

there is no prior history of toxicity to that drug, and (3) to elicit a complete and comprehensive history of all medical products used including prescription medications, herbal supplements, over-the-counter medication, and illegal drugs. In rare instances, rechallenge with the offending agent may be indicated to confirm a diagnosis of drug toxicity.

Helminthic infection should be considered in the differential diagnosis of chronic eosinophilic pneumonia. In the United States, *Strongyloides stercoralis, Ascaris lumbricoides,* and *Toxocara canis* are the most common parasitic infections associated with peripheral eosinophilia and pulmonary infiltrates, but other parasites, including *Ancyclostoma brasiliense, Ancyclostoma duodenale, Necator americanus,* and *Trichinella spiralis* have been implicated. In strongyloidiasis and ascariasis, the pulmonary infiltrates are often focal airspace densities that are fleeting. The infiltrates are caused by larval migration into the alveolar spaces causing a localized inflammatory reaction. The larvae enter the bloodstream by penetration of the skin after exposure via contaminated soil. Associated symptoms include cough, wheezing, and fever. Peripheral eosinophilia is a common finding in both strongyloidiasis and ascariasis. The demonstration of the parasite in feces, bronchoalveolar lavage fluid, or lung tissue establishes the diagnosis. Immunocompromised patients infected with *Strongyloides* are at risk for developing the hyperinfection syndrome. This potentially devastating complication has a case fatality rate of nearly 80%. In the normal life cycle of the helminth, the adult worms migrate to the gut by advancing up the respiratory tract and down the esophagus. The adult worms reproduce in the gut, causing the shedding of immature larval forms in the stool. In at-risk immunocompromised hosts, the larvae may penetrate the gut wall, directly entering the bloodstream. This breach of a critical barrier defense is associated with translocation of gram-negative bacteria into the bloodstream, leading to bacteremia, sepsis, and ARDS. Peripheral eosinophilia often is not present and the diagnosis is made incidentally or by a high index of suspicion in at-risk individuals.

Toxocara canis, the dog roundworm, causes visceral larva migrans. Pulmonary involvement is manifest by symptoms of cough and wheezing and patchy airspace infiltrates on chest radiograph. The diagnosis is established by the appropriate clinical presentation, history of dog exposure, and the presence of anti-*Toxocara* antibodies. Treatment is not indicated, as visceral larva migrans typically is a self-limited disease.

Idiopathic hypereosinophilic syndrome is a systemic disorder characterized by eosinophilic infiltration of multiple organ systems. In some cases, idiopathic hypereosinophilic syndrome represents a clonal disorder of T-lymphocytes resulting in exuberant expression of interleukin-5, a cytokine that promotes the differentiation of eosinophils. Most patients present with generalized symptoms of fever, anorexia, and weight loss. The diagnosis of idiopathic hypereosinophilic syndrome is established by the persistence of peripheral blood eosinophilia (1500 eosinophils/ mm³) for more than 6 months, absence of any secondary causes of eosinophilia, and end-organ damage related to eosinophilic infiltration. In particular, involvement of the heart, nervous system, intestine, skin, kidneys, joints, and muscles has been reported. Pulmonary disease is manifest by diffuse interstitial and airspace infiltrates, pleural effusions, and thromboembolic disease. Corticosteroids are used as first line therapy, although response rates are less than 50%. Other drugs that have been used include hydroxyurea, vincristine, cyclosporin, and etoposide. Recent reports suggest that interferon-α therapy may be effective.

Löeffler's syndrome was first described in 1932. It is characterized by migratory pulmonary infiltrates and peripheral blood eosinophilia. Symptoms include episodic cough, wheezing, and shortness of breath although many patients are asymptomatic. It is now believed that most cases represented pulmonary ascariasis, which was endemic at the time of the original description.

Tropical pulmonary eosinophilia (TPE) is a parasitic infection caused by both *Wucheria bancrofti* and *Brugia malayi* that is most commonly seen in residents of Southeast Asia. Clinically, patients present with generalized symptoms of fever, malaise, anorexia, and weight loss. Respiratory symptoms include cough (often nocturnal), wheezing, and dyspnea. Peripheral blood leukocytosis and eosinophilia are common laboratory findings along with elevated serum IgE antibody levels. Chest radiographic patterns in TPE include reticulonodular densities, hilar adenopathy, and pleural effusion. The diagnosis is often made on clinical grounds alone in a person with the appropriate exposure history of residence of at least several months in an endemic area. Microfilariae may be recovered from bronchoalveolar lavage fluid and lung or lymph node tissue, although most experts do not recommend such invasive measures. A favorable response to treatment with diethylcarbamazine (DEC) is accepted as confirmation of the diagnosis.

Treatment

Corticosteroids are first line therapy for chronic eosinophilic pneumonia with most patients enjoying complete or near complete responses. Initial dose recommendations are 1 mg/kg lean body weight per day for 2 weeks, followed by therapy every other day for 2 weeks.

The response to corticosteroids is often immediate and nearly complete within 2 weeks. After the first month, a slow taper should be initiated with a plan to discontinue therapy by 6 months. Up to 20% of patients will relapse while corticosteroids are being tapered. In some patients, it may be impractical to entirely discontinue corticosteroids and such patients should be maintained on therapy at the lowest effective therapeutic dose. Approximately another 40% of patients will relapse off corticosteroid therapy. In such cases, reinstitution of therapy remains highly effective. Leukotriene antagonists such as zileuton may have a role in the treatment of chronic eosinophilic pneumonia, but the clinical experience is lacking.

Prognosis

Chronic eosinophilic pneumonia is, in most cases, a benign disease that is readily responsive to therapy. Rarely, pulmonary fibrosis has been reported as a complication. The development of extrapulmonary disease or the failure to respond to corticosteroid therapy in a patient with chronic eosinophilic pneumonia should lead the clinician to reconsider the diagnosis.

There is minimal longitudinal data on mortality in chronic eosinophilic pneumonia. What is available suggests that there is no impact of the disease on long-term survival. However, nearly 50% of patients continue to have clinical asthma requiring treatment and 13% have fixed airflow limitation on pulmonary function testing. Further, 70% of patients remained on corticosteroid therapy more than 6 years after the onset of disease. It is likely that many of these patients have and will experience some of the late-term side effects of chronic corticosteroids, particularly truncal obesity, immunosuppression, and osteoporosis.

Allen JN, Davis WB: Eosinophilic lung diseases. Am J Respir Crit Care Med 1994;150:1423. [PMID: 7952571]. (A comprehensive review.)

Marchand E et al: Idiopathic chronic eosinophilic pneumonia. A clinical and follow-up study of 62 cases. Medicine 1998; 77:299. [PMID: 9772920]. (A long-term follow-up emphasizing a prolonged need for corticosteroids in the majority of patients.)

Ong RKC, Doyle RL: Tropical pulmonary eosinophilia. Chest 1998;113:1673. [PMID: 9631810]. (Discussion of this treatable eosinophilic condition.)

Vlahakis NE, Aksamit TR: Diagnosis and treatment of allergic bronchopulmonary aspergillosis. Mayo Clin Proc 2001;76: 930. [PMID: 11560305]. (Clinical spectrum of this poorly characterized disorder.)

Lung Transplantation

Mark R. Nicolls, MD, & Martin R. Zamora, MD

Lung transplantation has become a viable therapy for end-stage lung disease due to pulmonary parenchymal and vascular disease. Early results were suboptimal due to airway complications, the reimplantation response, and lack of effective immunosuppression. Improvements in surgical technique, perioperative care, immunosuppression, and recipient selection have led to better short- and long-term outcomes.

The modern era of lung transplantation began when Cooper's group at the University of Toronto in 1983 performed the first single-lung transplant resulting in long-term survival. Single-lung transplantation has become the most common procedure for emphysema and pulmonary fibrosis. Bilateral lung transplantation is currently performed for patients with cystic fibrosis and pulmonary hypertension. The number of lung transplant procedures reported to the International Society of Heart and Lung Transplantation (ISHLT) Transplant Registry during the past 7 years has quadrupled. In 2001, 1134 lung transplants were performed in North America and 1560 were done worldwide (ISHLT Transplant Registry Quarterly Reports, 2002; www.ishlt.org). This increased activity correlates with modestly improved survival rates at 3 months and 1, 3, and 5 years posttransplantation of 86.5%, 76.4%, 57.2% and 42.6%, respectively (ustransplant.org; Scientific Registry of Transplant Recipients; OPTN/SRTR Data as of August 1, 2001). Although the 5-year survival rate for lung transplantation lags behind that of other solid organ transplants, this therapy has quickly become a major treatment option for patients with terminal lung conditions.

General Considerations

The decision to refer a patient for lung transplantation should be made expeditiously, particularly in conditions associated with poor wait-list survival, such as cystic fibrosis and idiopathic pulmonary fibrosis, in which early evaluation and rapid placement on the transplant waiting list are critical. Patients being considered for lung transplantation are counseled that, in effect, they are exchanging one disease for another. They are "trading" their lung disease for a chronic immunosuppressed state. Too much immunosuppression can lead to infections and not enough predisposes the patient to rejection. Each of the immunosuppressive agents has a

unique side effect profile. It is not always possible to predict whether the patient will have a longer life with or without a transplant. Although surgical techniques and immunosuppressive regimens have generally improved since the 1980s, there remains substantial morbidity with lung transplantation. Strict compliance to immunosuppressive drugs and early medical intervention at the onset of symptoms of infection or rejection are of paramount importance in achieving long-term survival. What is clear is that successful lung transplantation allows patients to return to work, enjoy an active life, and be free from supplemental oxygen and dyspnea.

Indications for Transplantation

The leading indications for lung transplantation are outlined in Figure 17–1 and include emphysema (chronic obstructive pulmonary disease, COPD), cystic fibrosis, idiopathic pulmonary fibrosis, α_1-antitrypsin deficiency, primary pulmonary hypertension, retransplant/graft failure, and congenital heart disease. These indications vary for pediatric and adult lung transplant recipients. The type of transplant (ie, single-, double-, or heart–lung) that is appropriate for a given patient depends on several factors including the type of lung disease and patient age. Given that the survival rate for double-lung transplants is generally superior to that of single-lung transplants (62% versus 56% for 3-year survival; ISHLT Registry data, 2002; www.ishlt.org), double-lung transplants are preferentially offered to younger patients. Additionally, so-called "septic" or suppurative lung conditions that feature heavy bacterial loads due to bronchiectasis (eg, cystic fibrosis) are treated with double-lung transplants because of the risk of contralateral (nontransplanted lung) contamination in a single-lung transplant procedure. Starnes and colleagues, at the University of Southern California, have implemented a program performing living donor procedures. In this surgery, two donors are used with a right lower lobe or right middle lobe being removed from one donor and a left lower lobe from the other. These lobes respectively replace the right and left lungs of the lung transplant recipient. The appeal of this approach is the potential minimization of time prior to transplantation, and shorter ischemia times for the donated lung. Although early reports suggest a decreased

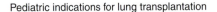

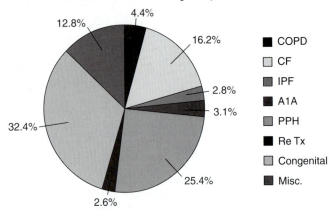

Pediatric indications for lung transplantation

4.4%
12.8%
16.2%
2.8%
3.1%
32.4%
25.4%
2.6%

- ■ COPD
- □ CF
- ▨ IPF
- ■ A1A
- ▨ PPH
- ■ Re Tx
- ▨ Congenital
- ▨ Misc.

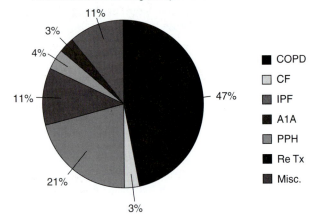

Adult indications for lung transplantation

11%
3%
4%
11%
47%
21%
3%

- ■ COPD
- □ CF
- ▨ IPF
- ■ A1A
- ▨ PPH
- ■ Re Tx
- ▨ Misc.

Figure 17–1. Pediatric and adult lung transplant recipients. Indications for transplantation. Data derived from ISHLT Registry (www.ishlt.org).

incidence of chronic rejection, whether this approach will lead to improved 5-year survival remains to be determined.

Organ Availability

Waiting time for lung transplantation varies widely among programs of different sizes and by region. Although the mean wait time at large centers (>30 transplants/year) may actually exceed that at smaller centers (ie, mean time to transplant >2 years at large centers versus <1.5 years at smaller centers), the death rate while on the wait list at smaller centers may exceed that at larger centers. The reason for this disparity in waiting list death rates is not known. Unfortunately, the rising number of patients awaiting lung transplantation has not matched the availability of organs (Figure 17–2). Accepting "marginal" lungs currently deemed unsuit-

able for transplantation may partially address this problem. Living donor procedures, artificial lungs, and xenotransplantation are modalities that may address this significant organ shortage in the future.

Recipient Criteria

A. CONTRAINDICATIONS

Guidelines published in 1998 by the American Thoracic Society (Tables 17–1 and 17–2) discuss general medical conditions that impact on the eligibility for lung transplantation. These conditions can be loosely divided into absolute and relative contraindications (as outlined in Table 17–1) although each candidate is considered on a case-by-case basis. Conditions that raise concern for eligibility of transplantation but will not necessarily exclude consideration for this procedure include symptomatic osteoporosis, musculoskeletal

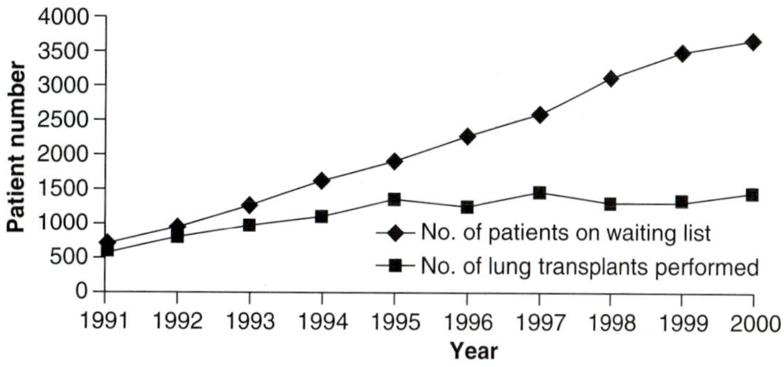

Figure 17–2. Number of patients awaiting lung transplants and number of lung transplants performed each year. Data derived from Scientific Registry of Transplant Recipients, 2002 (ustransplant.org).

Table 17–1. Selection criteria for lung transplantation.[1]

Suggested age limits for lung transplantation
  Heart–lung transplants, 55 years
  Single-lung transplants, 65 years
  Bilateral-lung transplants, 60 years
Contraindications
  Major organ dysfunction
    Creatinine clearance <50 mg/mL/min
    Unstable coronary artery disease
    Left ventricular dysfunction
  HIV infection
  Active malignancy (within the past 2 years)
    Excluding basal cell and squamous cell carcinoma of the
      skin
    Consider a waiting period of 5 years for other tumors
  Hepatitis B surface antigen positivity
  Hepatitis C with biopsy-proven histological evidence of
    liver disease
  Current smoking or alcohol or drug abuse
  Bone marrow failure
  Severe musculoskeletal disease
Relative contraindications
  Symptomatic osteoporosis
  Current use of corticosteroids (>20 mg prednisone/day)
Diagnostic and prognostic investigations
  Full pulmonary function tests
  Exercise performance measured by a standardized test
    (eg, 6-min walk)
  Electrocardiogram
  Echocardiogram
  High-resolution computed tomography
  Stress echocardiogram
  24-h creatinine clearance
  Liver function studies

[1]ATS Guidelines (1998).

Table 17–2. Disease-specific selection criteria.[1]

Nonbronchiectatic chronic obstructive lung disease
  FEV_1 <25% (without reversibility) and/or $Paco_2$ ≥55 mm Hg
    and/or elevated pulmonary artery pressures with pro-
    gressive deterioration
Cystic fibrosis and other bronchiectatic diseases
  Exclude presence of multiply resistant organisms (espe-
    cially *Burkholderia cepacia*)
  FEV_1 ≤ 30% predicted or rapid progressive respiratory de-
    terioration with FEV_1 ≤ 30% $Paco_2$ 50 mm Hg, Pao_2 <55
    mm Hg
  Young female patients (more prone to rapid deterioration)
**Idiopathic pulmonary fibrosis (cryptogenic fibrosing
alveolitis)**
  Resting or exertional oxygen desaturation (with failure of
    immunosuppressive therapy)
  Early referral for transplant evaluation
  Lung volumes <70% predicted
Pulmonary hypertension without congenital heart disease
  Symptomatic or progressive disease despite optimal med-
    ical/surgical management
  Cardiac index <2 L/min/m^2, right atrial pressure >15 mm
    Hg, and mean pulmonary artery pressure >55 mm Hg
**Pulmonary hypertension secondary to congenital heart
disease (Eisenmenger's syndrome)**
  Severe, progressive symptoms despite optimal medical
    management
**Pediatric lung transplantation: cardiopulmonary vascular
disease and other diseases**
  Disease that is nonresponsive to maximum medical/surgi-
    cal treatment
  Moderately severe or severe functional impairment
  Right ventricular failure, severe cyanosis, and low cardiac
    output

[1]ATS Guidelines (1998).

disease, and significant corticosteroid use. Osteoporosis becomes a relative contraindication for this procedure due to its high risk of acceleration while using chronic steroids following transplantation. Efforts should be made to document the extent of osteoporosis by bone densitometry and to initiate appropriate therapy prior to transplantation. Musculoskeletal diseases such as kyphoscoliosis that prevent proper thoracic mechanics may also impair recovery following transplantation. Progressive neuromuscular disease is an absolute contraindication for transplantation. Finally, a relatively common concern is steroid use prior to transplantation. Although recent reports suggest that preoperative steroids are less of a problem than originally suspected, efforts should be made to reduce the dose of prednisone to 20 mg/day given the deleterious effects of steroids on bronchial healing.

B. Disease-Specific Indications

Questions regarding the timing of transplantation for certain lung conditions arise frequently and must include relative rates of deterioration characteristic of different disease states (Table 17–2). The pace of decline is often difficult to predict but must take into account the estimated time on the waiting list, which can exceed 1–2 years. It should be noted that currently there is controversy on referring cystic fibrosis (CF) patients with a forced expiratory volume (FEV$_1$) <30%. One study suggested that the rate of decline and an age of <15 years should influence the decision to transplant. A recent analysis challenged the concept that the rate of decline of FEV$_1$ in CF was related to survival. Therefore, the guidelines provide only general parameters for the transplant physician, and each referred patient must be considered individually.

Donor Criteria

Thoughtful donor selection has improved outcomes following lung transplantation. Donors are typically accepted based on chest cavity size and ABO compatibility. Appropriate care of the lung donor includes minimizing high tidal volumes (target 8–10 mL/kg ideal body weight), airway pressures, and intravenous fluid administration before procurement. The standard criteria used to assess the suitability of donor lungs for transplantation are outlined in Table 17–3.

Given the shortage of donor organs, some of these criteria have been liberalized to include so-called "marginal donors" such as older patients or those with histories of limited smoking. Additionally, prospective donors with pulmonary contusions or a history of a traumatic pneumothorax can be considered acceptable if the contusion is not excessively large and a significant bronchopleural fistula is not evident. The "high risk" donor is

Table 17–3. Donor lung criteria.

1. po$_2$ >300 mm Hg with ventilator settings: Fio$_2$ of 1.0, PEEP of 5 cm H$_2$O, V$_T$ of 12 mL/kg
2. No CXR infiltrates (or infiltrates limited to a lung that will not be used)
3. Negative sputum gram stain for fungus and (preferably) gram-negative rods
4. Age <60 years
5. Negative serologies for HIV, hepatitis B and C antigens
6. Donor on ventilator for <1 week
7. No prior history of lung disease including asthma or emphysema
8. No prior "high-risk" behavior
9. Less than 30 pack-year smoking history
10. Chest circumference at the nipple line within 4–5 inches of the recipient's with reasonable matching of the height/weight dimensions (vertical dimension no less than 75% of the recipient's)
11. No gross purulence or evidence of aspiration from lobar or segmental bronchi orifices at the time of bronchoscopy

generally defined as one who has engaged in promiscuous sexual behavior, has been diagnosed with cancer in the remote past, has positive hepatitis serologies [without being human immunodeficiency virus (HIV) positive], or has a history of drug abuse or incarceration. Lungs from high-risk donors have been used when a patient is critically ill and no "low-risk" lungs are available. High-risk donors have also been used for ill patients awaiting lung retransplantation. Recent reports of use of organs from nonbeating heart donors for lung transplantation offer further hope of an expanded donor pool.

Surgical Techniques

A. Donor Technique

To procure lungs, a sternotomy and laparotomy are performed. The superior vena cava is ligated and divided, the aorta is cross-clamped, the left atrial appendage is amputated, the inferior vena cava is divided, and cardioplegia and pulmonoplegia are administered through the aorta and pulmonary arteries, respectively. A catheter in the pulmonary artery infuses 3 L of preservation solution (with concentrations similar to the extracellular space). The lungs are ventilated during the administration of pulmonoplegia, and the heart is subsequently excised. During removal of the heart, the pulmonary arteries, pulmonary veins, and main stem bronchi are isolated and dissected free. The bronchi are double-stapled just beyond the carina after the lung is fully inflated with the incision made between the staple lines. The lungs are then removed from the pleural space, bagged, and stored in ice saline slush.

B. RECIPIENT TECHNIQUE

For single-lung transplantation, the patient is ventilated through a double lumen endotracheal tube and placed in a lateral position with the opening incision being made in the fourth or fifth intercostal space. The main stem bronchus is identified and dissected free proximal to the upper lobe takeoff. The lung to be removed is collapsed. The pulmonary artery and veins are divided close to the lung parenchyma. The donor lung is brought into the field, the staple line is excised from the donor bronchus, and the left atrial donor cuff is anastomosed to the cuff of the recipient atrium. The bronchial anastomosis is then performed. For double-lung transplantation, a "clamshell" incision with or without sternal sparing is made going from one axillary line to the other. The patient is then placed in a lateral position and the same procedure is done as described for single-lung transplantation (usually right first followed by the left). After surgery, the endotracheal tube is replaced with a single lumen tube, and bronchoscopy is performed to examine the anastomosis.

Postoperative Period

A. VENTILATOR MANAGEMENT

For uncomplicated single-lung transplants, every effort is made to extubate patients within 8–24 h following transplantation. Double lung transplants or heart–lung transplants can suffer greater reperfusion injury and often require a longer period of mechanical ventilation. Prior to extubation, patients undergo bronchoscopy to reexamine the anastomosis site(s), and bronchoalveolar lavage is performed for culture. In the setting of vigorous diuresis, transient hypotension may result from intrinsic positive end-expiratory pressure (PEEP) (ie, autoPEEP). Temporarily disconnecting the patient from the ventilator circuit and noting a return to normal blood pressure can confirm the presence of intrinsic PEEP. Subsequently, appropriate adjustments of the ventilator settings, paralysis, and judicious liberalization of fluids may reverse the hypotension. Patients with pulmonary hypertension receiving a single lung are predisposed to developing pulmonary edema and may benefit from the addition of higher levels of PEEP in the immediate postoperative period.

The transplanted lung is generally kept at a higher elevation to minimize blood flow to the already hyperemic allograft (donated lung). With bilateral lung transplantation, alternating right-side-up with left-side-up supine positions can accomplish a similar result. Following liberation from the ventilator, patients may undergo postural drainage with chest percussion. Humidified air through a face tent prevents the mucous plugging that leads to impaired ventilation of the transplanted lung. Incentive spirometry or use of a positive expiratory pressure (PEP) valve can further facilitate sputum expectoration.

B. HEMODYNAMICS

To avoid pulmonary edema, efforts are made in the immediate postoperative period to normalize pulmonary artery pressures with diuresis and, if necessary, inhaled nitric oxide. Routine placement of a pulmonary artery catheter can assist with the maintenance of desired hemodynamics and guide fluid management. Given the disruption of pulmonary lymphatics, albumin has been a useful adjunct to diuretics. Albumin, administered as boluses, may work by transiently increasing intravascular oncotic pressures such that fluid is mobilized in the intravascular compartment to allow effective diuresis. Single-lung recipients with pulmonary hypertension are prone to episodic variability in blood pressure likely secondary to fluctuations in allograft pulmonary vascular resistance.

C. IMMUNOSUPPRESSION

Prior to transplantation, patients are given cyclosporine (5 mg/kg orally) and azathioprine (2 mg/kg orally). Intraoperatively, transplant recipients are administered 500 mg of methylprednisolone immediately before reperfusion of the transplanted lung. The use of induction therapy following transplantation with antilymphocyte globulin or anti-CD3 monoclonal antibodies has been associated with an increased risk of cancer and cytomegalovirus (CMV) infection. Many centers currently do not use induction therapy. For those centers that pursue induction therapy, antiinterleukin-2 receptor antibodies, basiliximab, and daclizimab are available, although their overall efficacy remains to be determined.

Methylprednisolone is administered 125 mg every 12 h for six doses and 1 mg/kg/day in divided doses for the first week. The patient is converted to an equivalent amount of prednisone that is tapered to 10–15 mg/day by 30 days posttransplantation. Intravenous cyclosporine is administered at 0.5–4 mg/h until the patient is converted to oral medications. In the face of early intravascular depletion, the introduction of cyclosporine can result in significant renal impairment. In this setting, intravenous cyclosporine is held or reduced until serum creatinine and urine output begin to normalize. Some centers start patients immediately on tacrolimus instead of cyclosporine with similar close monitoring of renal function.

Antimetabolites, such as azathioprine or mycophenolic acid, are administered and daily complete blood counts (CBCs) are monitored for the development of leukopenia. These agents, which function by inhibiting the purine analogue pathways of DNA synthesis, should be held or given at reduced doses if the white blood cell count falls below 4000 or if neutropenia develops. Because cyclosporine and tacrolimus are metabolized by the cytochrome P-450 enzyme system for drug metabolism, concomitantly administered drugs that induce or inhibit P-450 will alter blood levels of these calcineurin inhibitors (Table 17–4).

D. Reperfusion Injury

The reimplantation response occurs within hours to days following transplantation and is characterized by worsening gas exchange, infiltrates, and lung compliance. The lung injury pattern can resemble the adult respiratory distress syndrome and is likely secondary to reperfusion injury and lymphatic disruption in the perioperative period. Treatment strategies have included inhaled nitric oxide, paralysis, and independent lung ventilation. In severe cases, extracorporeal membrane oxygenation (ECMO) has been used with some success.

E. Primary Graft Failure

Acute graft dysfunction or primary graft failure is another cause of early morbidity following lung transplantation. This has been attributed to donor lung abnormalities such as aspiration, contusion, or inadequate lung preservation. It is characterized by pulmonary hypertension and rapidly progressive, noncardiogenic pulmonary edema. Treatment is largely supportive and patients may benefit from inhaled nitric oxide. In severe cases, ECMO therapy has been instituted and may lead to improved survival.

Table 17–4. Drugs that interfere with cyclosporine and tacrolimus metabolism.

Increases blood levels
  Methylprednisolone
  Macrolide antibiotics: azithromycin, erythromycin, clarithromycin
  Antifungal agents: ketoconazole > itraconazole > fluconazole
  Calcium channel blockers: diltiazem, verapamil, nicardipine
  Allopurinol
  Bromocriptine
  Danazol
  Metoclopramide
  Cimetidine
  Digoxin
  Whole grapefruit and grapefruit juice
Decreases blood levels
  Antibiotics: rifampin, rifabutin, nafcillin
  Anticonvulsants: phenytoin, carbamazepine, phenobarbital, primidone
  Ticlopidine
  Octreotide

F. Cardiac Dysrhythmias

Atrial flutter has been reported frequently in pediatric bilateral lung transplant recipients. Atrial flutter may, in part, be due to circus electrical movement around atrial cuff suture lines. The preponderance of atrial arrhythmias in the immediate postlung transplant period has prompted some centers to administer digoxin on a prophylactic basis.

G. Vascular Complications

Pulmonary vascular complications can be a cause of early graft dysfunction. Pulmonary artery stenosis and pulmonary venous obstruction are the prominent pathologies in this category. Although pulmonary artery stenosis can present with a clear chest x-ray, pulmonary venous obstruction can radiologically be similar to reperfusion injury. Both conditions present with pulmonary hypertension and can be distinguished from each other with a pulmonary arteriogram. The diagnosis of pulmonary venous obstruction is usually made by isotope perfusion scanning, pulmonary angiography (best for confirming anatomy), or transesophageal echocardiography. Pulmonary venous thrombosis is another potentially life-threatening early complication of lung transplantation. In one study, 87 consecutive adult lung transplant patients underwent transesophageal echocardiography within 48 h of surgery. Pulmonary vein thrombosis was diagnosed in 13 (15%) of these patients. Five of these patients subsequently died in the perioperative period resulting in a 38% mortality rate for pulmonary vein thrombosis in this study. Vascular complications carry a high mortality rate when undiagnosed. When recognized, reoperation is usually required with cardiopulmonary bypass, but in high-risk patients, vascular dilation or stent insertion can be a therapeutic option.

H. Airway Complications

In the initial weeks following transplantation, complications involving the airway anastomosis and the reimplantation response predominate. Airway complications represent a major morbidity following single- and double-lung transplantation. Bronchial dehiscence is a serious early airway complication. Telescoping anastomoses and improved preservation solutions have limited the degree to which this now occurs. Stenosis and/or bronchomalacia are often late sequelae of ischemic injury and early *Aspergillus* infection. Anastomotic stenosis is now the most common large airway complication and usually responds well to balloon dilatation or expanding metal stents. Stenosis may present for the first time in the months following transplantation. A decrease in spirometry, a palpable rumble on physical examination, and a history of intermittent hypoxemia resolved with coughing secretions all suggest the presence of physiologically significant bronchial stenosis.

Acute allograft rejection often occurs concurrently. For this reason, high-dose corticosteroids are often administered for several days at the time of bronchial dilation. Serial dilations may be required with certain patients. In this procedure, the bronchoscope is advanced orally, and under fluoroscopy, a wire is advanced beyond the stenotic area. The bronchoscope is slowly pulled out as the wire is being advanced. The balloon is advanced over the wire, and the balloon markers (radioopaque and visible by fluoroscopy) straddle the stenotic lesion. Bronchoscopy is used to confirm the correct position of the balloon, which is subsequently inflated to a predetermined pressure for about 20–30 s. Overdistention can rupture the bronchus and can cause hemorrhage.

I. PLEURAL COMPLICATIONS

Pleural effusions commonly occur in the first month following transplantation and can indicate poor pleural drainage (in the setting of low serum albumin and interrupted peribronchial lymphatics), rejection, or infection. These pleural fluid collections are generally serosanguineous, exudative, and neutrophil rich. Often responsive to diuresis with concomitant colloid administration, persistent effusion requires thoracentesis and potential bronchoscopy with bronchoalveolar lavage (BAL) and transbronchial biopsy (TBBx) to rule out empyema and/or rejection. Complicated parapneumonic effusions are more commonly seen in bilateral lung transplant recipients. More rarely, this effusion can be the result of a trapped lung, or increased right-sided pressures (eg, as in pericarditis with tamponade physiology). Other miscellaneous complications include chylothorax, subpleural hematoma, and hemothorax. Following lung transplantation, chest tubes are removed in a sequential fashion with care given not to remove bilateral chest tubes simultaneously unless one or more chest tubes remain. Given that the normally distinct and separate left and right pleural spaces are in communication following a double-lung transplant, a single chest tube is often adequate to drain both pleural spaces. Small air leaks are a common finding immediately following transplantation and can relate to an undersized donor lung. Approximately 10% of patients have a persistent air leak extending 2 weeks that generally resolves without surgical intervention, but airway dehiscence must be ruled out.

J. EARLY INFECTIOUS MORBIDITY

The infectious problems encountered early following transplantation are related to the surgical procedure and to ventilator dependence. In the perioperative period, donor intubation and ventilation put lungs at risk for colonization and aspiration just as recipient intubation will subsequently do. Bacterial pneumonia is the most common infection in the lung transplant recipient in the first month posttransplantation. Common pathogenic microorganisms and viruses encountered later following transplantation are described in greater detail later in this chapter. Patients undergoing lung transplantation receive broad spectrum antibiotics that empirically cover gram-positive and gram-negative organisms in the donor lung. Bacteria including *Pseudomonas* species, *Klebsiella* species, *Hemophilus influenzae*, and *Staphylococcus aureus* cause most postoperative infections. As results from donor-lung BAL cultures become available (pre- and posttransplant), antibiotics can be tailored for the individual recipient. In the absence of infection of the newly transplanted lung(s), empiric antibiotic therapy is usually discontinued after 48 h. Infection with *Burkholderia cepacia* in patients with cystic fibrosis is considered by some to be an absolute contraindication for lung transplantation because of the multidrug resistance of this bacterium. A recent report from the University of Toronto using an aggressive antibiotic regimen and a modified immunosuppressive regimen suggests that outcomes can be improved even for these patients.

K. PAIN CONTROL

Postoperative pain requires effective control to maximize ventilatory efforts and minimize basilar atelectasis. In some severe cases, placement of an epidural catheter can provide sufficient control of pain without the respiratory depression associated with excessive narcotic use. Nonsteroidal antiinflammatory drugs (NSAIDs) are avoided secondary to untoward renal effects in the face of other nephrotoxic agents that the patient is obliged to take such as cyclosporine.

L. HOSPITAL DISCHARGE

Following liberation from chest tubes, titration of oxygen, resumption of oral intake, and ambulation, patients are prepared for discharge. In optimal circumstances this can occur as soon as 5 days following transplantation. Patients who require daily intravenous infusions of antibiotics including ganciclovir use home-health care agencies or the hospital's ambulatory treatment unit.

Survival Rates

For data compiled between 1997 and 2001, survival rates at 1 month, 1 year, and 3 years for adult/pediatric recipients were reported as 93%/96%, 77%/86%, and

60%/52%, respectively (ustransplant.org, Scientific Registry of Transplant Recipients).

Transplant Monitoring

Patients are seen on a biweekly basis for the first month following transplantation. Efforts are made to taper prednisone to 10 mg/day by the end of the first month. The early examination consists of careful inspection of the surgical site and chest tube sites. Staples are removed at 21 days and the first posttransplant pulmonary function studies are obtained in the fourth week. Patients are required to stay with friends or family in the local area for the first 8 weeks to assist with home care and transportation. By the end of 6–8 weeks, if patients are making good progress, they are allowed to go home with close follow-up by a physician convenient to the patient. Patients are instructed to contact the lung transplant program nursing coordinators with all significant symptoms including upper respiratory tract infections. Lack of experience with this patient population in a facility can result in the misdiagnosis of significant rejection episodes or opportunistic infections.

The new lung transplant patient will often have improving pulmonary function tests for the first several months following transplantation, after which point airflows plateau to a new baseline. A typical clinic visit after 1 month posttransplantation begins with laboratories including CBC, a comprehensive chemistry panel, including serum magnesium, and trough cyclosporine or tacrolimus levels. Chest radiographs are obtained and compared with prior films to look for interval changes that indicate rejection, infection, or cancer. Spirometry is obtained and the FEV_1 and forced vital capacity (FVC) are compared with prior values.

A. SYMPTOMS AND SIGNS OF ACUTE ALLOGRAFT REJECTION

Hyperacute rejection is an antibody-mediated process occurring within minutes to hours of transplantation and has become an uncommon occurrence since the advent of screening for the presence of preformed antibodies (panel-reactive antibodies) in the transplant recipient. Acute rejection, a cellular-mediated immune process, is seen in up to 40% of patients in the first month following transplantation. The prevalence of early (1–12 weeks) acute rejection ranges between 60% and 75%. The following parameters suggest allograft rejection and/or infection: (1) a fall in the FEV_1 by >5–10%, (2) new pulmonary symptoms or signs (including O_2 desaturation at rest and/or with exertion), and (3) new radiographic findings. Symptoms of acute rejection are nonspecific and include fatigue, malaise, cough, fever, chest tightness, and dyspnea. Posttransplant pulmonary function tests are often not available in the first weeks to enable use of a decline in FEV_1 to assist diagnosis, but new or relative hypoxemia can be useful in this setting. The gold standard for acute allograft rejection is TBBx with BAL. The false-negative rate for TBBx is 15–28% and sensitivity for disease likely increases with the number of biopsies performed. Typically 6–10 pieces of lung tissue are obtained and sent to a pathologist skilled in reading lung transplant pathology. The ISHLT Guidelines provide a standard for interpreting the degree of allograft rejection (Table 17–5).

B. SURVEILLANCE BRONCHOSCOPY

It remains unclear whether monitoring clinically stable patients with scheduled, routine transbronchial biopsies is beneficial. It has been estimated that more than half

Table 17–5. Pathology of acute rejection.[1]

Grade (Description)	Pathology
0 (no acute rejection)	Normal pulmonary parenchyma.
A1 (minimal acute rejection)	Scattered infrequent perivascular mononuclear infiltrates in alveolated lung parenchyma that are not obvious at low magnification (ie, 40×). Blood vessels cuffed by small lymphocytes.
A2 (mild acute rejection)	Frequent perivascular mononuclear infiltrates surrounding vessels recognizable at low magnification consisting of lymphocytes, macrophages, and eosinophils. Subendothelial infiltration. Distinguished from minimal acute rejection by unequivocal mononuclear infiltrates.
A3 (moderate acute rejection)	Prominent cuffing of venules and arterioles by dense perivascular mononuclear infiltrates associated with endotheliatis. Eosinophils and neutrophils are sometimes present. Extension of inflammatory infiltrate into the perivascular, alveolar, and air spaces.
A4 (severe acute rejection)	Diffuse perivascular, interstitial, and air space infiltrates of mononuclear cells and prominent alveolar pneumocyte damage usually associated with intraalveolar necrotic cells, macrophages, hyaline membranes, hemorrhage, and neutrophils. Associated parenchymal necrosis, infarction, or necrotizing vasculitis.

ISHLT Guidelines (1996).

of lung transplant centers perform these and that 20% of asymptomatic patients have been found to have grade II or greater rejection. Usually this grade of rejection is treated, but it remains unclear if this has any long-term benefit compared with untreated patients. With current technologies, lymphocyte accumulations that are not necessarily harmful to the transplant cannot be distinguished from pathogenic alloreactive cells.

C. Immunosuppression for Acute Allograft Rejection

Patients diagnosed with acute rejection are given 3 days of high dose steroids (methylprednisolone 10 mg/kg intravenously every day). If patients have recently been treated with high dose steroids and have had little improvement (ie, steroid-resistant rejection), consideration is given to other therapeutic regimens. These include anti-CD3 monoclonal antibody (OKT3) or polyclonal antilymphocyte preparations such as antithymocyte globulin. Plasmapheresis may be a useful adjunctive therapy to mediate certain rejection processes such as capillaritis or hyperacute rejection. Additionally, when standard triple therapy (ie, calcineurin inhibitor, azathioprine, prednisone) does not prevent recurrent rejection episodes or if spirometry is not restored following standard treatment, other immunosuppressive agents can be tried. Methotrexate (given weekly and coadministered with daily folate), mycophenolic acid, and cyclophosphamide can be added to or substituted for azathioprine as an antimetabolite. Rapamycin, an antiproliferative agent, is being included in standard protocols for other solid organ transplants and has been used in lung transplantation. Rapamycin has been used as a substitute for calcineurin inhibitors or, more commonly, allows for reduced doses of the nephrotoxic calcineurin inhibitors. Concerns regarding wound healing and interstitial pneumonitis may limit the widespread use of rapamycin for lung transplantation.

Imaging Studies

Chest radiography is of central importance in the clinic visit of newly transplanted patients as well as patients bearing longer-term transplants. In the asymptomatic patient, the chest x-ray can be an early indication of acute rejection, infection, or cancer. In a symptomatic patient, the posteroanterior and lateral films can further direct bronchoscopic evaluation so that the appropriate lobes can be assessed. The appearance of acute rejection is radiologically inconsistent, sometimes appearing as an alveolar or interstitial infiltrate or as no infiltrate at all. By thin-section computed tomography (CT), rejection has a variable appearance presenting as a ground-glass opacity, consolidation, fissure thickening, pleural effusion, volume loss, septal thickening, peribronchovascular thickening, or a combination of the above findings. Expiratory thin-section CT is sensitive for depicting bronchiolitis obliterans syndrome (BOS)-related airway abnormalities such as regional air trapping.

Infectious Complications & Prophylaxis

Early infections in the first month following transplantation are usually bacterial and related to surgery and mechanical ventilation. Lung transplant recipients have numerous reasons for being at risk for infection including: (1) systemic immunosuppression, (2) denervation of the allograft that impairs the cough reflex and mucociliary clearance, (3) temporarily interrupted lymphatic drainage, and (4) an anastomotic site that may enhance colonization, may dehisce leading to mediastinitis, or may stenose leading to postobstructive infection. Some inactive infections or colonizations that occurred prior to transplantation may recur on immunosuppressive therapy (eg, tuberculosis, aspergillosis).

A. Bacterial Pneumonia

Bacterial pneumonia represents the most common infection in lung transplant recipients with reported incidences of 35-66%. In the early era of lung transplantation, bacterial pneumonia was frequent in the early postoperative period and was usually of donor origin. With the employment of prophylactic antibiotics and culture of donor lung BAL, these early pneumonias have become less common. The majority of bacterial pneumonias now arise in later postoperative periods and may be nosocomial. Infections with *Pseudomonas* species, Enterobacteriaceae, *Staphylococcus aureus*, *Enterococcus* species, and *Hemophilus influenzae* are noted in this setting.

B. Cytomegalovirus (CMV)

Although the second most common infection after bacterial pneumonia, CMV remains the single most important pathogen following solid organ transplantation. CMV is a significant cause of morbidity and mortality in patients receiving lung transplants. In addition to its acute effects of tissue injury and clinical illness, CMV may have important long-term sequelae in the lung transplant patient. With infection of the allograft, CMV may lead to enhanced allorecognition that subsequently leads to the development of acute and chronic rejection. The incidence of CMV infection ranges from 35% to 90% for lung transplant patients and is approximately 40% in heart–lung transplant recipients. As such, CMV is more severe in lung transplant recipients and has a higher rate of recurrence than that of any other solid organ transplant. CMV infection may also be associated with increased immunosuppression, leading to opportunistic infections with fungal or bacterial superinfections.

Primary infection is most severe in recipients negative for CMV who receive lungs from a CMV-positive donor. CMV infection may present with a constellation of nonspecific complaints including fever, malaise, myalgia, arthralgia, fatigue, and anorexia. New seroconversion from CMV-negative to CMV-positive status following transplantation is associated with more severe disease and higher mortality rates than reactivation of latent disease.

More than 50% of adults in the United States have serological evidence of prior CMV infection. Because CMV is so common in the general population, it is necessary to carefully distinguish CMV infection from CMV disease. The former can be defined as isolation of CMV in material obtained from any body site and identification of CMV by culture, immunohistology, cytology, and/or identification of genetic material in the absence of symptoms or histological changes associated with CMV. Currently available techniques include the shell vial assay, pp65 antigenemia, polymerase chain reaction, or hybrid capture assay for CMV DNAemia. CMV disease is associated with signs or symptoms of infection with histological evidence of tissue damage after exclusion of other etiologies in the presence of CMV infection.

Several studies suggest that CMV pneumonitis and positive CMV serology are risk factors for BOS, although this has not been a universal finding. Rapid and accurate diagnostic techniques are critical for the appropriate management of CMV. The issue of CMV prophylaxis and treatment remains as controversial as it is crucial. There is general consensus that a period of CMV prophylaxis with ganciclovir following transplantation should ensue. Generally, patients that are mismatched (ie, recipient CMV negative/donor CMV positive) will receive a longer period of prophylaxis with intravenous ganciclovir before being converted to oral acyclovir or an oral form of ganciclovir (eg, valganciclovir). In recent years, CMV immune globulin has been used as a monotherapy and in combination with ganciclovir to prevent and treat CMV.

C. Herpes Simplex Virus (HSV)

With acyclovir or valganciclovir prophylaxis, HSV pneumonia has diminished in incidence. Severe HSV pneumonia occurs in approximately 10% of patients not receiving prophylaxis with a fatality rate of 20%. Therefore, prophylaxis is imperative, especially in the first 3 months following transplantation. Of note, HSV

6, 7, and 8 related infections have all been reported following lung transplantation. These infections may be associated with encephalitis, bronchiolitis obliterans with organizing pneumonia (Boop), and Kaposi's sarcoma.

D. Other Viruses

It is likely that other respiratory viruses are epidemiologically relevant and may, in fact, have a role in triggering acute rejection. A peak incidence of BOS onset in the respiratory virus season suggests that common respiratory viral infections may trigger the complication. Commonly encountered pathogens include respiratory syncytial virus, adenovirus, influenza, parainfluenza infections, and rhinovirus. In a recent study, patients with infection of the lower respiratory tract were predisposed to high-grade BOS development, and patients with OB and BOS were predisposed to acquiring community respiratory viral infections. Because of the association between airway infection and rejection events, patients with symptoms of upper respiratory infections should be nasopharyngeally swabbed for virus.

Antiviral agents including amantidine, rimantidine, zanamivir, oseltamivir, inhaled ribavirin, and hyperimmune globulin have been utilized in the setting of acute infection. Amantidine and rimantidine are chemically related antiviral therapies active against influenza A (not B) viruses that inhibit the uncoating of virus by blocking viral ion channel activity. Zanamivir and oseltamivir are neuraminidase inhibitors active against both influenza A and B that function by inhibiting the release of progeny virus from infected cells. Immunoglobulin may be prepared from the serum of selected individuals who have high titers of antibody to particular viruses such as respiratory syncytial virus. This hyperimmune globulin has been used in conjunction with inhaled ribavirin, an agent that has activity against respiratory syncytial virus, influenza virus, and HSV. Ribavirin may work by acting as a cellular inhibitor of enzymes that act on guanosine and xanthosine. Although multicenter clinical trials have not been performed, some lung transplant programs are aggressively screening (with nasal washes) and treating community-acquired viral infections.

E. Fungal Infections

1. Aspergillus—Fungal infections are life threatening in all immunocompromised patients. *Aspergillus* species are of particular concern in patients with lung transplants. Invasive aspergillosis usually occurs in recipients who were previously colonized by *A. fumigatus* (also *A. niger* and *A. flavus*) and who undergo treatment for rejection, particularly with cytolytic therapy. Often, the infection arises in the native lung, which is more susceptible to infection due to decreased perfusion during transplantation. As the diagnosis and treatment of invasive *Aspergillus* can be difficult, many centers preemptively treat all *Aspergillus* airway isolates to prevent invasive disease. Bronchoscopy with cytological examination and fungal culture are not timely or sensitive predictors of invasive disease. In one study, invasive *Aspergillus* occurred only in patients initially colonized with *A. fumigatus* within the first 6 months posttransplant. Invasive disease requires treatment with intravenous amphotericin B. In cases in which only colonization is suspected, amphotericin B can also be administered in an inhaled form. Attention should be given to fungi that have inherent resistance to amphotericin B that may require therapy with newer classes of antifungal agents including the new triazoles and candins. Generally, *A. fumigatus* is the most susceptible to traditional therapies followed in order of decreasing susceptibility by *A. flavus, A. niger,* and *A. terreus.* Preemptive therapy of colonized patients with oral itraconazole is highly recommended and effectively prevents the development of invasive aspergillosis.

2. Candida—Most invasive infections with *Candida* species occur in the first month following transplantation, often being transmitted with the donor organ. This most commonly presents as a necrotic bronchial anastomotic infection, vascular anastomotic infection, or mediastinitis.

F. Pneumocystis carinii Pneumonia

The incidence of *Pneumocystis carinii* pneumonia varies greatly between transplant centers with a prevalence of up to 88% in patients not receiving prophylaxis. As up to one-third of infections with *P. carinii* pneumonias can occur after the first preoperative year, many centers maintain patients on life-long prophylaxis with trimethoprim-sulfamethoxazole or monthly-inhaled pentamidine for those patients with sulfa allergies. For some patients with sulfa-related allergies, a desensitization protocol often allows patients to start or resume trimethoprim-sulfamethoxazole.

G. Mycobacterial Infections

Mycobacterial infections following lung transplantation can occur at pulmonary and extrapulmonary sites. *Mycobacterium tuberculosis* is the most common infection and less commonly isolated organisms include *M. avium* complex, *M. kansasii, M. haemophilum, M. abscessus, M. asiaticum,* and *M. marinum.* Transient colonization with *M. avium* complex does not always necessitate therapy. Infected patients normally respond well to therapy. Complications, predominantly due to rifampin, include gastrointestinal distress and an increased likelihood of rejection. The latter phenomenon may be attributable to induction of the cytochrome P-450 pathway leading to low cyclosporine levels and a decreased bioavailability of prednisone.

Noninfectious Medical Complications

Medical complications related to a lung transplant patient's immunosuppressive regimen or the underlying illness that led to the transplant become more prominent over time as the acute issues of transplant surgery wane. Beyond the renal dysfunction that is chiefly attributable to calcineurin inhibitors, there are a myriad of potential side effects that prospective transplant recipients should be warned about prior to transplantation. A partial list of these side effects includes the following.

A. Renal Dysfunction

Renal dysfunction is an almost universal occurrence in lung transplant patients, although impairment in function can range from minimal to severe reduction in creatinine clearance. A sudden decrement in function is often associated with elevated levels of calcineurin inhibitors and will resolve with dose adjustment. During drug holidays off calcineurin inhibitors, patients can use nonnephrotoxic agents such as rapamycin to allow recovery of renal function. Because of the renal insufficiency that often accompanies lung transplantation, patients and their primary care providers are strongly encouraged to avoid NSAIDS.

B. Osteoporosis

Osteoporosis is a commonly encountered side effect in this patient population principally owing to chronic steroid use that may have preceded transplantation. Between 30% and 50% of patients coming to lung transplantation have osteoporosis. Postmenopausal women and all patients showing diminished bone density are treated with agents that increase calcium absorption including alendronate or pamidronate. Estrogen, supplemental calcium, and vitamin D are commonly employed. Alendronate can be associated with gastrointestinal side effects and must be taken at least one-half hour before the first food, beverage, or medication of the day. This is available as a once a day or once a week dose. Compression fractures are common and can cause significant distress. Physical therapy, TENS units, and nasal salmon calcitonin in conjunction with non-NSAID analgesia are useful treatment modalities.

C. Hyperlipidemia

Hyperlipidemia with accompanying accelerated atherosclerosis is commonly observed. Lipid-lowering agents can be employed, but care should be taken to monitor for myositis if statin drugs are used together with calcineurin inhibitors.

D. DIABETES

Patients commonly develop diabetes when being treated with high-dose steroids. This resolves, although not always completely, as steroids are being tapered. Additionally, tacrolimus, a commonly used calcineurin inhibitor, induces diabetes in a small subset of patients. Patients with CF can present a significant challenge, as their hyperglycemia may be most dramatic postprandially. As patients with CF age, there is a growing prevalence of diabetes. As survival in this patient group continues to improve, particular care of diabetes in both the transplanted and nontransplanted patient assumes greater importance.

E. NEUROTOXICITY

Neurotoxicity is chiefly attributable to tacrolimus and cyclosporine and can manifest centrally as posterior encephalopathy or vasculitis, with seizure activity, visual disturbance, headaches, confusion, and strokes. It can also present as peripheral neuropathy with paresthesias. Changing calcineurin inhibitors is usually warranted in these cases in addition to a full neurological evaluation.

F. GASTROINTESTINAL COMPLICATIONS

Gastrointestinal complications are more commonly encountered with lung transplantation than with other types of transplantation. Gastroesophageal reflux is frequently observed and responds well to H2 blockers, proton pump inhibitors, and motility agents. Diarrhea is often encountered, but an etiology may be difficult to determine. Multiple concomitant medications including immunosuppressives and supplemental magnesium are important noninfectious causes of diarrhea. Infectious causes of diarrhea include both normal and opportunistic pathogens and should be evaluated with appropriate stool studies. The cytokine storm associated with lytic T cell therapies such as OKT3 can be accompanied by diarrhea. Other gastrointestinal complications include diaphragmatic hernias, colonic perforation, ischemic bowel, and CMV colitis. Once identified, these conditions normally respond well to standard therapy. Because steroid use can mask symptoms that normally accompany an acute abdomen, the caring physician must have a high index of suspicion.

G. CANCER

Immunosuppression has been associated with increased risk of certain cancers, including non-Hodgkin's lymphoma, Kaposi's sarcoma, kidney and hepatobiliary tumors, and carcinoma of the vulva and perineum. Because of the increased risk of squamous cell cancers of the skin and lips, patients are encouraged to get thorough examinations by a dermatologist every 6–12 months. Other cancers that have been described in lung transplantation include acute myelogenous leukemia and recurrence of bronchoalveolar cell carcinoma.

Posttransplant lymphoproliferative disorder (PTLD) has been listed as the third leading cause of mortality outside of the immediate perioperative period with an incidence in one series of approximately 8%. Epstein–Barr virus (EBV) is associated with the polyclonal or monoclonal proliferation of B cells. Most adult recipients have serological evidence of prior exposure to EBV, but when a seronegative recipient receives an organ from a seropositive donor, the risk of primary infection is nearly 100%, and greater than half of these infections are associated with PTLD. In fact, most cases of PTLD in solid organ transplants are likely from EBV infections originating in the recipient rather than the donor.

Primary EBV infection causes fever, malaise, and fatigue, but PTLD can remain asymptomatic until tumor burden leads to pulmonary dysfunction or intestinal blockage. This disorder is often diagnosed radiographically before symptoms become apparent. Radiographically, PTLD commonly presents as a solitary pulmonary nodule. Other presentations include multiple nodules, multifocal alveolar infiltrates, and hilar and mediastinal adenopathy. CT scans may reveal additional nodules and lymph nodes.

Reactivation of latent virus occurs with periods of intense immunosuppression and, understandably, a primary treatment for PTLD is reducing the level of immunosuppression. Rituximab, a humanized anti-CD20 monoclonal antibody, is a promising new therapy for the treatment of PTLD. In one study, treatment with rituximab was effective for the treatment of PTLD without progression of transplant dysfunction.

Chronic Rejection (Bronchiolitis Obliterans)

Bronchiolitis obliterans syndrome (BOS) is defined by graft deterioration secondary to persistent airflow obstruction and does not necessarily require histological confirmation. By contrast, the term "bronchiolitis obliterans" is used for histologically confirmed diagnosis described further below. BOS has been classified into several stages (BOS 0–3) and has recently been defined as a 10–15% decrease in FEV_1 from a previous baseline. Additionally, evidence suggests that the forced expiratory flow (FEF_{25-75}) decreases before the FEV_1 in most bilateral and heart–lung transplant recipients with BOS. Therefore a reduction of FEF_{25-75} by ≥25% may also be an indicator of early BOS. Probable risk factors for BOS include acute rejection and viral infections.

Potential risk factors for BOS include bacterial, fungal, and non-CMV viral infections, older donor age, prolonged graft ischemic time, and donor-specific antigen reactivity. A peak incidence of BOS onset in the respiratory virus season suggests that common respiratory viral infections, such as respiratory syncytial virus infections, may trigger the complication.

The pathology of bronchiolitis obliterans (BO) is a cicatricial process involving the small airways of the transplanted lung. BO is thought to result from chronic lung rejection through a sequence of lymphocyte-mediated processes directed to the respiratory epithelium. In an animal model of bronchiolitis, BO was suggested to be a lymphocyte-dependent process when it was noted to be absent in lymphocyte-deficient mice. The initial process in BO is a lymphocytic infiltrate of the submucosa of the airways with migration of mononuclear cells through the basement membrane into the epithelium followed by epithelial cell necrosis and denudation. Fibroblasts and myofibroblasts migrate to the small airway lumen and intraluminal granulation tissue subsequently develops.

Unfortunately, treatment of BOS is unsatisfactory. By the time definitive diagnosis is made, the fibroproliferative process is relatively refractory to immunologically targeted therapies. Airflow obstruction, at this point, may stabilize or progressively deteriorate. Efforts are made to minimize excessive immunosuppression as opportunistic infections are poorly tolerated in this cohort of patients with diminished pulmonary function.

Retransplantation

In recent years, an increasing number of lung retransplantations have been performed for organ failure secondary to acute and chronic allograft rejection. The best results are achieved in experienced centers, in nonventilated patients, and in patients undergoing retransplantation more than 2 years after their first transplantation. The 1-year survival rate for this procedure is 47%. If subgroups are considered separately, ambulatory, nonventilated patients enjoy a 1-year survival rate of 64% versus 33% for nonambulatory ventilated patients. Consequently, in view of the scarcity of lung donors, patient selection for retransplantation should be considered carefully with a view to the outcome data described above.

Recurrence of the Primary Disease

Recurrence of the primary disease that originally led to lung transplantation has been described in sarcoidosis, alveolar proteinosis, eosinophilic granuloma, diffuse panbronchiolitis, talc granulomatosis, giant cell pneumonitis, and desquamative interstitial pneumonitis.

Additionally, with progression of obstructive lung disease, the native lung can compress and impair transplant lung function. Lung volume reduction surgery of the native lung can be therapeutic when this situation becomes severe.

American Society for Transplant Physicians (ASTP)/American Thoracic Society (ATS)/European Respiratory Society (ERS)/International Society for Heart and Lung Transplantation (ISHLT). International guidelines for the selection of lung transplant candidates. Am J Respir Crit Care Med 1998;158:335. [PMID: 9655748]. (The main governing bodies overseeing lung transplantation provide guidelines for lung transplantation.)

Armitage JM et al: Posttransplant lymphoproliferative disease in thoracic organ transplant patients: ten years of cyclosporine-based immunosuppression. J Heart Lung Transplant 1991;10:877. [PMID: 1661607]. (One center's experience with lymphoproliferative disease is chronicled during a decade of heart and lung transplantation.)

Augarten A et al: Prediction of mortality and timing of referral for lung transplantation in cystic fibrosis patients. Pediatr Transplant 2001;5:339. [PMID: 11560752]. (This study demonstrates that the current criterion of FEV$_1$ <30% predicted alone is not sufficiently sensitive to predict the mortality rate in CF patients.)

Billings JL et al: Community respiratory virus infections following lung transplantation. Transpl Infect Dis 2001;3:138. [PMID: 11493396]. (The current state of knowledge regarding the epidemiology, clinical manifestations, diagnosis, treatment, and outcomes associated with RSV, PIV, influenza virus, and adenovirus infections in lung transplant recipients is summarized.)

Billings JL et al: Respiratory viruses and chronic rejection in lung transplant recipients. J Heart Lung Transplant 2002;21:559. [PMID: 11983546]. [This study demonstrates that patients with community-acquired respiratory viral infections of the lower respiratory tract are predisposed to chronic rejection (BOS), and, conversely, patients with chronic rejection are predisposed to respiratory viral infections.]

Cahill BC et al: Aspergillus airway colonization and invasive disease after lung transplantation. Chest 1997;112:1160. [PMID: 9367451]. (This study demonstrates that Aspergillus colonization is common and that invasive Aspergillus is an important cause of morbidity and mortality among lung transplant recipients.)

Chaparro C et al: Infection with Burkholderia cepacia in cystic fibrosis: outcome following lung transplantation. Am J Respir Crit Care Med 2001;163:43. [PMID: 11208624]. (This study demonstrates that the mortality of patients with cystic fibrosis infected with B. cepacia is significantly higher than for those not infected with B. cepacia.)

Clark SC et al: Vascular complications of lung transplantation. Ann Thorac Surg 1996;61:1079. [PMID: 8607660]. (This retrospective study from one center examines the morbidity and mortality of vascular complications associated with lung transplantation.)

Cohen RG, Starnes VA: Living donor lung transplantation. World J Surg 2001;25:244. [PMID: 11338028]. (A pioneering program's experience with living donor lung transplantation is described.)

Duncan SR et al: Sequelae of cytomegalovirus pulmonary infections in lung allograft recipients. Am Rev Respir Dis 1992;146:1419. [PMID: 1333737]. (The deleterious effects of cytomegalovirus infections in lung transplant recipients are described.)

Estenne M et al: Bronchiolitis obliterans syndrome 2001: an update of the diagnostic criteria. J Heart Lung Transplant 2002;21:297. [PMID: 21895918]. (This article summarizes the updated classification for the bronchiolitis obliterans syndrome.)

Fishman J, Rubin R: Infection in organ-transplant recipients. N Engl J Med 1998;338:1741. [PMID: 9624195]. (This broad review of infections in transplantation focuses on prevention and early recognition of infection as well as common drug-related toxic effects.)

Grover FL et al: The past, present, and future of lung transplantation. Am J Surg 1997;173:523. [PMID: 9207168]. (The history and current status of lung transplantation are outlined along with a synopsis of the surgical technique.)

Herridge MS et al: Pleural complications in lung transplant recipients. J Thorac Cardiovasc Surg 1995;110:22. [PMID: 7541881]. (In a study involving 53 single- and 91 double-lung transplants, pleural complications were common, occurring in 22% of patients.)

Hosenpud JD et al: The Registry of the International Society for Heart and Lung Transplantation: Eighteenth Official Report—2001. J Heart Lung Transplant 2001;20:805. [PMID: 11502402]. (This article is a recent summary of transplant center statistics.)

Malouf MA, Glanville AR: The spectrum of mycobacterial infection after lung transplantation. Am J Respir Crit Care Med 1999;160:1611. [PMID: 10556129]. (In this retrospective study involving 261 lung and heart–lung transplant recipients, the incidence, etiology, and clinical outcome of mycobacterial infection after lung transplantation are detailed.)

Neuringer IP et al: Immune cells in a mouse airway model of obliterative bronchiolitis. Am J Respir Cell Mol Biol 1998;19:379. [PMID: 9730865]. (Results from this experimental model utilizing immunodeficient mice indicate that (1) obliterative bronchiolitis is predominantly an immunological airway injury and (2) CD4$^+$ and CD8$^+$ lymphocytes and macrophages play an important role in the evolution of airway inflammation and fibrosis.)

Novick RJ et al: Pulmonary retransplantation: predictors of graft function and survival in 230 patients. Pulmonary Retransplant Registry. Ann Thorac Surg 1998;65:227. [PMID: 9456123]. (This study describes factors that influence the outcomes of lung transplant recipients undergoing retransplantation.)

Pescovitz MD, Navarro MT: Immunosuppressive therapy and posttransplantation diarrhea. Clin Transplant 2001;15:23. [PMID: 11778784]. (This review assesses the overall incidence of posttransplantation diarrhea related to the various immunosuppressive medications currently in use.)

Pierson RN et al: Lung allocation in the United States, 1995–1997: an analysis of equity and utility. J Heart Lung Transplant 2000;19:846. [PMID: 11008073]. (A study of all U.S. lung transplant centers that examines the characteristics and mortality rates of patients on waiting lists for lung transplantation.)

Smith PC et al: Abdominal complications after lung transplantation. J Heart Lung Transplant 1995;14:44. [PMID: 7727475]. (This report reviews the incidence and spectrum of abdominal complications occurring in lung transplant recipients at a single institution.)

Speich R, van der Bij W: Epidemiology and management of infections after lung transplantation. Clin Infect Dis 2001;33(Suppl 1):S58. [PMID: 11389524]. (This review describes the infections in lung transplant recipients that represent the most common cause of early and late morbidity and mortality.)

Trulock EP et al: The role of transbronchial lung biopsy in the treatment of lung transplant recipients. An analysis of 200 consecutive procedures. Chest 1992;102:1049. [PMID: 1327662]. (Transbronchial lung biopsy is a useful and safe procedure that is sensitive for the diagnosis of acute rejection and pneumonia.)

Verschuuren EA et al: Treatment of posttransplant lymphoproliferative disease with rituximab: the remission, the relapse, and the complication. Transplantation 2002;73:100. [PMID: 11792987]. (In this article, rituximab, a humanized anti-CD20 monoclonal antibody, is shown to be an effective treatment of posttransplant lymphoproliferative disease.)

Yousem SA et al: Revision of the 1990 working formulation for the classification of pulmonary allograft rejection: Lung Rejection Study Group. J Heart Lung Transplant 1996;15:1. [PMID: 8820078]. (This article summarizes the updated classification for pulmonary allograft rejection.)

SECTION V

Diseases of the Pulmonary Vasculature

Pulmonary Arterial Hypertension | 18

Karen A. Fagan, MD

ESSENTIALS OF DIAGNOSIS

- *Common signs and symptoms: dyspnea on exertion, syncope–near syncope, chest pain.*
- *Accentuated second heart sound, systolic murmur of tricuspid regurgitation.*
- *Evidence of right heart failure: elevated jugular venous pressure, hepatic congestion, ascites, peripheral edema.*
- *Decreased diffusing capacity, hypoxemia.*
- *Cardiomegaly and enlarged central pulmonary arteries on chest radiograph.*
- *Enlarged right-sided cardiac chambers on echocardiography.*

General Considerations

The pulmonary circulation is usually a low-pressure, low-resistance, high-capacitance circuit that can accommodate large increases in blood flow during exercise without significant increases in pressure. Pulmonary arterial hypertension (PAH) is defined as a resting pulmonary artery mean pressure >25 or >30 with exercise. Previously, PAH had been defined as primary pulmonary hypertension (PPH) or secondary pulmonary hypertension (SPH), but the more general classification of PAH has now been adopted. PAH is a diagnosis of exclusion and treatment of PAH targets the underlying cause when present.

Approximately 300–1000 new cases of idiopathic PAH are diagnosed in the United States each year, al-though this may be increasing as a result of increased physician awareness. Women in the third and fourth decades of life are affected more frequently than men (1.7:1). Prior to development of effective treatment, median survival was estimated as 2.8 years from the time of diagnosis with a progressive decline in functional status until death.

PAH can occur in isolation (idiopathic Primary) or can be associated with a number of other diseases including connective tissue diseases (especially scleroderma), advanced parenchymal lung disease with hypoxemia (ie, interstitial pulmonary fibrosis, emphysema), sleep-disordered breathing, congenital heart disease, advanced liver disease (portopulmonary hypertension), human immunodeficiency virus (HIV), and chronic thromboembolic disease. PAH has also been associated with the use of appetite-suppressive agents, amphetamines, and intravenous drugs. These diseases are all associated with increases in precapillary pulmonary arterial pressure. Other very rare lung diseases cause PAH by increasing postcapillary pulmonary venous pressure, including pulmonary venoocclusive disease and pulmonary capillary hemangiomatosis (Table 18–1).

PAH is a common complication of connective tissue diseases, especially scleroderma and mixed connective tissue disease. PAH can be found in as many as 60% of patients with the *CREST* variant of limited scleroderma (*C*alcinosis cutis, *R*aynaud's phenomenon, *E*sophageal dysmotility, *S*clerodactyly, and *T*elangectasias). The presence of PAH with connective tissue disease significantly increases mortality, with a 40% survival at 2 years following the diagnosis of PAH in patients with scleroderma.

Approximately 5–15% of cases of PAH are familial and the gene responsible for familial PAH was recently identified by two separate investigators as the bone

Table 18–1. Conditions associated with PAH.

Idiopathic (primary)
Connective tissue disease
  Scleroderma
  Systemic lupus erythematosus
  Mixed connective tissue disease
  Dermatomyositis/polymyositis
  Rheumatoid arthritis
Parenchymal lung disease
  Emphysema
  Idiopathic pulmonary fibrosis
  Chronic obstructive pulmonary disease
Heart disease
  Congenital left-to-right shunts
    Atrial septal defect
    Ventricular septal defect
    Patent ductus arteriosus
Increased pulmonary venous pressure
  Pulmonary venoocclusive disease
  Pulmonary capillary hemangiomatosis
  Left ventricular dysfunction
    Congestive heart failure
    Diastolic dysfunction
  Increased left atrial pressure
    Mitral stenosis
    Mitral regurgitation
    Constrictive myocarditis/pericarditis
Pulmonary thromboembolic disease
HIV
Liver disease with portal hypertension
Sleep apnea
Intravenous drug use
Exposure to appetite suppressants/amphetamines

morphogenetic receptor protein 2 (BMPR2), a member of the transforming growth factor-β (TGF-β) superfamily. Abnormalities in this gene have also been found in up to 30% of patients with sporadic PAH. How abnormalities in the BMPR2 gene lead to PAH is not known.

Pathogenesis

The cause of idiopathic PAH is not known. The characteristic lesion found on biopsy or at the time of autopsy is the plexiform lesion. Thickening of medial and adventitial layers and proliferation of endothelial cells within the intima characterize the plexiform lesion. This results in obliteration of the pulmonary arteriole and is also associated with *in situ* thrombosis of the narrowed vascular channels. This lesion is found in patients with idiopathic PAH and may be found in patients with connective tissue disease-associated, appetite-suppressant-associated, HIV-associated congeni-

tal heart disease-associated, and advanced liver disease-associated PAH.

The recent identification of the gene for familial PAH, BMPR2, a member of the TGF-β superfamily, suggests that abnormal regulation of cell growth may be responsible for the plexiform lesion. Recently, it was reported that the proliferating endothelial cells in the plexiform lesion are monoclonal, suggesting expansion of a select population of cells.

Other possible etiologies such as an imbalance between endogenous vasodilators (ie, nitric oxide, prostacyclin) and vasoconstrictors (ie, endothelin-1, thromboxane) have been the rationale for the currently approved therapies. Although somewhat controversial, expression of the enzyme largely responsible for nitric oxide production in the vasculature may be decreased in the plexiform lesion. In contrast, endothelin-1 is increased in both the plexiform lesion and serum of patients with both idiopathic PAH and PAH in association with connective tissue disease (Table 18–2).

Use of appetite suppressants is associated with a small but significantly increased incidence of PAH. The mechanism is not clear but may be related to increased serotonin.

For patients with PAH in association with advanced cardiopulmonary disease, the etiology of the PAH is likely multifactorial (Table 18–2). In patients with severe emphysema, both loss of the vascular bed due to destruction of the lung parenchyma and vasoconstriction due to hypoxia contribute to the development of PAH. Hypoxia causes PAH by leading to sustained contraction of the pulmonary arteries and hypertrophy of vascular smooth muscle. It does so by stimulating smooth muscle cells directly and also by contributing to an imbalance between vasodilators and vasoconstrictors. Congenital left-to-right cardiac shunts increase pulmonary blood flow and can result in remodeling of the pulmonary circulation and narrowing of the pulmonary arteries. Pulmonary embolism, both acute and chronic, causes obstruction of pulmonary arteries.

Table 18–2. Potential mechanisms of PAH.

Mutations of bone morphogenetic receptor 2 gene
Proliferation of cells
  Monoclonal expansion of endothelial cells
  Vascular smooth muscle cell hypertrophy
Vasoconstriction
  Hypoxia
  Decreased vasodilators (nitric oxide, prostacyclin)
  Increased vasoconstrictors (endothelin-1, thromboxane)
Inflammation—relationship to connective tissue disease
Toxin exposure—amphetamines, appetite suppressants

Increased pulmonary venous pressure from a wide variety of causes also increases pulmonary arterial pressure and can produce pulmonary edema, which is not a feature of precapillary PAH. Pulmonary venoocclusive disease is a very rare idiopathic disease characterized by fibrosis and thrombosis of the pulmonary veins, which leads to pulmonary edema and can cause hemoptysis. There is no effective therapy. Currently available treatments for PAH may lead to severe pulmonary edema and death in patients with postcapillary PAH (ie, pulmonary venoocclusive disease and pulmonary capillary hemangiomatosis).

Prevention

Unfortunately, there are few preventive measures for idiopathic PAH. Avoidance of agents associated with the development of PAH such as appetite suppressants and amphetamines is important. Family members of patients with PAH should strongly consider performing screening echocardiography (perhaps with exercise), which may identify familial cases before the onset of disabling symptoms. Although a gene responsible for familial PAH has been identified, genetic screening is not available.

Although complicated, adequate treatment of underlying diseases associated with PAH with underlying diseases, may prevent or improve PAH. For example, in patients with severe lung disease associated with hypoxemia, treatment with supplemental oxygen may improve PAH. A more detailed discussion regarding treatment options is discussed below.

Clinical Findings

Figure 18–1 presents an algorithm for evaluating patients with suspected PAH.

A. SYMPTOMS AND SIGNS

The symptoms of idiopathic PAH are insidious and are usually present for some time prior to the diagnosis. Dyspnea on exertion is the most common presenting symptom and is often attributed to deconditioning, asthma, etc. Chest pain, described as angina-like in quality, is also a frequent complaint. The cause of the pain is not known but may reflect ischemia of the strained and hypertrophied right ventricle. Patients with advanced disease may have signs of right heart failure such as jugular venous distention, hepatic congestion, ascites, and lower extremity edema. Syncope may also occur, as the cardiac output in advanced PAH is low and unable to increase during changes in position (ie, sitting to standing) or with physical exertion. In pa-

tients with PAH in association with other diseases, the symptoms of PAH are similar but are often attributed to the underlying disease and not PAH. Unfortunately, none of the symptoms of PAH is specific to this disease. Thus, many patients remain undiagnosed until the condition is advanced.

Assessment of functional status is important in directing therapy for patients with PAH. The New York Heart Association (NYHA) functional status classification is widely used to characterize functional limitation in patients with PAH (Table 18–3).

The clinical history is an important tool in determining if suspected PAH is idiopathic or is associated with other cardiopulmonary or systemic diseases. Identifying possible causative diseases may influence therapeutic options for patients. Specifically, a history of heart murmurs may suggest congenital heart disease as a potential cause of PAH. A history of deep venous thrombosis (DVT) and/or pulmonary embolus (PE) may suggest chronic thromboembolic pulmonary hypertension as a cause. The presence of Raynaud's phenomenon, arthritis, and/or rash may suggest an underlying connective tissue disease. Headache, snoring, and daytime somnolence may suggest sleep-disordered breathing. A history of ethanol use and/or hepatitis may suggest underlying liver disease and portopulmonary hypertension. A history of exposure to medications or illicit drugs should also be obtained, as use of certain drugs has been associated with an increased risk of developing PAH. Lastly, a careful family history should also be obtained to look for evidence of familial disease.

A physical examination may be very helpful in establishing the diagnosis of PAH and suggesting other associated conditions. Findings associated with PAH include an accentuated second heart sound, systolic murmur consistent with tricuspid regurgitation, palpable pulmonic valve closure, right ventricular heave, jugular venous distention, hepatomegaly, ascites, and peripheral edema. Patients frequently have low systemic blood pressures from compromised cardiac output. Findings of other systemic diseases such as connective tissue disease and liver disease may also be present during the physical examination.

B. LABORATORY FINDINGS

The laboratory evaluation in patients with suspected PAH should include routine blood counts, electrolytes, renal function, hepatic function, and coagulation studies. Polycythemia may suggest chronic, severe hypoxemia while a prolonged partial prothrombin time (PTT) might suggest a lupus anticoagulant and hypercoagulable state. Abnormal liver function might suggest underlying hepatocellular disease. Arterial blood gases may reveal hypoxemia with a respiratory alkalosis. All

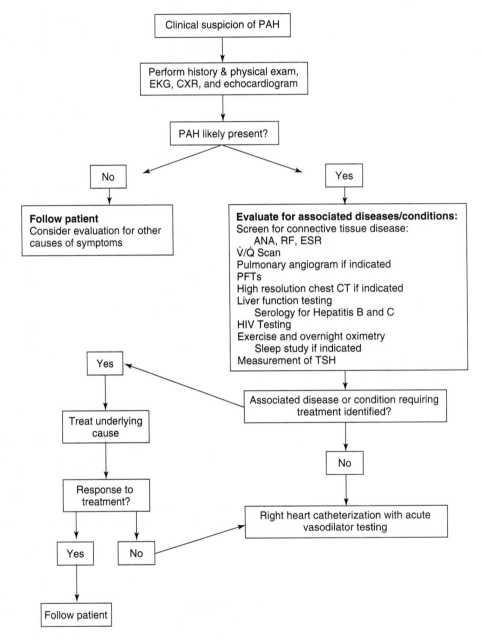

Figure 18-1. General approach for evaluating suspected PAH.

patients should undergo screening tests for collagen vascular disease including an antinuclear antibody (ANA), sedimentation rate erythrocyte (ESR), rheumatoid factor (RF), and more specific tests such as for scleroderma if clinically suggested. These tests may identify patients with previously undiagnosed connective tissue disease for which PAH is a presenting sign. All patients should also be tested for HIV. Lastly, patients with PAH should have thyroid-stimulating hormone (TSH) measured, as thyroid dysfunction has been associated with idiopathic PAH.

Electrocardiography may demonstrate right ventricular hypertrophy and a rightward axis in patients with PAH.

Table 18–3. New York Heart Association heart failure functional classification.

Class I:	Asymptomatic
Class II:	Symptoms with moderate activity
Class III:	Symptoms with mild activity
Class IV:	Symptoms at rest

An isolated decrease in diffusing capacity is the most common abnormality found during pulmonary function testing in patients with idiopathic PAH. In patients with underlying parenchymal lung disease, additional abnormalities attributable to the underlying process are found. Exercise testing may reveal a decrease in exercise tolerance and impaired gas exchange with an abnormal increase in dead space ventilation with exercise.

C. IMAGING STUDIES

Chest radiography frequently demonstrates cardiomegaly with enlarged central pulmonary arteries. If present, parenchymal lung disease such as emphysema or interstitial fibrosis may be present and should prompt evaluation with high-resolution computed tomography (CT). The presence of pulmonary edema should suggest the possibility that pulmonary venous pressure is increased as in valvular heart disease or in rare diseases such as pulmonary venoocclusive disease.

Ventilation perfusion scanning or CT angiography should be performed in all patients with PAH to evaluate for possible occult thromboembolic disease. If the scan is positive or inconclusive, pulmonary angiography should be performed to confirm or exclude the diagnosis and anatomically identify the lesions. This may be helpful in determining if the patient might be a candidate for surgical treatment of the chronic thromboembolic disease.

D. SPECIAL TESTS

Echocardiography is usually the first test suggesting the presence of PAH in patients referred for evaluation. Enlargement of the right ventricle and atrium with tricuspid regurgitation are the most common findings. In addition, left heart function and potential valvular disease can be assessed. When performed with agitated saline contrast, echocardiography may also identify right-to-left intracardiac shunting. Identification of a left-to-right shunt may require a cardiac catheterization. Echocardiography may also be a useful tool to follow response to treatment for patients with PAH, although it may not be accurate in patients without a suitable echocardiographic window.

Overnight oximetry should be performed in all patients to determine if hypoxemia worsens with sleep and requires treatment with supplemental oxygen.

Polysomnography should be performed in patients with symptoms consistent with sleep-disordered breathing and in patients with a suggestive overnight oximetry.

E. SPECIAL EXAMINATIONS

Ultimately, all patients with suspected idiopathic PAH should undergo a right heart catheterization with vasodilatory testing. Right heart catheterization allows pulmonary arterial pressure, cardiac output, and pulmonary vascular resistance to be accurately measured and also detects left-to-right shunts and evidence of left heart dysfunction. An elevated pulmonary capillary wedge pressure may suggest the presence of pulmonary venous disease (ie, pulmonary venoocclusive disease).

Acute pulmonary vasoreactivity can also be determined at the time of right heart catheterization and may ultimately direct therapy. A variety of agents have been used to test vasoreactivity including nitric oxide, adenosine, and prostacyclin. A favorable response is defined as a $\geq 10\%$ decrease in mean pulmonary artery pressure, $\geq 30\%$ increase in cardiac output, and a $\leq 30\%$ decrease in calculated pulmonary vascular resistance. A favorable response to acute administration of vasodilators may predict a response to chronic treatment with oral vasodilators such as calcium channel blockers.

Treatment

Recent advances in the treatment of patients with idiopathic PAH have dramatically improved survival and functional status. At one time, aggressive therapy for PAH was considered a bridge to transplantation. However, aggressive medical therapy extends lives and is increasingly being considered as primary therapy for these patients (Figure 18–2).

The goal of identifying a potentially treatable cause of PAH is to treat the underlying condition with the expectation that the PAH may improve. For example, in patients with severe sleep-disordered breathing or with HIV, PAH may significantly improve with continuous positive airway pressure therapy or with highly active antiretroviral therapy, respectively. Improvement in PAH following liver transplantation has been reported in patients with portopulmonary hypertension. Patients with PAH due to chronic thromboembolic disease have demonstrated marked improvement with surgical removal of lesions during pulmonary thromboendarterectomy.

A. OXYGEN

Because hypoxemia can contribute to pulmonary vasoconstriction, PAH patients with hypoxemia should be treated with supplemental oxygen to maintain an arterial oxygen saturation of >90% at all times. Patients who do not need oxygen during waking hours may still need supplemental oxygen at night and should be tested with

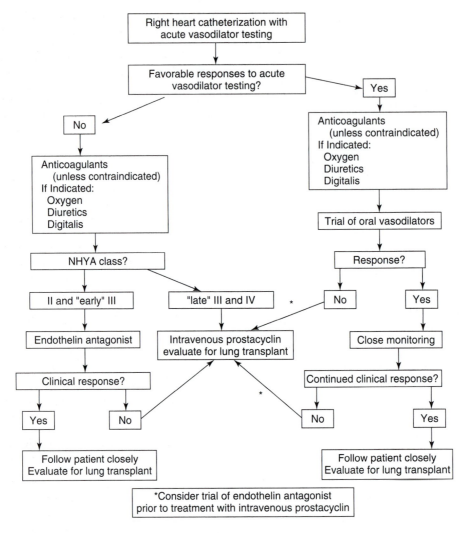

Figure 18–2. General approach to management of PAH.

overnight oximetry. In patients for whom the etiology of pulmonary hypertension is advanced lung disease with hypoxemia, supplemental oxygen is the mainstay of treatment.

B. DIURETICS

In patients with advanced PAH, either idiopathic or due to underlying disease, development of right heart failure is an ominous sign. Diuretic therapy combined with sodium and fluid restrictions may improve the peripheral edema and ascites. Choice of diuretic agents must be individualized to each patient and can include loop diuretics, thiazide diuretics, aldactone, and metolazone in refractory cases. Maintenance of normal intravascular volume is the goal of therapy.

C. ANTICOAGULATION

Idiopathic PAH has been associated with *in situ* thrombosis of the small pulmonary arterioles as well as with increased risk for thromboembolism. Thus, treatment with warfarin sodium is indicated. For patients with chronic thromboembolic PAH, life-long anticoagulation and possibly placement of an inferior vena cava filter are necessary even if the patient undergoes pulmonary thromboendarterectomy.

D. DIGITALIS

Digitalis may be indicated in patients with evidence of right ventricular failure and/or atrial dysrhythmias but requires close monitoring of levels.

E. ORAL VASODILATORS

Because approximately 25% of patients with PAH have a favorable response to vasodilators, a trial of oral vasodilators may be indicated. Calcium channel blockers (especially nifedipine and diltiazem) have been useful in treating some patients with PAH. Many centers will perform a hemodynamically monitored trial of calcium channel blockers after a favorable short-term response to determine efficacy and optimal dose. Other vasodilators with case reports of efficacy include angiotensin-converting enzyme inhibitors, α-adrenergic blockers, and hydralazine. For patients who fail to improve with oral vasodilators, treatment with other agents (see below) may be indicated.

F. PROSTACYCLIN

Prostacyclin, a metabolite of arachidonic acid, is produced by vascular endothelium and is a potent vasodilator with antimitogenic, antiplatelet aggregatory effects, as well as other effects. The more stable derivative of prostacyclin, epoprostenol, when administered by continuous intravenous infusion, is effective in treating patients with idiopathic PAH and PAH in association with scleroderma. Treatment with epoprostenol improves hemodynamics, functional status, and short- and long-term survival in patients with idiopathic PAH and likely improves survival in patients with scleroderma when compared to historical controls. Case reports have suggested improvement in epoprostenol-treated patients with congenital heart disease, HIV, and portopulmonary hypertension.

However, administration of epoprostenol is complex requiring placement and management of an indwelling intravenous catheter, reconstitution of the drug every 24–48 h, and operation of a portable infusion pump. Frequent complications are related to the presence of an indwelling catheter with insertion site infections, deep tunnel infections, and sepsis. Other less common complications include both over- and underdosing of drug, drug boluses, pump malfunction, catheter damage, catheter occlusion, thrombosis around the catheter, air embolus, and sudden death with the abrupt termination of the drug.

Thus, careful consideration regarding patient selection must be undertaken prior to initiation of intravenous epoprostenol. Patients with idiopathic PAH who do not have a favorable response to vasodilators and who have functional limitation (NYHA class III and IV symptoms) and no contraindication to treatment should be considered for intravenous epoprostenol. Patients with connective tissue disease and PAH without favorable vasodilator testing should also be considered for therapy. The presence of significant parenchymal lung disease is problematic as epoprostenol is a nonselective vasodilator and could worsen ventilation–perfusion ($\dot{V}/\dot{Q}$) mismatch by increasing perfusion to poorly ventilated areas of the lung.

Despite these limitations, treatment with continuously infused epoprostenol remains the mainstay of treatment of patients with advanced idiopathic and connective tissue disease- related PAH. For patients whose symptoms progress despite this therapy, some centers consider the addition of endothelin antagonists and lung transplant as the only remaining options.

G. ENDOTHELIN ANTAGONISTS

Recently, the endothelin-1 antagonist bosentan (Tracleer) was approved for treatment of patients with moderate to severe PAH. Studies in patients with idiopathic PAH and PAH in association with connective tissue disease demonstrated improvement in hemodynamics and functional status over a period of 16 weeks. The study was not powered to detect improvement in survival. Long-term follow-up is not yet available as this treatment has been available only since late 2001, although preliminary reports suggest a survival benefit to patients enrolled in juried studies compared to historical controls. Many centers are using this agent as first line therapy for patients with NYHA class II and early class III symptoms. For patients whose symptoms progress despite this treatment, addition or substitution of therapy with prostacyclin is the next option.

Hepatotoxicity appears to be the most limiting adverse drug reaction with bosentan thus far. Approximately 10–15% of patients treated with this agent develop a significant (more than threefold) increase in transaminases requiring either a decrease in dosage or termination of the drug. It also has been associated with a mild anemia. Teratogenicity and decreased sperm count have been reported in laboratory animals. Thus, monthly monitoring of liver function and pregnancy status as well as adequate pregnancy prevention methods are required. Sperm banking for male patients desiring future fertility is suggested.

H. TRANSPLANTATION

For patients with idiopathic PAH that progresses despite aggressive medical therapy, lung transplantation may be the only remaining option. The choice of single, double, or heart–lung transplantation remains controversial, with most centers preferring bilateral lung transplantation. In cases with severe heart disease or uncorrectable congenital heart disease, heart–lung transplantation is necessary, as the right heart is not likely to recover function after transplantation. Lung transplantation in patients with PAH has a higher operative and immediate posttransplant mortality than transplantation for other reasons. This is likely due to the severely compromised hemodynamics at baseline.

Prognosis

Prior to the development of specific therapy for idiopathic PAH, the prognosis was poor, with a median survival of less than 3 years from time of diagnosis. However, long-term treatment success has been reported with calcium channel blockers and prostacyclin in many patients, whereas the experience with endothelin antagonists is too recent to know conclusively if survival is improved. Without treatment, and in some cases despite aggressive treatment, patients may ultimately succumb to progressive right heart failure and death unless transplantation occurs.

The prognosis for patients with PAH due to underlying cardiopulmonary disease depends on successful treatment of the underlying disorder. Generally, PAH due to underlying disease carries a poor prognosis.

Badesch DB et al: Continuous intravenous epoprostenol for pulmonary hypertension due to the scleroderma spectrum of disease. A randomized, controlled trial. Ann Intern Med 2000;132:425. [PMID: 10733441]. (Randomized study of intravenous epoprostenol in patients with scleroderma-associated PAH demonstrating short-term efficacy and safety of this treatment.)

Barst RJ et al: A comparison of continuous intravenous epoprostenol (prostacyclin) with conventional therapy for primary pulmonary hypertension. The Primary Pulmonary Hypertension Study Group. N Engl J Med 1996;334:296. [PMID: 8532025]. (Report of a randomized trial of epoprostenol in patients with idiopathic PAH demonstrating short-term improvement in hemodynamics, exercise, and survival compared to conventional treatment.)

D'Alonzo GE et al: Survival in patients with primary pulmonary hypertension. Results from a national prospective registry. Ann Intern Med 1991;115:343. [PMID: 1863023]. (Results of a national registry of patients with idiopathic PAH demonstrating female predominance and poor survival.)

Deng Z et al: Familial primary pulmonary hypertension (gene PPH1) is caused by mutations in the bone morphogenetic protein receptor-II gene. Am J Hum Genet 2000;67:737. [PMID: 10903931]. (Report of the identification of BMPR2 as the gene responsible for familial PAH. Reported at the same time as Lane below.)

Lane KB et al: Heterozygous germline mutations in BMPR2, encoding a TGF-β receptor, cause familial primary pulmonary hypertension. The International PPH Consortium. Nat Genet 2000;26:81. [PMID: 10973254]. (Report of the identification of BMPR as the gene responsible for familial PAH. Reported at same time as Deng above.)

Rich S, Kaufmann E, Levy PS: The effect of high doses of calcium-channel blockers on survival in primary pulmonary hypertension. N Engl J Med 1992;327:76. [PMID: 1603139]. (Report of long-term improvement in a subgroup of patients with idiopathic PAH treated with calcium channel blockers.)

Rich S et al: Anorexigens and pulmonary hypertension in the United States: results from the surveillance of North American pulmonary hypertension. Chest 2000;117:870. [PMID: 10713017]. (Report of increased incidence of PAH in persons who took appetite-suppressant medications.)

Rubin LJ: Primary pulmonary hypertension. N Engl J Med 1997;336:111. [PMID: 8988890]. (Review article.)

Rubin LJ et al: Bosentan therapy for pulmonary arterial hypertension. N Engl J Med 2002;346:896. [PMID:11907289]. (Report of improvement on exercise and functional classification in patients in a randomized trial of endothelin antagonist with PAH.)

Thomson JR et al: Sporadic primary pulmonary hypertension is associated with germline mutations of the gene encoding BMPR-II, a receptor member of the TGF-beta family. J Med Genet 2000;37:741. [PMID: 11015450]. (Report of a high prevalence of mutations in BMPR2 in patients with sporadic, not familial PAH.)

Pulmonary Thromboembolism

19

Patrick Nana-Sinkam, MD

ESSENTIALS OF DIAGNOSIS

- *Clinicians should be aware of individual risk factors for development of pulmonary embolism.*
- *Pulmonary embolism should be considered in cases of unexplained hypoxemia.*
- *Limitations exist for all current diagnostic studies.*
- *All clinicians should have a diagnostic algorithm in cases of suspected pulmonary embolism.*

General Considerations

Venous thromboembolism (VTE), a common medical problem, is the third most common vascular disease and carries a high morbidity and mortality. It is characterized by intravenous thrombus formation either as a deep venous thrombosis (DVT) in leg veins or as a pulmonary embolism (PE), a thrombus migrating to the lung circulation from proximal leg veins or the pelvis. Risk of venous thromboembolism rises with increasing age, up from 1:10,000 in childhood to 1:100 in the elderly. It is estimated that DVT occurs in 1 of 1000 adults and PE in 10–25% of these patients. Both conditions are difficult to diagnose due to their nonspecific symptoms and signs. As a result, many cases are recognized only postmortem or after a thrombus has migrated to the lung circulation. Therefore, it is extremely important to identify patients at risk to facilitate prompt diagnosis and management (Table 19–1). An algorithm can be instrumental in doing this. Because the thrombi originate in the legs, PE is potentially avoidable if preventive therapy, such as anticoagulation or compression stockings, is used in high-risk situations.

Clinical Findings

A. Symptoms and Signs

Presenting signs and symptoms for pulmonary embolism are nonspecific, which makes clinical diagnosis difficult. The most common presenting symptoms noted in the patients from the Prospective Investigation of Pulmonary Embolism Diagnosis (PIOPED) study who had angiographically confirmed PE were dyspnea, pleuritic chest pain, and tachypnea. The findings on physical examination included increased respiratory rate, rales, tachycardia, a loud second heart sound, deep venous thrombosis, temperature above 38.5°C, wheeze, Homan's sign (pain on palpation of the calf), pleural friction rub, an S3 gallop, and cyanosis. Syncope or hypotension may uncommonly be the presenting symptoms of pulmonary embolism and suggests severe hemodynamic compromise. The presence of the above clinical findings can heighten concern for PE but does not constitute a diagnosis.

Although clinical symptoms and signs are nonspecific, clinical models using findings from history and physical examination help focus clinical suspicion for PE. Recent clinical models use weighted clinical scores to assign low, moderate, or high clinical probability of a PE. Some use clinic assessment plus a noninvasive diagnostic test, such as the d-dimer assay that measures active fibrinolysis. Wells reports an example of such a score for DVT tested prospectively on a large number of patients. This model, which includes nine findings from history and physical examination, weighs these features into a clinical score of low, moderate, or high likelihood of DVT. The features included are leg swelling, pain to palpation, heart rate greater than 100 beats/min, immobilization, surgery in the previous 4 weeks, prior PE or DVT, hemoptysis, malignancy, and likelihood of PE greater than likelihood of other diagnoses. A low probability clinical score coupled with a negative d-dimer assay gave a negative predictive value of 99.5% (CI 99.1–100%) for PE. Clinical tools such as this combined clinical/laboratory assessment protocol are useful in stratifying information obtained from the history and physical examination to decide on further diagnostic testing.

B. Laboratory Findings

1. Arterial blood gas (ABG)—ABG is of limited use in assessment of pulmonary embolism. Although respiratory alkalosis and hypoxemia are common findings, they should not be used in isolation to detect PE. In the prospective PIOPED trial, 8–23% of patients with PE confirmed by angiography had normal alveolar–arterial (A–a) oxygen gradients and 7% had completely normal ABG results. Although ABG findings should not be

Table 19–1. Risk factors for venous thromboembolism.

Immobility
Cancer
Prior VTE
Venous insufficiency
Obesity
Prolonged air travel
Major surgery
   Hip
   Knee
   Abdominal
   Neurosurgery
Pregnancy
Congestive heart failure
Myocardial infarction
Fractures of the lower extremities
Femoral catheters/other central venous catheters
Hypercoagulable conditions (malignancy, oral contraceptives,
   Protein C and S deficiency, Factor V Leiden mutation, anti-
   thrombin III deficiency)
Age
Chronic respiratory failure

---

used to confirm a diagnosis of PE, profound hypoxemia without clear explanation should raise suspicion for possible PE.

2. D-dimer—D-dimer, a product of the fibrinolytic degradation of cross-linked fibrin, has emerged as a potentially useful serological marker in the assessment of PE. Its current use is to rule out pulmonary embolism in the appropriate clinical setting; sensitivity rates are in the mid-90% range. Fibrinolytic markers including d-dimer are, however, elevated in many other medical disorders including cancer, hepatic and renal insufficiency, septicemia, stroke, and major trauma, thus limiting specificity in these situations. Five methods have been developed for detecting elevations in d-dimer: (1) enzyme-linked immunosorbent assay (ELISA) testing, which has the highest sensitivity but low specificity, (2) latex agglutination testing, which has improved specificity but lower sensitivity, (3) the immunofiltration assay, (4) an immunoturbidometric assay, and, more recently, (5) the SimpliRED d-dimer agglutination assay, which uses a biospecific antibody directed against d-dimers and red blood cells. ELISA appears to have a high negative predictive value (91–100%) but is limited by longer testing time and lack of widespread availability. Latex agglutination testing is more readily available and requires less time, but is limited by a negative predictive value between 67 and 97%. To interpret these studies, it is important to know which test is used by the local clinical laboratory. Currently, although a neg-

ative d-dimer may be used to prevent further testing in the setting of low pretest probability and low probability imaging, it does not provide full assurance of the absence of a PE.

C. IMAGING STUDIES

1. Chest radiograph—Findings on chest x-ray are rarely diagnostic for pulmonary embolism. Radiographs may often look completely normal. When abnormal, radiographs show infiltrates, pleural effusion, or atelectasis. Less common abnormalities include unilateral enlargement of a pulmonary artery, and the Westermark sign, which is the asymmetry of lung markings due to absence of perfusion distal to a clot; the hemithorax without the thrombus appears denser. Hampton's hump describes a pleural-based wedge-shaped infiltrate/atelectasis from an infarct. Chest radiography is most useful in diagnosing other processes that may present with a similar clinical picture such as pneumonia or pneumothorax. Often, the presence of a chest film showing little abnormality for a patient with new onset hypoxemia is a clue to the presence of pulmonary vascular disease such as PE.

2. Ventilation–perfusion scanning—The ventilation-perfusion scan ($\dot{V}/Q$) has been the most common diagnostic test for suspected pulmonary embolism. ^{99}Tc-radiolabeled albumin is injected intravenously into the pulmonary capillary bed followed by inhalation of a radioactive gas to assess ventilation. A diagnosis of pulmonary embolism is based on the pattern of ventilatory and perfusion defects with PE causing large segmental decrease in perfusion with preserved ventilation. Major disadvantages of this test are the limitations posed by the presence of comorbid lung disease and the test's lack of sensitivity for small clots. These result in underdiagnosis of PE. Therefore nondiagnostic or negative $\dot{V}/Q$ scanning must be considered in each clinical risk setting: high, moderate, or low likelihood of PE. PIOPED data have indicated that ventilation–perfusion scanning has a high positive predictive value (96%) in the setting of a high pretest clinical suspicion and a high probability scan (Figure 19–1). However, a low probability scan with the same high clinical suspicion still has an associated 40% incidence of pulmonary embolism (Table 19–2). Scans appear to be of particular use when they are either normal or high probability rather than low or indeterminant probability; in PIOPED the majority (75%) were nondiagnostic.

Commonly, physicians need to choose a diagnostic test for pulmonary embolism for a patient with significant pulmonary disease such as chronic obstructive pulmonary disease (COPD). Data suggest that the positive predictive value of $\dot{V}/Q$ scanning remains the same, but that the incidence of indeterminant scans is much higher among those with COPD due to underlying

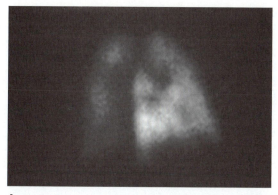

A

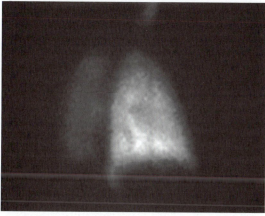

B

Figure 19–1. High-probability ventilation/perfusion images (***A, perfusion; B, ventilation***) revealing several mismatched defects in the left lung. (Courtesy of Marcus Chen, MD, Department of Nuclear Medicine, University of Colorado Health Sciences Center.)

Table 19–2. V̇/Q scan usefulness varies with high, uncertain, and unlikely clinical estimates.

V̇/Q scan	Clinical estimate of probability		
	High (80–100%)	**Uncertain (20–79%)**	**Unlikely (0–19%)**
High	28/29 (96%)	70/80 (88%)	5/9 (56%)
Indeterminate	27/41 (66%)	66/236 (28%)	11/68 (16%)
Low	6/15 (40%)	30/191 (16%)	4/90 (4%)
Near normal/ normal	0/5 (0%)	4/62 (6%)	1/61 (2%)
Total	61/90 (68%)	170/569 (30%)	21/228 (9%)

From ATS Consensus Statement (1999).

ventilation abnormalities. In the setting of a nondiagnostic study, examination of lower extremity for thrombus may be used to assist in reaching a diagnosis.

3. Lower extremity doppler—Because pulmonary thromboemboli originate primarily in the legs, lower extremity (LE) Doppler and ultrasound studies are an alternative strategy for diagnosing suspected venous thromboembolic events, particularly in the setting of nondiagnostic V̇/Q scans. Venous ultrasonography is a noninvasive and relatively inexpensive test that is useful in identifying proximal venous thrombosis. Doppler examination entails placement of an external probe for flow assessment. Patients with negative LE Dopplers and nondiagnostic V̇/Q scan may be followed with serial Doppler/ultrasound examinations. Other modalities used to examine the lower extremities include impedance plethysmography and contrast venography. Lower extremity imaging, especially if positive for clot, may complement other diagnostic tests, especially indeterminate V̇/Q scanning, even without direct visualization of the lung circulation.

4. Pulmonary angiography—Pulmonary angiography remains the gold standard for the diagnosis of pulmonary embolism. Diagnosis is based on pulmonary artery occlusion or the presence of intraluminal filling defects in two views. Other suggestive findings include asymmetrical blood flow, slow filling of the artery, and arterial cutoff. Pulmonary angiography is invasive; access is achieved via the femoral, basilic, or internal jugular vein. Angiography is reserved for a setting of high clinical suspicion when nondiagnostic testing is provided by the less invasive studies, since it has a higher complication rate due to the dye load and need for central vein catheter placement. It is important to recognize risks of angiography including bleeding risk and dye-induced nephropathy. Death has been reported in 0.2–0.5% of studies. Complications include arrhythmias and groin hematomas. Even high-risk patients, though, can safely undergo angiography if the platelet count is at least 75,000 µL, coagulation studies are only minimally elevated, and adequate prestudy hydration is provided.

5. Helical computed tomography (CT) scan—Recently, helical or spiral CT scanning has received attention as a primary diagnostic tool for acute pulmonary embolism. Helical CT scanning constructs a two-dimensional lung image over a brief period of time after injection of contrast dye. Defects in dye penetration of a vessel diagnostic of thrombus may be detected centrally or peripherally (Figure 19–2). Helical CT scanning has the advantage of being minimally invasive, similar to V̇/Q scanning. To date, there is no consensus on the role of helical CT scanning in the diagnosis of acute PE. Prospective studies have reported sensitivities

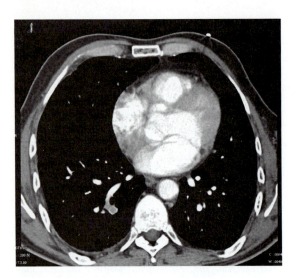

Figure 19–2. CT angiogram revealing right lower lobe intravascular filling defect with expansion consistent with acute thrombus. (Courtesy of Debra Dyer, MD, Department of Radiology, University of Colorado Health Sciences Center.)

of 53–100% and specificities ranging from 81 to 100%. There are data in selected case series revealing a low incidence of PE among patients up to 3 months after a negative helical CT scan. However, studies have been limited by several features including small sample size, bias in patient selection, retrospective selection, presence or absence of comorbid conditions, and lack of angiography as the reference standard. Interobserver variation among radiologists remains a potential problem in scan interpretation. Although helical CT is effective in imaging main, lobar, and subsegmental emboli, it generally lacks resolution for detecting subsegmental (small) emboli. Some believe that it should be a first-line replacement for V̇/Q scans and angiography, while others have suggested reserving it for selected patients in whom V̇/Q scanning is nondiagnostic or unavailable. Currently, CT scanning appears useful in identifying central emboli, an area of weakness for V̇/Q scans. It also identifies previously undetected parenchymal, pleural, and mediastinal abnormalities that could be alternate explanations for patient symptoms. A large multicenter trial is under way nationwide to assess the role of CT scanning prospectively. A promising extension of CT scanning is scanning of the pelvic and leg veins during the same injection protocol as CT of the chest to identify vena caval, iliac, or femoral venous thrombosis.

6. Magnetic resonance angiography—Magnetic resonance angiography (MRA) is an alternative method for diagnosing pulmonary vascular disease. To date, only small studies have examined the role of MRA in the diagnosis of acute PE with reports of sensitivities as high as 86% in main arteries and as low as 50% in lobar arteries. Earlier reports were limited technically by lack of contrast enhancement. Current studies using contrast-enhanced methods report slightly better results for this unproven test.

7. Electrocardiograms (ECGs)—ECGs are of limited use in diagnosing acute PE. Most commonly, patients present with sinus tachycardia. Although patterns of right ventricular strain may be evident, these are often absent, especially for small emboli. Findings of right ventricular strain include right bundle branch block (RBBB), incomplete RBBB, T wave inversions in V1–V4 or III, S wave in I, Q wave in III, and S1Q3T3 complexes. In a prospective assessment of ECGs in patients with suspected pulmonary embolism, only sinus tachycardia [positive predictive value (PPV) 38%, negative predictive value (NPV) 81%] and incomplete RBBB (PPV 100%, NPV 77%) were significantly more frequent in patients with confirmed PE.

8. Echocardiogram—For the majority of patients, echocardiography adds little to diagnosis or treatment. In submassive PE, however, right ventricular electrocardiographic strain patterns vary with the severity of the pulmonary artery pressure estimated by echocardiogram. These patterns help estimate the extent of PE in clinically severe cases. Some authors have suggested that echocardiogram may identify right ventricular dysfunction in the suspected massive pulmonary embolism and guide a decision for use of thrombolytic therapy.

9. Diagnostic algorithm—At present, there is no perfect algorithm for PE assessment. Experts have endorsed strategies such as the one outlined in Figure 19–3. Helical CT scans are playing an increasing role in diagnosis despite the lack of wide-based prospective testing. Their current use should probably be similar to the V̇/Q scan with pursuance of low probability or negative results using a pulmonary angiogram as clinically indicated. Negative d-dimer assays may be added to a clinical algorithm to minimize further scanning in the low likelihood clinical settings.

Differential Diagnosis

Given the frequently nonspecific symptoms observed in pulmonary embolism, multiple diagnoses are often considered. Chest radiograph is performed to rule out pneumonia, pleural effusion, pneumothorax, or congestive heart failure, all of which can have chest pain or shortness of breath. Cardiac ischemia presents with acute onset chest pressure or shortness of breath and can be initially assessed by electrocardiogram. Based on the previous clinical history, exacerbations of COPD,

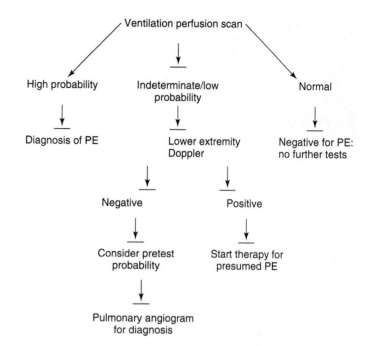

Figure 19–3. Clinical presentation and suspicion for pulmonary embolism. D-dimer can be used at the time of presentation to help interpret V̇/Q scan.

asthma, gastroesophageal reflux with aspiration, esophageal spasm, and unusual presentations of high-altitude pulmonary edema or drug reactions are considered. Very rarely, interstitial lung disease has an acute presentation.

Treatment

PE and DVT comprise a systemic disease with similar therapeutic strategies. Treatment options are growing due to new pharmaceutical developments and are outlined below.

A. UNFRACTIONATED HEPARIN

Heparin is considered by most to be first line therapy in confirmed PE, and low-molecular-weight heparin is currently first line therapy for DVT. Heparin acts by enhancing the effect of antithrombin III, which results in inactivation of thrombin (factor IIa), factor Xa, factor V, and factor VIII. Heparin is effective in reducing mortality among patients with PE. Initial dosing is best achieved via a weight-based nomogram using an initial bolus of 80 U/kg followed by a continuous infusion of 18 U/kg/h and monitored by following the activated partial thromboplastin time (PTT). Several retrospective and randomized trials have concluded that the risk of recurrent venous thromboembolism is reduced if the PTT is maintained at levels between 1.5 and 2.3 times normal. However, circulating factors such as heparin-

binding proteins can decrease the effect of heparin. Therefore, some advocate monitoring of plasma heparin levels (goal of 0.2-0.4 IU/mL) in the treatment of acute thrombosis. It is important to avoid underanticoagulation as inadequate heparinization in the first 24 h heightens the risk of recurrent PE. The minimum duration of heparin administration in the setting of acute thrombosis appears to be 5 days. Oral warfarin should be started in this time window. Heparin may be discontinued 24–48 h after an international normalized ratio (INR) of >2.0 is reached on the PT test used to monitor warfarin effect.

There is a 1% incidence of heparin-induced thrombocytopenia (HIT) with heparin use, which can lead to paradoxical arterial or venous thrombus formation (heparin-induced thrombocytopenia and thrombosis, HITT). In this setting in the presence of heparin, platelet factor 4/heparin complexes induce platelet aggregation. Reduction in platelet count is seen in the first 5–7 days of therapy and is unusual beyond 2 weeks. Because of this, the American College of Chest Physicians (ACCP) guidelines recommend checking a platelet count between Days 3 and 5 of therapy. Should the platelet count drop below 100,000/μL or by 50%, heparin should be discontinued and alternative therapy chosen. Diagnostic tests for heparin-induced antibodies are notoriously inaccurate and include a high rate of false negative results. Thus, clinical suspicion should drive cessation of heparin even when the assay is nondiagnostic. Other heparin-associated complications include bleeding and osteoporosis. Contraindications to anticoagulation include recent major bleeding including cerebral hemorrhage or gastrointestinal bleed. Heparin induces osteopenia, which poses problems for the postmenopausal or pregnant patient.

B. Low-Molecular Weight Heparin

Therapy for venous thromboembolic disease has recently expanded to include low-molecular-weight heparins (LMWH). Several options are available (Table 19–3). These molecules have a mean molecular weight of 4000–5000 Da, compared to unfractionated heparin, with a higher mean molecular weight of 15,000 Da. Advantages of LMWH are a subcutaneous route of administration, lack of need for laboratory monitoring or dose adjustment, and reduction in length of required hospitalization. Several randomized controlled trials have successfully compared the efficacy of LMWH to unfractionated heparin in the setting of acute thrombosis and concluded that LMWH appears to be at least as effective as unfractionated heparin in DVT and stable pulmonary embolism. However, ACCP guidelines have suggested these minimal requirements for use of LMWH, particularly in the outpatient setting: DVT or PE without evidence of hemodynamic instability, hypoxemia, absence of severe renal insufficiency, appropriate support for outpatient administration and surveillance, and low bleeding risk.

C. Alternate Anticoagulant Drugs

For acute anticoagulation, there are new anticoagulant options under development including a pentasaccharide Fondaparinux that is a Factor x inhibitor with even smaller molecular size than LMWH, and possibly less toxicity. The direct thrombin inhibitors lepirudin, hirudin, and argatroban are currently available for use in HIT or HITT when heparin is contraindicated.

Table 19–3. Low-molecular-weight heparin and heparin treatment dosing.

Unfractionated heparin	80 U/kg bolus and 18 U/kg/h intravenously
Enoxaparin (Lovenox)	1 mg/kg subcutaneously twice a day or 1.5 mg/kg subcutaneously daily
Dalteparin (Fragmine)	200 anti-Xa IU/kg subcutaneously daily
Tinzaparin	175 anti-Xa IU/kg daily
Nadroparin (Innohep)	86 anti-Xa IU/kg subcutaneously twice a day for 10 days
(Fraxiparin)	

There is also clinical experience with dextran and danaparoid for those patients who cannot use heparin or LMWH. Therapy with danaparoid is monitored by an antifactor xa assay.

D. Warfarin Sodium (Coumadin)

Coumadin is the common coumarin derivative used in the United States. Coumarins function by inhibiting several vitamin K-dependent proteins including factors II, VII, IX, and X and two anticoagulant factors: protein C and S. Overlap therapy with heparin in the setting of acute VTE is needed to avoid a paradoxical procoagulant effect in early warfarin therapy. Coumadin must be administered for several days in order to reach therapeutic levels. Therapy is monitored by checking the INR, which represents a standardization of the prothrombin time. Effective therapy for VTE is usually achieved with an INR of 2.0–3.0. Warfarin is potentially teratogenic and should not be used during pregnancy.

E. Thrombolytic Therapy

Although first used 30 years ago, thrombolytic therapy including streptokinase, urokinase, and tissue plasminogen activator followed by heparin therapy remains a limited part of treatment for PE (Table 19–4). This is due to the marginal improvement over heparin or LMWH alone, and the risk of intracerebral bleeding. Use in PE has been limited to the hemodynamically unstable patient. Recently, a trial of treatment of the hemodynamically stable patient with acute right heart failure demonstrated by echocardiogram has suggested that the bleeding risk can be lowered by changing the dose and duration of the thrombolytic agent. The role of thrombolytic treatment in improving outcome in PE still, however, remains controversial.

F. Vena Caval Filters

In clinical practice, vena caval interruption is accomplished by surgery or a placement of a filter. The purpose is to prevent embolization of venous thromboses to the lung when the risk of anticoagulation is high, such as for a person with a recent gastrointestinal bleed, or when anticoagulation in therapeutic doses has failed to prevent a pulmonary embolism. The data on use of vena caval filters are mixed. A randomized controlled

Table 19–4. Thrombolytic agents.

Streptokinase	250,000 IU load followed by 100,000 IU/h for 24 h
Urokinase	4400 IU/kg body weight load followed by 2200 IU/kg/h for 12 h
Tissue plasminogen activator (tPA)	100 mg infusion over 2 h

trial in Europe compared filter use to no filter in 400 patients with DVT. Although acute risk of PE was lower for those receiving a filter (1.1% vs. 4.8%), outcomes at 2 years demonstrated a 1.87-fold increase in risk of recurrent DVT for persons with the filter. There was no difference in 2-year mortality between groups. Thus the frequent use of filters should probably be minimized, especially as sole treatment for pulmonary embolism. ACCP guidelines recommend the placement of filters in cases of acute thrombus when anticoagulation is contraindicated and cases in which there is recurrent thrombus despite adequate anticoagulation.

G. Direct Vascular Infusion of Thrombolytic Agents/Embolectomy

Data on the use of both direct thrombolytic infusion into the pulmonary circulation and embolectomy are limited. However, for patients with pulmonary embolism and hemodynamic instability who fail to respond to thrombolysis or have contraindications these options may be considered.

Duration of Therapy

For pulmonary embolism in the setting of an identified risk situation such as trauma, myocardial infarction, or surgery, total anticoagulation duration is recommended at 3–6 months. For patients with recurrent venous thrombosis, some experts would consider life-long therapy if the risk of bleeding is not high. Duration of therapy for idiopathic venous thrombosis, defined as thrombosis without a recognizable clinical risk event, is at least 6 months, with longer duration or even life-long therapy recommended by some experts. Inclusion of genetic risk information in treatment decisions is not standardized, but it is likely that those with genetic risk factors may be those who present with VTE without recognizable risk factors. In a recent randomized trial, authors concluded that low-intensity anticoagulation with coumadin (INR 1.5 to 2.0) beyond standard duration of therapy is effective in preventing recurrent thromboembolism.

Other Considerations

A. Prophylaxis

Clearly, prevention of thrombus is preferred to treatment, as the sequelae of PE include pulmonary hypertension, hypoxemia, and death. Identification of high-risk conditions or diseases should be pursued whenever possible. Causal factors for VTE can be determined for a majority of cases. The ACCP guidelines note conditions of high risk and make recommendations for prevention in surgical settings such as general surgery, hip and knee surgery, hip fracture, and neurosurgery. Medical conditions are less well studied but myocardial in-

farction, congestive heart failure, stroke, malignancy, pregnancy and the postpartum period, and intensive care unit illness also pose high risk. Oral contraceptive pills and hormone replacement therapy confer a mild increase in risk, which may be higher in those with underlying genetic risk factors. Risk of thrombosis also increases with age, obesity, and prolonged travel.

Absolute criteria for preventive therapy for situations other than surgery are not straightforward. Prevention includes heparin, 5000 U subcutaneously twice a day, LMWH, and compressive pneumatic stockings. A combination of the anticoagulant with compression stockings may be better than one or the other alone in certain high-risk situations. Recommendations for surgical prophylaxis are outlined by the ACCP consensus conference on antithrombotic therapy as summarized in Table 19–5.

B. Hypercoagulable/Genetic Risk Factor Assessment

The growing knowledge of genetic risk factors for VTE has captured the imagination but outstrips knowledge of clinical application. Many identified risk factors involve the activated protein C endogenous anticoagulant system, including the factor V Leiden (FVL) mutation where FVL fails to bind to the activated protein C complex and switch off thrombosis. Genetic polymorphisms such as FVL lead to underactivity of this endogenous anticoagulant system, as do high levels of factor VIII and low levels of protein C or protein S. Other well-characterized procoagulant conditions associated with higher risk of venous thromboembolism include the antithrombin (AT) deficiency, formerly called AT III. High levels of homocysteine and the prothrombin 20210 G-A point mutation are moderate risk factors. Abnormalities of the fibrinolytic system that are not yet fully characterized likely enhance risk as well. These include high levels of or mutations in fibrinogen and the plasminogen activator inhibitor, PAI-1.

Although there is much interest in the inherited genetic polymorphisms, acquired conditions often pose a hypercoagulable risk. The lupus anticoagulant, measured as an elevated anticardiolipin antibody, is a common example. There is growing recognition that hypercoagulability risks may be acquired rather than only inherited. Acquired inflammatory conditions, including malignancy, infection, and collagen vascular disease, may induce a hypercoagulable state and thrombus formation. Combinations of genetic and acquired risk may result in a synergistic increase in thrombosis risk. In addition to heightened risk from a genetic plus an acquired risk factor, two or more genetic risk factors also appear to act synergistically to increase risk of VTE.

A genetic panel of tests is frequently ordered at the time of clinical diagnosis of PE. Assessment for a hyper-

Table 19–5. Prophylaxis recommendations from ACCP consensus conference on antithrombotic therapy, 2001, based on thromboembolism risk for surgical patients.

Risk	Proximal DVT	PE	Prevention
Low risk Early mobilization Minor surgery for patients under age 40 and no other risk factors	0.4%	0.2%	None
Moderate risk Minor surgery with other risk factors: nonmajor surgery for patients ages 40–60 without risk factors, major surgery patients under age 40 without risk factors	2–4%	1–2%	Low dose heparin (5000 U subcutaneously every 12 h), or LMWH, or elastic stockings, or pneumatic compression stockings
High risk Nonmajor surgery in patients over age 60 or with risk factors; major surgery for patients over age 40 or with risk factors	4–8%	2–4%	Low dose heparin every 8 h, LMWH, or pneumatic compression stockings
Highest risk Major surgery in patients over age 40 plus prior thrombosis, cancer, or identified hypercoagulable risk; hip or knee arthroplasty, hip fracture surgery, major trauma, spinal cord injury	10–20%	4–10%	LMWH, oral anticoagulants, pneumatic compression + LMWH/low-dose heparin, or full dose heparin

coagulable state should be considered in persons younger than age 45 with thrombosis, for those with a positive family history, and/or in the setting of recurrent VTE. For genetic testing, the timing of sample accrual is not important, however, factor levels, antithrombin, and protein S and protein C activity are affected by disease and use of anticoagulant drugs. Patients may be inappropriately labeled protein C deficient, for example, if samples are taken during presentation with an acute clot. Optimal timing of samples is at least 3 weeks after stopping all anticoagulant medications. Although debatable, a standard hypercoagulable work-up should start with prothrombin time (PT), activated partial thromboplastin time (PTT), and anticardiolipin antibody (aCL) or lupus anticoagulant, using the latter to assess for antiphospholipid syndrome, which is relatively common in adults with unexplained thrombosis. For persons younger than age 45, with multiple recurrent thromboses or thrombosis in the absence of clinical risk factors, where there is a higher likelihood of inherited risk, a genetic work-up may be slightly more extensive and include antithrombin, protein C, protein S, and factor V Leiden. Good outcome data are, however, lacking for this recommendation.

C. SUSPECTED PULMONARY EMBOLISM IN PREGNANCY

In the evaluation of suspected pulmonary embolism, ventilation–perfusion scanning appears to be a safe diagnostic study and may be used in conjunction with lower extremity ultrasound in the setting of a nondiag- nostic scan. Regarding therapy for acute venous thromboembolism, unfractionated heparin or LMWH should be utilized as warfarin clearly has teratogenic effects.

Prognosis

Approximately 1% of pulmonary emboli result in death. Patients may be left with debilitating symptoms of shortness of breath and chronic pulmonary hypertension, although most have resolution of the majority of their symptoms. Postphlebitic syndrome causes symptoms for approximately 20% of those with DVT. A person with a single PE or DVT in a high clinical risk setting may never have a recurrence. If an event is idiopathic or if there are multiple events, the clinical risk of recurrent thrombosis versus the risk of anticoagulant-induced bleeding should be weighed to see if there is reason for life-long anticoagulation therapy.

Adcock DM, Fink L, Marlar RA: A laboratory approach to the evaluation of hereditary hypercoagulability. Am J Clin Pathol 1997;108:434. [PMID: 9322598]. (One view of hypercoagulable assessment.)

American Thoracic Society Committee on Venous Thromboembolism: The diagnostic approach to acute venous thromboembolism, Clinical Practice Guideline. Am J Respir Crit Care Med 1999;160:1043. [PMID: 10471639]. (This is an extensive compilation of detailed information on diagnostic testing.)

Chan WS et al: Suspected pulmonary embolism in pregnancy. Arch Intern Med 2002;162:1170. [PMID: 11530132]. (This cohort study of 120 pregnant women undergoing evaluation for suspected pulmonary embolism addresses ventilation–perfusion scans and safety.)

Dalen JE, Hirsh J, Guyatt G (eds): Sixth ACCP Consensus Conference on Antithrombotic Therapy. Chest 2001;119(Suppl): 1S. (This document is the consensus of experts and has an extensive bibliography and treatment recommendations.)

Decousus H et al: A clinical trial of vena caval filters in the prevention of pulmonary embolism in patients with proximal deep-vein thrombosis. Prevention du Risque d'Embolie Pulmonaire par Interruption Cave Study Group. N Engl J Med 1998;338:409. [PMID: 9459643]. (The only randomized trial using vena caval filters.)

Goldstein N et al: The impact of the introduction of a rapid d-dimer assay on the diagnostic evaluation of suspected pulmonary embolism. Arch Intern Med 2001;161:567. [PMID: 11252116]. (Randomized prospective trial examining the impact of a rapid d-dimer assay on diagnostic testing.)

Ost D et al: The negative predictive value of spiral computed tomography for the diagnosis of pulmonary embolism in patients with nondiagnostic ventilation-perfusion scans. Am J Med 2001;110:16. [PMID: 11152860]. (Results are reassuring but patient selection may have biased these results.)

PIOPED Investigators: Value of the ventilation/perfusion scan in acute pulmonary embolism. Results of the prospective investigation of pulmonary embolism diagnosis (PIOPED). JAMA 1990;263:2753. [PMID: 2332918]. (This is a comprehensive study comparing ventilation–perfusion scanning to the "gold standard" pulmonary angiography.)

Rathbun S, Raskob G, Whitsett T: Sensitivity and specificity of helical computed tomography in the diagnosis of pulmonary embolism: a systematic review. Ann Intern Med 2000;132:227. [PMID: 10651604]. (This is a review of the case series that use helical CT scanning for PE diagnosis. Many design flaws are revealed.)

Ridker, P etal: Long-term, low intensity warfarin therapy for the prevention of recurrent venous thromboembolism. N Engl J Med 2003;348:1425 [PMID 126010175]. (Randomized trial that concludes that in cases of idiopathic venous thromboembolism, long-term, low-intensity warfarin therapy is beneficial.)

Stein PD, Henry JW: Clinical characteristics of patients with acute pulmonary embolism stratified according to their presenting syndromes. Chest 1997;112:974. [PMID: 9377961]. (Study evaluating presenting clinical symptoms.)

Wells PS et al: Excluding pulmonary embolism at the bedside without diagnostic imaging: management of patients with suspected pulmonary embolism presenting to the emergency department by using a simple clinical model and d-dimer. Ann Intern Med 2001;135:98. [PMID: 11453709]. (An excellent method of combining a clinical index with d-dimer levels to minimize use of ventilation–perfusion scanning.)

Vasculitis & the Diffuse Alveolar Hemorrhage Syndromes

20

Gregory P. Cosgrove, MD, & Marvin I. Schwarz, MD

PULMONARY VASCULITIDES

 ESSENTIALS OF DIAGNOSIS

- Subacute–acute onset.
- Anorexia.
- Fever.
- Multisystem involvement.

General Considerations

The pulmonary vasculitides are a heterogeneous group of systemic disorders (Table 20–1) characterized by vascular inflammation leading to tissue necrosis and subsequent end-organ dysfunction. Pulmonary vasculitis may be a manifestation of an underlying connective tissue disease, such as systemic lupus erythematosus, or may occur in the absence of any other associated, underlying disease, as is the case in microscopic polyangiitis or Goodpasture's syndrome.

In general, the systemic vasculitides are uncommon and involve the lung with variable frequency. Pulmonary involvement occurs in up to 70–90% of patients with Wegener's granulomatosis (WG) but is rare in several other disorders such as giant cell arteritis, Behçet's syndrome, polyarteritis nodosa, cryoglobulinemia, and Kawasaki's disease. The incidence varies from two to three cases per million people per year for microscopic polyangiitis to 12–13 cases per million people per year for vasculitis associated with the collagen vascular diseases. Recent studies suggest that the incidence of systemic vasculitis is increasing. However, this increase likely reflects the recent availability and widespread use of testing for antineutrophil cytoplasmic antibodies (ANCAs), autoantibodies commonly found in WG, microscopic polyangiitis, polyarteritis nodosa (PAN), and Churg–Strauss syndrome (CSS).

Vasculitis is defined as inflammation of a vessel involving small, medium, or large arteries or veins. If medium- or large-diameter vessels are involved, infarction, necrosis, and end-organ dysfunction result. In contrast, involvement of small-diameter vessels (ie, capillaries, arterioles, and venules) results in the loss of vascular integrity and leakage of blood into the tissue. Small-diameter vessel involvement in the lung is termed pulmonary or alveolar capillaritis and manifests as diffuse alveolar hemorrhage (DAH). The analogous lesions in the skin and kidney appear as leukocytoclastic vasculitis with visible, raised palpable purpura, and sometimes as petechiae and focal, segmental, necrotizing glomerulonephritis. Although the focus of this chapter is on the pulmonary manifestations of vasculitides, it should be noted that any organ system can be affected.

Several of the systemic vasculitides can be further subclassified based on their histopathology. WG, CSS, necrotizing sarcoid granulomatosis, giant cell arteritis, and Takayasu's arteritis all share the similar histological features of granulomatous inflammation.

Granulomatous inflammation involving small- and medium-diameter blood vessels is characteristic of WG. Concomitant with vascular inflammation and tissue necrosis, a necrotizing granulomatous process is present in the tissue adjacent to and within the wall of the affected blood vessel. An area of central necrosis, surrounded by mixed acute and chronic inflammatory cells, palisading histiocytes, and giant cells is seen in WG. These changes are most apparent in tissue obtained from the lung. Samples from other sites such as the kidney may reveal nonspecific changes that can be seen in a variety of systemic vasculitides. Focal, segmental necrotizing glomerulonephritis, often with crescent formation, may be present not only in WG but in many different vasculitides and is therefore limited in differentiating the exact nature of the illness.

In CSS, granulomatous inflammation of medium- and small-diameter vessels is associated with an eosinophilic cellular infiltration of vessel walls and an eosinophilic pneumonia. Giant cell arteritis, the most common type of vasculitis, and Takayasu's arteritis also present with granulomatous inflammation; however, giant cell arteritis rarely involves the lung. Takayasu's arteritis affects large- and medium-diameter vessels and may lead to major pulmonary artery occlusion.

Table 20–1. Systemic vasculitides.

Small-diameter vessel vasculitis
    Behçet's syndrome
    Wegener's granulomatosis
    Churg–Strauss syndrome
    Collagen vascular diseases
    Polyarteritis nodosa
    Microscopic polyangiitis
    Isolated pauci-immune capillaritis
    Henoch–Schönlein purpura
    Mixed cryoglobulinemia
    Goodpasture's syndrome
Medium-diameter vessel vasculitis
    Takayasu's arteritis
    Giant cell arteritis
    Behçet's syndrome
Large-diameter vessel vasculitis
    Takayasu's arteritis
    Giant cell arteritis
    Behçet's syndrome

Sullivan, EJ, Hoffman GS: Pulmonary vasculitis. Clin Chest Med 1998;19:759. [PMID: 9917965]. (Overview of the pulmonary vasculitides.)

Pathogenesis

The pathogenesis of this group of diseases remains unknown. Recent evidence suggests that certain ethnicities are more predisposed to a vasculitide; concurrent infections may also predispose patients to develop one of the several different vasculitides. WG is more likely in patients whose upper respiratory tract is chronically colonized by staphylococci. PAN, cryoglobulinemia, and microscopic polyangiitis are associated with chronic hepatitis B and C viral infections. Takayasu's arteritis occurs in young women of Asian descent. CSS follows a several year prodrome of allergic rhinitis and asthma.

Two different immunological processes have been implicated in the pathogenesis of vasculitis: (1) pathogenetic autoantibodies to neutrophil cytoplasmic components and (2) immune complex deposition.

The development of ANCAs occurs in 85% of patients with WG, 70% of patients with microscopic polyangiitis (MPA), 45% of patients with CSS, and 10–20% of patients with PAN. PAN, however, rarely affects the lung. The autoantibodies are directed against neutrophil cytoplasmic components. By utilizing indirect immunofluorescent staining techniques, two distinct staining patterns are commonly seen. A cytoplasmic-staining pattern (c-ANCA) occurs most commonly in WG. Autoantibodies are directed against a serine

proteinase, proteinase-3. A perinuclear-staining pattern (p-ANCA) most commonly occurs in MPA, CSS, and PAN where the autoantibodies are directed against myeloperoxidase. Autoantibodies to several other antigens may result in a positive p-ANCA. However, the clinical significance of antibodies to these different epitopes has yet to be determined.

In contrast to other autoantibodies, it is believed that ANCAs actively participate in the pathogenesis of the vasculitides. One proposal is that activated, circulating neutrophils express proteinase-3 and/or myeloperoxidase on their cell surfaces. ANCAs bind to the target sites on an activated neutrophil cell membrane, proteinase-3 or myeloperoxidase, and initiate the respiratory burst, degranulation, neutrophil fragmentation, and subsequent apoptosis (cell death). Toxic oxygen radicals and cytoplasmic proteolytic enzymes are thereby released into the surrounding tissue, causing endothelial and tissue injury. The ANCAs additionally inhibit the naturally occurring antiinflammatory α_1-antiprotease inhibitor, and thereby enhance the enzymatic injury caused by serine proteases. Direct endothelial-cell cytotoxicity and the release of chemokines that are able to attract inflammatory cell populations have also been associated with ANCAs. However, similar vasculitic changes can occur in patients who do not have circulating ANCAs and ANCA levels do not necessarily correlate with clinical activity. Therefore, additional pathogenetic mechanisms are likely present.

The second proposed pathogenetic mechanism in vasculitis involves immune complex deposition. Immune complex deposition has been found in the kidney and lungs of patients who have systemic lupus erythematosus (SLE), mixed connective tissue disease (MCTD), rheumatoid arthritis (RA), Henoch-Schönlein purpura (HSP), and Goodpasture's syndrome. In all of these conditions, pulmonary capillaritis and/or a focal segmental necrotizing glomerulonephritis may develop.

Immune complexes attach to vascular endothelium and activate complement, which results in chemotaxis of inflammatory cells and subsequent vascular necrosis. In Goodpasture's syndrome, a specific antibody to basement membrane is found in both the lung and kidney. This antibody is directed against an antigen found in type IV collagen, the major component of basement membranes. In the majority of cases of Goodpasture's syndrome, the antibody is found in serum and in continuous, linear patterns of staining in the lung and/or kidney using direct immunofluorescence. In contrast, immune complex deposition in SLE, MCTD, RA, and HSP produces a granular, interrupted pattern of immunofluorescence, which indicates immunocomplex formation in the circulation and subsequent attachment to the tissue. Despite being ANCA positive, WG,

MPA, and CSS are not associated with immune complex deposition, and are referred to as pauci-immune.

Viral infections have been implicated in the development of vasculitic syndromes. Up to one-third of patients who have PAN show evidence of prior hepatitis B virus infection. Human immunodeficiency virus (HIV), cytomegalovirus, parvovirus B19, and hepatitis C virus have also been associated with vasculitis.

Weidebach W et al: C-ANCA-positive IgG fraction from patients with Wegener's granulomatosis induces lung vasculitis in rats. Clin Exp Immunol 2002;129:54. [PMID: 12100022].

Xiao H et al: Antineutrophil cytoplasmic autoantibodies specific for myeloperoxidase cause glomerulonephritis and vasculitis in mice [comment]. J Clin Invest 2002;110:955. [PMID: 12370273]. (Both articles provide insight into the pathogenesis of the ANCAs.)

Clinical Findings

The systemic nature of the vasculitides that affect the lung frequently results in nonspecific symptoms such as fever, malaise, anorexia, and weight loss. With respiratory tract involvement, cough, dyspnea, and hemoptysis are reported. Multiorgan involvement is common and the pattern of involvement varies with the different vasculitides. Several systemic vasculitides more commonly affect the lung, have characteristic pulmonary manifestations, and therefore deserve specific mention.

A. Wegener's Granulomatosis

WG affects the upper and lower respiratory tracts early in the course of the disease in over 70% of patients. Involvement of the upper and/or lower respiratory tract may be isolated and this is referred to as limited WG. Upper airway involvement manifests as sinus, nasal, or otic disease. Pansinusitis, involvement of the nose with crusting, nosebleeds, and septal perforation that results in saddle nose deformity are often initial manifestations of the disease. Complications occasionally include chronic otitis media and mastoiditis. Ocular involvement occurs in up to 50% of patients including conjunctivitis, episcleritis, uveitis, and retinal artery occlusion.

Tracheal and/or major bronchial involvement can result in tracheobronchial inflammation, ulceration, and malacia, which ultimately leads to stenosis and causes fixed airflow limitation. Parenchymal involvement typically manifests as single or multiple nodules with or without cavitation. Atelectasis and postobstructive pneumonias secondary to primary endobronchial obstruction may also occur. A potentially catastrophic presentation of WG is hemoptysis with diffuse pulmonary infiltrates due to DAH resulting from capillaritis. Pulmonary capillaritis may be the sole manifestation

of WG or may precede, follow, or occur with the more typical single or multiple cavitary nodules. Pleural effusions and hilar lymphadenopathy occur in a small percentage of patients.

Extrapulmonary manifestations of WG may precede or appear subsequent to the development of lung disease. Cutaneous involvement is manifest as palpable purpura (leukocytoclastic vasculitis) whereas neurological involvement presents as mononeuritis multiplex or cranial neuropathies. Diabetes insipidus has been documented as a complication of WG in which vasculitic involvement of the pituitary gland occurs. Glomerulonephritis (focal, segmental necrotizing glomerulonephritis) is a common manifestation of the generalized forms of WG. It occurs in < 40% of patients at the time of presentation but subsequently develops in more than 85% of patients. Severe renal impairment, which may require chronic dialysis, occurs.

B. Churg–Strauss Syndrome

CSS, unlike other vasculitides, follows chronic atopy (ie, rhinitis, nasal polyps, asthma, peripheral eosinophilia, and sometimes chronic eosinophilic pneumonia). Sinus disease, in the form of allergic rhinitis, and asthma are present in all affected individuals. Parenchymal lung disease is present in over 70% of cases and may occur with or without pleural effusions. Differentiating CSS from chronic eosinophilic pneumonia is often difficult as more than 50% of patients with chronic eosinophilic pneumonia also have an allergic prodrome. Additionally, chronic eosinophilic pneumonia may subsequently develop into overt CSS. Cutaneous and neurological involvement, manifest as subcutaneous skin nodules and mononeuritis multiplex, are seen in at least 60% of patients. Unlike WG, cardiac involvement occurs in up to 50% of patients, presenting as congestive heart failure, pericardial effusion, a restrictive cardiomyopathy, or dysrhythmias. Cardiac involvement portends a significantly worse prognosis with considerable morbidity and increased mortality. Vasculitic involvement of the gastrointestinal tract causes abdominal pain, gastrointestinal bleeding, and diarrhea. Glomerulonephritis (focal, segmental necrotizing glomerulonephritis) occurs less commonly in CSS than in WG.

Choi YH et al: Thoracic manifestation of Churg-Strauss syndrome: radiologic and clinical findings. Chest 2000;117:117. [PMID: 10631208]. (Review of the pulmonary manifestations of CSS.)

C. Polyarteritis Nodosa

The clinical manifestations of PAN are similar to those of CSS. However, atopy is not a feature of PAN and the incidence of glomerulonephritis is higher. As a consequence of renal involvement, hypertension is commonly seen in PAN. In contrast to WG and CSS, in which pulmonary involvement is frequent, parenchymal lung disease is rarely seen in PAN.

D. MICROSCOPIC POLYANGIITIS

MPA, thought to represent a small-diameter vessel variant of PAN, is discussed with the alveolar hemorrhage syndromes in the next section.

E. NECROTIZING SARCOID GRANULOMATOSIS

Necrotizing sarcoid granulomatosis is an uncommon primary lung disease affecting young individuals. It is a granulomatous vasculitis involving the medium-diameter vessels, and pulmonary involvement manifests as nodules, which are often discovered only following routine chest radiography. It is thought by some to be a variant of sarcoidosis. However, it is restricted to the lung and its associated histopathological features of a granulomatous vasculitis help differentiate it from sarcoidosis.

Chittock DR et al: Necrotizing sarcoid granulomatosis with pleural involvement. Clinical and radiographic features. Chest 1994;106:672. [PMID: 8082336]. (Case series describing the clinical presentation and treatment of necrotizing granulomatosis.)

Diagnosis

Common to all of the vasculitic syndromes is an elevated erythrocyte sedimentation rate (ESR), often exceeding 75 mm/h, and an increased serum C-reactive protein. Antinuclear antibodies and rheumatoid factor titers may be elevated. Leukocytosis is common. Peripheral eosinophilia may sometimes occur in WG, but is most commonly associated in CSS. Renal involvement may initially manifest as microscopic hematuria but progresses to active glomerulonephritis producing red cell casts and proteinuria.

c-ANCA seropositivity suggests a diagnosis of WG. c-ANCA is highly specific for WG and present in 90% of patients during the active disease. The sensitivity decreases when the disease is limited to the respiratory tract. In this situation, a definitive diagnosis depends on distinguishing the characteristic histopathological changes. Nonspecific signs of inflammation and necrosis are commonly found on nasal, sinus, and even endobronchial biopsies. Therefore, a surgical lung biopsy, preferable via video-assisted thoracoscopy, is recommended for a definitive diagnosis. A positive serum p-ANCA supports the diagnosis of CSS, PAN, or MPA. It may also be positive in up to 15% of patients who have WG. Necrotizing sarcoid granulomatosis is typically diagnosed as part of the surgical evaluation of asymptomatic pulmonary cavities.

Treatment & Outcome

The therapy for Wegener's vasculitis is immunosuppression using a combination of corticosteroids and cyclophosphamide (eg, prednisone 1 mg/kg ideal body weight per day and cyclophosphamide 2 mg/kg ideal body weight per day). If symptomatic control is achieved, the prednisone is tapered after the first month and discontinued over a period of 2–3 months. Full-dose cyclophosphamide is continued for 6–12 months after symptomatic remission. Cyclophosphamide therapy is then gradually tapered over the ensuing 2–6 months as long as the patient remains asymptomatic. Small prospective trials and retrospective analyses suggest that > 75% of patients with WG respond to the combined oral prednisone/cyclophosphamide regimen. However, side effects occurred in > 45% of patients. A slightly lower response rate has been reported with a methotrexate-based regimen of weekly methotrexate (MTX) and daily oral prednisone. Significant treatment-related side effects occurred in approximately 46% of patients. Severe, life-threatening *Pneumocystis carinii* pneumonia occurred in up to 10% of patients treated with the MTX/prednisone-based regimen.

In the event of diffuse alveolar hemorrhage or rapidly progressive acute renal failure, intravenous therapy (methylprednisolone, 1000 mg daily in divided doses, and cyclophosphamide, 2–4 mg/kg ideal body weight) is recommended. The remission rate in intravenous therapy is significantly less than that of an oral-based regimen. This may be somewhat misleading as those patients who seem to respond to therapy have less aggressive disease. The utility of daily trimethaprim/sulfamethoxazole (TMP/SMX) for the treatment of WG is controversial. Several reports document excellent remission rates when TMP/SMX is used in the treatment of the limited form of WG. Its efficacy in the generalized form of the disease is limited, but it may reduce disease recurrence following the induction of remission.

Therapy for MPA is similar to that for WG. A combined regimen of an oral corticosteroid preparation and cyclophosphamide is recommended since several reports suggest improved remission rates using a combined regimen compared to oral corticosteroids alone. In the majority of patients with CSS, oral corticosteroids provide adequate symptomatic control. The role of cyclophosphamide in CSS is not well established. However, it is occasionally used for symptomatic control. Necrotizing sarcoid granulomatosis resolves in all patients after treatment with corticosteroids alone and, as opposed to other vasculitic syndromes, recurrences are rare.

Therapy with cyclophosphamide has significantly decreased the mortality rate in WG. The medication does, however, have a number of potential complications including sterility, alopecia, bone marrow suppression, and an increased incidence of opportunistic infections, bladder cancer, and lymphoma. TMP/SMX prophylaxis is recommended to reduce the incidence of *Pneumocystis carinii* pneumonia for patients treated with corticosteroids, cyclophosphamide, or other immunosuppressive agents.

Prognosis

Complete remission in more than 90% of patients and a greater than 80% survival after 8 years can be achieved in WG using standard therapies. This is in contrast to its uniformly fatal course prior to aggressive immunosuppressive therapy. Relapses occur, however, and it is advisable to monitor the urine, ESR, and possibly the c-ANCA levels. The titer of ANCAs poorly correlates with disease activity and, therefore, the utility of routine testing is unclear. Limited data are available concerning patients with CSS.

DIFFUSE ALVEOLAR HEMORRHAGE SYNDROMES

 ESSENTIALS OF DIAGNOSIS

- *Cough with or without hemoptysis.*
- *Diffuse alveolar infiltrates.*
- *Falling hematocrit.*
- *Sequentially hemorrhagic bronchoalveolar lavage.*

General Considerations

Diffuse alveolar hemorrhage (DAH) is a clinical syndrome characterized by diffuse alveolar bleeding due to disruption of the alveolar capillaries. Less commonly, the injury occurs within the arterioles or venules. The hallmarks of the disease are intraalveolar accumulation of red blood cells, fibrin, and hemosiderin-laden macrophages. Several different etiologies exist and are summarized in Table 20–2.

Pathogenesis

The etiologies of DAH represent a broad spectrum of diseases caused by one of three different histologies: pulmonary capillaritis, bland pulmonary hemorrhage, or diffuse alveolar damage.

A. Pulmonary Capillaritis

Pulmonary (alveolar) capillaritis is a small-diameter vessel vasculitis of the lung, which may occur in isolation as in isolated pauci-immune capillaritis, in lung transplant rejection, or as part of a systemic vasculitis or collagen vascular disease. A distinctive histological finding is neutrophil accumulation within the alveolar walls. The cells are fragmented, pyknotic, and undergoing apoptosis (cell death) with subsequent release of nuclear debris into the surrounding tissue. The alveolar interstitium is also affected and becomes broadened by neutrophilic infiltration, edema, and fibrinoid necrosis of the capillary walls. Fibrinoid necrosis may be secondary to the release of cytoplasmic proteases and oxidative damage following a neutrophilic oxidative burst. Capillary damage ensues leading to the exudation of red blood cells, fibrin, and the fragmented neutrophils into the alveolar spaces and the histological appearance of DAH.

B. Bland Alveolar Hemorrhage

Bland alveolar hemorrhage is a form of DAH in which capillary endothelial injury occurs in the absence of overt inflammation or necrosis. In Goodpasture's syndrome, for example, the alveolar-capillary basement membrane is affected with immunoglobulin deposition, complement activation, and injury.

C. Diffuse Alveolar Damage

The third histopathological entity resulting in DAH is diffuse alveolar damage (DAD). DAD can follow a variety of disorders such as viral or opportunistic infections, inhalational injuries, drug toxicity, or an acute immunological pneumonia occurring with a collagen vascular disease. It is this histological entity that is seen in the acute respiratory distress syndrome. Histologically, interstitial and alveolar edema occurs with subsequent accumulation of proteinaceous exudates and hyaline membrane formation within alveoli.

Specks U: Diffuse alveolar hemorrhage syndromes. Curr Opin Rheumatol 2001;13:12. [PMID: 11148710]. (General overview of DAH.)

Clinical Findings

A. Symptoms and Signs

Hemoptysis, the hallmark of DAH, occurs in at least two-thirds of patients. The severity and duration vary considerably. Hemoptysis may be trace or massive, intermittent or continuous, and precedes the fulminant presentation by weeks, days, or, in the case of crack cocaine inhalation, hours. Nonspecific symptoms of

Table 20–2. Etiologies and underlying histologies for diffuse alveolar hemorrhage.

Pulmonary capillaritis
  Wegener's granulomatosis
  Microscopic polyangiitis
  Isolated pulmonary capillaritis (ANCA[1] positive)
  Isolated pulmonary capillaritis (ANCA negative)
  Systemic lupus erythematosus[2]
  Rheumatoid arthritis
  Mixed connective tissue disease
  Scleroderma
  Polymyositis
  Primary antiphospholipid syndrome
  Henoch–Schönlein purpura
  Behçet's disease
  IgA nephropathy
  Goodpasture's syndrome[2]
  Idiopathic glomerulonephritis (pauci-immune or immune complex related)
  Acute lung transplant rejection
  Idiopathic pulmonary fibrosis
  Diphenylhydantoin
  Retinoic acid toxicity
  Autologous bone marrow transplantation
  Myasthenia gravis
  Cryoglobulinemia
  Ulcerative colitis
  Propylthiouracil
Bland pulmonary hemorrhage
  Idiopathic pulmonary hemosiderosis
  Goodpasture's syndrome[2]

  Systemic lupus erythematosus[2]
  Coagulation disorders
  Trimellitic anhydride
  Isocyanate exposure
  Penicillamine
  Amiodarone
  Nitrofurantoin
  Mitral stenosis
  Subacute bacterial endocarditis
  Polyglandular autoimmune syndrome
  Multiple myeloma
Diffuse alveolar damage
  Bone marrow transplantation (idiopathic pneumonia syndrome)
  Crack cocaine inhalation
  Cytotoxic drug therapy
  Systemic lupus erythematosus[2]
  Radiation therapy
  Acute respiratory distress syndrome
  Miscellaneous histologies
  Lymphangioleiomyomatosis and tuberous sclerosis
  Pulmonary venoocclusive disease
  Pulmonary capillary hemangiomatosis
  Fibrillary glomerulonephritis
  Metastatic renal cell carcinoma
  Epithelioid hemangioepithelioma
  Angiosarcoma
  Choriocarcinoma syndrome

Adapted from Schwarz MI: Diffuse alveolar hemorrhage. In: *Interstitial Lung Diseases,* ed 3. Schwarz MI, King TE (editors). BC Decker, 1998, p 535.
[1]ANCA, antineutrophil cytoplasmic antibody.
[2]Entities with several underlying histologies possible.

cough, progressive dyspnea, malaise, and low-grade fevers may accompany the hemoptysis. Depending on the underlying etiology, other systemic symptoms such as a cutaneous rash, visual disturbances, myalgias, arthralgias, and peripheral neuropathy (mononeuritis multiplex) may also be present. In severe cases, gas exchange abnormalities leading to acute respiratory failure may occur requiring mechanical ventilation. Significant intraalveolar bleeding, as evidenced by sequentially hemorrhagic bronchoalveolar lavage fluid and an acute fall in hematocrit, may occur in 33% of patients without hemoptysis. On auscultation, diffuse crackles or signs of consolidation may be present, however, these do not differentiate DAH from other air space filling disorders.

A prior history of hemoptysis should be elicited from all patients, as DAH is often recurrent in the vasculitic syndromes, collagen vascular diseases, mitral stenosis, idiopathic pulmonary hemosiderosis, and venoocclusive disease. DAH may also be the initial and/or only manifestation of a vasculitis or collagen vascular disease. As DAD is one of the common pathological entities underlying DAH, a thorough review of current and prior medications, prescription and nonprescription, should be obtained. D-Penicillamine, crack cocaine, diphenylhydantoin, amiodarone, propylthiouracil, nitrofurantoin, and several cytotoxic drugs have all been associated with DAH. Penicillamine, propylthiouracil, and diphenylhydantoin can also produce a hypersensitivity vasculitis with skin and renal involvement. Signs or symptoms to suggest a coagulopathy should be investigated as anticoagulation, thrombocytopenia, and antiplatelet therapy predispose patients to spontaneous hemorrhage and should be considered in all patients regardless of the site of hemorrhage. Mitral stenosis, although relatively rare in the postantibiotic era, may manifest as DAH, which may be the initial presentation of the disease.

Extrapulmonary physical findings are often helpful in delineating the etiology of DAH. Signs and symptoms such as conjunctivitis, iridocyclitis, episcleritis, palpable purpura, or active synovitis suggest an underlying collagen vascular disease. Valvular heart disease, such as mitral stenosis, may become evident on examination based on an accentuated second heart sound with a characteristic diastolic murmur.

Radiographic studies in DAH are nonspecific, revealing alveolar infiltrates that initially may be focal, but rapidly progress to a diffuse alveolar filling pattern. In chronic DAH, signs of fibrosis may develop. Left atrial enlargement, Kerley B lines, and dilation of the main and central pulmonary arteries suggestive of pulmonary hypertension may occur in DAH associated with mitral stenosis. Kerley B lines may also be seen in pulmonary venoocclusive disease. High-resolution computed tomography is of limited utility in DAH.

Diffuse alveolar hemorrhage is characterized by a falling hematocrit in the setting of diffuse alveolar infiltrates. Leukocytosis and thrombocytosis occur but are nonspecific. Thrombocytopenia may accompany DAH secondary to bone marrow suppression from a myeloproliferative disorder or cytotoxic therapy, idiopathic thrombocytopenic purpura, thrombotic thrombocytopenic purpura, or disseminated intravascular coagulopathy. SLE and primary antiphospholipid syndrome should also be considered in patients presenting with DAH and thrombocytopenia. In the setting of a systemic vasculitis, focal segmental necrotizing glomerulonephritis is suggested by the presence of proteinuria, microscopic hematuria, and red blood cell casts in the face of renal insufficiency.

B. CLINICAL FEATURES

1. Wegener's granulomatosis—Diffuse alveolar hemorrhage, secondary to pulmonary capillaritis, is the initial manifestation of WG in up to 10% of patients. The more typical features of a systemic vasculitis may develop in the ensuing months to years following the initial episode of DAH. DAH may also represent an exacerbation of previously established WG. In patients who develop DAH as the initial manifestation of WG, a focal, segmental necrotizing glomerulonephritis occurs concomitantly in all reported cases. Differentiating between WG and MPA in these patients is often difficult. c-ANCA positivity differentiates the two diseases if present. However, several cases of p-ANCA-positive WG have been reported adding more difficulty to the diagnostic evaluation in patients with acute onset DAH and glomerulonephritis. In some cases, an accurate diagnosis can be attained only after the more typical clinical–radiographic–histological features of WG develop.

2. Microscopic polyangiitis—MPA is a systemic, necrotizing vasculitis that affects the small-diameter vessels. It is considered to be a variant of PAN. It is a systemic disease causing arthritis, myositis, gastrointestinal bleeding, polyneuropathy, and sinusitis. MPA is differentiated from PAN by its lack of medium-vessel involvement, a relatively high incidence of lung involvement manifested as DAH secondary to pulmonary capillaritis (33% of cases), and the absence of systemic hypertension. All patients who have MPA have a focal segmental necrotizing glomerulonephritis and > 90% demonstrate p-ANCA positivity. As in PAN, up to one-third of patients are seropositive for hepatitis B or C. Elevated antinuclear antibodies and rheumatoid factors occur in 30–40% and 20–30% of patients, respectively.

Lauque D et al: Microscopic polyangiitis with alveolar hemorrhage. A study of 29 cases and review of the literature. Groupe d'Etudes et de Recherche sur les Maladies "Orphelines" Pulmonaires (GERM"O"P). Medicine 2000;79(4):222. [PMID: 10941351]. (Decriptive case series and review of MPA.)

3. Pauci-immune idiopathic glomerulonephritis—Pauci-immune idiopathic glomerulonephritis is a rapidly progressive focal segmental glomerulonephritis. It is considered to be a localized form of renal vasculitis. In contrast to Goodpasture's syndrome or Henoch–Schönlein purpura, linear or coarse immune complex deposition cannot be detected and it is therefore termed pauci-immune. An immune-mediated process is inferred, however, based on the high incidence of p-ANCA positivity. Half of these patients will develop DAH, making it difficult to differentiate from Goodpasture's syndrome or MPA.

4. Isolated pulmonary capillaritis—Isolated pulmonary capillaritis represents a small vessel vasculitis limited to the lung resulting in DAH. In one case series, it was found to be the most common cause of pulmonary capillaritis. It is not associated with any other clinical or serological features of an underlying systemic disease. It is considered to be a pauci-immune capillaritis, as immunofluorescent studies fail to demonstrate linear or coarse immune complex deposition. Isolated pulmonary capillaritis may occur with or without p-ANCA positivity and therefore may represent a limited form of MPA. Longitudinal studies have yet to determine if patients subsequently develop features of an underlying systemic disease.

Schwarz MI et al: Isolated pulmonary capillaritis and diffuse alveolar hemorrhage in rheumatoid arthritis and mixed connective tissue disease. Chest 1998;113:1609. [PMID: 9631801]. (Interesting case report of isolated capillaritis associated with a connective tissue disease without systemic vasculitis.)

5. Collagen vascular diseases—Clinically significant pulmonary involvement in SLE occurs in over 70% of patients. DAH occurs in only 3–4% of patients but is often a devastating complication with a mortality rate approaching 50%. It may appear as the initial manifestation of SLE in up to 10% of patients, most of whom have concomitant lupus nephritis. The majority of patients are young women in whom the diagnosis is already established. Hemoptysis is reported in up to 65% of patients initially but virtually all patients report hemoptysis during subsequent evaluation. Bland pulmonary hemorrhage and DAD were initially thought to be responsible for the majority of cases of DAH in SLE. More recently, capillaritis has been reported as the underlying histology in most cases.

DAH has also been reported in several other collagen vascular diseases including polymyositis, RA, MCTD, as well as primary antiphospholipid syndrome. DAH may occur in the absence of a systemic vasculitis and most often appears to result from pulmonary capillaritis. Immune complex deposition is often present, as it is in SLE-related DAH. In contrast to patients with SLE, DAH secondary to other collagen vascular disease appears to be responsive to standard immunosuppressive therapy.

6. Goodpasture's syndrome—Goodpasture's syndrome [antibasement membrane disease (ABMD)] is the prototypical pulmonary–renal syndrome. The disease is limited to the kidney and lung. Simultaneous lung and kidney disease occurs in up to 60–80% of patients. Isolated glomerulonephritis occurs in 10–30%. In up to 5–10% of patients, DAH occurs in the absence of any renal disease. The disease predominantly occurs in young adults, with men more often affected. Smoking appears to have a significant impact on the development of DAH. In one study, all smokers with Goodpasture's syndrome went on to develop DAH, whereas only 20% of nonsmokers developed this complication. Recent viral infections or exposure to volatile chemicals may also precede an episode of DAH.

In 90% of patients with Goodpasture's syndrome, antibodies to the α-3 chain of type IV basement membrane collagen are detected, hence the term antibasement membrane disease. The antibody appears to be directly involved in the pathogenesis, since renal disease develops in mice exposed to the human antibody. A characteristic continuous, linear antibody deposition can be detected by immunofluorescence in both the lung and kidney in affected patients. Serum antibasement membrane antibody (ABMA) levels appear to correlate with the extent of renal disease, but not with the development of DAH. It is not surprising, therefore, that plasmapheresis is useful in the treatment of progressive renal disease, but not in the treatment of DAH. ANCA seropositivity may

occur in up to 40% of patients with Goodpasture's syndrome. These patients with ANCA may have subtle signs of a systemic vasculitis and represent an overlap between Goodpasture's syndrome and either WG or MPA. Bland pulmonary hemorrhage and pulmonary capillaritis have both been reported in Goodpasture's syndrome. In cases of pulmonary capillaritis, the alveolar wall necrosis commonly seen in capillaritis associated with systemic vasculitis is not present. In contrast to most other causes of DAH, recurrences are less common in Goodpasture's syndrome and plasmapheresis has been demonstrated to be an effective form of therapy, at least for the treatment of glomerulonephritis.

Ball JA, Young KR Jr: Pulmonary manifestations of Goodpasture's syndrome. Antiglomerular basement membrane disease and related disorders. Clin Chest Med 1998;19:777. [PMID: 9917968]. (Descriptive review of Goodpasture's syndrome.)

7. Henoch–Schönlein purpura—Henoch–Schönlein purpura is a systemic, necrotizing vasculitis causing leukocytoclastic vasculitis (palpable purpura), arthralgias, gastrointestinal bleeding, and a focal segmental necrotizing glomerulonephritis. Children are more commonly affected than adults. Pulmonary capillaritis and DAH have been documented but are rare complications. The disease is characterized by circulating and tissue immunoglobulin A (IgA) immune complexes without ANCA positivity.

Vats KR et al: Henoch-Schönlein purpura and pulmonary hemorrhage: a report and literature review. Pediatr Nephrol 1999;13(6):530. [PMID: 10452284]. (Pediatric review of the systemic manifestations including pulmonary hemorrhage.)

8. Idiopathic pulmonary hemosiderosis—Idiopathic pulmonary hemosiderosis (IPH) is a rare, recurrent form of DAH most often reported in children. Twenty percent of patients are adults and men are affected twice as frequently as women. Due to the recurrent episodes of DAH, iron-deficiency anemia may develop. Pulmonary fibrosis with restrictive physiology and chronic obstructive lung disease have been reported as long-term complications from the DAH. Because the disease is idiopathic, it is a diagnosis of exclusion established by tissue evaluation.

Cohen S: Idiopathic pulmonary hemosiderosis. Am J Med Sci 1999;317:67. [PMID: 9892276]. (Longitudinal evaluation of two children with IPH.)

9. Pulmonary venoocclusive disease—Pulmonary venoocclusive disease (PVOD) is a rare disease that results from fibrous obliteration of the postcapillary venules and pulmonary veins and causes severe, progressive pulmonary and left atrial hypertension. DAH may also occur. Most cases of PVOD are idiopathic. It may also occur as a complication of chemotherapy (bleomycin and carmustine), thoracic radiation, HIV infection, and collagen vascular diseases such as RA and SLE.

Holcomb BW Jr et al: Pulmonary venoocclusive disease: a case series and new observations [comment]. Chest 2000;118:1671. [PMID: 11115457]. (Case series describing the relevant clinical and radiographic findings as well as prognosis for VOD.)

Diagnosis

In patients with hemoptysis, establishing the diagnosis of DAH is relatively straightforward. Hemoptysis, diffuse alveolar filling opacities on radiograph, a falling hematocrit, and sequentially hemorrhagic lavageate on bronchoalveolar lavage confirm the diagnosis. In patients who present with acute to subacute respiratory symptoms in the presence of diffuse radiographic abnormalities but without hemoptysis, DAH may be more difficult to diagnose and therefore a high index of suspicion must be maintained. Bronchoalveolar lavage in these patients will also serve to evaluate for infectious processes as well as assess for occult intraalveolar hemorrhage. The exact etiology for the DAH may require more invasive testing such as surgical lung biopsy. A definitive diagnosis should be pursued as the therapeutic armamentarium varies depending on the underlying etiology. Immunofluorescence studies should be performed on all patients in whom DAH is suspected.

Complications

Pulmonary fibrosis and emphysema are potential complications of recurrent DAH. In IPH, patients may develop progressive pulmonary fibrosis with restrictive lung disease. The pathophysiology responsible for the progressive fibrosis is unclear. It does not appear that pulmonary hemosiderosis, secondary to recurrent hemorrhage, is necessarily responsible as pulmonary fibrosis does not occur in other diseases that produce iron overload in the lung. Obstructive lung disease due to the secondary development of emphysema may follow recurrent episodes of DAH and capillaritis. One potential mechanism for this is excessive neutral protease activity within the lung due to release from degranulating neutrophils, as well as antibody-mediated inactivation of antiproteases by ANCAs.

Infectious complications and drug toxicity must be considered in all patients undergoing therapy for vasculitis and/or DAH. Up to 10% of patients receiving therapy develop a secondary infection, most often sepsis and/or pneumonia, even in the absence of drug-induced leukopenia. Drug-related toxicity should also be considered in all patients, as multiorgan toxicities have

also been described for cyclophosphamide, azathioprine, and methotrexate.

Treatment

Cyclophosphamide and oral corticosteroids are the mainstay of therapy for DAH with an underlying histology of capillaritis and bland pulmonary hemorrhage, working under the assumption that DAH is a manifestation of a vasculitic process. In patients with Goodpasture's syndrome without renal involvement, there may be a response to corticosteroids alone. However, in the presence of glomerulonephritis, plasmapheresis and cytotoxic therapy are more effective for the prevention of permanent renal dysfunction. Plasmapheresis is not recommended for any of the other known causes of DAH. In patients who develop DAH secondary to diffuse alveolar damage, high-dose intravenous corticosteroids are recommended. Several reports suggest a benefit from activated Factor VIIa in the treatment of DAH. It has been used successfully to treat idiopathic pneumonia related to bone marrow transplantation as well as a case of MPA. Its role is unclear, but it may facilitate the restoration of endothelial–platelet interaction by bypassing the tissue factor pathway in the coagulation cascade.

Prognosis

Morbidity and mortality are adversely affected following the development of DAH in patients with a systemic vasculitis. Mortality is either secondary to progressive respiratory failure or a secondary opportunistic infection. In the presence of DAH, mortality approaches 40% in WG and 25% in MPA. Five-year survival is also reduced as recurrence is common. In patients with SLE-induced DAH, initial mortality approaches 50% and is further influenced by coexisting infection and the need for mechanical ventilation. Furthermore, 5-year survival is also reduced (65%). The prognosis for isolated pauci-immune pulmonary capillaritis is more favorable than that seen in DAH associated with the systemic vasculitides. Longitudinal follow-up is required to adequately assess the natural history of the disease. To date, signs of an underlying systemic vasculitis or connective tissue disease have not been documented in these patients. In Goodpasture's syndrome, the 2-year survival is 50%. In patients with severe renal dysfunction or recurrent DAH, the prognosis falls to 50% survival at 6 months. IPH may follow several different courses. Up to 25% of adults are disease free after their initial episode. It may progress to fibrosis and restrictive physiology in another subset of patients or persist with recurrent episodes of hemorrhage and respiratory failure, leading to death. The 5-year mortality for IPH approaches 50%.

SECTION VI
Diseases of the Pleura

Pneumothorax/Hemothorax	21

Michael E. Hanley, MD, & Michael P. Gruber, MD

■ PNEUMOTHORAX

Michael E. Hanley, MD

 ESSENTIALS OF DIAGNOSIS

- *The most common symptoms of pneumothorax are chest pain and dyspnea.*
- *Physical signs include hyperresonant percussion, diminished tactile and vocal fremitus, and decreased or absent breath sounds.*
- *Laboratory abnormalities include hypoxia and a widened $P(A-a)O_2$ gradient. P_{CO_2} may be either decreased or increased.*
- *Radiographic signs include the peripheral absence of lung markings and the presence of a pleural "stripe" that is strictly intrathoracic.*

General Considerations

Pneumothorax, defined as the presence of air within the pleural space, is classified as either spontaneous or traumatic. Spontaneous pneumothorax occurs without obvious cause and is subclassified as either primary or secondary. Primary spontaneous pneumothorax occurs in the absence of underlying lung disease. Secondary spontaneous pneumothorax occurs as a complication of underlying lung disease. The incidence of primary and secondary pneumothorax is similar, with both conditions

being more common in males than females. The incidence of primary spontaneous pneumothorax in a longitudinal health study in Olmsted County, Minnesota was 7.4/100,000/year in males and 1.2/100,000/year in females. It is more common in younger persons, with a peak incidence in the third decade of life, and is rare after age 40. The incidence of secondary spontaneous pneumothorax in the Olmsted County, Minnesota study was 6.3/100,000/year in males and 2.0/100,000/year in females. Secondary spontaneous pneumothorax is more commonly associated with severe respiratory compromise due to lack of significant respiratory reserve from the underlying lung disease.

Traumatic pneumothorax, which results from direct or indirect trauma to the chest, is subclassified as either iatrogenic or noniatrogenic. Iatrogenic pneumothorax is the most common type of pneumothorax.

Tension pneumothorax occurs when intrapleural pressure exceeds atmospheric pressure throughout expiration. Although any pneumothorax can cause this, the most common cause of tension pneumothorax is barotrauma from positive pressure mechanical ventilation. Tension pneumothorax is a medical emergency that is frequently associated with hemodynamic instability and considerable mortality.

Barton ED: Tension pneumothorax. Curr Opin Pulmon Med 1999;5:269. [PMID: 10407699]. (Good review of the clinical manifestations and pathophysiology of tension pneumothorax.)

Pathogenesis

Primary spontaneous pneumothorax results from rupture of subpleural emphysematous blebs. The blebs tend to occur more commonly in lung apices. Although the etiology of the blebs is unknown, epidemiological observations that identify risk factors for primary spontaneous pneumothorax offer clues to processes that may contribute to their development. These studies indicate that tobacco use, body habitus, and family history are risk factors for this condition. For example, primary spontaneous pneumothorax is more common in tall, thin males. There is also a familial tendency to this type of pneumothorax; up to 11% of patients with primary spontaneous pneumothorax have a family history of spontaneous pneumothorax. Patients with primary spontaneous pneumothorax are also more likely to have bronchial abnormalities such as narrowed airways and missing or accessory bronchi. These abnormalities are present in over 90% of nonsmoking patients with primary spontaneous pneumothorax. Airway inflammation, especially due to tobacco use, also appears to contribute to development of blebs. Of primary spontaneous pneumothoraces 90% occur in cigarette smokers with the greatest incidence occurring in the heaviest smokers. The risk of pneumothorax in one study was seven times higher in male patients who smoked less than 12 cigarettes per day compared to nonsmokers but 80-fold higher in those who smoked more than 22 cigarettes per day. Taken in total, these observations suggest that the pathogenesis of primary spontaneous pneumothorax is likely dependent on both airway inflammation and a hereditary predisposition to bleb formation. Airway inflammation is probably the more important of these mechanisms.

Secondary spontaneous pneumothorax may occur in almost any lung disease. Some of the more common causes are listed in Table 21–1. Although chronic obstructive pulmonary disease (COPD) and *Pneumocystis carinii* pneumonia are the most common causes in more recent studies, the incidence of pneumothorax from the various causes depends in part on the frequency of the underlying conditions in the population being studied.

Noniatrogenic traumatic pneumothorax results from both penetrating and blunt chest trauma. Penetrating trauma may cause pneumothorax by either entry of atmospheric air directly into the pleural space through chest wall wounds or leakage of intrapulmonic air from injury to the visceral pleura. Some pneumothoraces due to blunt trauma result from rib fractures with subsequent visceral pleura injury. The more common mechanism of injury, however, involves alveolar rupture due to a sudden increase in alveolar pressure related to chest compression. Alveolar air then enters the interstitial space, dissects toward the visceral pleura or mediastinum, and ruptures through either the visceral or mediastinal pleura.

Iatrogenic pneumothorax is a frequent but preventable problem. Table 21–2 lists common causes of iatrogenic pneumothorax.

Liman ST et al: Chest injury due to blunt trauma. Eur J Cardiothorac Surg 2003;23:374. [PMID: 12614809]. (Review of risk factors associated with pneumothorax in 1490 trauma patients.)

Prevention

Efforts to prevent pneumothorax focus on reducing the risk of iatrogenic pneumothorax and preventing recurrence of spontaneous pneumothorax. Numerous factors that increase the risk of iatrogenic pneumothorax have been identified. Prevention emphasizes teaching proper technique through formal procedure training programs, avoiding procedures if the risk is too great, or modifying technique to minimize risk. For example, some studies suggest the risk of pneumothorax following transthoracic needle aspiration depends upon the depth of the lesion being aspirated, the presence of COPD, and whether the needle must traverse aerated lung. Avoidance of transthoracic needle aspiration by pursuing other approaches to biopsy is preferable if all of these risk factors are present. This is especially true in patients with significant respiratory compromise. The incidence of pneumothorax following thoracentesis is increased in patients with COPD and those with small effusions. Performing the procedure under ultrasound

Table 21–1. Common causes of secondary spontaneous pneumothorax.

Chronic obstructive pulmonary disease
Pneumocystis carinii pneumonia (AIDS)
Tuberculosis
Necrotizing pneumonia
Cystic fibrosis
Asthma
Idiopathic interstitial pneumonia
Connective tissue disease
Pneumoconiosis
Lung cancer

Table 21–2. Common causes of iatrogenic pneumothorax.

Percutaneous transthoracic needle aspiration and/or biopsy
Subclavian and supraclavicular central venous catheterization
Thoracentesis
Positive pressure mechanical ventilation
Transbronchial biopsy
Closed pleural biopsy
Tracheostomy
Cardiopulmonary resuscitation

guidance reduces this risk. In contrast, placement of subclavian catheters under ultrasound guidance does not decrease the rate of pneumothorax from this procedure. However, instituting formal training programs that emphasize proper catheterization technique does.

The other approach to prevention is minimizing the risk of recurrence of primary and secondary spontaneous pneumothorax. The rate of recurrence following an initial primary spontaneous pneumothorax is controversial, ranging from 28% to 52%, but increases with each subsequent pneumothorax. In one study the rate of recurrence was 83% in untreated patients who previously had three primary spontaneous pneumothoraces. Although the majority of recurrences occur in the first year, risk likely remains increased for many years after the first event. There is no reliable method to predict which patients are more likely to have a recurrence after an initial primary spontaneous pneumothorax, but in one study the incidence of recurrence was higher in taller, thinner patients. Recurrence rates following secondary spontaneous pneumothorax are slightly higher than those in primary spontaneous pneumothorax, ranging from 39% to 47%.

Sclerosis and subsequent obliteration of the pleural space prevent recurrence. Methods available to achieve this goal include mechanical scarification by either open thoracotomy or video-assisted thoracoscopic surgery (VATS) and chemical pleurodesis during either surgery or via installation of a sclerosing agent through a thoracostomy tube. A number of different sclerosing agents have been used, including talc, tetracycline derivatives, quinacrine, and bleomycin. Talc and tetracycline derivatives are the most efficacious. Talc may be superior to the tetracyclines but isolated case reports of acute respiratory distress syndrome following talc-induced sclerosis of malignant pleural effusions and concerns regarding contamination with asbestos have tempered its use. It may also be associated with chronic pleural fibrosis and restrictive lung disease years after its use. Recurrence rates following pleurodesis with these agents range from 9% to 25% for tetracycline and 10% for talc. Parenteral tetracycline is no longer available, however, minocycline and doxycycline appear to be equally effective. Use of bleomycin has been limited due to significant expense compared to other agents and limited effectiveness in animal models.

VATS and open thoracotomy are the most effective approach to prevent recurrence but are associated with increased morbidity and some mortality. These procedures allow both elimination of blebs and bulla as well as creation of a pleurodesis. Bullectomy is performed in thoracotomy by either wedge resection or direct suturing. VATS can eliminate bulla by either wedge resection with endoscopic stapling or ablation with an Nd-YAG laser. The two methods appear to be equally

effective although wedge resection may be more expensive. Pleurodesis can be performed with either surgical approach (open thoracotomy or VATS) through either application of talc or tetracycline, laser abrasion of the parietal pleura, parietal pleurectomy, or simple scarification by direct abrasion with dry surgical gauze. The latter is likely the best approach given the concerns regarding talc exposure mentioned above. Recurrence of pneumothorax after VATS or open thoracotomy does occur but is quite rare. Most published series describe recurrence rates of less than 3%.

The timing, indication, and best method to achieve sclerosis are unclear. Although VATS and open thoracotomy are nearly 100% effective in preventing recurrence, a surgical approach may be overly aggressive considering 50% of initial spontaneous pneumothoraces never recur. This has led some authorities to advocate chemical pleurodesis as the preferred method of sclerosis despite its inferior efficacy. A recent Delphi analysis of management of spontaneous pneumothorax by the American College of Chest Physicians (ACCP) recommended VATS or open thoracotomy as the preferred approach to prevent recurrence due to higher efficacy rates and relative safety; the timing of sclerosis depends on the type of pneumothorax (Table 21–3). Chemical pleurodesis is indicated in those patients who refuse surgery or are not operative candidates. There was not, however, 100% consensus regarding these recommendations.

Saji H et al: The incidence and the risk of pneumothorax and chest tube placement after CT-guided lung lung biopsy: the angle of the needle trajectory is a novel predictor. Chest 2002;121:1521. [PMID: 12006438]. (The authors retrospectively review their experience in 289 patients and discuss approaches to reduce risk of pneumothorax.)

Clinical Findings & Diagnosis

A. SYMPTOMS AND SIGNS

Symptoms of primary and secondary spontaneous pneumothorax are very similar. Almost all patients complain of either chest pain or dyspnea and two-thirds have both symptoms. Dyspnea is more common and severe in patients with secondary spontaneous pneumothorax due to their underlying lung disease. Both dyspnea and chest pain tend to be acute in onset. The chest pain is usually pleuritic and localized to the side of the pneumothorax.

Patients with primary spontaneous pneumothorax frequently have normal vital signs except for tachycardia. Secondary spontaneous pneumothorax is more likely to be associated with respiratory distress, cyanosis, and anxiety. All classes of pneumothorax are associated with physical signs on chest examination that are localized to the side of the pneumothorax. These

Table 21-3. Management of spontaneous pneumothorax.

Pneumothorax	Clinical Scenario	Primary Treatment	Comments	Secondary Treatment[1,2]
Primary	Small, clinically stable[3]	Emergency department observation	Discharge home if pneumothorax is radiographically stable after 3–6 h Obtain follow-up radiograph 12–48 h postdischarge Hospitalize if lives distantly from emergency department or follow-up is unreliable Tube thoracostomy if enlarges on radiograph	Consider after first recurrence or if patient has occupation/avocation in which pneumothorax could be life-threatening
Primary	Large, clinically stable	Hospitalize, reexpand lung with small-bore (<14F) catheter or small (16–22F) chest tube	Connect thoracostomy tube to either Heimlich valve or underwater seal Apply suction if lung does not reexpand quickly	Consider after first recurrence or if patient has occupation/avocation in which pneumothorax could be life-threatening
Primary	Large, clinically unstable	Hospitalize, reexpand lung with either a small-bore (≤14F) catheter or small (16–22F) chest tube (latter preferred in more unstable patients)	Larger (24–28F) chest tube preferred if mechanical ventilation is required or large air leak is anticipated Connect chest tube to underwater seal (preferable) Heimlich valve acceptable if clinical stability is obtained after immediate reexpansion of lung Apply suction if lung does not immediately reexpand and patient remains clinically unstable	Consider after first recurrence or if patient has occupation/avocation in which pneumothorax could be life-threatening
Secondary	Small, clinically stable	Hospitalize with observation[4] or insertion of chest tube	Small (16–22F) chest tubes preferable Small-bore (<14F) catheter may be acceptable if small pneumothorax Use large (24–28F) tube if large air leak is anticipated or mechanical ventilation is required Connect to underwater seal; apply suction if lung does not expand	Perform after first episode
Secondary	Large, clinically stable	Hospitalize and insert chest tube	Small (16–22F) chest tubes preferable Use large (24–28F) tube if large air leak is anticipated or mechanical ventilation is required Connect to underwater seal; apply suction if lung does not expand	Perform after first episode
Secondary	Clinically unstable, any size	Hospitalize and insert chest tube	Small (16–22F) chest tubes preferable Use large (24–28F) tube if large air leak is anticipated or mechanical ventilation is required Connect to underwater seal; apply suction if lung does not expand	Perform after first episode

[1]Secondary treatment consists of a definitive procedure to prevent recurrence.
[2]The decision should be considered carefully if the patient is a lung transplant candidate.
[3]A small pneumothorax is a pneumothorax that is less than 3 cm from the cupola to the lung apex. Clinically stable is defined as *all* of the following: respiratory rate < 24, 60 < pulse < 120, normal blood pressure, room air arterial O_2 saturation > 90%, and a patient able to speak in complete sentences.
[4]Rare case reports of death with this approach have been reported.

typically include decreased tactile and vocal fremitus, hyperresonant percussion, and decreased or absent breath sounds. Physical signs of COPD-related pneumothorax may be difficult to appreciate due to preexisting hyperresonance and diminished breath sounds from the underlying obstructive lung disease.

Patients with tension pneumothorax frequently present with cardiopulmonary collapse and hemodynamic instability. This form of pneumothorax most commonly occurs in mechanically ventilated patients. Patients typically develop sudden respiratory distress and agitation and appear to "fight the ventilator." Physical signs may include marked tachycardia, tachypnea with labored breathing, hypotension, and cyanosis. In addition to the usual physical signs on chest examination there is commonly hyperexpansion of the ipsilateral hemothorax and deviation of the trachea toward the unaffected lung.

Signs and symptoms of pneumothorax in mechanically ventilated patients are also occasionally very subtle. Symptoms are usually undetectable as patients are intubated and frequently sedated. Subtle signs of pneumothorax in this setting include unexplained agitation, tachypnea, tachycardia, respiratory distress, hypoxia, and a sudden increase in peak inspiratory and plateau airway pressures.

B. LABORATORY FINDINGS

Laboratory abnormalities in primary spontaneous pneumothorax are usually mild. They include hypoxia, increased $P(A–a)O_2$ gradient, and hypocapnea with respiratory alkalosis. These abnormalities are typically more severe in secondary spontaneous pneumothorax; a significant number of these patients have hypercapnea with respiratory acidosis. Respiratory failure is also more common in this subset of patients. Tension pneumothorax is commonly associated with profound, refractory hypoxia.

C. IMAGING STUDIES

A diagnosis of pneumothorax is confirmed by demonstrating a pleural line on chest radiograph. Pleural lines may not be readily apparent in mechanically ventilated patients. Radiographs in these patients are frequently obtained in the supine position; air in this position collects anteriorly. Radiographic clues suggesting pneumothorax in this setting include relative lucency over the upper abdominal quadrants, visualization of the anterior costophrenic sulcus resulting in a curvilinear change in density over the ipsilateral upper quadrant, sharp definition of the diaphragm despite lung consolidation, the deep sulcus sign, unilateral increase in hemithorax volume, and relative lucency in one lung or part of a lung. Expiratory chest radiographs or computed tomography are useful in clarifying the diagnosis

in patients with suspicious but inconclusive routine radiographs.

Hyperexpansion of the ipsilateral hemithorax, specifically a tracheal and/or mediastinal shift toward the contralateral hemithorax or depression of the ipsilateral hemidiaphragm, suggests tension pneumothorax.

Sahn SA, Heffner JE: Spontaneous pneumothorax. N Engl J Med 2000;342:868. (Concise but thorough review of spontaneous pneumothorax including clinical manifestations.)

Schramel FM et al: Current aspects of spontaneous pneumothorax. Eur Respir J 1997;10:1372. [PMID: 9192946]. (Includes a discussion of the value of expiratory radiographs in diagnosis.)

Differential Diagnosis

The differential diagnosis of pneumothorax includes those conditions that are associated with acute pleuritic chest pain and dyspnea. This includes musculoskeletal disorders such as costochondritis and rib fracture, pulmonary embolism, infectious pneumonia, viral pleuritis, empyema, and occasionally myocardial ischemia or infarction. Although chest radiographs usually easily distinguish pneumothorax from these other conditions, pleural lines are occasionally confused with soft tissue shadows that overlie the chest. Typical findings that differentiate these two abnormalities and identify the pleural line include absence of lung markings between the line and chest wall and presence of the line strictly within the thorax. Shadows that extend beyond the chest wall or diaphragm are not of intrathoracic origin. Pleural lines may also occasionally be confused with the thin walls of bulla, indwelling catheters, intrathoracic loops of bowel, and dilated bowel loops interposed between the hemidiaphragm and liver. Observing the angle created between the line and lateral chest wall helps differentiate pneumothorax and bulla. This angle is usually concave with bulla and convex with pneumothorax.

Complications

Complications of pneumothorax include bronchopleural fistula and reexpansion pulmonary edema. Bronchopleural fistula is a pleural air leak that persists after placement of tube thoracostomy. It is uncommon after primary spontaneous pneumothorax but occurs more frequently with secondary spontaneous and traumatic pneumothorax, and in mechanically ventilated patients. Bronchopleural fistula should be initially managed conservatively with only tube thoracostomy drainage, as many close spontaneously. Direct surgical closure and pleurodesis to prevent recurrence by either VATS or open thoracotomy is indicated for fistulas that persist beyond 4–7 days. Management with chemical pleurodesis is reserved for patients with persistent fistulas who refuse surgery or are not operative candidates.

Reexpansion pulmonary edema is an uncommon complication of the treatment of pneumothorax. It is characterized by unilateral pulmonary edema that develops within 48 h after reexpansion of the collapsed lung. Involvement of the contralateral lung occurs but is rare. The pulmonary edema is due to increased permeability of the pulmonary vasculature and may result from oxidant-mediated reperfusion injury. Risk factors for development of edema appear to include the duration of pneumothorax prior to tube thoracostomy and application of negative pressure to the pleural space following tube placement. Almost all cases have occurred in patients whose symptoms suggest the pneumothorax was present at least 3 days prior to drainage. Management is supportive, including mechanical ventilation for acute respiratory failure.

Treatment

Several treatment options are available to manage pneumothoraces, including observation, simple aspiration, tube thoracostomy with either small-bore catheters or smaller chest tubes, VATS, and open thoracotomy. Remarkably few studies have evaluated the appropriateness of specific options in different clinical settings. General guidelines based on the recent ACCP Delphi analysis of management of spontaneous pneumothorax are summarized in Table 21–3. It should be emphasized that none of the treatment recommendations was supported by perfect consensus from the expert panel involved in the analysis and there was significant disagreement regarding some recommendations. A few additional recommendations should be highlighted. The rate of spontaneous absorption of pleural air increases 4- to 6-fold if high flow oxygen is administered. Patients managed with observation alone should also receive this therapy. Thoracostomy tubes should be removed after there is complete reexpansion of the lung with no evidence of persistent air leak and stability has been demonstrated on radiographs obtained with the tube connected to an underwater seal. The timing of the follow-up radiograph is controversial, ranging from 4 to 24 h after conversion to a water seal.

The ACCP panel did not review management of traumatic pneumothorax, however, some general comments can be made. Management of iatrogenic pneumothorax depends upon the need for mechanical ventilation and degree of physiological impairment from the pneumothorax. Iatrogenic pneumothorax in mechanically ventilated patients should be managed with tube thoracostomy due to the high risk for development of tension pneumothorax. Furthermore, chest tubes should not be removed for at least 48 h following resolution of the pleural air leak if the patient remains ventilated. Noniatrogenic traumatic pneumothorax and ia-

trogenic pneumothorax in patients not receiving mechanical ventilation may be managed conservatively with either observation and supplemental oxygen or simple aspiration if the pneumothorax is small and the patient is minimally symptomatic. Tube thoracostomy is indicated in patients with larger pneumothoraces, significant physiological impairment, or enlarging air collections identified on subsequent radiographs. Pleurodesis is not indicated for either type of traumatic pneumothorax as recurrence is unlikely.

Tension pneumothorax should always be managed with a large tube thoracostomy.

Baumann MH et al: Management of spontaneous pneumothorax: an American College of Chest Physicians Delphi consensus statement. Chest 2001;119:590. [PMID: 11171742]. (A must read for providers who manage pneumothorax.)

Kurihara Y et al: The utility of the frontal chest radiograph in the evaluation of chest drain placement. Clin Radiol 1996;51: 350. [PMID: 8641099]. (Review of radiographic features of anterior, posterior, and interlobar thoracostomy tubes.)

Yamagami T et al: Management of pneumothorax after percutaneous CT-guided lung biopsy. Chest 2002;121:1159. [PMID: 11948047]. (Forty-three of 46 patients with pneumothorax following lung biopsy were successfully managed with either simple aspiration or observation.)

Prognosis

Death has been reported with every class of pneumothorax, including primary spontaneous pneumothorax. However, mortality directly attributable to pneumothorax is difficult to estimate as pneumothorax may go undiagnosed as the immediate cause of death and death in a patient with pneumothorax may not be related to the pneumothorax. In the absence of definitive data it is presumed that prognosis is likely related to the degree of prior lung dysfunction, the degree of physiological impairment from the pneumothorax itself, and the underlying condition. Using this model the prognosis of primary spontaneous pneumothorax following treatment is quite good. Secondary spontaneous pneumothorax is more life threatening. Early studies reported mortality in patients with COPD and spontaneous pneumothorax was as high as 17%, but recent studies suggest it is closer to 1%. *Pneumocystis carinii* pneumonia-related pneumothorax in human immunodeficiency virus (HIV) seropositive persons has been associated with 34% mortality. Mortality from iatrogenic pneumothorax depends on the cause of the pneumothorax and was as high as 2% in a VA Medical Center 5-year review. The worst prognoses are associated with tension pneumothorax and pneumothorax that develops in critically ill patients. Mortality from tension pneumothorax in early studies was reported at 7%; mortality increased to 31% if diagnosis was delayed. Mortality in a recent study of critically ill patients who developed pneumothorax while in the intensive care unit was 60%; the highest mortality occurred in patients whose pneumothorax was associated with barotrauma or tension physiology. Patients in this study with procedure-related pneumothorax had better outcomes.

Afessa B: Pleural effusions and pneumothoraces in AIDS. Curr Opin Pulmon Med 2001;7:202. [PMID: 11470975]. (Good review, emphasizing management and prognosis.)

Chen KY et al: Pneumothorax in the ICU: patient outcomes and prognostic factors. Chest 2002;122:678. [PMID: 12171850]. (Retrospective study of outcome in patients who develop pneumothorax while in the ICU. Pneumothorax due to barotrauma and tension pneumothorax were independently associated with death.)

■ HEMOTHORAX

Michael Gruber, MD, & Michael E. Hanley, MD

ESSENTIALS OF DIAGNOSIS

- *The most common cause of hemothorax is chest trauma. Iatrogenic and nontraumatic causes are uncommon.*
- *Suspect hemothorax in any trauma patient with a pleural effusion.*
- *Hemothorax may not be apparent on initial chest radiograph in trauma patients.*
- *The diagnosis is confirmed by a pleural fluid hematocrit >50% that of peripheral blood.*
- *Diagnosis in nontrauma patients mandates a thorough evaluation for underlying etiology, especially those conditions associated with high morbidity and mortality.*
- *Management usually requires drainage with tube thoracostomy.*

General Considerations

Hemothorax is the presence of blood in the pleural space. It is strictly defined as a pleural effusion with a hematocrit greater than 50% of that of peripheral blood collected simultaneously. True hemothorax must be distinguished from hemorrhagic effusion. The latter is defined by a pleural fluid red blood cell count greater than 100,000/μL but a pleural fluid to peripheral hematocrit ratio less than 50%. Hemothorax is catego-

rized as either traumatic or nontraumatic. Traumatic hemothorax is subcategorized as either iatrogenic or noniatrogenic. Most hemothoraces are traumatic, whereas hemorrhagic effusions occur more commonly in nontraumatic settings. A thoracostomy tube should be inserted to evacuate unclotted blood and monitor further bleeding once a hemothorax has been confirmed by thoracentesis. Hemothorax in nontraumatic circumstances mandates thorough etiological evaluation with a high index of suspicion for conditions associated with significant morbidity and mortality.

Pathogenesis

Table 21–4 lists causes of hemothorax. Traumatic hemothorax results from both penetrating and blunt chest trauma. Up to 30–40% of patients with chest trauma develop hemothorax. Rib fractures do not appear to increase the incidence of hemothorax unless they are displaced. Blood can enter the pleural space from injury to the lung, mediastinum, diaphragm, or chest wall. Subsequent coagulation with clot organization, adhesion formation, and loculation occurs early after blood entry and can result in fibrothorax.

Iatrogenic and nontraumatic hemothoraces are infrequent. Iatrogenic hemothorax is the more common of these types. It is a complication of many common procedures including thoracentesis, closed pleural biopsy, transbronchial biopsy, and transthoracic aortography, but the most common cause is vascular injury related to central venous catheterization. Nontraumatic hemothoraces are quite rare.

Ruesch S et al: Complications of central venous catheters: internal jugular versus subclavian access—a systematic review. Crit Care Med 2002;30:454. [PMID: 11889329]. (The incidence of hemothorax or pneumothorax was only 1.4%.)

Yeam I, Sassoon C: Hemothorax and chylothorax. Curr Opin Pulmon Med 1997;3:310. [PMID: 9262119]. (General review of causes and management of hemothorax.)

Clinical Findings

A. SYMPTOMS AND SIGNS

Symptoms of hemothorax are nonspecific and are similar to pleural effusions of other causes. Patients typically have chest pain or dyspnea following blunt or penetrating chest trauma. The history of trauma, however, may be subtle. Patients with multisystem trauma may not complain of chest symptoms if other distracting injuries are present. Dyspnea and chest discomfort are also common in nontraumatic hemothorax. However, nontraumatic hemothorax may also be associated primarily with nonrespiratory complaints related to the underlying problem. Unilateral or bilateral effusions in this setting are often found incidentally on chest radiography.

Table 21–4. Causes of hemothorax.

Traumatic
  Penetrating
    Stab/knife
  Blunt
    Rib fractures/flail chest
    Lung contusion
    Diaphragmatic rupture
    Thoracic spine fractures
  Iatrogenic
    Subclavian or internal jugular vein central line placement
    Percutaneous liver or kidney biopsy
    Anticoagulation therapy
    Thoracentesis
    Cardiothoracic surgery
    Implantable pacemaker/defibrillator placement
    Thoracic epidural anesthesia
    Thrombolytic therapy
    Chest tube placement
Vascular
    Thoracic aortic aneurysm
    Bronchial artery aneurysm
    Pulmonary artery aneurysm
    Internal thoracic artery aneurysm
    Arteriovenous fistula
Carcinoma
  Primary
    Mediastinal malignancies (parathyroid, thyroid, thymo-
      mas, teratomas, schwannomas, hemangiopericytomas)
    Malignant mesothelioma
    Malignant fibrous histiocytoma
    Angiosarcoma
    Osteosarcoma
    Angiomyolipoma
    Chronic myelogenous leukemia
    Chronic lymphocytic leukemia
  Metastatic
    Hepatocellular carcinoma
Spontaneous
    Exercise-induced
    Neurofibromatosis type I (von Recklinghausen's disease)
    Hemophilia (inherited coagulopathies)
    Connective tissue disease, Ehlers–Danlos
    Osler–Weber–Rendu syndrome
    Costal exostosis
    Pulmonary sequestration
Gynecological
    Ectopic pregnancy
    Pleural endometriosis
    Catamenial hemothorax

Common physical findings are those associated with pleural effusions and include decreased breath sounds with dullness to percussion and diminished tactile and vocal fremitus over the hemothorax.

B. LABORATORY STUDIES

Pleural fluid analysis is nonspecific except for elevated red blood cell counts. True hemothorax is associated with a pleural fluid hematocrit that is 50% or greater than that of peripheral blood.

C. IMAGING STUDIES

Typical findings of hemothorax on chest radiography are those associated with pleural effusions. The effusions may be unilateral or bilateral. Radiographic evidence of a pleural effusion in patients with significant chest trauma is virtually diagnostic of hemothorax. However, up to 25% of patients with traumatic hemothorax have no apparent effusion on initial radiograph, especially if it is obtained with the patient in a supine position. Films should be obtained with the patient in an upright position and/or a repeat evaluation in 3–6 h should occur if there is strong suspicion for the condition. Computed tomography (CT) is more sensitive than plain radiography in detecting traumatic effusions. Radiographs and CT may also hold clues to the etiology of the hemothorax such as rib fractures, widened mediastinum suggesting aortic injury, misplaced central venous catheters, or the presence of a lung mass. Air in the pleural space is often detected; 62–83% of traumatic hemothorax have a concurrent pneumothorax.

Martinez FJ et al: Spontaneous hemothorax. Report of six cases and review of the literature. Medicine 1992;71:354. [PMID: 1435230]. (Comprehensive review of hemothorax.)

Differential Diagnosis

Pleural fluid appears bloody when it has a hematocrit of less than 5%. The differential diagnosis of bloody appearing pleural fluid includes hemothorax, hemorrhagic effusion, and traumatic thoracentesis. All bloody effusions should be analyzed for cell count and pleural fluid hematocrit to differentiate among these conditions (Figure 21–1). Distinguishing between true bloody effusion and traumatic thoracentesis can be challenging. Traumatic thoracentesis is suggested by nonuniform color of the fluid during aspiration, clotting within minutes of aspiration, and absence of pleural hemosiderin-laden macrophages. The differential diagnosis of hemorrhagic effusion includes trauma, neoplasm, pulmonary embolism, postcardiac injury/ surgery, and asbestosis.

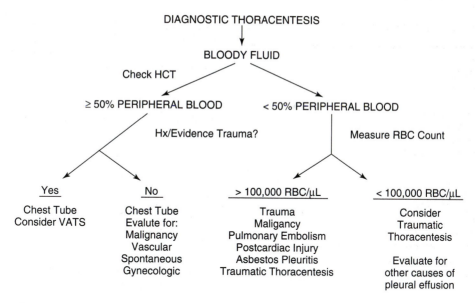

Figure 21–1. Algorithm for the evaluation of bloody effusions.

Complications

Complications of hemothorax include infection, fibrothorax, inadequate removal of clotted blood, and pleural effusion. Empyema occurs in up to 5% of hemothoraces. Empiric antibiotics, generally first-generation cephalosporins, decrease the incidence of empyema in patients with traumatic hemothorax managed with tube thoracostomy. Conditions associated with an increased risk of empyema following hemothorax include contamination of the pleural space at the time of initial injury, circulatory shock on presentation, concomitant abdominal injury, and prolonged chest tube drainage. Fibrothorax is diffuse pleural thickening that occurs as a result of an inflammatory reaction to blood in the pleural space. It is rare and typically develops weeks to months after initial injury. Fibrothorax requires surgical decortication for definitive management. Pleural effusions occur in 10–30% of patients with hemothorax following removal of thoracostomy tubes. Diagnostic thoracentesis for culture is recommended in patients who develop a postthoracostomy tube pleural effusion to exclude underlying infection. Clinical observation is appropriate if no infection is present.

Treatment

Hemothorax is best managed by timely drainage with thoracostomy tubes and parenteral antibiotics. Large-bore (36–40F) tubes are indicated to minimize clotting within the tube. Advantages to immediate tube thoracostomy include improved evacuation of blood from the pleural space, the ability to quantitate and monitor the extent of bleeding, and a decreased rate of associated complications, including empyema and fibrothorax. Most hemothoraces can be managed with this approach. Surgical evacuation is recommended if there are retained collections of blood or persistent pleural hemorrhage. The rate of pleural hemorrhage that should prompt surgical exploration is unclear, however, surgery should be strongly considered for bleeding >200 mL/h that does not appear to be diminishing. Evidence supports early surgical intervention to prevent further clot organization and adhesion formation as well as to permit less invasive surgical procedures. Many complicated hemothoraces can be managed effectively with video-assisted thoracoscopic surgery (VATS) if intervention occurs early, thus avoiding a more invasive thoracotomy. The best timing for successful VATS procedures is generally 2–5 days after initial injury. Complications increase and technical difficulties develop if VATS is delayed beyond 7 days.

Ambrogi MC et al: Videothoracoscopy for evaluation and treatment of hemothorax. J Cardiovasc Surg 2002;43:109. [PMID: 11803341]. (Review of 33 patients with hemothorax managed with VATS; includes recommendations for thoracotomy.)

Carrillo EH, Richardson JD: Thoracoscopy in the management of hemothorax and retained blood after trauma. Curr Opin Pulmon Med 1998;4:243. [PMID: 10813242]. (This reviews the role of VATS, especially for posttraumatic hemothorax.)

Landreneau RJ et al: Thoracoscopy for empyema and hemothorax. Chest 1996;109:18. [PMID: 8549184]. (The authors review their experience managing hemothorax with VATS.)

Pleural Effusions, Excluding Hemothorax

22

Benjamin T. Suratt, MD

ESSENTIALS OF DIAGNOSIS

- *Asymptomatic in many cases; pleuritic chest pain if pleuritis is present; dyspnea if effusion is large.*
- *Diminished breath sounds; decreased tactile fremitus; dullness to percussion; egophony if effusion is large.*
- *Radiographic evidence of pleural effusion.*
- *Diagnostic findings on thoracentesis.*

General Considerations

In the healthy human being the surfaces of the pleural cavity are coated with a surfactant-containing, hypooncotic fluid that lubricates, allowing frictionless apposition of the parietal and visceral pleura during the respiratory cycle. Under normal conditions approximately 0.2–0.3 mL/kg of pleural fluid is present in the pleural space. Its continuous turnover represents a balance between production by the systemic vessels of the pleura (primarily the capillaries of the less dependent portions of the parietal pleura) and removal by the pleural lymphatics (largely in the more dependent portions of the parietal pleura). The rate of production of pleural fluid under homeostatic conditions is estimated to be 0.01 mL/kg/h and is governed by the permeability of the pleural vessels and the balance of hydrostatic and oncotic gradients across the pleural surfaces. Normal pleural fluid is low in protein (~1 g/dL), slightly alkaline compared to serum, and relatively hypocellular with approximately 2000 white blood cells (WBC)/ μL in a monocyte/macrophage predominance with 10–20% lymphocytes and a few granulocytes and erythrocytes.

Pathogenesis

Pleural effusion is an abnormal collection of fluid in the pleural space. Effusions, which may arise from a wide variety of pathological conditions, are typically classified as empyematous, hemorrhagic, chylous, exudative, or transudative. Whereas the first three categories denote collections of pus (from thoracic infection), blood (as in hemothorax), or lipid-rich chyle (from the chylous duct), the last two represent broader categories of pathogenesis. Exudative effusions are protein rich and often quite cellular, typically reflecting inflammatory or infiltrative processes directly affecting the pleura (such as pneumonia or cancer), whereas transudative effusions are low-protein, acellular filtrates that usually arise from imbalances in the body's hydrostatic and/or oncotic forces in the setting of otherwise normal pleura (such as occur in congestive heart failure or nephrotic syndrome). Causes of transudative and exudative effusions are listed in Table 22–1.

Clinical Findings

A. SYMPTOMS AND SIGNS

The hallmarks of pleural effusion on physical examination are diminution of breath sounds, dullness to percussion, and decreased tactile fremitus over the area of the effusion, but such physical findings generally occur only with effusions > 300 mL. Other findings such as a friction rub may accompany the development of pleural effusion secondary to pleuritis, and are dependent on the underlying pathology. In cases of large effusions, egophony and crackles may be heard above the effusion, reflecting compressed lung overlying the effusion. Signs of tension (increased pressure affecting one hemithorax) such as midline shift of the trachea and bulging of the intercostal spaces may accompany massive effusions (see Table 22–2).

Symptoms of pleural effusion may be absent, but often include dyspnea, cough, or pleuritic chest pain. Interestingly, dyspnea is often disproportionate to measurable hypoxemia or reduction in lung volume, and appears to result more from mechanical inefficiency of the respiratory muscles due to distortion of the chest wall and diaphragm by the effusion. Dyspnea markedly out of proportion to the size of the effusion should suggest the possibility of pulmonary embolism as the underlying diagnosis.

Table 22–1. Causes of transudative and exudative pleural effusions.

Transudates	Exudates
Congestive heart failure	Infection
Cirrhosis with ascites	Bacterial
Nephotic syndrome	Viral
Peritoneal dialysis	Fungal
Myxedema	Tuberculosis
Acute atelectasis	Parasitic
Constrictive pericarditis	Actinomycosis/nocardia
Superior vena cava syndrome	Cancer
Fontan procedure	metastatic or primary
Sarcoidosis	Pulmonary embolism
Urinothorax	PostCABG
Pulmonary embolism	Postmyocardial infarction
	syndrome
	Gastrointestinal disease
	Pancreatic disease
	Esophageal perforation
	Intraabdominal abscess
	Postsurgical/variceal
	sclerosis
	Collagen vascular disease
	Rheumatoid disease
	Lupus
	Sjögren's syndrome
	Wegener's granulomatosis
	Churg–Strauss syndrome
	Immunoblastic lympha-
	denopathy
	Asbestos
	Sarcoidosis
	Uremia
	Meigs' syndrome
	Yellow nail syndrome
	Drug reaction
	Nitrofurantoin
	Dantrolene
	Methylsergide
	Bromocriptine
	Procarbazine
	Amiodarone
	Chronic atelectasis/trapped
	lung
	Radiation therapy
	Chylothorax
	Hemothorax

B. IMAGING STUDIES

1. Conventional radiography—Although as little as 5 mL of pleural fluid can be detected using lateral decubitus position chest radiography, the more traditional posteroanterior and lateral views are significantly less sensitive. At least 50–75 mL of fluid must accumulate

Table 22–2. Causes of massive effusion with mediastinal shift.

Metastatic disease of the pleura (75% of massive effusions)
Tuberculosis
Empyema
Hepatic hydrothorax
Chylothorax
Hemothorax
Congestive heart failure

before blunting of the posterior costophrenic angle may be identified on the lateral view, and > 175–200 mL must be present to cause visible blunting of the lateral costophrenic angles on the posteroanterior view. With greater accumulation, the apex of the hemidiaphragm may be laterally displaced, then obscured (>500 mL), with subsequent opacification of the lung base. The appearance of a fluid meniscus along the chest wall or mediastinum is frequently seen, as is thickening of the major and minor fissures, indicative of superior tracking fluid.

Trapping or loculation of pleural fluid may lead to the appearance of pleural or even parenchymal lung masses. These have a typically lenticular or rounded appearance and smooth-contoured interface with the lung. Such collections usually appear along the chest wall or within the major or minor fissures of the lung, and lack air bronchograms within the "mass." Loculations are best identified by either ultrasound or computed tomography (CT) scan.

2. Ultrasound—Ultrasound may be very useful in two situations: (1) diagnosis and sampling of loculated fluid collections and (2) guided sampling of small effusions or those difficult to tap (failing two or three attempts). Ultrasound is not generally warranted for the routine diagnosis/sampling of moderate or large effusions and has not been shown to decrease the incidence of pneumothorax as a complication of the procedure.

3. Computed tomography—CT is the most sensitive radiographic study for the detection and delineation of pleural fluid collections. Free flowing fluid appears as a sickle-shaped opacity in the most dependent part of the thorax posteriorly, whereas loculations appear as lenticular or rounded opacities in a fixed position (nonflowing). CT may be extremely useful in the sampling of loculated fluid or the placement of drainage catheters in complex collections. Although CT is also helpful in distinguishing pleural fluid from parenchymal and extrapleural disease due to its ability to distinguish these anatomic compartments, CT density coefficients are not specific enough to definitively discriminate among parenchymal lesions, solid pleural masses, and pleural collections of serous fluid, blood, or pus.

4. Magnetic resonance imaging—Magnetic resonance imaging is of limited use at present in the evaluation of pleural effusions, with CT being the preferred modality.

C. LABORATORY FINDINGS

1. Thoracentesis versus observation—It has been said that "the sun should never set on an undiagnosed effusion." Although this imperative continues to be largely true when evaluating new pleural effusions, exceptions have been suggested. First, in cases of negligible pleural fluid volume (< 1 cm of fluid present on lateral decubitus film or the absence of blunting of the posterior costophrenic angles on lateral chest radiograph) sampling may be deferred. In the case of suspected pneumonia, a more aggressive approach may be warranted, as detailed in Chapter 23. Second, patients with congestive heart failure and bilateral pleural effusions of similar size, in the absence of chest pain or fever, may be observed during a 72-h trial of diuresis, after which those with persistent effusions should undergo prompt thoracentesis. Otherwise, new effusions should be sampled on presentation. If the patient is dyspneic at rest, therapeutic drainage should be performed to alleviate symptoms. This may be done as one or more thoracenteses of 1–1.5 L each (or more in the case of massive effusion), as long as the patient does not develop worsening dyspnea, chest pain, or severe cough during fluid removal. Although relative contraindications to thoracentesis including bleeding diathesis [as indicated by platelets <50,000, prothrombin time (PT) or partial thromboplastin time (PTT) >2 mid-normal range, or serum creatinine >6] and mechanical ventilation should be weighed, no absolute contraindication exists. Small or loculated effusions may require ultrasound- or CT-guided thoracentesis.

2. General appearance—Important clues to the cause of pleural effusion may be gained by simple inspection of the fluid. Frank pus indicates a pleural space infection, or empyema, the management of which is detailed in Chapter 23. Bloody fluid raises the possibility of hemothorax, and a spun fluid hematocrit should be performed. A fluid hematocrit >50% of the measured peripheral blood hematocrit is diagnostic of hemothorax (Chapter 21), whereas a fluid hematocrit 1–50% of the peripheral blood typically suggests cancer. An elevated hematocrit may also occur with pulmonary embolism, trauma, or even pneumonia. A fluid hematocrit <1% of peripheral blood is considered insignificantly bloody. Milky or turbid pleural fluid should also be spun: clearing indicates the presence of cellular debris, whereas continued turbidity suggests chylous effusion (lipid-containing lymph from an obstructed or disrupted thoracic duct) or pseudochylous effusion (cholesterol-rich fluid forming in a chronic setting). Fluid triglycerides and cholesterol should be sent for testing to pursue these diagnoses (see below). Clear yellow pleural fluid, particularly with an odor of urine, suggests urinary obstruction with urinothorax, and fluid creatinine (Cr) confirms this diagnosis (pleural fluid Cr > serum Cr).

3. Transudate versus exudate—Essential to the diagnosis of pleural effusions is the distinction between exudative effusions (those arising from disease affecting the pleura and leading to increased vascular permeability and/or decreased lymphatic drainage of the pleural space) and transudative effusions (those arising from derangement of hydrostatic and oncotic forces within the thorax in the setting of normal pleura). This distinction is best made using pleural fluid (PF) and serum lactate dehydrogenase (LDH) and total protein measurements to apply "Light's criteria." Pleural fluid is likely exudative if one or more of the following criteria are met:

1. PF protein/serum protein ratio > 0.5.
2. PF LDH/serum LDH RATIO > 0.6.
3. PF LDH > two-thirds the upper limits of the normal serum range.

Occasionally, these criteria may be met in the setting of strong clinical evidence to suggest a transudative etiology (most commonly in the setting of recent diuretic therapy). In this situation, determination of the PF–serum albumin gradient is useful: a gradient >1.2 g/dL is indicative of a transudate.

Examination of pleural fluid may be limited to LDH and total protein (± albumin, as above) in the setting of a presumed transudative etiology [eg, congestive heart failure (CHF)]. Once established as a transudate, diagnosis and treatment of the underlying condition, such as CHF (>90% of cases), cirrhosis, or nephrotic syndrome, should be pursued. Further evaluation is warranted for exudative effusions, however (Figure 22–1). This should include fluid cell count and differential, glucose, Gram stain and culture (best sent in bedside-inoculated blood culture bottles), and cytology (several hundred milliliters, if a malignancy is suspected). Findings in the most common causes of pleural effusion are listed in Table 22–3. Other, specialized tests are indicated by the clinical setting, as noted in Table 22–3 and discussed below.

D. SPECIAL TESTS

1. Cell count and differential—Although fluid cell count is relatively nonspecific, the cell type predominance and pattern may be helpful in establishing a diagnosis.

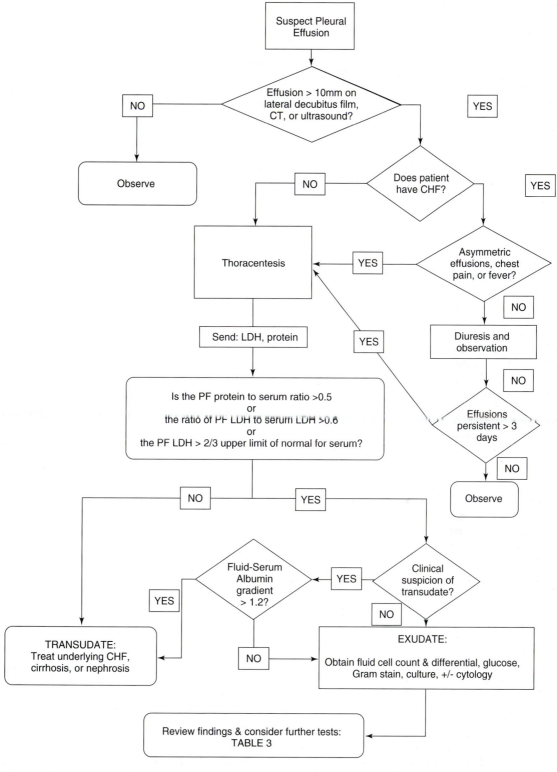

Figure 22–1. Algorithm for the initial evaluation of pleural effusion. (Modified from Light RW: Pleural effusion. N Engl J Med 2002;346:1971.)

Table 22–3. Causes of pleural effusions and their typical findings (ranked by relative incidence).[1]

Etiology	Gross Appearance	Exudative (Ex)/ Transudative (Trans)	White Blood Cell Count and Differential	Red Blood Cell Count	Glucose
Congestive heart failure	Serous	Trans	<1k, lymphocytes and mesothelial cells	<1k	Serum
Pneumonia Uncomplicated parapneumonic	Serous to turbid	Ex	5k–25k, PMNs; mononuclear in viral disease	<5k	Serum
Empyema	Turbid to purulent (pus)	Ex	25k–100k, PMNs (may be < 1k due to lysis)	<5k	Low
Cancer (other than mesothelioma)	Turbid to bloody; may be serous	Ex	1k–10k, lymphocytes or mesothelial cells predominantly; eosinophilia rare	100–100k	Usually serum; < 60 mg/dL in 15%
Pulmonary embolism	Serous to grossly bloody	Ex > trans	1k–100k, PMNs and lymphocytes; often > 10% eosinophils and/or mesothelial cells	100–100k	Variable
PostCABG Acute (< 30 days)	Bloody	Ex	Frequently eosinophilic	>100k	Serum
Chronic	Serous > bloody	Ex	Lymphocytic	<5k	Serum
Cirrhosis with ascites	Serous	Trans	<1k, lymphocytes and mesothelial cells	<1k	Serum
Gastrointestinal Pancreatitis	Serosanguineous to turbid	Ex	1k–50k, PMNs	1k–10k	Serum
Esophageal rupture	Turbid to purulent; red-brown	Ex	1k–50k, PMNs; squamous epithelial cells	1k–10k	Usually low
Connective tissue disease Rheumatoid disease	Turbid—greenish-yellow	Ex	1k–20k, mononuclear cells or PMNs, multi-nucleated macrophages	<1k	< 40 mg/dL
Lupus (systemic or drug induced)	Serosanguineous/ yellow	Ex	1k–20k, mononuclear cells or PMNs	<1k	Usually serum
Tuberculosis	Serous to serosanguineous	Ex	1k–10k, lymphocytic (PMNs if early); eosinophils >10% or mesothelial cells >5% make TB an unlikely diagnosis	<10k	May be serum or low
Asbestos	Serous to serosanguineous	Ex	1k–20k, mononuclear cells or PMNs; often (25–50%) of patients eosinophilic	< 10k	Serum
Mesothelioma	Serous to bloody; may be viscid	Ex	1k–5k; mesothelial cells (normal and malignant) and varying PMNs and lymphocytes	100–100k	May be serum or low (33%)

(continued)

Chest Radiograph	Comment
Most often (80–90%) bilateral and symmetric; pulmonary vascular congestion, pulmonary edema	May appear "exudate" by Light's criteria, especially after ≥ 3 day diuresis
Loculated or large effusions (>50% hemithorax) may require thoracostomy (see Chapter 23)	Fluid **pH** <7.30 or glucose <60 suggest complicated parapneumonic, whereas frank pus, positive Gram stain or culture is diagnostic of empyema (see Chapter 23)
May cause massive effusion with mediastinal shift	
Effusion ipsilateral to cancer in lung ± breast cancer; effusions typically moderate/large; 10% have massive effusion	Lung > breast > lymphoma; low glucose and pH may correlate with large tumor burden and poor prognosis; fluid **cytology ± amylase** should be obtained
30–40% PE have effusion, usually small; >50% have concomitant parenchymal infiltrate	55% of all patients with pleuritic chest pain and effusion have PE; 25% of patients with PE and effusion have no chest pain
Usually small and left-sided	Up to 90% of postCABG patients; resolves spontaneously
Larger than acute; 40% bilateral or right-sided	10% of patients; no correlation to history of acute effusion; ?autoimmune
70% are right-sided, but may be left (15%) or bilateral (15%); small to massive (10%); may have small pneumothorax after paracentesis	5–10% of patients with ascites develop hepatic hydrothorax; may be hemorrhagic in setting of coagulopathy; detectable ascites may be absent; may be complicated by spontaneous bacterial pleuritis (see text)
Typically small and bilateral; left-sided predominance in larger effusions	High **amylase** in fluid; persistent effusions (> 2 weeks) suggest pseudocyst or abscess
Usually left-sided; pneumothorax in 25%; occasionally mediastinal widening and/or pneumomediastinum	Uncommon, but a surgical emergency; high **amylase** (salivary), low **pH,** sometimes food particles; esophagogram to diagnose
Small/moderate effusion; 25% bilateral; may wax/wane and/or alternate sides over time	5% RA pts: 80% male, 80% have subcut nodules; usually older with longstanding RA; may have chest pain ± fever; fluid **pH** < 7.20, high **RF** (>1:320) and LDH, often cholesterol crystals
Small effusion; 50% bilateral; may wax/wane and/or alternate sides over time	40–50% develop effusion; most have chest pain ± fever; may precede other lupus findings; **pH** > 7.35 (80%); fluid ANA or LE cell preparation not helpful in diagnosis
Small/moderate effusion, almost always unilateral; one-third with concomitant parenchymal infiltrate (ipsilateral)	Two-thirds of patients have acute illness with cough and chest pain, one-third chronic with low grade fever, weakness and weight loss; fluid protein >5.0 g/dL suggests diagnosis; see text for other tests
Small/moderate unilateral (90%) effusion; often with pleural plaques and/or parenchymal asbestosis (50%)	Diagnosis of exclusion; one-half to two-thirds are asymptomatic; chest pain most common complaint (one-third); may develop within years to decades following exposure to asbestos; 80% benign/recurrent but 20% develop massive pleural fibrosis (and ~5% mesothelioma)
Effusion present in 75–90% of mesothelioma patients; often large (and obscuring tumor); one-third have evident pleural plaques in opposite hemithorax; may produce ipsilateral mediastinal shift and loculation as encases lung; CT scan useful in evaluation	Most patients experience insidious onset chest pain or dyspnea; 10–70% with history of asbestos exposure; although fluid **cytology** may indicate malignancy, VATS is often required to establish diagnosis of mesothelioma

[1]Common etiologies of pleural effusion, in descending order of incidence. Suggested additional testing to establish diagnoses **bolded** in comments section. CABG, Coronary artery bypass grafting; PMNs, polymorphonuclear cells; k, 1000; PE, pulmonary embolism; RA, rheumatoid arthritis; RF, rheumatoid factor; ANA, antinuclear antibody; LE, lupus erythematosus; LDH, lactate dehydrogenase; VATS, video-assisted thoracic surgery.

Neutrophilic effusions [>50% polymorphonuclear cells (PMNs)] indicate an acute process affecting the pleural surfaces. In association with infiltrates, a neutrophilic effusion typically reflects a parapneumonic response (including early viral, early tuberculous, or more commonly bacterial infections) or pulmonary embolism. In the absence of infiltrates, pulmonary embolism, acute viral infection, or pancreatitis should be considered. Cancer and acute tuberculous pleuritis are rare causes of neutrophilic effusions.

A mononuclear predominance usually accompanies chronic processes of the pleura. Such processes include cancer, resolving viral pleuritis, tuberculosis, or pulmonary embolism (20%). A predominance of small lymphocytes on differential (>50%) is nearly always secondary to tuberculosis, cancer, or the occasional chronic postcoronary artery bypass grafting (CABG) effusion, whereas the presence of fluid eosinophils (>10%) or more than a few mesothelial cells makes tuberculosis a less likely diagnosis and may suggest a diagnosis of pulmonary embolism (PE).

Fluid eosinophilia (>10% eosinophils) is most often secondary to air or blood in the pleural space following trauma or other intrathoracic insult, and can confound interpretation of the fluid differential following repeated thoracentesis. It may also arise from drug-induced pleuritis (dantrolene, bromocriptine, or nitrofurantoin), asbestos-related effusion, paragonimiasis, or Churg–Strauss syndrome. Concomitant low fluid pH and glucose suggest the latter two diagnoses. Frequently, no diagnosis is established in the setting of eosinophilic effusion.

2. Glucose—Pleural fluid glucose may be significantly lower than serum due to impairment of glucose diffusion through the pleura and/or increased consumption of glucose by cells within the pleural space. Causes of low fluid glucose (<60 mg/dL) include complicated parapneumonic effusion/empyema, cancer, tuberculous pleuritis, and rheumatoid disease. Less common causes include esophageal rupture, hemothorax, Churg–Strauss syndrome, paragonimiasis, and occasionally lupus pleuritis. Although fluid pH is currently preferred over fluid glucose in the evaluation of parapneumonic effusions, in its absence a fluid glucose of <60 mg/dL is useful in suggesting a complicated parapneumonic effusion that possibly requires chest tube drainage (see Chapter 23).

Causes of elevated pleural fluid glucose are few and result almost exclusively from the leakage of high glucose solutions into the pleural space either via a diaphragmatic defect (peritoneal dialysis with high glucose dialysate) or iatrogenic misadventure (such as a misplaced central venous line).

3. Amylase—Although no longer recommended for the routine evaluation of exudative pleural effusions,

fluid amylase level is extremely useful in the rapid detection of esophageal perforation and the diagnosis of pancreatitis-related effusions. Elevated fluid amylase levels (greater than the upper limit of normal serum) occur in esophageal perforation (salivary), acute pancreatitis (pancreatic), chronic pancreatitis with fistula (pancreatic; >4000 IU/mL), and about 10% of malignant effusions (salivary), most commonly from adenocarcinoma. Elevated fluid amylase may rarely be seen in tuberculous pleuritis, parapneumonic effusion, and cirrhosis, as well. Effusions secondary to acute pancreatitis occur in approximately 50% of cases and tend to correlate with attack severity and subsequent development of pancreatic pseudocysts.

4. pH—Fluid pH (by blood gas machine) is indicated in the assessment of parapneumonic effusions (see Chapter 23), and may be useful in malignant effusion. Causes of low fluid pH (<7.20) include complicated parapneumonic effusion/empyema, esophageal perforation, rheumatoid pleuritis, tuberculosis, cancer, hemothorax, paragonimiasis, urinothorax, systemic acidosis, and occasionally lupus pleuritis. The finding of low pH in malignant effusion indicates extensive pleural disease and correlates with a high likelihood of fluid cytological diagnosis, but poor response to chemical pleurodesis and poor overall prognosis (life expectancy less than 3 months from thoracentesis). Acidic malignant effusion alone should not, however, preclude therapeutic pleurodesis in otherwise appropriate patients.

5. Cultures, stains, and other microbiological tests—Gram's stain and culture (aerobic and anaerobic) should be sent on all exudative effusions for two important reasons: First, a Gram's stain or culture positive for organisms is diagnostic of empyema, which most often requires immediate interventions (see Chapter 23). Second, stain and culture are necessary to exclude pleural space infection in the setting of existing (and often confounding) pleural disease, such as for rheumatoid pleuritis in which the fluid glucose and pH are typically low even in the absence of infection. Other microbial stains and cultures, such as mycobacterial or fungal, typically have low yields and should be sent only when a specific diagnosis is suspected.

The diagnosis of tuberculous pleuritis should be pursued in all patients with unexplained pleural fluid lymphocytosis, yet establishing this diagnosis remains difficult. Stains for acid-fast bacilli are positive in < 10% of cases, whereas mycobacterial culture of fluid takes weeks and lacks sensitivity (<40%). Even a positive skin test (purified protein derivative, PPD) may initially be absent in up to 30% of patients with tuberculous pleuritis. Several other tests have been evaluated for the diagnosis, including fluid adenosine-deaminase (ADA), interferon-γ levels, and polymerase chain reaction to detect mycobacterial DNA. These tests remain controversial and unavailable at many centers. In the absence of positive fluid acid-fast bacillus (AFB) or culture, and lacking access to competent assays of these newer markers, the use of pleural needle biopsy should be considered. Pleural biopsy is diagnostic in 50–80% of patients, with subsequent mycobacterial culture increasing diagnostic yield to >90%.

6. Cytology and other approaches to the diagnosis of cancer —Although variably successful in diagnosing cancer, pleural fluid cytology is minimally invasive and may yield a ready diagnosis. Cytology yield ranges from 40 to 87% and is influenced by tumor type (adenocarcinomas highest) and extent of disease. Large tumor burden, as indicated by low fluid pH and glucose, has cytological yields approaching 95%. The collection of one or two additional fluid samples for cytology several days after an initial large volume (>300 mL) thoracentesis increases the diagnostic yield, as well. Unfortunately, even the presence of malignant cells on cytology may be insufficient to establish a specific diagnosis of cancer. The use of a variety of immunohistochemical stains may be helpful in this situation, whereas flow cytometry may detect clonal cell populations and establish the diagnosis of lymphoma.

If no diagnosis can be established through repeated fluid cytology, fiberoptic bronchoscopy may be considered if the patient has findings of an airway lesion such as hemoptysis or atelectasis on imaging. Either bronchoscopic or CT-guided biopsy may be appropriate if an accessible lesion is present on chest radiography or CT. In the absence of such a lesion, pleural needle biopsy (although of lower yield than fluid cytology) may have a role, particularly if tuberculous effusion is a consideration. However, thoracoscopic biopsy offers the most definitive approach and should be considered both to establish the diagnosis and possibly to perform palliative pleurodesis (see below).

7. Lipids and cholesterol—Measurement of pleural fluid lipids and cholesterol is generally reserved for cases of suspected chylothorax or pseudochylothorax, usually on the basis of milky effusions that remain turbid even after centrifugation. Often, the distinction between chylous and pseudochylous effusions may be made on clinical history: pseudochylous fluid is usually found in the setting of chronic pleural effusion with pleural fibrosis, whereas chylous effusions are most often acute in nature. Although the most definitive approach to diagnosing chylothorax is the demonstration of chylomicrons in the pleural fluid by lipoprotein analysis, a simpler and less costly initial approach employs measurement of triglycerides (TG) and cholesterol. Chylothorax is diagnosed when fluid TG is >110 mg/dL, fluid TG/serum TG is >1, and fluid cholesterol/serum

cholesterol is <1. Fluid TG <50 mg/dL effectively rules out the diagnosis of chylothorax, and in the presence of a fluid cholesterol >250 mg/dL identifies pseudochylothorax. Fluid TG of 50–110 mg/dL (or >110 in the setting of a fluid/serum cholesterol ratio >1) warrants lipoprotein analysis for a definitive assessment. Fluid glucose and potassium should be sent when central venous total parenteral nutrition (TPN) is in use and leakage into the thorax is suspected.

Differential Diagnosis

For differential diagnosis of pleural effusions, see Table 22–3 and Figure 22–1.

Treatment & Prognosis

In general, the treatment (and prognosis) of pleural effusion centers on treatment of the causative disease process. Pulmonary embolism with effusion should be treated as pulmonary embolism (bloody effusion does not contraindicate anticoagulation), whereas tubercular pleuritis typically resolves after 6 weeks of standard treatment of tuberculosis (TB). Acute effusion following CABG usually resolves spontaneously, although chronic effusions may require therapeutic thoracentesis (one or two times) with or without nonsteroidal antiinflammatory drugs (NSAIDs). Lupus effusion typically mandates steroid therapy, but rheumatoid effusion most often spontaneously resolves within 3 months. Many cases of pleural effusion require a more complex approach due to either the persistence of effusion despite therapy for the underlying illness, or to complications of the effusion itself. Several of the more important instances include parapneumonic effusion/ empyema (detailed in Chapter 23) and hemothorax (detailed in Chapter 21), as well as the following.

A. MALIGNANT EFFUSION

Effusion is an unfortunate and not uncommon complication of cancer, occurring in approximately 15% of all cancer patients. Although most result from direct infiltration of the pleura by tumor cells, some occur due to other complications, such as pulmonary embolism or postobstructive pneumonia. Such effusions are referred to as "paramalignant effusions," and are best addressed based on their immediate cause (eg, pulmonary embolism or pneumonia).

A general approach to the management of malignant effusion begins with assessment of the patient. In addition to appropriate management of the patient's cancer, some additional form of palliative therapy is indicated for those who are dyspneic and experience relief following thoracentesis. To this end, large volume thoracentesis should be performed (as described above) to remove as much effusion as possible in all dyspneic patients.

Patients whose dyspnea is not improved by thoracentesis should be evaluated for other causes of their symptoms (such as pulmonary embolism or lymphangitic spread of tumor), whereas patients in whom complete reexpansion of the lung is unsuccessful should be evaluated for possible bronchial occlusion or trapped lung due to bulky pleural tumor. In symptomatically improved patients in whom effusion returns slowly after thoracentesis, or in whom poor performance status or life expectancy preclude more aggressive management options, a conservative approach of repeated therapeutic thoracentesis as needed for symptoms may be the most appropriate plan. Otherwise, patients with rapid return of symptomatic effusion warrant consideration of a more aggressive approach with pleurodesis to obliterate the pleural space.

Although controversy exists over the best method for pleurodesis, the use of sterile talc, either by poudrage or instilled slurry, appears to be the most effective and economical approach, with a success rate >90% in some series. Following appropriate narcotic and sedative premedication of the patient, poudrage is achieved by insufflating talc under direct observation with thoracoscopy, while slurry (4–5 g talc in 50 mL saline) is instilled via an inferoposteriorly directed chest tube. In the slurry approach, the patient's chest tube is clamped after instillation and the slurry dwells in the pleural space for 1 h while the patient rotates position in bed to effect even distribution of the talc. After either procedure, the chest tube is left to suction (20 mL water), and is not removed until drainage has fallen below 100–150 mL/day. If drainage continues to exceed 250 mL/day after 3 days, pleurodesis may be repeated. Common complications of this procedure include fever and chest pain that may last up to 72 h. These are treated symptomatically. Rarely, empyema or acute respiratory distress syndrome (ARDS) may develop following talc pleurodesis, although the relationship of these complications to the procedure and their true incidence remain controversial.

Options for treatment after failure of pleurodesis include surgical pleurectomy, placement of a pleuroperitoneal shunt, or a more conservative approach with chronic thoracostomy drainage catheter and bag.

B. Hepatic Hydrothorax

Although treatment of hepatic hydrothorax is primarily directed at controlling the patient's ascites through the use of sodium restriction and diuretics, such effusions may become refractory despite therapy, or become infected, much like ascitic fluid. The approach to recurrent effusion in such patients is controversial and frequently unsuccessful. Following initial therapeutic thoracentesis and aggressive medical therapy for ascites, careful, repeated large volume paracentesis may slow the reaccumulation of pleural fluid. However, this may not be effective if minimal drainable ascites is present (with the fluid rapidly translocating to and collecting in the chest) or complications of large volume paracentesis arise, such as hypotension or electrolyte abnormalities.

Simple pleurodesis is rarely successful in these patients. Thus chest tube thoracostomy should generally be avoided, as it is at best temporizing and may lead to rapid fluid loss with hypotension, hypoalbuminemia, and renal dysfunction or pleural infection. Pleurodesis in conjunction with thoracoscopic repair of the diaphragmatic defects that typically lead to hydrothorax is a promising approach, but is not widely performed, and surgical peritoneal-venous shunting is controversial. Transjugular intrahepatic portosystemic shunt (TIPS) is effective in >75% of cases, but may be complicated by worsening encephalopathy and liver function. The most definitive approach to the problem is liver transplantation, which should be a serious consideration in appropriate candidates given the >50% 1-year mortality experienced by patients developing hepatic hydrothorax.

Bacterial infection of hepatic hydrothorax in the absence of underlying pneumonia [spontaneous bacterial empyema (SBE)] occurs in 13% of patients with such effusions, often in the absence of bacterial peritonitis (40%), and may in fact occur without appreciable ascites. The diagnosis is established by positive fluid cultures [typically with organisms found in spontaneous bacterial peritonitis (SBP)] or by a pleural fluid neutrophil count >500 (culture negative SBE). Such infections are treated with culture-directed antibiotics (or empiric coverage appropriate for SBP), without need for chest tube thoracostomy.

C. Chylothorax and Pseudochylothorax

Most important in the treatment of chylothorax is the diagnosis of the underlying cause. As chylothorax results from leakage of lipid-rich lymph (or chyle) from the thoracic duct either due to disruption or obstruction of the duct, its causes generally fall into one of two categories: traumatic/surgical and nontraumatic. An important exception to this is chylothorax due to transdiaphragmatic movement of chylous ascites. Although any trauma or surgery resulting in damage or stretching of the chest wall or thoracic spine and mediastinum may result in disruption of the thoracic duct, thoracic and head and neck surgery as well as esophageal sclerotherapy appear to be the most common traumatic causes. The list of nontraumatic causes is extensive (including cancer, thrombosed left subclavian central venous catheter, mediastinal irradiation, congenital abnormalities, and a variety of other infrequent causes), yet the single most common cause is lymphoma (50%), typically non-Hodgkins. If no traumatic or surgical cause can be identified in the workup of chylothorax, attention should turn to lymphoma, and a CT of the chest and upper abdomen should be performed to identify lymphadenopathy or abnormality of the lung parenchyma. If this is unrevealing, lymphangiogram may localize a lesion for video-assisted thoracic surgery (VATS) or open lung biopsy. Often no diagnosis is made, and the effusion is labeled idiopathic. Because such effusions may be the presenting finding in lymphoma, the patient should be closely followed for this diagnosis.

Regardless of underlying cause, rapidly reaccumulating chylothorax should be treated, as patients are not only symptomatic but lose substantial protein and nutrients with the chyle. Treatment of the underlying disease often improves chylothorax, but even good response to therapy (particularly in the case of lymphoma) may not improve chylothorax. Conservative measures to reduce the amount of chyle produced should follow, including a low fat diet with medium-chain triglycerides or, failing this, complete bowel rest with TPN alimentation. Although >50% of traumatic/surgical cases will respond to this approach, failure (>1.5 L/day drained for 5 days or 2 weeks without improvement) is more common in nontraumatic cases, and may be addressed with talc pleurodesis, pleuroperitoneal shunt implantation, or surgical ligation of the thoracic duct.

Pseudochylous (or chyliform) effusion, although appearing similar to chyle on thoracentesis, is a completely different entity, resulting from the collection of cholesterol in a chronic effusion. Such effusions usually occur in the setting of chronically thickened pleura due to, for example, tuberculous or rheumatoid pleurisy, or poorly treated hemothorax or empyema, and do not warrant intervention if stable. Growing effusions should be evaluated with AFB stain and culture, as well as chest CT, to search for an active process.

Special Circumstances

A. Pleural Effusion in Acquired Immunodeficiency Syndrome (AIDS)

Pleural effusions occur in up to 27% of hospitalized patients with AIDS, with more than half of these being parapneumonic. Other common causes of effusion include tuberculosis, Kaposi's sarcoma (KS), renal failure, and hypoalbuminemia. Although management of parapneumonic effusions in these patients is similar to that in immunocompetent patients, early empiric staphylococcal coverage should be considered until an organism has been identified, given the high incidence of *Staphylococcus aureus* pneumonia among AIDS patients. Tuberculosis may be an important cause of effusion depending on local epidemiology. Interestingly, as CD4

counts fall below 200, the incidence of tuberculous effusion decreases, and yet the rate of positive acid-fast stains on pleural fluid increases. The diagnosis of KS should be entertained in the setting of bilateral effusions with focal air space consolidation, intrapulmonary nodules, and hilar lymphadenopathy. Such effusions are typically serosanguineous or bloody exudates with a mononuclear predominance. Although the definitive diagnosis of KS effusion requires thoracoscopic identification of the lesions on the pleura, a presumptive diagnosis may be made in the setting of identified lesions on bronchoscopy and exclusion of other etiologies.

B. Nonresolving and Idiopathic Effusions

The time course of resolution for nonmalignant effusions, although variable, may be roughly predicted based on the underlying cause. This can a useful gauge for the clinician both in monitoring response to therapy and in ensuring diagnostic accuracy. Rapidly resolving effusions (<2 months) include CHF, parapneumonic, acute pancreatitis, postCABG (acute), pulmonary embolism, SLE, and traumatic chylothorax. Effusions that resolve more slowly (2–6 months) include tuberculous, postCABG (chronic), and chronic pancreatitis. Rheumatoid and benign asbestos effusions can last from 2 months to 1 year before resolving, and trapped lung, along with some causes of chylothorax, can cause persistent, unresolving effusions.

Persistent, undiagnosed effusions occur in up to 20% of patients evaluated for pleural effusion, despite aggressive workup. Common causes of the difficult to diagnose effusion include cancer, tuberculosis, and pulmonary embolism. Other, less common causes are subclinical ascites, chronic pancreatitis, and granulomatous infections such as fungi and atypical mycobacterial disease. If diagnosis of effusion remains elusive despite multiple thoracenteses, further evaluation might best focus on these diagnoses. Tuberculosis should be pursued aggressively in patients with lymphocytic effusions by sending fluid and needle pleural biopsy stains and cultures, and placing serial PPDs (with anergy panel) separated by 6–8 weeks. If the patient has a positive skin test, empiric therapy for TB should be strongly considered despite negative cultures and stains. Otherwise, for patients with constitutional symptoms or large effusions, thoracoscopic examination and biopsy should be considered. Watchful waiting may be appropriate in cases in which treatable causes have been excluded, as conservative management of untreatable (malignant) or undiagnosable effusions is often preferable to invasive tests.

Afessa B: Pleural effusions and pneumothoraces in AIDS. Curr Opin Pulmon Med 2001;7:202. [PMID: 11470975]. (Succinct, well- referenced review.)

American Thoracic Society: Management of malignant pleural effusions. Am J Respir Crit Care Med 2000;162:1987. [PMID: 11069845]. (Exhaustive review of options for the management of malignant effusions.)

Ansari T, Idell S: Management of undiagnosed persistent pleural effusions. Clin Chest Med 1998;19:407. [PMID: 9646991]. (Thorough discussion of the diagnosis and treatment of persistent effusions of unknown etiology.)

Cohen M et al: Resolution of pleural effusions. Chest 2001;119:1547. [PMID: 11348966]. (Very useful review of more than 30 years of published reports and series of pleural effusions, broken down by etiologies.)

Lazaridis K et al: Hepatic hydrothorax: pathogenesis, diagnosis, and management. Am J Med 1999;107(3):262. [PMID: 10492320]. (Good review of hepatic hydrothorax and proposed algorithm for its management.)

Light R, Sahn S: Am J Respir Crit Care Med 2000;162:2023. [PMID: 11112103]. (Informative pro/con editorials by Light and Sahn on talc pleurodesis.)

Noppen M et al: Volume and cellular content of normal pleural fluid in humans examined by pleural lavage. Am J Respir Crit Care Med 2000;162:1023. [PMID: 10988124]. (An examination of normal pleural fluid in humans.)

Romero-Candeira S et al: Influence of diuretics on the concentration of proteins and other components of pleural transudates in patients with heart failure. Am J Med 2001;110:681. [PMID: 11403751]. (Interesting study examining the changes in CHF pleural effusion chemistry following diuresis. Suggests that fluid protein and albumin gradients are the most useful determinants of transudative effusion in the setting of diuretic use.)

Valdes L et al: Tuberculous pleurisy: a study of 254 patients. Arch Intern Med 1998;158:2017. [PMID: 9778201]. (Case series describing the radiological and biochemical characteristics of tuberculous effusions, as well as the utility of ADA, interferon-γ, and other tests in establishing the diagnosis. Good overview of testing modalities provided by Light's accompanying editorial.)

Villena V et al: Amylase levels in pleural effusions: a consecutive unselected series of 841 patients. Chest 2002;121:470. [PMID: 11834659]. (Study of the causes and relative frequency of amylase-rich pleural effusions. Given the increased incidence of malignant effusion compared to pancreatitis-related effusion, amylase-rich effusion is more often malignant, and in the absence of clinical pancreatitis should be considered.)

Empyema

John E. Heffner, MD

ESSENTIALS OF DIAGNOSIS

- *Parapneumonic effusions are pleural effusions that occur in association with pneumonia.*
- *If inadequately treated, parapneumonic effusions progress through the exudative, fibrinopurulent, and organized phases of empyema formation.*
- *All hospitalized patients with pneumonia should be evaluated by imaging studies for the presence of a parapneumonic effusion.*
- *Pleural fluid analysis establishes the diagnosis and aids in determining management.*
- *Early diagnosis and prompt thoracentesis decrease morbidity and mortality for patients with parapneumonic effusions.*

General Considerations

Parapneumonic effusions occur in 20–60% of patients with pneumonia that is sufficiently severe to require hospitalization. Although most of these effusions are sterile and resolve with antibiotic therapy for the underlying pneumonia, 5–10% of patients hospitalized for pneumonia develop intrapleural infection. These patients require prompt pleural fluid drainage to prevent the formation of an empyema, which is characterized by the presence of intrapleural pus. Because of the significant morbidity and mortality associated with empyema, the primary focus of managing parapneumonic effusions centers on early detection and urgent evaluation to identify those patients who require pleural fluid drainage to prevent or treat an empyema.

Heffner JE: Infection of the pleural space. Clin Chest Med 1999;20:607. [PMID: 10516908]. (General review of parapneumonic effusions and empyema with a discussion of the value of biochemical tests to guide drainage decisions.)

Pathogenesis

Parapneumonic effusions occur when regions of pneumonia abut pleural surfaces and alter pleural membranes. Mesothelial cells line the visceral pleura and form a semipermeable membrane that prevents free diffusion of fluid and passage of circulating cells from the bloodstream into the pleural space. When stimulated by an adjacent pneumonia, mesothelial cells alter their membrane characteristics and permit fluid and high-molecular-weight compounds, such as protein and lactic dehydrogenase (LDH), to enter the pleural space. Activated mesothelial cells also release cytokines and other proinflammatory mediators that recruit inflammatory cells and fibroblasts. Progressive pleural inflammation promotes the deposition of fibrin onto pleural surfaces, which forms a latticework for fibroblasts to deposit collagen and form intrapleural loculations and pleural peels. Pleural peels can encase the lung and prevent lung reexpansion (trapped lung) when an intrapleural catheter is placed to drain a parapneumonic effusion.

The progression of a parapneumonic effusion to an established empyema has three distinct phases, each of which has therapeutic implications. Free-flowing nonviscous fluid and the absence of a pleural peel characterize the *exudative* phase. Most but not all exudative effusions respond to antibiotic therapy. The development of more viscous fluid and the early formation of intrapleural loculations and pleural peels characterize the *fibrinopurulent* phase. The *organizing* phase of empyema formation is characterized by established fibrotic peels, viscous pleural pus, and loculations. Management of organized empyema requires thoracotomy with decortication or other extensive surgical procedures.

Nearly all bacterial and fungal pathogens that cause pneumonia can also cause parapneumonic effusions and empyemas. The relative frequency of different pathogens varies by their distribution as a cause of pneumonia in a community. *Streptococcus pneumoniae*, *Staphylococcus aureus*, *Hemophilus influenzae*, and *Klebsiella pneumoniae* are the pathogens that most commonly cause parapneumonic effusions. Multiple fungal pathogens cause empyema and fungal empyema is becoming more common in clinical practice. Atypical bacteria, parasites, and viral agents are rare causes of infected pleural effusions.

An established empyema often results from anaerobic lung infections that progress in an indolent manner, which allows extensive pleural infection to develop before patients present for antibiotic therapy. Most empyemas have a mixed population of aerobic and anaerobic bacterial pathogens detected with the culture of pleural pus.

Antony VB et al: Pathophysiology of pleural space infections. Semin Respir Infect 1999;14:9. [PMID: 10049988]. (Overview of the pathophysiological events that initiate and perpetuate pleural inflammation.)

Bryant RE et al: Pleural empyema. Clin Infect Dis 1996;22:747. [PMID: 8722927]. (Large patient series that describes the pathogens that cause empyema.)

Chen KY et al: A 10-year experience with bacteriology of acute thoracic empyema: emphasis on Klebsiella pneumoniae in patients with diabetes mellitus. Chest 2000;117:1685. [PMID: 10858403]. (Case series that emphasizes the importance of gram negative pathogens in causing empyema.)

Ko SC et al: Fungal empyema thoracis: an emerging clinical entity. Chest 2000;117:1672. [PMID: 10858403]. (This study reports the clinical characteristics and outcome of patients with fungal empyemas.)

Prevention

Empyemas most often are a consequence of delayed antibiotic therapy for lung infections. The most important preventive measure, therefore, is prompt evaluation and initiation of appropriate antibiotics for patients who present with acute signs and symptoms of pneumonia. Some patients with empyema due to anaerobic bacteria, however, may follow an indolent course with early symptoms of chest infection misdiagnosed as a "chest cold" or "bronchitis." These patients may later present with an established empyema that requires surgical drainage. Most of these patients, however, have risk factors for aspiration (altered mentation, alcoholism, or poor dentition). Recognition of these risk factors allows clinicians to identify patients who would benefit from a chest radiograph at the onset of new respiratory symptoms, even when the respiratory symptoms are otherwise mild and nonspecific.

When patients present with a parapneumonic effusion, the most important strategy for preventing the formation of a frank empyema is prompt thoracentesis to determine the need for pleural fluid drainage. Delayed drainage of infected pleural fluid is associated with an increase in mortality, morbidity, and duration of hospitalization.

Clinical Findings

The symptoms associated with parapneumonic effusion and empyema merge with those of the underlying pneumonia. Patients present with fever, cough with purulent sputum, various degrees of shortness of breath, occasionally diaphoresis and rigors, and pleuritic chest pain, which is a more specific feature. Chest pain may resolve or become dull as patients in the acute exudative phase progress to a frank empyema. Failure to respond to antibiotics directed toward pneumonia also suggests the possibility of empyema. Patients with anaerobic pleuropulmonary disease may follow an indolent course and present with weight loss, foul breath, fatigue, and inanition, thereby simulating the presentation of a patient with cancer.

Signs of a parapneumonic effusion include decreased breath sounds, dullness, egophony, and decreased fremitus over the region of pleural fluid collection. Detection of decreased fremitus is especially important because the absence of fremitus differentiates dullness to percussion related to a pleural fluid collection from dullness due to consolidated lung, which has increased fremitus. A pleural friction rub indicates the presence of pleurisy, which occurs most commonly during the early exudative phase of empyema. Friction rubs diminish when increasing pleural fluid separates the inflamed visceral from the parietal pleura.

The standard radiograph may demonstrate obvious evidence of pleural fluid if the effusion is large (>200–500 mL), but may not be sensitive enough to detect smaller parapneumonic effusions. Extensive regions of lung consolidation may obscure the presence of an adjacent free-flowing or loculated parapneumonic effusion. Lower lobe consolidation commonly obscures free-flowing effusions because both of these conditions produce a silhouette sign with the diaphragm.

Differential Diagnosis

Because the clinical and radiographic presentation of a patient with a parapneumonic effusion merges with the clinical features of pneumonia, clinicians should carefully examine every patient hospitalized with pneumonia for the presence of a pleural effusion. The algorithm in Figure 23–1 is one evaluative approach that relies on a sequenced imaging strategy for hospitalized patients with pneumonia.

As shown in Figure 23–1, evidence of pleural fluid on a standard radiograph or obscuration of the diaphragm warrants right and left decubitus radiographic views to determine if the fluid is free flowing or if the obscured diaphragm is due to adjacent consolidated lung or a subpulmonic effusion. Layering of pleural fluid 1 cm or greater against the dependent chest wall on the decubitus view is considered by most experts to warrant thoracentesis.

If the standard radiograph suggests the presence of a loculated parapneumonic effusion, chest ultrasonography can localize the fluid, determine the presence of septated loculations, and guide thoracentesis. Ultrasonography is also indicated to exclude a loculated effusion if a patient with obscuration of the diaphragm on a standard radiograph does not demonstrate layering fluid on a decubitus view.

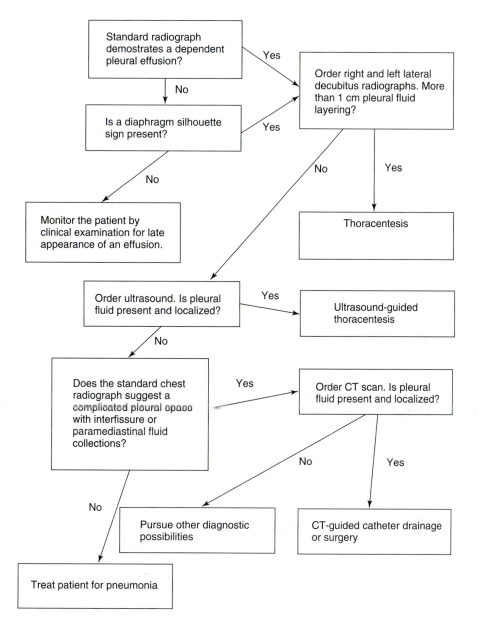

Figure 23–1. Algorithm for directing the chest imaging evaluation of patients with parapneumonic effusions.

Patients with standard radiographs that suggest multiple loculations can be evaluated by chest computed tomography (CT) with intravenous contrast. Chest CT can show a "split pleurae" sign wherein the visceral and parietal pleura enhance with contrast and separate in the region of a loculated pleural effusion. This sign distinguishes lung consolidation and peripheral lung abscesses from loculated parapneumonic effusions. Chest

CT can also detect paramediastinal loculations better than chest ultrasonography. Chest CT is not as sensitive as ultrasonography, however, for establishing the presence of septae within monolocular fluid collections.

Thoracentesis is indicated for hospitalized patients with parapneumonic effusions that are either loculated or free flowing with more than 1 cm of layering detected on a decubitus chest radiograph. Appropriate studies with their clinical significance are listed in Table 23–1.

Thoracentesis has several purposes in evaluating and managing patients with parapneumonic effusions. So that the procedure serves a therapeutic purpose as much fluid as possible should be drained with the initial thoracentesis. Pleural fluid test results can (1) establish the infectious nature of the pleural effusion, (2) identify an etiological pathogen for the underlying pneumonia, (3) categorize the exudative, fibrinopurulent, or organizing phases of the effusion, and (4) assist in determining whether pleural fluid drainage is needed.

Table 23–1. Pleural fluid tests to assist the evaluation of patients with parapneumonic effusions.

Test	Clinical Significance
Complete cell count and differential	White blood count—marginal value. Noninfectious effusions may have high leukocyte counts (eg, lupus pleurisy); empyema may have low leukocytes counts (< 1000/μL) due to cell lysis. Differential—neutrophil predominance establishes acuity of infection.
pH, glucose, LDH	Provides some assistance with decision for drainage; pH < 7.00 suggests a ruptured esophagus as cause of empyema.
Amylase (order if ruptured esophagus suspected)	Elevated salivary amylase establishes ruptured esophagus.
Aerobic/anaerobic cultures	Identifies etiological pathogen, directs antibiotics, establishes need for drainage.
Gram stain	Identifies pathogen morphology, establishes need for drainage.
Special studies in selected patients Mycobacterial stains and cultures Fungal stains and cultures Special stains and culture techniques for *Nocardia* spp.	Establish presence of unusual pathogens.
Cytology	Identifies underlying malignancy or presence of food particles suggesting ruptured esophagus.

Levin DL et al: Imaging techniques for pleural space infections. Semin Respir Infect 1999;14:31. [PMID: 10197395]. (Review of the clinical utility of various imaging studies in evaluating patients with pleural space infections.)

Complications

Prompt diagnosis and early initiation of appropriate therapy promote the resolution of a parapneumonic effusion and the reexpansion of the lung against the chest wall. Delays in therapy allow the formation of loculations and thick pleural peels. These peels produce a trapped lung that cannot reexpand against the chest wall even if the pleural fluid is drained. This complication requires extensive chest surgery to promote pleural fluid drainage and remove the pleural peel.

Another complication of empyema is persistent fever and failure of a patient with pneumonia to respond to appropriate antibiotics. More chronic and extensive pleural infections may progress to an empyema necessitans, wherein pleural pus erodes through the chest wall causing spontaneous pleural drainage. This complication of empyema has become rare in the era of antibiotics.

Treatment

Therapy for parapneumonic effusions includes initiating appropriate antibiotics for the underlying pneumonia and determining if the effusion requires drainage. Except for aminoglycosides, which are inactivated in the presence of low pH pus, nearly all antibiotics that enter the bloodstream penetrate to the pleural space and maintain activity in pleural fluid. The underlying pneumonia, therefore, dictates the antibiotic regimen for most patients. If a parapneumonic effusion does not require drainage or if it is completely drained, patients can be treated with the usual 7–10 days of antibiotics prescribed for pneumonia. If the patient has an established empyema, antibiotics are continued for several weeks until pleural purulence is either completely drained or until chronic drainage is established with resolution of tissue infection.

Establishing the need for draining a parapneumonic effusion rests largely on clinical judgment because of the absence of valid prospective randomized studies. Most clinicians retain a bias toward draining all parapneumonic effusions because of the morbidity and mortality attached to delays in drainage of infected pleural fluid.

The American College of Chest Physicians (ACCP) recently published guidelines developed by an expert consensus panel for managing parapneumonic effusions. They proposed a staging system for selecting patients for pleural drainage (Table 23–2) that includes

Table 23–2. The American College of Chest Physician staging schema of parapneumonic effusions.

Pleural Space Anatomy		Pleural Fluid Bacteriology		Pleural Fluid Chemistry	Category	Risk of Poor Outcome	Drainage
A0: Minimal, free-flowing effusion (< 10 mm on lateral decubitus)	and	BX: Culture and Gram stain results unknown	and	CX: pH unknown	1	Very low	No
A1: Small to moderate free-flowing effusion (> 10 mm and < 1/2 hemithorax)	and	B0: Negative culture and Gram stain	and	C0: pH > 7.20	2	Low	No
A2: Large, free-flowing effusion (50% hemithorax), loculated effusion or effusion with thickened parietal pleura	or	B1: Positive culture or Gram stain	or	C1: pH < 7.20	3	Moderate	Yes
		B2: pus			4	High	Yes

the microbiological, anatomic, and biochemical characteristics of pleural fluid.

The microbiological indications for pleural fluid drainage are the least controversial of the ACCP guidelines. Most experts agree that parapneumonic effusions that have identifiable pathogens by Gram stain or culture of pleural fluid require drainage.

The anatomic components of the ACCP staging system are less certain. Some observational studies support the impression that larger parapneumonic effusions (>50% of the hemithorax) are less like to respond to antibiotics alone. No prospective data, however, provide the relative risk of antibiotic failure for different volumes of pleural fluid collections. Clinical experience indicates that multiple loculations establish the need to drain the pleural space.

The biochemical components of the ACCP staging systems also require further investigation. Multiple studies have indicated that low pleural fluid pH, low glucose, and high LDH effusions require pleural drainage. A meta-analysis of these studies, however, found multiple flaws in their study design. Despite these limitations, the meta-analysis determined that based on available data pH is the preferred pleural fluid test because it had a diagnostic accuracy higher than pleural fluid LDH and glucose. Moreover, no single cutoff point identified with confidence patients who require pleural fluid drainage. The meta-analysis recommended a Bayesian approach by which patients at high risk for having infected pleural fluid or a complicated course if an empyema occurred would undergo drainage with a pH at or below 7.30. Lower risk patients would undergo drainage with a pH at or below 7.20. Pleural fluid LDH and glucose were recom-

mended only if a pH were not available. Reliability of pleural fluid pH depends on performing the test with a blood gas analyzer.

Several approaches are available for patients who require pleural fluid drainage. As mentioned, patients with free-flowing parapneumonic effusions may respond to complete drainage performed during the initial diagnostic thoracentesis. Worrisome pleural fluid test results and recurrence of pleural fluid justify either a repeat thoracentesis or placement of a chest catheter. Some radiologists routinely perform diagnostic thoracentesis with a small pigtail catheter that they leave in the pleural space of hospitalized patients overnight. The catheter is pulled if the effusion and catheter drainage resolve or is left in place if pleural fluid test results establish a need for further drainage.

If a small volume diagnostic thoracentesis is performed and pleural fluid test results indicate a need for drainage, one or more therapeutic thoracenteses may be performed with careful patient follow-up. Alternatively, a chest catheter can be inserted, which is what we prefer.

Patients who present in the fibrinopurulent phase of empyema formation typically fulfill ACCP criteria for pleural fluid drainage. Because pleural fluid is not too viscous to drain and extensive loculations have not developed in these patients, small (8- to 16-Fr) catheters usually suffice. Patients who fail catheter drainage or who at initial evaluation have a greater degree of loculations with more viscous pleural fluid may require surgical drainage, although these clinical features do not exclude the possibility of success with catheter drainage. Video-assisted thoracoscopic surgery (VATS) has emerged as a highly successful procedure for most of these patients. A muscle-sparing limited thoracotomy with partial decortication, however, remains an effective approach in the absence of expertise for performing VATS. Patients can be converted to a limited thoracotomy during the performance of VATS if thoracoscopic inspection of the pleural space demonstrates dense peels or loculations that cannot be lysed with a thoracoscope.

Traditionally, when patients underwent thoracostomy tube drainage for parapneumonic effusions, a standard chest tube was used. Blind insertion of a large-bore chest tube, however, has a low success rate (50–60%) for completely draining parapneumonic effusions, primarily due to errant placement distant from loculated effusions. Moreover, blind chest tube insertion is associated with complications that include perforated lungs, liver, spleen, and diaphragm.

Image-guided placement of small-bore catheters is associated with a higher rate of success (~90%) because of better patient selection and use of imaging modalities that allow accurate insertion of catheters into pleural loculums. Small-bore, image-guided catheters are routinely placed as the initial drainage procedure for exudative and fibrinopurulent effusions. An imaging study (chest radiograph, ultrasound, or chest CT) is then repeated to ensure complete pleural fluid drainage and correct catheter placement. Patients who fail to experience effective, early drainage are evaluated for additional drainage procedures.

One such procedure is the instillation of a fibrinolytic drug into the pleural space to lyse fibrin adhesions and break down loculations to promote drainage. Multiple observational studies have reported enhanced pleural fluid drainage after a period of failed chest tube drainage in patients with multiloculated parapneumonic effusions. Small prospective, randomized trials have demonstrated benefits of fibrinolytic therapy in terms of increased success of chest tube drainage, increased volume of chest tube drainage, shorter time to defervescence, and decreased length of hospital stays. A recent Cochrane Collaboration systematic review, however, concluded that insufficient data were available to recommend intrapleural fibrinolytic therapy for parapneumonic effusions.

The ACCP expert panel, however, recommends the instillation of fibrinolytic agents for all patients who undergo drainage by a chest catheter. We have taken a middle ground and recommend fibrinolytic therapy for patients who fail to drain pleural fluid loculations after 24 h when imaging studies demonstrate correct catheter placement. Some imaging experts suggest that chest ultrasonography can assist in selecting patients for fibrinolytic therapy by detecting the presence of pleural septation.

Streptokinase (250,000 units/dose) and urokinase (100,000 units/dose) are the two fibrinolytic drugs used for patients with parapneumonic effusions. Either drug is instilled in 30–100 mL of saline through the chest tube with a 1–2 h dwell time. One to three instillations a day may be required with frequent chest imaging to determine the adequacy of drainage. Intrapleural instillation of fibrinolytic drugs has not been reported to induce systemic fibrinolysis and is considered a generally safe off-label use of these drugs. There are anecdotal reports of cardiac arrest, hemothorax, and aortic rupture, however.

Patients treated by chest catheter drainage with or without fibrinolytic therapy who fail to respond are promptly referred (within 2–3 days) for VATS or thoracotomy. Delayed referral for definitive surgery prolongs hospitalization and exposes patients to complications related to poor nutrition. Prolonged chest tube drainage is indicated only for patients who are poor surgical candidates.

Most patients with organized empyemas require a formal thoracotomy with decortication to drain pleural pus, remove pleural peels, and allow the lung to reexpand against the chest wall and thereby obliterate the empyema cavity. Lung function improves dramatically in most patients after decortication, although some long-term measurable impairment of lung function remains. Some recent reports support a role for VATS in selected patients with chronic empyema. Patients with comorbid respiratory conditions, such as chronic obstructive pulmonary disease or lung cancer, may be poor surgical candidates for decortication. These patients may benefit from open window thoracostomy with an Eloesser flap. These procedures remove one or two ribs overlying the empyema cavity and allow purulent material to drain through the chest wall window into a collection bag. Over time, the lung may reexpand against the chest wall as the empyema cavity granulates and becomes sterile. Occasional patients may then undergo closure of the chest wall window.

Cameron R, Davies H: Intra-pleural fibrinolytic therapy for parapneumonic effusions and empyema (Cochrane review). Cochrane Library 2003;1. [PMID: 10908554]. (Systematic review of fibrinolytic therapy for empyema. The reviewer concludes that insufficient evidence exists to support the use of fibrinolytic therapy in this clinical setting.)

Colice GL et al: Medical and surgical treatment of parapneumonic effusions: an evidence-based guideline. Chest 2000;118:1158. [PMID: 11035692]. (Consensus-based clinical practice guideline that proposes a staging system for classifying parapneumonic effusions.)

Heffner J: Indications for draining a parapneumonic effusion. An evidence-based approach. Semin Respir Infect 1999;14:48. [PMID: 10197397]. (Evidence-based review that presents an approach to using pleural fluid tests in guiding therapy.)

Heffner JE et al: Pleural fluid chemical analysis in parapneumonic effusions. A meta-analysis. Am J Respir Crit Care Med 1995;151:1700. [PMID: 7767510]. (A meta-analysis of primary data that establishes the role of pleural fluid pH, glucose, and LDH in selecting patients for pleural fluid drainage.)

Klein JS et al: Interventional radiology of the chest: image-guided percutaneous drainage of pleural effusions, lung abscesses, and pneumothorax. Am J Radiol 1995;164:581. [PMID: 7863875]. (Review of the role of interventional radiology in managing patients with pleural disease.)

Lackner RP et al: Video-assisted evacuation of empyema is the preferred procedure for management of pleural space infections. Am J Surg 2000;179:27. [PMID: 10737573]. (Balanced recommendations for the role of thoracoscopy in managing patients with empyema.)

Maruyama R et al: Clinical course and management of patients undergoing open window thoracostomy for thoracic empyema. Respiration 2001;68:606. [PMID: 11786716]. (Clinical study that defines the role of open window thoracostomy in managing patients with chronic empyema.)

Moulton JS: Image-guided management of complicated pleural fluid collections. Radiol Clin North Am 2000;38:345. [PMID: 10765394]. (Focused review on the pragmatic aspects of image-guided percutaneous catheter drainage of parapneumonic effusions.)

Okada M et al: Surgical treatment for chronic pleural empyema. Surg Today 2000;30:506. [PMID: 10883469]. (Overview of the surgical management of empyema.)

Sahn SA: Use of fibrinolytic agents in the management of complicated parapneumonic effusions and empyemas. Thorax 1998;53:S65. [PMID: 10193351]. (Practical review of the clinical utility and practice of intrapleural instillation of fibrinolytic agents for managing parapneumonic effusions.)

Prognosis

Empyema is associated with a mortality of 5–20% in general patient populations. The mortality is greater than 50% in elderly patients and patients with comorbid conditions, such as lung cancer. Insufficient data exist to develop models that allow clinicians to estimate the short-term and long-term outcome of individual patients with parapneumonic effusions.

Mwandumba HC et al: Pyogenic lung infections: factors for predicting clinical outcome of lung abscess and thoracic empyema. Curr Opin Pulmon Med 2000;6:234. [PMID: 10782709]. (Expert review of clinical factors associated with outcome experienced by patients with empyema.)

SECTION VII

Diseases of the Mediastinum

Diseases of the Mediastinum	24

Robert S. Crausman, MD MMS, Vera A. De Palo, MD, & Randy L. Sid, MD

 ESSENTIALS OF DIAGNOSIS

- *Most mediastinal abnormalities are benign and asymptomatic.*
- *Division into anterior, superior, middle, and posterior "compartments" facilitates differential diagnosis.*
- *More than 60% of lesions in adults are in the anterior-superior mediastinum, whereas more than 60% in children are in the posterior mediastinum.*
- *Of masses, 75% in adults and 50% in children are benign.*
- *The most common malignant masses of the anterior-superior mediastinum are thymoma, Hodgkin's disease (HD), non-Hodgkin's lymphoma (NHL), and germ cell tumors.*
- *Neurinomas are the most frequent tumor in the posterior mediastinum and are often recognizable by their classic dumbbell-shaped contour*

General Considerations

The finding of an abnormality on chest radiograph or chest computed tomography (CT) most often prompts consideration of diseases of the mediastinum. Findings may be incidental on a radiograph obtained as part of the evaluation of an unrelated clinical issue (eg, suspected pneumonia) or may be recognized on a study obtained to evaluate a specific complaint, symptom, or sign directly referable to potential mediastinal pathology (eg, swallowing difficulty) or after chest trauma (eg,

risk of dissection of the thoracic aorta). When present, symptoms are related either to the primary disease process or to associated compressive effects on regional anatomy. Thus, a symptom or sign referable to a particular organ system may not be indicative of primary disease in that system. For example, dysphagia may result from either esophageal pathology or an extrinsic compressing mass.

Although there are no reliable estimates of prevalence, abnormalities of structures within the mediastinum are varied and common. Many abnormalities, such as courses or dilatations of otherwise normal blood vessels, are benign structural variants, which are of no pathological significance. Many nonmalignant lesions occur including pericardial or bronchogenic cysts, aneurysmic dilatations of the aorta and great vessels, benign tumors, and substernal goiters. Such lesions are generally, but not always, asymptomatic. Malignant lesions may be either primary or metastatic, and are equally likely to be symptomatic or asymptomatic. Symptomatic lesions are most often malignant. Thymoma, germ cell tumors, lymphoma, and neurinoma are the most common tumors of the mediastinum.

Anatomically, the mediastinum is the region of the body bounded by the thoracic inlet superiorly, the diaphragm inferiorly, the sternum anteriorly, the vertebral column posteriorly, and the pleura bilaterally (Figure 24–1). Core elements of the respiratory, digestive, and cardiovascular systems are located in this central area as are elements of the neurological, lymphatic, and endocrine systems.

Separation of the mediastinum into anterior, superior, middle, and posterior subdivisions, although not arbitrary, is somewhat misleading in that there are no clear boundaries that separate one division from another (eg, there are no fascial planes that define these

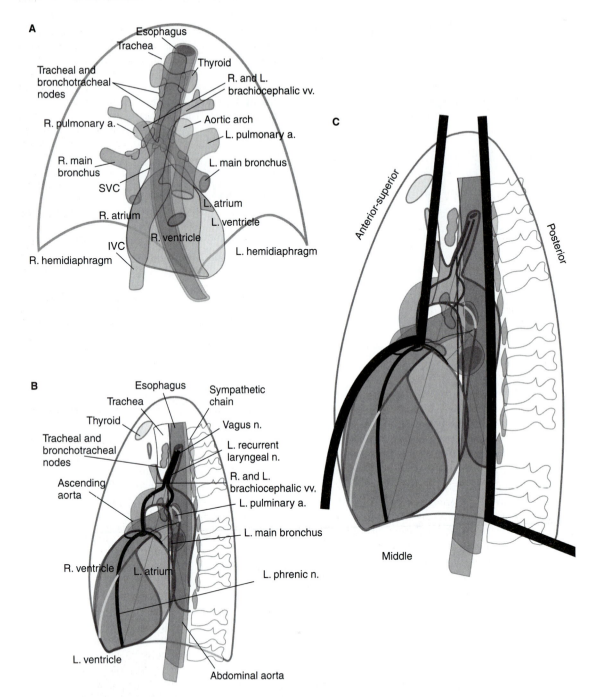

A

Esophagus
Trachea
Thyroid
Tracheal and bronchotracheal nodes
R. and L. brachiocephalic vv.
R. pulmonary a.
Aortic arch
L. pulmonary a.
R. main bronchus
L. main bronchus
SVC
L. atrium
R. atrium
L. ventricle
IVC
R. ventricle
R. hemidiaphragm
L. hemidiaphragm

B

Esophagus
Sympathetic chain
Trachea
Thyroid
Vagus n.
Tracheal and bronchotracheal nodes
L. recurrent laryngeal n.
Ascending aorta
R. and L. brachiocephalic vv.
L. pulminary a.
L. main bronchus
R. ventricle
L. atrium
L. phrenic n.
L. ventricle
Abdominal aorta

C

Anterior-superior
Posterior
Middle

Figure 24–1. Basic anatomy of the mediastinum. ***A***: Anterior view. ***B***: Lateral view. ***C***: Mediastinal divisions.

compartments). Further, the location of the mediastinum within the chest may vary, as processes in either hemithorax (eg, tension pneumothorax or pleural effusion) may cause mediastinal deviation and shift of its contents to one side or the other. Of note, combining the anterior and superior divisions for description as the anterior-superior mediastinum is sometimes clinically useful as processes often extend from one to the other.

The **anterior-superior mediastinum** contains several important structures including the great vessels and aortic root, the thymus gland, inferior aspects of the trachea, and esophagus (Figure 24–2A). In addition, a substernal thyroid and parathyroids are common variants. Lymphatic tissue is also present (Figure 24–2B). The most common mass in the superior mediastinum is a substernal thyroid (goiter). The most common masses in the anterior mediastinum are germ cell tumors, Hodgkin's disease, and non-Hodgkin's lymphoma. The **posterior mediastinum** interfaces with the paravertebral sulci and anterior vertebral column and includes the spinal nerve roots, which combine to form the intercostal nerves, the sympathetic chain, and the thoracic duct as well as the inferior portion of the descending aorta. Neurinomas, tumors of peripheral nerves, which are almost always benign, are the most common mass lesions found in this compartment. The **middle mediastinum,** which includes that space bounded by the pericardium anteriorly, the vertebral bodies posteriorly, the diaphragm inferiorly, and the pleura laterally, contains within its confines the only true mediastinal compartment, the pericardial sac. Lymphatics, proximal airways, the esophagus, the vagus (including the recurrent laryngeal branch) and phrenic nerves, and blood vessels including the pulmonary arteries and the superior and inferior vena cavae are also present (Figure 24–2C). Tumors and cysts of the heart, pericardium, trachea, proximal airways, and esophagus may all occur. Fat deposition (mediastinal lipomatosis), which may be associated with exogenous steroid therapy, can affect all mediastinal compartments and presents as a mass lesion causing mediastinal widening with characteristic smooth margins.

There are marked differences between children and adults regarding the relative frequency of abnormalities in the various mediastinal subdivisions. In adults approximately 65% of lesions are found in the anterior mediastinum, 25% in the posterior mediastinum, and 10% in the middle mediastinum. In children only about 25% of lesions are in the anterior mediastinum and the majority (65%) are in the posterior mediastinum. Most mass lesions in adults are benign (75%), whereas slightly more than half in children are malignant.

Pathogenesis

Although separation of the mediastinum into different compartments facilitates developing practical differential diagnoses, a systems-oriented approach is helpful

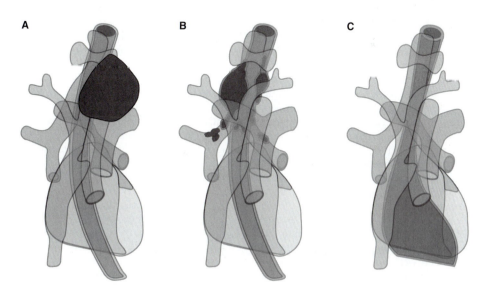

Figure 24–2. A: Thymoma presenting as an anterior mediastinal mass. **B:** Lymphadenopathy presenting as a middle mediastinal mass. **C:** Paraesophageal hernia presenting as a posterior mediastinal mass.

for understanding the pathogenesis of common mediastinal pathology.

A. Respiratory

The trachea, mainstem bronchi, and draining lymphatics are contained in the mediastinum. The recurrent laryngeal and phrenic nerves course through the superior and middle mediastinum. Tracheal and bronchial tumors may be either benign or malignant. Malignant tumors may be primary or metastatic. The mediastinal lymph nodes are frequently involved in the spread of bronchogenic cancer. Small cell lung cancer, in particular, is often associated with bulky hilar and mediastinal lymphadenopathy. Adenoid cystic carcinoma and squamous cell carcinoma are the most common primary cancers of the trachea. The trachea and proximal airways may also be secondarily involved in bronchogenic, laryngeal, esophageal, thyroid, and lymphoproliferative cancers. Finally, malignant pleural disease such as mesothelioma or metastatic adenocarcinoma may occur medially along the mediastinal pleural reflections and present radiographically as a mass-like lesion.

Bronchogenic cysts are common congenital abnormalities and may account for more than 50% of resected mediastinal tumors. They are epithelial-lined structures that typically lay in close proximity to the carina, mainstem bronchi, or hila and arise during embryonic lung development. The presence of an air–fluid level on plain radiograph suggests an anatomic connection to an airway or superimposed infection. They frequently produce symptoms in neonates owing to compression of adjacent large airways causing dyspnea, respiratory distress, or cough. Lobar or complete lung collapse may occur. Symptomatic lesions in older patients are much less common. Surgical resection, which may be done with the videothoracoscope, is generally recommended for bronchogenic cysts, although observation may be appropriate for relatively small, asymptomatic lesions. Symptomatic patients who are not operative candidates may be treated with fine-needle aspiration to confirm that the lesion is benign and instillation of a sclerosing agent such as bleomycin.

Air in the mediastinum, pneumomediastinum, most frequently results from pulmonary barotrauma with air subsequently dissecting medially toward the hilum. Pneumothorax may variably also occur. From the mediastinum, air may then dissect superiorly into the neck and subcutaneous tissues and inferiorly into the retroperitoneum. If not accompanied by a pneumothorax most patients do well and do not require specific therapy beyond supplemental oxygen. Less frequently gas in the mediastinum may arise from esophageal rupture. This condition is a surgical emergency as patients typically develop an infectious necrotizing mediastinitis

and have a high mortality rate without urgent surgical repair and broad spectrum antibiotics.

Lobar collapse, for example, collapse of the left lower lobe of the lung, may abut the mediastinum and mimic the radiographic appearance of a paramediastinal mass. An extrapulmonary sequestration may present similarly.

B. Cardiovascular

The pericardial sac surrounding the heart is the only true compartment of the mediastinum. Pericardial cysts, much more common in adults than children, typically occur at the cardiophrenic angle. These simple cysts are benign and generally do not require surgical removal. Uncommonly these cysts may be associated with arrhythmia, atelectasis, or erosion into vital structures and may necessitate surgical resection. Cardiomegaly may occasionally be so severe as to widen the mediastinum. Alternatively, valvular disease such as mitral stenosis may lead to massive enlargement of one chamber such as the left atrium, which may compress the esophagus.

Common vascular abnormalities include aneurysms of the thoracic aorta and, less frequently, the pulmonary arteries, pulmonary veins, coronary arteries, superior vena cava, or azygous vein. An anomalous right-sided aortic arch is a common variant. Coarctation of the aorta may be associated with poststenotic dilatation of the descending aorta in the posterior mediastinum. A mediastinal hematoma may occur after chest surgery, cardiac transplantation, trauma, or spontaneously.

C. Gastrointestinal

Esophageal abnormalities are the most common of gastrointestinal mediastinal conditions and include megaesophagus, esophageal diverticuli, duplications (enterogenous cysts), achalasia, and carcinoma. In addition, hiatal and paraesophageal hernias may present as mediastinal masses and must be distinguished from malignant disease. Herniation of abdominal viscera through defects in the diaphragm may be congenital or acquired, often after abdominal trauma, and generally require surgical repair. Herniation of the small or large bowel through the foramen of Morgagni through which the internal mammary arteries pass may present as an inferior-anterior mediastinal mass. Pancreatic pseudocysts may also rarely erode into the mediastinum.

D. Lymphatic

Hodgkin's disease (HD) and non-Hodgkin's lymphoma (NHL) can occur in the mediastinum and together comprise approximately 10–15% of mediastinal masses. They are much more common in the anterior mediastinum and rare in the posterior mediastinum.

Despite their malignant nature, one-third of patients are asymptomatic at diagnosis. B-symptoms of fever, weight loss, or night sweats occur in one-third, and symptoms due to local disease such as airway involvement (eg, dyspnea, wheeze, or stridor) in two-thirds. Lymphadenopathy may be bulky and bilateral but is always asymmetric. This helps to distinguish it from pulmonary sarcoidosis-associated lymphadenopathy that is usually symmetric. HD has a bimodal peak incidence first in young adulthood (ages 20–30) and then again in late middle age (ages 50–60). HD is less common than NHL, accounting for only 25% of cases of lymphoma overall, but disproportionately causing 70% of mediastinal lymphomas. Mediastinal involvement is frequent and occurs in 75% of patients with HD. Half are limited to the mediastinum. Nodular sclerosing disease is the dominant histological subtype (90%). Radiotherapy and chemotherapy are very effective treatments for HD with an overall 5-year survival of 80%.

NHL involves the mediastinal lymph nodes much less frequently (5–10%) than does HD. Airways involvement, pulmonary infiltrates, and pleural and pericardial effusions may occur. Therapy and prognosis depend upon stage and grade of disease, but NHL generally responds to radiation and chemotherapy, although patients with low-grade lymphoma may not require treatment.

Sarcoidosis is a systemic granulomatous disorder that characteristically affects the mediastinal lymph nodes. Associated lymphadenopathy may be bulky but is also typically symmetrical. Pulmonary parenchymal involvement may be absent at presentation (stage I disease). The overall prevalence is thought to be 10–20 per 100,000 but is much more frequent in African-Americans and those of Mediterranean descent. Prognosis of stage I disease is excellent with 75% of patients demonstrating significant regression of their hilar lymphadenopathy in 3 years. Treatment, when necessary, for more severe disease is generally with systemic corticosteroids.

Mediastinal lymphadenopathy may also be a manifestation of infectious disease and may occur with bacterial or viral pneumonia, tuberculosis, or fungal disease.

E. ENDOCRINE

A substernal thyroid goiter is the most common superior mediastinal mass, and cervical goiters extend into the superior or anterior mediastinum in 20% of cases. Ninety percent of thyroid masses are benign.

Thymomas are the most common mediastinal cancer and affect both men and women equally with a peak incidence in middle age. More than 80% occur in the anterior-superior mediastinum. Two-thirds of pa-

tients are asymptomatic at diagnosis. On chest CT thymomas appear as a well-defined, encapsulated soft-tissue mass that may have cystic changes. Histologically they appear benign, are composed of epithelial and lymphoid cells, and may be difficult to distinguish from thymic lymphoma. Of note, benign-appearing, well-encapsulated thymoma may be invasive in 30% of patients. "Invasive" or "malignant" thymoma is usually locally invasive and affects adjacent mediastinal structures and pleura, but does not metastasize. Only 10% of well-encapsulated thymomas recur, but invasive thymoma recurs much more commonly. Locally invasive disease is associated with a 67% 5-year survival after treatment. Treatment for thymoma usually requires surgical resection, sometimes followed by postoperative radiation and chemotherapy. Most recurrences occur locally, but many patients (20%) subsequently develop second malignancies. Patients who are unresectable or poor surgical candidates may benefit from chemotherapy. Diagnostic fine needle aspiration (FNA) should be avoided owing to the risk of mechanically spreading tumor cells along the needle tract. Thymomas are frequently associated with myasthenia gravis (33–50%) and, less often, pure red cell aplasia (5%) or acquired hypogammaglobulinemia (5%). Benign hyperplasia may lead to enlargement of the thymus and may be associated with Grave's disease.

Thymic lymphoma may be difficult to distinguish from thymoma. Thymic carcinoma is a very uncommon and aggressive malignancy that primarily affects middle-aged adults. It typically has many malignant histopathological features, tends to metastasize widely, and commonly causes pleural effusions. Five-year survival with aggressive multimodality therapy is only about 33%. Thymic carcinoid is rare and may be associated with carcinoid syndrome, Cushing's syndrome, or multiple endocrine neoplasia (MEN) 1 syndrome.

Thymolipomas are rare, benign fatty tumors. Benign cysts of the thymus are usually incidental and do not require treatment. Parathyroid adenomas may arise in the anterior or middle mediastinum and may be difficult to identify. Rarely, pheochromocytoma may also present in the mediastinum.

F. NEUROLOGICAL

Neurogenic tumors are the most common mediastinal tumor in children and rank third behind thymomas and lymphomas in adults in terms of frequency. They occur almost exclusively in the posterior mediastinum. Of such lesions 50% in children and 90% in adults are benign. These lesions often present as a dumbbell-shaped tumor posteriorly in the paravertebral sulci owing to their growth from the spinal ganglia and may extend into the spine along the spinal nerve roots. They are typically diagnosed incidentally, but may uncommonly produce symptoms due to cord involvement, compression, or destruction of the sympathetic ganglia (Horner's syndrome). Schwanomas and neurofibromas of the peripheral nerves originate from nerve sheaths and are most often benign. Of patients with neurofibromas 25% have von Recklinghausen's disease; the incidence of malignant schwanomas and neurogenic carcinoma is markedly increased in this disorder. Malignant nerve sheath tumors are otherwise very rare.

G. Infectious

Infection of the mediastinum, mediastinitis, may mimic a mediastinal mass radiographically. Pyogenic infection can result from extension of an infectious focus from a contiguous extramediastinal space. For example, oral or retropharyngeal abscesses may extend inferiorly into the mediastinum (Ludwig's angina) or an intraabdominal focus, such as an infected pancreatic pseudocyst, may extend superiorly. Esophageal perforation within the mediastinum, which can result from retching or instrumentation, typically causes necrotizing mediastinitis. Patients with necrotizing mediastinitis may appear toxic with a widened mediastinum on radiographic imaging. Air–fluid levels suggest the presence of abscesses, and pneumomediastinum suggests infection with a gas-forming organism such as clostridial species. Etiological organisms reflect oropharyngeal flora and thus Gram-positive and anaerobic organisms (*Peptostreptococcus*, *Bacteroides fragilis*) are most common. However, Gram-negative organisms are also important and aggressive use of broad-spectrum antibiotics is vital to effective treatment. Surgical drainage is indicated once mediastinal involvement occurs. Despite aggressive therapy mortality can be high. Postoperative infections of the sternum may also extend into the mediastinum. They are typically caused by *Staphylococcus aureus* and streptococcal species and generally respond well to antibiotic therapy. Methicillin-resistant *S aureus* is being increasingly encountered in hospitalized patients and is an added consideration. The development of mediastinitis in this setting is also an indication for surgical debridement and drainage. Because the different "compartments" of the mediastinum are not actual anatomic divisions there are few barriers to prevent spread of infection from one mediastinal division to another. Purulent pericarditis is the exception because the pericardium does define an actual mediastinal compartment that serves as an effective barrier.

Some parenchymal pulmonary infections, such as *Mycobacterium tuberculosis* (MTB), histoplasmosis, coccidioidomycosis, or anthrax also cause mediastinitis. The clinical presentations vary depending upon both host factors and invading organism, but in general me-diastinitis caused by histoplasmosis or tuberculosis is chronic and indolent whereas that caused by anthrax is acute and fulminant. It is important to distinguish infectious causes of chronic mediastinitis from noninfectious causes such as sarcoidosis or Wegener's granulomatosis, as treatments differ. It may also be idiopathic. Long-term sequelae of chronic infection include mediastinal fibrosis and superior vena cava (SVC) syndrome, hemoptysis, and bronchiolithiasis. The erosion of densely calcified lymph nodes into an airway lumen causes bronchiolithiasis. Patients may actually expectorate stones. Mediastinal fibrosis (chronic fibrosing or sclerosing mediastinitis) can be severe and progressive, resulting in obliteration of mediastinal blood vessels, compromise of airways, and compression of the esophagus. There is almost always serological evidence of histoplasmal infection, but unfortunately the response to antifungal or corticosteroid therapy is poor. Antifungal therapy is usually attempted prior to consideration of surgery owing to poor surgical outcomes as well. Rarely, chronic mediastinal fibrosis may be part of a broader disease process that includes retroperitoneal fibrosis.

H. Oncological

Neoplastic disease may occur in any mediastinal division and in any age group. However, only 25% of mediastinal lesions in adults and 50% in children are malignant. Lymphoma, thymoma, germ cell tumors, and neurinomas are the most common mediastinal tumors. With the exception of neurinomas, most cancers are in the anterior-superior mediastinum. Mesenchymal soft-tissue tumors (eg, sarcomas) also occur, but are uncommon.

Germ cell tumors and teratomas (benign germ cell tumors) are derived from primitive cell types and combine elements of the embryonic ectoderm, mesoderm, and endoderm. They can therefore incorporate elements of bone, teeth, muscle, skin, cartilage, or fat. These tumors can be either benign or malignant and account for 10–15% of tumors in the anterior mediastinum. If malignant, germ cell tumors are seminomatous, nonseminomatous, or mixed. Seminomatous and nonseminomatous tumors occur with about equal frequency. They tend to be midline in location and are thought to arise from primitive rests of embryonal cells. Benign teratoma occurs in both adults and children and is more common (60%) than malignant germ cell tumors. Malignant germ cell tumors may arise in the mediastinum primarily, or more commonly may result from metastatic disease. Ninety percent of malignant mediastinal germ cell tumors occur in males. Less than 5% of germ cell tumors arise in the mediastinum, so evaluation should always include assessment for a potential testicular primary or other extragonadal site (retroperitoneal or cranial) of origin. The mediastinum is rarely the only site of metastasis from a testicular primary. The same spectrum of histopathology that characterizes testicular cancer is present in mediastinal germ cell tumors, including seminoma, choriocarcinoma, yolk-sac carcinoma, and embryonal cell carcinoma. Tumor markers α-fetoprotein (AFP) and human chorionic gonadotropin (β-HCG) may be elevated in patients with nonseminomatous germ cell tumors and when elevated confirm a diagnosis of cancer. AFP is elevated in 70% and β-HCG in 50% of nonseminomatous germ cell tumors. β-HCG, but never AFP, may be elevated in seminomatous disease. Surgical resection and radiotherapy may be curative for seminomatous disease limited to the anterior mediastinum. Chemotherapy is reserved for those with more widespread disease. Nonseminomatous malignant germ cell tumors occur primarily in children and young men. Choriocarcinomas typically secrete β-HCG and gynecomastia is common. Yolk-sac (endodermal sinus) tumors also occur in both adults and children and secrete AFP. Mixed-cell tumors, teratocarcinomas, are also common. Radiation and chemotherapy are the primary treatments, and the role for surgery is limited to treating select patients, such as those whose tumor markers have returned to normal but who still have residual tumor mass after initial treatment. Primary mediastinal tumors are less responsive to therapy than testicular tumors and aggressive therapeutic regimens are associated with only approximately 50% 5-year survival rates.

Prevention

There are no routine screening recommendations to assess for the presence of mediastinal pathology in asymptomatic individuals from the general population. It is likely that screening chest or total body CT, which is being popularized in the lay press, will lead to the increased recognition of mediastinal abnormalities. The value of incidental recognition of asymptomatic mediastinal disease identified from mass screening of a general population is a matter of speculation.

Screening, or surveillance, of certain high-risk subgroups of the population for specific diseases such as lung cancer that can affect the mediastinum may soon be recommended. There is renewed interest in the use of the yearly screening chest radiograph and probably chest CT for cigarette smokers, particularly if chronic obstructive pulmonary disease (COPD) is also present.

Patients with a history of treated lymphoma or bronchogenic lung cancer generally have periodic chest imaging with either plain chest radiograph or CT to assess for recurrent disease.

Clinical Findings

The clinical findings of patients with mediastinal disease vary depending upon the specific underlying diagnosis and possible involvement of adjacent mediastinal structures. In general, benign lesions are asymptomatic, malignant lesions are equally likely to be symptomatic or asymptomatic, and symptomatic lesions are likely to be malignant.

Certain symptoms strongly suggest mediastinal pathology. Development of hoarseness implies compression of the recurrent laryngeal nerve by tumor, lymph node, aneurysm, or dilated left atrium. Isolated facial and upper extremity swelling are signs of the SVC syndrome, which can result from compression of the SVC by tumor or chronic mediastinal fibrosis (Figure 24–3). Localized chest pain suggests chest wall invasion or may be neuropathic in origin. Cough, hemoptysis, bronchiolithiasis, wheeze, or dyspnea indicates airways involvement. Regurgitation, reflux, dysphagia, or odynophagia raises suspicion for esophageal pathology. The presence of B-symptoms such as weight loss, fever, or night sweats raises the possibility of lymphoma. Hypotension and tearing chest pain suggest aortic dissection. Hypotension and pulsus paradoxicus suggest pericardial tamponade. Chest pain may be from chest wall extension of a mediastinal disease process or may be neuropathic. Paroxysms of hypertension characteristically result from pheochromocytoma. These symptoms may also be due to extramediastinal disease as well and are of limited specificity.

Differential Diagnosis

Pathology generally found in one mediastinal subdivision may variably occur in another. Localization of a lesion to a particular mediastinal subdivision should guide, but not limit, the development of a differential diagnosis. In the anterior mediastinum the most common disease processes producing mass lesions on radiograph are lymphoma, thymoma, and germ cell tumors. HD is much more common than NHL. Less commonly bronchogenic lung cancer and other mesenchymal soft tissue tumors may arise. Mass lesions in the superior mediastinum are frequently due to the thyroid. Posterior mediastinal masses are almost always neurogenic in origin. The middle mediastinum has a wide spectrum of pathology. However, apart from lymphoma, lymph node enlargement, and rare soft-tissue sarcomas, most abnormalities are benign cysts or vascular aneurysms.

After history and physical examination, routine chest radiography with frontal and lateral projections is the first step in identifying a mediastinal mass. Projection in two views allows for localization to a particular

A

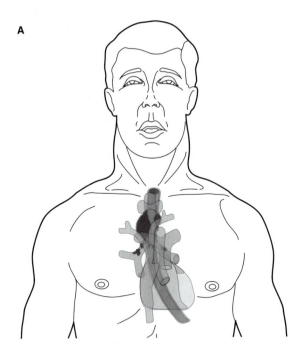

B

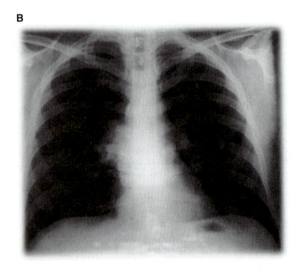

Figure 24–3. Superior vena cava syndrome. ***A:*** Clinical signs include swelling of the head and neck, engorgement of neck veins, and development of collateral circulation in the chest wall. ***B:*** Chest radiograph demonstrating mediastinal widening.

mediastinal compartment and a more focused differential diagnosis. Chest CT is now routinely employed as the next diagnostic test for suspected mediastinal masses. It provides an excellent means to specifically localize lesions anatomically, to separate cystic from solid lesions, to identify fatty structures (eg, pericardial fat pad), and, with intravenous contrast, to differentiate lymphadenopathy and vascular abnormalities. Masses that are not diagnosed definitively on chest CT require further study. CT or ultrasound-guided needle biopsy is a useful approach that often obviates the need for more invasive strategies. If surgery is required for further characterization or treatment, chest CT is useful in guiding the selection of approach. Chest magnetic resonance imaging (MRI) is useful for patients who cannot tolerate intravenous contrast because of contrast allergy or renal insufficiency or for those with suspected vascular, chest wall, or extrathoracic invasion.

Transthoracic or transesophageal echocardiography can be very useful in assessment of cardiac structures, the pericardium, and aortic root. It may also characterize a mass as cystic. Transthoracic or endoscopic ultrasound may also be used to guide needle biopsy. Radionuclide scintigraphy is useful for the evaluation of substernal goiter (^{131}I or ^{123}I), pheochromocytoma ($[^{131}$I]metaiodobenzylguanine), or lymphoma (gallium). The role of positron emission tomography (PET) scanning has yet to be determined, but will likely prove useful in the evaluation of metastatic and inflammatory lesions.

Measurement of serum biochemical markers is useful in several conditions. Serum determinations of AFP and β-HCG should be done in patients suspected of having germ cell tumors. Urinary catecholamines, vanillylmandelic acid, and homovanillic acid may be elevated with pheochromocytoma or neurogenic tumors.

Decisions to biopsy for suspected cancer must be individualized. Relevant considerations include the presence of symptoms, clinical status of the patient, elevation of serum markers, evidence of invasion on imaging studies, and presence of extrathoracic disease, which may offer alternative sites for biopsy. Full resection is favored over tissue biopsy if pheochromocytoma is likely as tumor manipulation may precipitate a hypertensive crisis. Resection is also favored with suspected thymoma as FNA may cause tumor spread.

Tissue specimens may be obtained via CT or ultrasound-guided FNA prior to a definitive surgery. CT-guided FNA is well tolerated and is diagnostic in 75% of patients. Biopsy of hilar or mediastinal lymph nodes may also be done transbronchially. Surgical approaches that may be used to provide for either tissue biopsy or possible resection of a mediastinal mass include anterior mediastinotomy, cervical mediastinoscopy, and videothoracoscopy.

Complications

Complications of mediastinal pathology reflect both the primary pathology and the relationship of anatomic structures within the mediastinum. Tumors or infection within the mediastinum may produce complications through direct extension and involvement of adjacent structures, by compression of adjacent structures, by causing paraneoplastic syndromes, or by metastasis elsewhere. Four dreaded complications of mediastinal disease are (1) tracheal obstruction, (2) SVC syndrome, (3) vascular invasion and catastrophic hemorrhage, and (4) esophageal rupture.

Treatment

Treatment recommendations regarding mediastinal disease in most cases is predicated upon a specific clinical and pathological diagnosis as well as knowledge of a particular patient's overall medical and functional status. Thus, imaging and tissue biopsy precede treatment; there is only a limited role for empiric therapies. In general, malignant disease of the mediastinum due to lymphoma, germ cell tumor, or thymoma responds well to aggressive therapy, which may be multimodal involving surgery, radiation, and chemotherapy. Acute necrotizing infection most often requires surgical intervention and broad-spectrum intravenous antibiotics. Chronic infections may respond to antibiotic therapy alone. Benign disease may sometimes be managed expectantly if the patient is asymptomatic. Bronchogenic cysts should generally be removed despite their benign nature. Patients with mediastinal masses are at significant risk of airway collapse or obstruction and hemodynamic compromise when undergoing general anesthesia and may require preoperative bronchoscopy as a component of their perioperative assessment.

Prognosis

The prognosis of benign mediastinal disease is good, particularly if the patient is asymptomatic. The outlook for patients with malignant disease is variable depending upon specific diagnosis, stage of illness, and other patient-specific characteristics. Most mediastinal malignancies respond well to conventional therapies. Most patients with infectious disease do well with timely institution of broad-spectrum antibiotics and surgical intervention when indicated. Modern vascular surgical techniques are very effective at treating many vascular lesions. There is, however, great individual variation owing to the broad spectrum of pathology present.

Hudson MM, Donaldson SS: Hodgkin's disease. Pediatr Clin North Am 1997;44:891. [PMID: 9286290]. (An overview of HD in pediatric patients.)

Maki DD, Gefter WB, Alavi A: Recent advances in pulmonary imaging. Chest 1999;116:1388. [PMID: 10559104]. (An update on emerging pulmonary imaging techniques.)

Narang S, Harte BH, Body SC: Anesthesia for patients with a mediastinal mass. Anesthesiol Clin North Am 2001;19:559. [PMID: 11571906]. (A pathophysiological review of the anesthesia-associated risks for surgery.)

Sawin RS: Pediatric chest lesions. Pediatr Clin North Am 1998;45:861. [PMID: 9728192]. (A review of pediatric intrathoracic cancer for the generalist.)

Shad A, Magrath I: Non-Hodgkin's lymphoma. Pediatr Clin North Am 1997;44:863. [PMID: 9286289]. (An overview of NHL in pediatric patients.)

Strollo DC, Rosado-de-Christenson ML, Jett JR: Primary mediastinal tumors. Part 1. Tumors of the anterior mediastinum. Chest 1997;112:511. [PMID: 9266892]. (An excellent overview of anterior mediastinal tumors.)

Strollo DC, Rosado-de-Christenson ML, Jett JR: Primary mediastinal tumors. Part II. Tumors of the middle and posterior mediastinum. Chest 1997;112:1344. [PMID: 9367479]. (An excellent overview of middle and posterior mediastinal tumors.)

Swartz MN: Recognition and management of anthrax—an update. N Engl J Med 2001;345:1621. [PMID: 11704686]. (A concise, post 9/11, review that underscores the importance of early diagnosis.)

Wood DE: Mediastinal germ cell tumors. Semin Thorac Cardiovasc Surg 2000;12:278. [PMID: 11154723]. (A recent review of the biology and epidemiology of germ cell tumors.)

Relevant Web Sites

www.emedicine.com

A web-based, peer-reviewed electronic resource for physicians.

www.chestnet.org

The American College of Chest Physicians.

www.cancer.org

The American Cancer Society.

SECTION VIII

Disorders of Ventilatory Control

<table>
<tr><td>

Acute Ventilatory Failure

</td><td>

25

</td></tr>
</table>

James P. Maloney, MD

Principles of Ventilation & Gas Exchange

The two major functions of the lungs are to supply oxygen to blood for delivery to tissues and to clear blood of carbon dioxide produced during tissue metabolism. When the lungs fail to provide adequate oxygenation of blood, Type I respiratory failure, also known as hypoxemic respiratory failure, is present. Hypoxemic respiratory failure occurs only when a significant amount of intrapulmonary shunt is present. When the lungs fail to provide an adequate clearance of carbon dioxide, Type II respiratory failure, also known as ventilatory failure, is present. Some patients suffer from both ventilatory failure and hypoxemic respiratory failure, for example, a patient intubated for severe emphysema with bilateral pneumonia. However, most patients with respiratory failure will display predominant features of only one of these mechanisms. This chapter will discuss ventilatory failure.

It is important to understand that ventilatory failure can occur even with a normal arterial partial pressure of carbon dioxide ($PaCO_2$); ventilatory failure is not synonymous with elevated $PaCO_2$. For instance, a patient may have status asthmaticus with severe bronchospasm and impending respiratory arrest, yet have a normal $PaCO_2$. Likewise, a patient with a high bicarbonate level of 35 mEq/L due to diuretic therapy will usually have a compensatory elevation in $PaCO_2$ to buffer pH, but ventilatory failure is not present. Ventilatory failure is not synonymous with a requirement for mechanical ventilation either, as many patients with ventilatory failure are effectively managed without mechanical ventilatory support. Ventilatory failure can be acute, chronic, or acute superimposed on chronic.

The balance of tissue CO_2 production and its subsequent excretion through the lungs determines the arterial carbon dioxide level ($PaCO_2$). $PaCO_2$ is thus dependent on the production of carbon dioxide ($\dot{V}CO_2$), minute ventilation ($\dot{V}E$), and the fraction of tidal volume (VT) that encounters unperfused alveoli, known as dead space (VD):

$$PaCO_2 = \dot{V}CO_2 \times k / [\dot{V}E \times (1 - VD/VT)] \qquad (1)$$

where k is a constant of 0.863 if $\dot{V}CO_2$ is in milliliters per minute.

As carbon dioxide is transferred from blood across alveolar membranes, the airways and unperfused alveoli are useless in removing carbon dioxide. Dead space has a fixed component that is "anatomic" due to the conducting airways (trachea and airways proximal to respiratory bronchioles) and a variable "physiological" component due to the fraction of alveoli that are ventilated but unperfused. In reality, increased dead space is often due to areas of lung that receive minimal perfusion (as opposed to none) but have normal or near normal ventilation. This creates high ventilation-to-perfusion ratio alveolar units, or $\dot{V}/Q$ mismatching. It is crucial to note that hypoventilation in a normoxic environment must lead to a higher $PaCO_2$ (hypercarbia) and a lower arterial PaO_2 (hypoxemia), yet the alveolar to arterial difference of the partial pressure of oxygen (A–aDO$_2$, or "A–a" gradient) will usually remain unchanged if hypoventilation is the only event. This interdependence of PaO_2 and $PaCO_2$ is represented mathematically by the alveolar gas equation:

$$PAO_2 = FIO_2 \times (PB - 47) - PaCO_2/RQ \qquad (2)$$

where RQ is the respiratory quotient of $\dot{V}CO_2/\dot{V}O_2$, estimated as 0.8; PB is barometric pressure (usually 760 mm Hg at sea level), P_A denotes alveolar partial pressure, P_a denotes arterial pressure, and 47 mm Hg is water vapor pressure at 37°C.

Conceptually, this can be understood, as the partial pressures of all dry gases in the alveoli (nitrogen, carbon dioxide, and oxygen) must equal the prevailing barometric pressure minus the water vapor pressure. The alveolar partial pressure of water due to airway humidification is constant at 47 mm Hg (at a temperature of 37°C), whereas the partial pressure of nitrogen varies inversely with that of oxygen—thus the alveolar partial pressures of oxygen ($P_{A}O_{2}$) and carbon dioxide ($P_{A}CO_{2}$) must be interrelated. For instance, a patient with obesity hypoventilation breathing room air at sea level has a normal $P_{a}O_{2}$ of $(760 - 47) \times 0.21 = 150$ mm Hg, has an elevated $P_{a}CO_{2}$ of 70 mm Hg, and a low $P_{a}O_{2}$ of 50, but the A–aDO_{2} [as calculated by Eq. (2)] is normal at 12, as hypoventilation is the only problem in this patient.

In this scenario, provision of only a small amount of oxygen, such as raising the fraction of inspired oxygen ($F_{I}O_{2}$) to 28% with a nasal cannula, will yield a $P_{A}O_{2}$ of $0.28 \times (760 - 47) = 200$ mm Hg (where P_{B}, or barometric pressure, is 760 mm Hg at sea level) and thereby increase $P_{a}O_{2}$ by 50 mm Hg ($200 - 150$) to a final 100 mm Hg, sufficient to maintain adequate $P_{a}O_{2}$ for tissue oxygenation. The ability of a small increase in $F_{I}O_{2}$ to overcome the mild hypoxia of hypoventilation is characteristic of acute ventilatory failure. In contrast, the large amount of intrapulmonary shunt inherent in hypoxemic respiratory failure often makes sources that deliver very high $F_{I}O_{2}$ necessary to maintain adequate tissue oxygenation. A high $\dot{V}CO_{2}$ may occur from overfeeding or during acute illnesses with increased tissue metabolism, such as infections. For example, with each 1°C of fever, $\dot{V}CO_{2}$ increases by 13%. Thus reduction of a fever of 42°C to 38°C is associated with a 52% reduction in $\dot{V}CO_{2}$, leaving less CO_{2} for the lungs to clear.

The Ventilatory Pathway

Ventilation is achieved through a complex pathway that starts in the brain and ends when the respiratory muscles expand the lungs. Ventilation is a coordinated action of the brain stem, efferent nerves, anterior horn cells, neuromuscular junctions, muscles of respiration, the lungs, and chest wall. An interruption of any component of this pathway can lead to ventilatory failure. Efferent information from the medullary respiratory center in the brain stem [which receives input from cerebrospinal fluid (CSF) pH, carotid and aortic chemoreceptors, and lung stretch receptors] supplies efferent impulses to anterior horn cells in the cervical spinal cord and thoracic spinal cord. Anterior horn cells in the spinal cord send impulses via the phrenic nerves

(C3–C5) to the diaphragm, the crucial muscle of respiration. The accessory muscles of respiration are utilized during times of higher ventilatory demands during illness. Accessory muscles include the intercostal muscles (T1–T12), sternocleidomastoids and trapezoids (C1–C2, CN XI), and scalenes (C4–C8). Abdominal muscles and muscles of the upper airway also have important roles in ventilation. Efferent neural impulses are then coupled through neuromuscular junctions to the respiratory muscles.

Respiratory muscles change the respiratory rate or V_T through the rate and strength of muscle contraction. The ventilatory efficiency of the lungs depends on the maximal $\dot{V}E$ achievable and the V_D volume/tidal volume (V_D/V_T) ratio. The evaluation of ventilatory failure is best conducted (and best classified) based on an evaluation of the fidelity of each component of these pathways for a given patient (Figure 25–1). For instance, a teenager with acute ventilatory failure who is comatose from a heroin overdose has lost brain stem drive to breathe due to direct suppression of the medullary respiratory center by heroin, but he may also have aspirated while unconscious and have an increased work of breathing even after the overdose is reversed. A woman with acute ventilatory failure due to Guillain–Barré syndrome (GBS) has lost efferent nerve impulses to the muscles of respiration and suffers from a neuromuscular coupling defect. A patient with emphysema who develops ventilatory failure during an upper respiratory infection has high V_D, a decrease in maximal $\dot{V}E$, possible respiratory muscle fatigue, and increased work of breathing. In these cases, the other components of the ventilatory pathway are intact.

Figure 25–1 provides an anatomic classification of the six major mechanisms of ventilatory failure: disruption of central drive, disruption of neuromuscular coupling due to anterior spinal cord processes, disruption of neuromuscular coupling due to nerve conduction processes, disruption of neuromuscular coupling due to neuromuscular junction processes, respiratory muscle failure, and increased work of breathing due to lung or chest wall disease. Lung disease increases V_D, alters $\dot{V}/\dot{Q}$ matching, increases work of breathing, and decreases minute ventilation. Respiratory muscle failure occurs from excessive work of breathing typically due to either excessive airway resistance loads [eg, asthma or chronic obstructive pulmonary disease (COPD) exacerbation] or excessive chest wall resistance loads (eg, severe kyphoscoliosis or large pleural effusions).

Although the treatment of ventilatory failure also varies based on the illness and the component of the ventilatory pathway affected, the treatment of any acute ventilatory failure centers on improving $\dot{V}E$, decreasing V_D created by $\dot{V}/\dot{Q}$ mismatching, reversing the cause of the increased work of breathing, and providing rest to

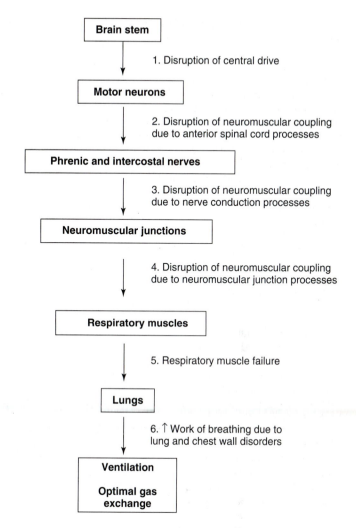

Figure 25–1. The ventilatory pathway and the six major mechanisms of acute ventilatory failure.

fatigued respiratory muscles. In some patients, therapy should also be directed at decreasing carbon dioxide production ($\dot{V}CO_2$). In practice it is simpler to first evaluate whether the primary abnormality is in the lungs or elsewhere. A mechanistic approach should then be used to dissect possible contributions from each component of the ventilatory pathway.

A Mechanistic Approach to Acute Ventilatory Failure

A. FAILURE OF CENTRAL DRIVE

Table 25–1 lists the main illnesses that cause acute loss of central respiratory drive. A mild acute loss of drive may cause acute ventilatory failure if it is superimposed on a larger but chronic loss of drive. Central drive problems without depressed mental status are less common,

but are seen in obesity hypoventilation or rare "primary" hypoventilation syndromes. A failure in central drive is often due to the effects of substances of abuse (including alcohol) or to prescription drugs with inhibitory effects on the medullary respiratory center. Respiratory suppression by drugs may be iatrogenic or intentional. Unresponsive patients with ventilatory failure in the community must be presumed to have a substance overdose until proven otherwise. Brain injuries sufficient to cause ventilatory failure must involve the brain stem directly, or increase intracranial pressure enough to affect brain stem function. Patients may lose all cortical function from an anoxic injury, but if brain stem function is intact, ventilatory failure does not ensue unless other components of the ventilatory pathway are affected. Likewise, a patient with a unilateral hemispheric stroke will usually have a normal respira-

Table 25–1. Illnesses that decrease central respiratory drive.

Acute conditions
 Substance overdose
  Alcohol, opiates, benzodiazepines, barbiturates
 Brain stem injury
  Trauma
  Stroke
  Subarachnoid hemorrhage
  Multiple sclerosis
  Increased intracranial pressure: tumors, trauma, hydro-
   cephalus, hematomas
  Poliomyelitis[1]
 Metabolic encephalopathies
  Anoxia, sepsis, hypoglycemia, hypermagnesemia
  Postictal state
  Severe hepatic and renal failure (usually increased drive)
 Toxic encephalopathies: carbon monoxide, drugs
 Nonconvulsive status epilepticus
 CNS infections
  Encephalitis
  Meningoencephalitis
  Meningitis
  Poliomyelitis[1]
Chronic conditions
 Obesity hypoventilation (Pickwickian syndrome)
 Other alveolar hypoventilation syndromes[1]
  Ondine's curse
  Myxedema

---

[1]Rare.

tory drive. Any metabolic or toxic encephalopathy can decrease central drive. Although hepatic or septic encephalopathies usually increase V̇E, they may decrease central drive when severe. Severe hypoglycemia can decrease central drive as well. The chronic loss of central drive in obesity hypoventilation syndromes usually will not lead to acute ventilatory failure unless other components of the ventilatory pathway become deranged, such as onset of acute respiratory muscle fatigue due to an excessive work of breathing during an infection.

B. FAILURE OF NEUROMUSCULAR COUPLING

Other than traumatic quadriplegia, this is an uncommon cause of acute ventilatory failure (Table 25–2). With traumatic quadriplegia, most patients who have injuries below C4 will retain enough diaphragmatic function to live without a ventilator. Neuropathies in efferent neurons and nerves that innervate the respiratory muscles may be idiopathic, toxic, infectious, and traumatic. Involvement of the diaphragm (phrenic nerve) is universal if respiratory failure occurs. Common illnesses include the acute ascending inflammatory polyneuropathy of GBS (yearly incidence 10/100,000 in U.S. populations), and high cervical spinal cord in-

Table 25–2. Illnesses that disrupt neuromuscular coupling.

Motor neuron diseases (with C3–C5 involvement)
 Acute myotrophic lateral sclerosis (ALS)
 Spinal cord trauma
 Multiple sclerosis
 Acute poliomyelitis[1] (may involve respiratory center)
 Enterovirus 71 (polio-like)[1]
 Postpolio syndrome[1]
 Transverse myelitis[1]
Motor neuropathies
 Guillain-Barré syndrome
 Critical illness polyneuropathy
 Bilateral phrenic nerve injury[1]
 Diphtheria[1]
 Acute intermittent porphyria[1]
Neuromuscular junction processes
 Neuromuscular blocking drugs (iatrogenic)
 Eaton–Lambert syndrome (paraneoplastic)
 Myasthenia gravis
 Tick paralysis[1]
 Poisonings
  Botulism[1]
  Paralytic shellfish (saxitoxin)
  Pufferfish (saxitoxin, tetrodotoxin)
  Pacificreef fish (ciguatoxin)
  Insecticides
  Nerve gases (sarin)[1]
  Arsenic, mercury, buckthorn plant[1]
  Snakebites (cobra)
  Black widow spider bite[1]
  Aminoglycosides and procainamide (not in isolation)

---

[1]Rare.

juries. Less common illnesses include delayed presentations of amyotrophic lateral sclerosis (ALS), multiple sclerosis with high cervical cord involvement, and the sensorimotor neuropathy of critical illness. Rare neuropathies occur from arsenic and mercury poisonings, acute poliomyelitis, and bilateral phrenic neuropathy. Processes that do not primarily affect nerve transmission but instead disrupt the neuromuscular junction include myasthenia gravis, Eaton–Lambert syndrome (due to paraneoplastic proteins that block synaptic transmission), the descending paralysis of botulism (due to a potent toxin that decreases acetylcholine in presynaptic vesicles), the ascending weakness of tick paralysis (synaptic location unclear), and poisonings from insectides, sarin (a nerve gas; used by terrorists in the Japanese subway poisonings of 1995), saxitoxin or tetrodotoxin (ingestion of pufferfish), ciguatoxin (ingestion of reef fish and diphtheria. Myasthenia gravis is the most common disorder of the neuromuscular junction. Botulism occurs in three forms: food borne (ingestion of *Clostridium botulinum* toxin), infant (due to intestinal colonization with *C. botulinum* and toxin production), and wound. Adults are fortunately not susceptible to gut colonization with *C. botulinum*. Infant botulism is the most common, although only 62 cases of botulism were reported to the Centers for Disease Control (CDC) in 2002. Diphtheria is now rare due to use of vaccination, with only one case reported to the CDC in 2002.

C. FAILURE OF RESPIRATORY MUSCLES

In contrast to failure of neuromuscular coupling, this is a common cause of acute ventilatory failure (Table 25–3). Chronic respiratory muscle fatigue is common in severe cases of lung disease, particularly COPD (including emphysema) and obesity hypoventilation. In severe COPD, respiratory muscles may consume more than 30% of the body's $\dot{V}O_2$ as they work to match an increased work of breathing. The lung hyperinflation characteristic of COPD also flattens the normal dome shape of the diaphragm and puts these muscles at an inefficient position of function. Many acute conditions that affect muscle function can exacerbate chronic respiratory muscle fatigue and lead to decompensation and acute ventilatory failure. For example, the higher the site of an abdominal surgery in a patient with COPD, the more likely it is to lead to postoperative respiratory complications by affecting diaphragm function. Profound hypophosphatemia and hypokalemia may decrease diaphragm strength and push a borderline

compensated patient with an emphysema exacerbation into ventilatory failure.

D. INCREASED WORK OF BREATHING DUE TO LUNG, CHEST WALL, AND PLEURAL PROCESSES

This is the most common cause of acute ventilatory failure (Table 25–4). These processes often cause respiratory muscle fatigue as well. It is useful to think of an increased work of breathing as being due to a lung process (most common) or a chest wall process (less common) that increases the respiratory workload. Exacerbations of chronic lung diseases such as asthma and COPD primarily act to increase work of breathing and represent a large subset of acute ventilatory failure.

1. Exacerbations of COPD (including emphysema)—COPD is the fourth leading cause of death in the United States, with many deaths being related to acute ventilatory failure. COPD exacerbations are characterized foremost by an increased work of breathing due to increased airway resistance, a load that the respiratory muscles must overcome with each breath. Respiratory muscle fatigue, $\dot{V}/Q$ mismatching, and increased V_D are also present in COPD exacerbations. Patients with COPD often have subtle respiratory muscle fatigue that predisposes to acute ventilatory failure in the

Table 25–3. Causes of respiratory muscle failure.

Acute or chronic (acute processes are rare in isolation)
  COPD exacerbation
  Obesity hypoventilation
  Muscular dystrophies
  Primary myopathies
    Myositis[1]
    Steroid myopathy
  Congenital metabolic disease
    Mitochondrial myopathies[1]
    Acid maltase deficiency[1]
    Carnitine palmitoyltransferase deficiency[1]
  Conditions that aggravate underlying muscle fatigue
    Malnutrition
    Electrolyte disorders (hypokalemia, hypophosphatemia)
    Acidosis
    Hypoxia
    Hypoperfusion/shock
Acute
  Hypokalemic periodic paralysis (familial or thyrotoxic)[1]
  Poor respiratory muscle oxygenation (hypoxemia, shock)
  Acute myositis[1]

[1]Rare.

Table 25–4. Lung, chest wall, and pleural processes that increase work of breathing.

Increased airways resistance load
  Upper airway: tumor, infection, foreign body, obesity, edema due to allergic reactions, angioedema
  Asthma exacerbation
  COPD exacerbation
  Congestive heart failure (typically hypoxic respiratory failure)
Increased minute ventilation load
  Sepsis
  Metabolic acidosis
  Lung disorders that increase dead space, $\dot{V}/Q$ mismatch
    COPD
    Interstitial lung disease
    Any parenchymal lung disease
Increased chest wall resistance load
  Multiple rib fractures
  Pleural processes
    Large effusions
    Hemothorax
    Pneumothorax
  Abdominal effects on diaphragms
    Massive ascites
    Ileus
    Abdominal compartment syndrome
  Kyphoscoliosis

setting of any acute illness that further increases the work of breathing, such as systemic infection (high $\dot{V}E$ requirements), pneumothorax, or bronchospasm.

2. Asthma exacerbations—Asthma exacerbations that lead to acute ventilatory failure usually occur in a patient with poor baseline pulmonary function due to severe disease, noncompliance with medication, or poor living and working environments. Asthma exacerbations are characterized by increased work of breathing due to increased airway resistance. Respiratory muscle fatigue, $\dot{V}/Q$ mismatching, and increased VD occur late in asthma exacerbations, which is quite different than in COPD exacerbations. Patients with asthma usually do not have chronic respiratory muscle fatigue.

3. Other lung and chest wall diseases—In less common diseases such as pulmonary fibrosis, the work of breathing is increased due to the need for each breath to overcome the elastic load of expanding fibrotic lungs. Patients with pulmonary fibrosis may also present with hypoxemic respiratory failure due to progressive alveolar wall thickening and intrapulmonary shunting. Any process that leads to a less compliant chest wall or lung compression will increase the work of breathing as well. Thus a large pneumothorax, a large hemothorax due to trauma, massive pleural effusions, and multilevel rib fractures will all increase the work of breathing and in some settings may trigger acute ventilatory failure, particularly if other components of the ventilatory pathway are disrupted.

4. Severe kyphoscoliosis—These patients often develop acute ventilatory failure during pulmonary infections or otherwise mild respiratory illnesses. Dyspnea typically occurs late in these patients, occurring at 100° of scoliotic angulation, measured as the Cobb angle. The Cobb angle is calculated as the posterior angle defined by the axis of the primary (lumbar) scoliotic curve and the secondary (thoracic, or "compensatory") scoliotic curve. Patients with severe kyphoscoliosis with a Cobb angle beyond 120° often develop chronic respiratory acidosis, pulmonary hypertension, and right heart failure. The degree of restrictive impairment on pulmonary function tests typically does not correlate with the severity of scoliosis defined by the Cobb angle.

Clinical Findings

A. Symptoms and Signs

The signs and symptoms of ventilatory failure reflect the sites at which the ventilatory pathway is disrupted. Physical examination and the history will disclose the pathway disruptions that underlie the mechanism of ventilatory failure in almost all cases (Table 25–5).

Dyspnea and anxiety are near-universal symptoms if mental status is not depressed. With a loss of central

Table 25–5. Symptoms and signs of acute ventilatory failure.

Nonspecific
  Symptoms: dyspnea, fatigue, mood alterations, cough
  Signs: tachypnea, tachycardia, anxiety, cyanosis, labored respiration
Pathway specific
  Central drive
    Symptoms: sleepiness, substance abuse
    Signs: lethargy, confusion, obtundation, seizures, miosis, hypoventilation
  Neuromuscular coupling (see also Table 25–6)
    Motor neuron disease
      Symptoms: neck pain (if traumatic), limb muscle weakness
      Signs: diffuse weakness, sensory level (cord injury), fasciculations (ALS)
    Neuropathy
      Symptoms: paresthesias, weakness; porphyria: onset after anesthesia/drugs, abdominal pain, rash
      Signs: diminished sensation, weakness, diminished reflexes, dysautonomia
    Synaptic processes (see also Table 25–6)
      Symptoms: weakness, no paresthesias; insecticide exposure: excessive salivation, weakness
  Respiratory muscle failure
    Symptoms: dyspnea chief complaint, lung disease, muscle pain (myositis)
    Signs: morbid obesity, accessory muscle use, abdominal paradox
  Disorders that increase work of breathing
    Airway obstruction: drooling, dysphagia, sore throat, choking, stridor
    Lung disorders
      Symptoms: wheezing, dyspnea, cough, fatigue, chest pressure
      Signs: rales, rhonchi, wheezing, poor air movement, pulsus paradoxus
    Chest wall and pleural disorders
      Kyphoscoliosis: bent posture; Cobb angle more than 100°
      Pneumothorax: pleurisy, dyspnea, smoking history; hyperresonance
      Hemothorax/rib fractures: chest trauma; percussed dullness, tenderness
      Pleural effusion: subacute dyspnea, cough, chest pain, pleurisy; dullness
    Increased $\dot{V}E$ load: fever, ongoing acute infections and other catabolic states

drive, lethargy is typical. Such patients are often unable to provide a history, so a history from family and friends is sought. Sleep disruption, mood alteration, hallucinations, and fatigue often occur with chronic respiratory muscle fatigue and hypercarbia. Acute onset of dyspnea, stridor, and lip and tongue edema in the setting of certain drugs [angiotensin-converting enzyme (ACE) inhibitors, antibiotics] or foods suggests allergic upper airway edema or angioedema (which may be hereditary and associated with abdominal pain) and impending airway obstruction. In patients with asthma and COPD exacerbations, recent sick contacts, acute upper respiratory infections (URIs), fever, wheezing, exposure to known individual triggers of bronchospasm (aeroallergens, animals, smoke, extremes of temperature), noncompliance with medications, and drug abuse are common precipitants of exacerbations. Diarrhea, emesis, and dysphagia are common with botulism. Diarrhea, upper respiratory infections, or recent surgery are common associations of GBS. Neuromuscular coupling defects due to neuropathy may be divided into strictly motor (myasthenia gravis, tick paralysis) and sensorimotor (GBS, critical illness polyneuropathy, many toxins) based on symptoms. Numbness, tingling, or other paresthesias occur if sensory nerves are affected. The pattern of muscle involvement is often helpful. Botulism and GBS both present with bulbar weakness (diplopia, swallowing difficulty), but GBS is an ascending paralysis whereas botulism is descending—bulbar symptoms, drooling, and blurred vision are present from the outset in botulism but occur later in GBS. Botulism occurs in less than 72 h in most cases, whereas GBS is often subacute over weeks. Tick paralysis is ascending, with rare bulbar involvement. Motor neuron diseases such as amyotrophic lateral sclerosis (ALS) usually cause an insidious onset of weakness that may progress acutely during illnesses that increase the work of breathing (such as infection). Acute ventilatory failure occurs in < 10% of patients with myasthenia gravis, is rare in Eaton–Lambert syndrome, but is common in GBS.

The physical examination (Table 25–5) should include the following.

1. Vital signs and inspection—The first steps in the care of patients with acute ventilatory failure are to ascertain the patient's vital signs, level of responsiveness, patency of the airway, and adequacy of respiration. Foreign body obstruction of the larynx such as by food must be ruled out. Fever, tachycardia, and tachypnea suggest infection. Fever and lethargy suggest central nervous system (CNS) infection or septic encephalopathy. An elevated pulsus paradoxus of more than 10 mm Hg suggests lung overdistention due to expiratory airflow obstruction, such as in asthma or COPD exacerbations. Depressed mental status, low respiratory rate, and diminished chest excursion are easy to detect by inspection and auscultation, and typify failure of central drive. For instance, a patient with GBS syndrome may have poor air movement, but will be alert and often have a normal or high respiratory rate. The preference for a patient to sit upright, to appear anxious, with shoulders hunched forward, and to refuse to lie flat is typical of COPD and asthma exacerbations. Morbid obesity suggests a potential for chronic hypoventilation. The odor of ethanol is readily detectable in cases of intoxication, but needs laboratory validation.

2. Neurological examination—Depressed mental status such as lethargy or coma is typical of central drive failure. Failure of central drive can often thus be diagnosed from the foot of the bed. Pupil size and reactivity must be assessed, as opiate overdoses will cause pupillary constriction (miosis). Severe hypercarbia will cause miosis as well. A lack of response to noxious stimuli suggests a failure of central drive. Muscle fasciculations in the tongue and limbs occur in ALS and other motor neuron diseases. Sensory deficits suggest a polyneuropathy [GBS or intensive care unit (ICU) polyneuropathy]. Bulbar weakness is common in both botulism and GBS. Nuchal rigidity suggests meningitis. The less common Miller–Fisher variant of GBS is characterized by ataxia and areflexia. Ataxia may also occur with other neuropathies and myopathies.

3. Head and neck—Inspiratory stridor with or without drooling suggests upper airway obstruction. However, vocal cord dysfunction is often mistaken for upper airway obstruction or airflow obstruction, but rarely causes respiratory failure. The pharynx and tonsillar areas need inspection. Pharyngeal membranes occur in the cases of diphtheria. Lip, tongue, or pharynx edema suggests allergic reactions to drugs or foods, or angioedema. A weak or absent gag reflex may be normal, but when combined with lethargy suggests a high risk for aspiration. Note should be taken of retrognathia, obesity, or a poorly visible posterior pharynx, which will make intubation difficult. Copious saliva and sputum, mydriasis, flushing, and other cholinergic signs are characteristic of insecticide-mediated cholinesterase inhibition.

4. Chest—The pattern of respiratory muscle contraction will readily separate failure of central drive from other mechanisms—breathing will usually be infrequent and unlabored, except in obesity hypoventilation. An increased anteroposterior chest diameter, hyperinflation and hyperresonance to percussion, and diminished breath sounds suggest COPD. The recruitment of normally inactive intercostal, scalene, and sternocleidomastoid muscles suggests increased work of breathing is present. Decreased airflow with or without wheezing in an alert patient suggests airflow obstruction, as does a prolonged expiratory phase. Rhonchi suggest infection or edema. Rales suggest heart failure, pulmonary fibrosis, atelectasis, or pneumonia. However, many patients with COPD will have basilar rales chronically. Massive pleural effusions or hemothoraces can usually be defined by percussed dullness, decreased fremitus, and diminished breath sounds. A large pneumothorax will diminish breath sounds but is associated with increased resonance to percussion. A strong cough suggests reasonable preservation of respiratory muscle strength.

5. Cardiac—Tachycardia and hypertension are common in acute ventilatory failure. Signs of right heart failure may be present in COPD or pulmonary fibrosis. Heart sounds are usually diminished in COPD and in asthmatic hyperinflation.

6. Abdomen—Normal abdominal wall movement is outward with inspiration; inward movement with inspiration is paradoxical and suggests diaphragmatic fatigue. Ascites, ileus, and abdominal distention may cause upward diaphragm displacement. Diarrhea and emesis are common in botulism.

7. Extremities—Edema suggests cor pulmonale due to chronic lung disease. Clubbing is uncommon with COPD, but occurs with pulmonary fibrosis and bronchiectasis.

8. Skin—Track marks should be sought if intravenous opiate abuse is suspected. Diaphoresis is common in opiate overdose or infection. Flushing is common with insecticide poisoning. All patients with apparent neuromuscular coupling defects or muscle weakness should have their skin and hair inspected for ticks in nonwinter months. Botulism may occur from wounds, typically in feet and hands.

B. LABORATORY TESTING

Although the part of the ventilatory pathway that is disrupted in acute ventilatory failure is usually discernible from the history and physical examination, the exact process causing that disruption needs to be clarified by laboratory, physiological, and imaging tests to provide optimal therapy.

1. Arterial blood gas (ABG)—The ABG is essential in the evaluation of acute ventilatory failure. The severity of respiratory acidosis is determined first and may in itself dictate the need for intubation and mechanical ventilation if severe. The "50–50 rule" of intubating a patient based on either a PaO_2 of < 50 mm Hg or a $PaCO_2$ or > 50 mm Hg is antiquated and should be discarded. For instance, even moderate hypercarbia does not predict the eventual need for mechanical ventilation in status asthmaticus, and a $PaCO_2$ of 70 mm Hg may not be far from the baseline of a patient with se-

vere COPD. A decrease in arterial pH below 7.20–7.25 due to an acute respiratory acidosis will usually require ventilatory support. Interpretation of an inadvertent venous blood gas (VBG) must be avoided. Although the $PaCO_2$ and PaO_2 on a VBG are not helpful, the pH may be valuable as it is reliably 0.04 pH units lower than arterial pH. Evidence for chronic compensation of a respiratory acidosis based on a high bicarbonate provides clues to the presence of chronic lung disease. A separation of the calculated hemoglobin saturation (based on pH and PaO_2) and measured saturation may provide clues to the presence of carbon monoxide poisoning or methemoglobinemia. Serial ABGs are used to guide ventilatory support and reassess adequacy of ventilation.

2. Complete blood count (CBC)—Leukocytosis suggests infection. Anemia can be associated with dyspnea, and worsens oxygen transport to tissues, but in isolation is not a cause of ventilatory failure.

3. Lumbar puncture (LP)—An LP is essential in cases of suspected CNS infection or GBS. A high CSF protein in the setting of a normal white cell count and CSF glucose is characteristic of GBS. CSF leukocytosis with or without high CSF protein and low CSF glucose may suggest bacterial meningitis (neutrophil predominant), viral or tubercular meningitis (mononuclear predominant), or viral encephalitis (mononuclear predominant).

4. Serum chemistries—Potassium, phosphate, and magnesium levels should be determined, as low levels may contribute to respiratory muscle fatigue. Iatrogenic hypermagnesemia may lead to a decrease in central drive. A suppressed thyroid-stimulating hormone (TSH) may be seen with thyrotoxic hypokalemic periodic paralysis. Alterations in anion gap, glucose, blood urea nitrogen (BUN), creatinine, sodium, and liver function tests may provide clues to metabolic encephalopathies affecting central drive and loss of ability to protect the airway.

5. Toxicology tests—Urine toxicology screens are rapid and screen for the most common drugs of abuse. A serum toxicology screen may be needed to detect less common drugs. Some drugs that cause respiratory suppression cannot be screened easily (such as γ-hydroxybutyrate). Serum ethanol levels are needed in suspected cases, and must be evaluated in the context of other concurrent drug abuse. Evaluation for suspected arsenic or mercury overdoses and other unusual ingestions should be done with the guidance of a toxicologist or poison control center.

6. Pulmonary function tests—Bedside testing of respiratory muscle strength by respiratory therapists with handheld equipment can be easily obtained by measuring negative inspiratory force (NIF) and positive expiratory force (PEF), and vital capacity (VC). Diminutions in the expected values signal respiratory muscle fatigue and/or lung disease. The normal values for NIF, PEF, and VC are −50 to −100 cm H_2O, +50–100 cm H_2O, and 65 mL/kg (all values 25% less for women). When monitoring patients with acute neuromuscular coupling defects, such as GBS or myasthenia gravis, a decrease in VC to < 20 mL/kg correlates with impending CO_2 retention and ventilatory failure, particularly if the fall is rapid. Patients with these illnesses lose their ability to protect their airway and universally retain CO_2 at VC <10 mL/kg. They should be electively intubated before reaching this stage. Careful observation and repetitive respiratory strength testing are crucial during these illnesses to prevent avoidable deaths due to aspiration, pneumonia, and sepsis. Airflow obstruction can be evaluated by a handheld peak flow meter. Serial peak flow measurements are useful in evaluating the response to therapy during asthma exacerbations. Peak flow measurements are less helpful in patients with COPD due to a greater degree of airway collapse on forced exhalation. It is often not practical to obtain bedside spirometry in acute ventilatory failure due to the cooperation required for sustained exhalation.

7. Microbiological and immunological tests—Infection as a precipitant of ventilatory failure should be evaluated by cultures of suspected sites. A lumbar puncture will help determine the likelihood of suspected acute viral or bacterial CNS infections. Stool analysis may uncover *Campylobacter* infection that is often associated with GBS. *C. botulinum* may be cultured from stool or wounds. Serum antibodies to the gangliosides GM1, GM2, GD1a, GD1b, and GQ1b and anti-*Campylobacter* antibodies are associated with GBS. Anticalcium channel antibodies occur with Eaton–Lambert syndrome. Antiacetylcholine receptor antibodies occur with myasthenia gravis. Of botulism cases 35% will have positive antibodies to the botulinum toxin, yet these laborious tests usually require state health agency assistance.

C. IMAGING AND OTHER TESTS

1. Thoracic imaging—A chest radiograph is essential in the evaluation of acute ventilatory failure. Pneumonia, atelectasis, pulmonary edema, evidence of chronic lung disease, tumors, chest wall abnormalities, and pleural abnormalities can all be screened by a chest radiograph. Most patients with asthma and COPD exacerbations will not have acute changes on a chest radiograph. Although more commonly presenting as hypoxic respiratory failure, large pulmonary emboli create V_D and $\dot{V}/Q$ mismatch and are best evaluated by ventilation–perfusion lung scanning or chest computed tomography (CT) scan protocols. Noncontrast chest CT scans can clarify tumors, pleural and chest wall disease, and parenchymal lung disease. Thymomas, present in 10–15% of cases of myasthenia gravis, are often detected on a chest CT scan.

2. Neurological imaging—Brain and spinal cord magnetic resonance imaging (MRI) is useful to screen for encephalitis, brain stem pathology, and spinal cord injury. An emergent noncontrast head CT scan is an essential evaluation of any patient with unexplained lethargy, focal neurological signs, or trauma that leads to ventilatory failure.

3. Cardiac testing—Electrocardiograms may show evidence of chronic lung disease (P pulmonale, right ventricular strain) and will screen for acute myocardial infarction. Even if a primary myocardial infarction is not suspected, the stress of ventilatory failure in older patients with potential coronary disease may precipitate coronary ischemia. Echocardiography is easily available in many intensive care units and can help guide therapy if left ventricular failure or valve disease is suspected of contributing to the ventilatory failure.

4. Neurological testing—Failure of central respiratory drive may be due to global encephalopathy or nonconvulsive status epilepticus. A neurologist should evaluate any patient with an unexplained depressed sensorium who has a known seizure disorder, or signs of tonic, clonic, myotonic, or posturing events. Emergent electroencephalography (EEG) to evaluate for nonconvulsive status epilepticus may be necessary. Diffuse slowing on EEG is seen with anoxic or metabolic encephalopathies. Neuromuscular coupling defects such as GBS, myasthenia gravis, Eaton–Lambert syndrome, and tick paralysis are characterized by reliable patterns on electromyography (EMG) and nerve conduction velocity (NCV) studies that help differentiate them (Table 25–6). An intravenous edrophonium chloride (Tensilon) test, used to inhibit anticholinesterases, is used when myasthenia gravis is suspected and will lead to transient but diagnostic improvement of weakness in most patients with myasthenia gravis.

Prevention

A. VACCINES

Vaccines are among the best preventative measures. Polio and diphtheria have been vaccinated out of existence in the United States—cases are very rare, although these diseases persist in developing countries that do not provide vaccinations. Pneumonia and influenza are the sixth leading cause of death in the United States. Pneumococcal vaccination will provide protection against 23 common *Streptococcus pneumo-*

Table 25–6. Signs, symptoms, and treatment of select neuromuscular coupling process.[1]

	Guillain–Barré Syndrome	Critical Illness Polyneuropathy	Myasthenia Gravis	Eaton–Lambert	ALS	Tick Paralysis
History	Recent GI or URI illness; surgery; rapid, any age	Recent prolonged ICU stay	Insidious onset; adults	Older age, smoker, at risk for cancer, subacute	Insidious; older adults	Rapid; travel in woods; any age
Symptoms	Ascending paresthesias and weakness	Weakness	Diffuse weakness, diplopia	Diffuse weakness	Diffuse weakness	Ascending weakness
Signs	Sensorimotor; bulbar	Sensorimotor; unable to wean from ventilator	Motor; bulbar early, thymoma on imaging	Motor, limb early, bulbar late	Motor, fasciculations	Motor, ptosis, neck weakness
EMG/NCV findings	Demyelination; sensorimotor neuropathy; usually not axonal	Motor more than sensory, diaphragms often involved	Motor; decremental response to a repetitive stimulation	Motor; incremental response to a repetitive stimulation	Motor; axonal	Motor; low-amplitude and slowed motor potentials
Specific therapies	IV-Ig; plasmapheresis; may need ventilation for weeks	None	Steroids; plasmapheresis; thymectomy	Treat cancer	Home NPPV or mechanical ventilation; riluzole	Find and remove tick
Specific tests	Ab to gangliosides, *Campylobacter*	None	Acetylcholine; receptor Ab in 90%; positive neostigmine tests	Ab to calcium channels	None	Tick identification

[1] Ab, antibody; NPPV, noninvasive positive pressure ventilation; IV-Ig, intravenous immunoglobulin; GI, gastrointestinal; URI, upper respiratory infection.

niae strains, including those with increased penicillin resistance. Pneumococcal vaccination should be given to at-risk groups such as those age 65 years or older and patients with diabetes, chronic renal and hepatic failure, asthma, emphysema, and many other comorbidities, as outlined by the CDC (http://www.cdc.gov). For hospitalized patients who have illnesses targeted for pneumococcal vaccination, the CDC recommends vaccination before hospital discharge. This is recommended even if the patient was hospitalized for pneumococcal pneumonia but belongs to a targeted vaccination group. Pneumococcal vaccination decreases mortality from invasive pneumococcal disease in most of these targeted groups. Influenza vaccination is essential to provide protection against influenza A and B during the fall and winter months in patients with chronic lung disease or diseases that impair immunity. Influenza vaccinations decrease overall mortality in many populations, and an unvaccinated person is much more likely to die of complications of influenza than they are from complications resulting from the very rare cases of GBS linked to the vaccine.

B. Antismoking Measures

The prevention of tobacco-related lung disease and cessation of smoking in patients with established lung disease, particularly in asthma and COPD, are key measures to decrease the incidence of ventilatory failure due to lung diseases.

C. Trauma Prevention

Seatbelt use decreases the incidence of neck trauma and quadriplegia, and patients should be questioned and counseled on the subject.

D. Medical Compliance

Regular outpatient clinic visits for patients with asthma, COPD, and other chronic diseases that cause ventilatory failure are essential to minimize exacerbations of those diseases. Too many of these patients rely on emergency rooms as their caregivers. A dedicated primary care physician working in partnership with the patient is the best preventative strategy. Patients often cannot afford medications; in such cases the clinic physician should consult a social worker and/or work to secure free samples from pharmaceutical company programs for such individuals.

E. Environment

Patients with asthma, COPD, and other chronic lung disease benefit from clean, aeroallergen, and temperature-controlled environments. A patient suffering acute ventilatory failure from status asthmaticus who has cats and dust as triggers will do poorly if discharged to a poorly kept home with cats. Aeroallergen control measures are essential for patients with asthma. Patients with asthma and chronic lung disease should minimize time outside on high pollution days.

F. Drug Abuse and Toxin Avoidance

Prevention of street drug abuse and alcohol abuse is essential. Crack cocaine use is a common precipitant of status asthmaticus. Current food control measures have made cases of botulism rare, although home canning of food must be done with assiduous care. Hikers should screen each other and their children for ticks after travel in wooded or natural areas in warm seasons. The eating of puffer fish should be avoided, and public education of populations that live near coastal areas can decrease shellfish ingestion at times of toxin algae blooms. Patients with anaphylactic food and bee allergies should be given automatic delivery epinephrine syringes to carry at all times when they are at risk, as many patients can develop airway edema and respiratory failure. An allergist should evaluate these patients.

G. Prevention of Atelectasis

Optimizing secretion clearance with suctioning and bronchodilators, positioning in standard or rotational beds, chest physiotherapy, and intermittent positive pressure breathing (IPPB) treatments are useful.

H. Early Recognition of Loss of Airway Protection

Illnesses that cause lethargy or bulbar muscle weakness predispose to aspiration and should lead to early airway protection measures, such as intubation. Elevation of the head of the bed is important in reducing aspiration risk. Such patients should be monitored in a setting that allows for sufficient observation and intervention, such as in a step-down unit or intensive care unit.

I. Avoiding Medication Side Effects

The respiratory suppressant effects of opiates and benzodiazepines often cause acute ventilatory failure in the hospital setting, and they must be used cautiously in patients with any perturbation of the ventilatory pathway, particularly in patients with chronic lung disease and resting hypercarbia. The use of aspirin, nonsteroidal antiinflammatory drug (NSAID) agents, and mucomyst (*N*-acetylcysteine) in patients with severe asthma should be administered cautiously, if at all, due to a potential to precipitate bronchospasm.

J. Advance Directives

Many elderly and chronically ill patients have never discussed advanced directives for times of severe illness. Because of this, many individuals who want to avoid aggressive life-sustaining measures are intubated and ventilated for respiratory failure. Initiation and documentation of these discussions of advanced directives are important, as is provision of the often necessary bracelet or displayable home documentation needed by emergency providers to verify and honor the patient's wishes.

Treatment

The treatment of acute ventilatory failure is discussed below in the context of specific diseases and location of abnormalities in the ventilatory pathway.

A. MONITORING

All patients with acute ventilatory failure should be monitored in an intensive care unit or intermediate care unit if they do not quickly improve with simple measures in an emergency room, clinic, or hospital ward setting.

B. GENERAL MEASURES

Inhaled bronchodilators should be administered to all patients with bronchospasm. Fever reduction with acetaminophen will decrease CO_2 production, and decrease the $\dot{V}E$ load upon the lungs. Sedation in select patients will decrease the excess $\dot{V}CO_2$ due to muscle activity. Attention to avoiding excessive caloric intake (which increases $\dot{V}CO_2$) in patients with COPD is practical, although a true impact is controversial. Cervical collars are needed in patients with suspected cervical spine trauma. Drainage and preventive measures for massive ascites or pleural effusions will decrease work of breathing.

C. FAILURE OF CENTRAL DRIVE

Patients who present from the community with obtundation should receive 0.4–2 mg of naloxone and 50% dextrose intravenously for potential opiate overdose or hypoglycemia. Patients with narcotic overdoses will often need repeat doses of naloxone, as its half-life is shorter than that of most opiates of abuse. Care must be taken in reversing benzodiazepines with flumazenil in the setting of chronic benzodiazepine use, as seizures may occur. All patients with depressed mental status, respiratory muscle weakness, or weakness of pharyngeal muscles during acute illness need to have measures instituted to protect the airway. These range from good oral care and frequent suctioning of oropharyngeal secretions, frequent nursing observation, decubitus or nonrecumbent positioning, use of nasogastric tubes during abdominal distention, to tracheal intubation and mechanical ventilation. Mistakes are often made by withholding intubation and mechanical ventilation to patients with obtundation or rapidly progressive neuromuscular syndromes. Such patients may later require

emergent intubation or develop pneumonia or acute lung injury from aspiration, with an attendant increase in mortality.

D. STATUS ASTHMATICUS

Asthma exacerbations are a frequent cause of acute ventilatory failure. The treatment employed for asthma (Table 25–7) are similar to the treatment for COPD exacerbations (Table 25–7) with important caveats emphasized below. The treatment for asthma exacerbations is reviewed elsewhere in this text. The most important step is to provide rapid administration of bronchodilators. Patients can often be discharged to home with or without oral corticosteroids. Patients who

Table 25–7. Treatment of acute ventilatory failure due to asthma or COPD.[1]

Treatment	Asthma	COPD
Oxygen (titrate to saturation 92–94%)	X	X
Inhaled bronchodilators (usually by nebulizer)		
β2-agonists (albuterol)	X	X
Ipratropium	Limited data	X
Subcutaneous β-agonists		
Epinephrine	X	Avoid
Terbutaline	X	X[2]
Intravenous methylxanthines	X[2]	X[2]
Intravenous corticosteroids	X	X
Intravenous magnesium	X[2]	No support
Antibiotics (for purulent sputum, usually oral)	X[2]	X[2]
Noninvasive ventilation	Limited data	X
Mechanical ventilation	X	X
Neuromuscular blocking agents (when intubated)	X[2]	Anecdotal
Inhaled anesthetics (when intubated)	Anecdotal	Anecdotal
Inhaled helium–oxygen mixture	Limited data	No support
Inhaled N-acetylcysteine	Avoid	Limited data
Oral mucolytics	Limited data	Limited data

[1]X, accepted efficacy; X[2], second-line therapy, to be considered only after other therapies are optimized.

do not clear their bronchospasm or improve their bedside peak expiratory flow rates sufficiently will need admission to the hospital.

1. Oxygen—$\dot{V}/\dot{Q}$ mismatching and mild hypoxemia are common in asthma exacerbations. Oxygen therapy can be empiric using 1–2 L/min by nasal cannula or guided by pulse oximetry. Most nebulizers are given with a driving flow of 6–12 L/min of oxygen rather than air. If mechanical ventilation is required for ventilatory failure, a high FIO_2 is rarely needed.

2. Bronchodilators—Bronchodilators are the most important initial therapy of asthma exacerbations. Selective β_2-adrenergic agonists (albuterol) are the preferred therapy. Inhaled anticholinergic agents are often provided, but evidence is limited as to any additional benefit they confer. Bronchodilators are usually given as inhaled treatments by nebulizer, usually every 15–30 min. Clinical trials of asthma exacerbations have also proven that the use of inhaled β_2-agonists by metered dose inhaler (MDI) with a spacer and a larger number of puffs (five or six) is comparable to the response achieved with nebulizers. However, most patients find nebulizers easier to use during exacerbations. In severe exacerbations, continuous nebulization of β_2-adrenergic agonists is often performed. Continuous nebulizers may cause a lactic acidosis, and thus require more frequent ABG monitoring. It is unclear whether isomeric β_2-adrenergic agonists (levalbuterol) offer any meaningful benefit over standard (racemic) preparations. Inhaled β_2-agonists should be given until a patient feels sufficiently improved, until wheezing is resolved or greatly improved, and until air movement is improved.

3. Corticosteroids—Steroids are a first-line therapy. All patients with frank or impending ventilatory failure due to asthma should be treated with corticosteroids. Although these agents are highly bioavailable orally, the high dosages employed can cause nausea and emesis, and intravenous therapy is best until the patient improves. Then, doses of 60 mg or less of prednisone are prescribed. The frequently employed dose of 125 mg of methylprednisolone intravenously every 6 h was found in a small clinical trial to be more efficacious than two lower dose regimens, and has since been embraced. Smaller initial doses in less-ill hospitalized patients are often used to avoid steroid side effects. Conversion to oral prednisone therapy occurs when patients have cleared their bronchospasm, and prednisone is then tapered off or reduced to prior baseline level over several weeks based on response. Side effects include hyperglycemia, mood alteration, and fluid retention.

4. Parenteral β_2-agonist therapy—Subcutaneous β_2-agonists are a second-line therapy. In patients with severe asthma exacerbations who are unable to inhale β_2-agonists sufficiently, subcutaneous epinephrine or terbutaline may be given as single or multiple doses. These agents offer little benefit to patients unless inhaled β_2-agonist therapy is delayed or suboptimal due to severe airflow obstruction with respiratory failure. Side effects include tremor, anxiety, tachycardia, nausea, and emesis.

5. Intravenous magnesium—Magnesium is a second-line therapy. Although controversial, sufficient data exist for the use of one or two doses of intravenous magnesium sulfate in status asthmaticus requiring mechanical ventilation. As the main side effect is respiratory suppression, this is irrelevant in a newly intubated patient. The use of intravenous magnesium in less severe asthma exacerbations is often of benefit, but must be balanced against the risk of respiratory suppression.

6. Methylxanthines—Methylxanthines are a second-line therapy. Intravenous aminophylline or theophylline may be of benefit in status asthmaticus for patients who are not on these agents. If patients are on these agents chronically, therapeutic levels should be targeted with supplemental oral or intravenous medication. Clinical trials vary as to the effectiveness of intravenous methylxanthines in acute asthma. Because of marginal data for efficacy and frequent side effects (tremor, tachycardia, drug interactions) they are usually reserved for intubated patients or patients who are not improving despite use of other therapies.

7. Antibiotics—Antibiotics are not usually required in asthma exacerbations, as bacterial bronchitis is uncommon. Nonetheless, they are frequently prescribed for URI symptoms, although they offer only the risk of side effects to most patients. In severe asthma exacerbations, discolored sputum is often sterile and may be due to eosinophils. Antibiotics are indicated for bacterial sinusitis and pneumonia. Antiinfluenza agents such as neuraminidase inhibitors are indicated for the first 48 h of flu-like illness during times of active influenza in the community.

8. Anxiolytics—Benzodiazepines must be used with caution in a monitored setting or not at all in patients not on mechanical ventilation due to their potential for respiratory suppression. Patients on chronic benzodiazepine therapy should in most cases have their daily dose administered to avoid withdrawal. In intubated patients with status asthmaticus, large doses of benzodiazepines are often needed for sedation to permit effective ventilation. Morphine should be avoided due to histamine release. In intubated patients, fentanyl is a good choice for pain control and sedation.

9. Neuromuscular blocking agents—In mechanically ventilated patients with severe status asthmaticus, neuromuscular blocking agents are often needed to facilitate patient–ventilator interactions in the setting of high airway resistance. These can be used only in intubated patients, and for as brief a time as possible. They may be given as a bolus initially, but thereafter heavy sedation must be delivered and attempts should be made the first day to remove neuromuscular blockers if patient improvement permits. Because chronic myopathy due to the interaction of neuromuscular blocking agents and corticosteroids is common, the optimal goal is to minimize use of neuromuscular blockers to less than 24–48 h. Atracurium in particular should be avoided due to histamine release; *cis*-atracurium does not have this property.

10. Noninvasive ventilation—Noninvasive positive pressure ventilation (NPPV) is a means of providing ventilatory support by a nasal mask or full facemask without the use of an endotracheal tube. NPPV may be done with a ventilator or a bilevel-pressure (BiPAP) apparatus. NPPV is not commonly employed in status asthmaticus due to limited validation in clinical trials, patient anxiety and claustrophobia requiring sedation, need for frequent nebulizer therapy, and the often precipitous development of respiratory failure. For acute respiratory failure in asthma, NPPV should be used only in ICU or ER settings. The settings are adjusted to provide an adequate exhaled VT, respiratory rate, and subjective improvement. NPPV is generally reserved for alert patients who can protect their airway. Barotrauma appears less commonly with this modality than with endotracheal intubation and ventilation.

11. Mechanical ventilation—Patients with asthma who present in respiratory failure or who progress to respiratory failure after medical therapy require endotracheal intubation and ventilation. The process of ventilating these patients is difficult due to severe elevations in airway resistance. The periintubation period requires extensive sedation and often neuromuscular blockade. Large endotracheal tubes should be used to minimize resistance to airflow (8–9 mm internal diameter). Bronchodilators and other medications need to be maximized. Selected VTs are often small (5–8 mL) and rates are less than 25 to increase expiratory time and minimize intrinsic positive end-expiratory pressure (PEEP) ("autoPEEP"). Peak airway pressures are targeted at < 60 cm H_2O (less than 45 is ideal), mean airway pressures < 25 cm H_2O, and inspiratory plateau pressures < 30 cm H_2O to minimize barotrauma and volutrauma to the alveoli. Volume-cycled ventilation is typically preferred, although other ventilation modes are frequently employed. The technique of permissive hypercapnea is often helpful. In this the clinician lets the $PaCO_2$ rise (typically above 60 mm Hg, often to above 80 mm Hg) and the pH fall, with the emphasis on providing the minimal ventilation necessary for oxy-

genation and hemodynamic stability, while minimizing barotrauma. A pH > 7.1–7.2 is sought. Sodium bicarbonate may or may not be supplemented in this strategy. Frequent ABG monitoring is necessary and may be simplified by the insertion of an arterial monitoring line (radial artery preferred). The patient is assessed for liberation from mechanical ventilation when bronchospasm has improved, sedation needs are minimal, and respiratory muscle strength is adequate. Early extubation is desirable and feasible in asthma.

12. Other therapies—Helium gas increases laminar flow, thereby improving airway resistance, and can be provided as mixtures of helium and oxygen (such as 40% oxygen, 60% helium) in most hospitals. It has been useful in small clinical trials in nonintubated as well as in intubated patients, but remains an unproven therapy. Anecdotal reports indicate that inhalational anesthetic agents provide bronchodilation in mechanically ventilated patients unresponsive to conventional therapy. No prospective clinical trials have validated this technique.

E. Exacerbations of Chronic Obstructive Pulmonary Disease

Exacerbations of COPD are a frequent cause of acute ventilatory failure. Unlike patients with asthma, patients with COPD often have chronic respiratory muscle fatigue and need mechanical ventilation to rest these muscles as much as for treatment of increased airway resistance. The treatments employed for COPD exacerbations are similar to the treatments for asthma (Table 25–7) with important caveats emphasized below. The most important step is to provide rapid administration of bronchodilators. Intravenous corticosteroids are efficacious and evidence based. Bedside peak expiratory flow rates are less useful than in asthma. Frequent ABG monitoring is necessary and may be simplified by the insertion of an arterial monitoring line (radial artery preferred).

1. Oxygen—Patients with COPD are often on chronic oxygen therapy. Worsened $\dot{V}/\dot{Q}$ mismatching and mild hypoxemia are the rule in COPD exacerbations. Oxygen therapy should be guided by pulse oximetry and ABG. If mechanical ventilation is required for ventilatory failure, a high FIO_2 is rarely needed. The provision of an adequate PaO_2 is essential and is best achieved with an oxygen saturation above 90% and a PaO_2 above 55 mm Hg. Hypoxemia and saturations < 90% may contribute to encephalopathy, worsen respiratory muscle fatigue, worsen pulmonary hypertension and right heart failure, and decrease tissue oxygenation. Withholding oxygen to achieve a lower $PaCO_2$ at the cost of providing inadequate tissue oxygenation should be avoided. Respiratory acidosis may worsen even in patients receiving the necessary level of oxygenation, so $PaCO_2$ should be monitored. Excessive oxygenation should be prevented, although the respiratory acidosis that results is due more to $\dot{V}/\dot{Q}$ mismatching than to hypoventilation.

2. Bronchodilators—Bronchodilators are the most important initial therapy for COPD exacerbations. Selective β_2-adrenergic agonists in conjunction with anticholinergic agents (ipratropium) are preferred. Bronchodilators are usually given as inhaled treatments by nebulizer, usually every 15–30 min. Use of MDIs with a spacer and a larger than usual number of puffs (five or six) may yield comparable responses. Continuous nebulization of β_2-adrenergic agonists is performed less often due to side effects (tachycardia). It is unclear whether isomeric β_2-adrenergic agonists offer any meaningful benefit over standard (racemic) preparations. Tachycardia is more common in COPD exacerbations and may worsen with bronchodilators.

3. Corticosteroids—Steroids are a first-line therapy. All patients with frank or impending ventilatory failure due to COPD should be treated with intravenous corticosteroids until they improve. Then, doses of 60 mg or less of prednisone are prescribed. Dosing with 125 mg of methylprednisolone intravenously every 6 h was found in a large clinical trial to be efficacious. Smaller initial doses in less-ill hospitalized patients are often used to avoid steroid side effects. Conversion to oral prednisone therapy occurs when patients have cleared their bronchospasm, and prednisone is then tapered off or reduced to prior baseline level over 2 weeks based on response.

4. Parenteral β_2-agonist therapy—Parenteral β_2-agonists are a second-line therapy. Subcutaneous epinephrine is usually avoided due to the age of most patients and the risk of precipitating hypertension or coronary ischemia. Subcutaneous terbutaline may be given in single or multiple doses, although it offers little benefit over maximal inhaled β_2-agonist therapy. Side effects include tremor, anxiety, tachycardia, nausea, and emesis.

5. Intravenous magnesium—Because of lack of data, magnesium is not a recommended therapy in COPD exacerbation.

6. Methylxanthines—Methylxanthines are a second-line therapy. Intravenous aminophylline or theophylline may be of benefit for patients who are not on these agents. If patients are on these agents chronically, therapeutic levels should be targeted with supplemental doses as needed. Clinical trials vary as to the effectiveness of intravenous methylxanthines in COPD exacerbations. Because of marginal data for efficacy and frequent side effects (tremor, tachyarrhythmias, drug interactions), methylxanthines are usually reserved for intubated patients or patients who are not improving despite use of other therapies.

7. Antibiotics—Antibiotics are a first- to second-line agent in COPD exacerbations associated with increase in quantity or purulence of sputum. Their efficacy has been documented in clinical trials and suggested by meta-analysis reports. Patients with COPD often have chronic bronchitis, and bacterial "bronchitis" may represent chronic airway colonization rather than acute infection. However, there is a lower rate of hospitalization in patients with acute exacerbations of chronic bronchitis treated with empiric oral antibiotics. Standard agents such as sulfonamides, β-lactams, and macrolides should be employed first. Second-line agents (quinolones) should be reserved for known *Pseudomonas* or other resistant gram-negative organisms, when other regimens have failed, or based on drug interactions and allergies. Intravenous antibiotics may be needed for patients who have poor absorption due to acute illness. Oral agents can still be given through nasogastric tubes in intubated patients. Antiinfluenza agents such as neuraminidase inhibitors are indicated for the first 48 h of flu-like illness during times of active influenza in the community.

8. Anxiolytics—Benzodiazepines must be used with caution in a monitored setting as delineated for patients with asthma. Compared to these patients, intubated patients with COPD need large doses of benzodiazepines for sedation less often and histamine release from morphine is also less often an issue.

9. Neuromuscular blocking agents—In mechanically ventilated patients with COPD exacerbations, neuromuscular blocking agents are infrequently needed due to more profound typical respiratory muscle fatigue.

10. Noninvasive ventilation—NPPV is an evidence-based method of providing ventilatory support to patients with COPD exacerbations. Because of frequent do-not-intubate advanced directives for many of these patients, a noninvasive method is of particular use. Efficacy has been demonstrated in numerous clinical trials, with lower rates of infection and improved mortality compared to intubation and mechanical ventilation. Because of patient anxiety, mask discomfort, claustrophobia, requirements of sedation, and confusion, NPPV should be done only in monitored settings. NPPV is adjusted to provide an adequate V_T, respiratory rate, improvement of respiratory acidosis, and subjective improvement as previously described. In the setting of do-not-intubate advanced directives, NPPV may be provided to lethargic or obtunded patients as an alternative, although this should be avoided in patients with asthma (who rarely have do-not-intubate directives).

11. Mechanical ventilation—Patients with COPD who are in respiratory failure may require endotracheal intubation and mechanical ventilation. Compared to patients with asthma, ventilation is less difficult due to less severe elevations in airway resistance and more profound respiratory muscle fatigue. Large endotracheal tubes should be used to minimize resistance to airflow (7.5–9 mm internal diameter). Bronchodilators and other medications need to be maximized. Selected VTs, rates, and other settings are similar to those used in asthma and again are chosen to increase expiratory time and minimize intrinsic PEEP ("autoPEEP") and barotrauma. Permissive hypercapnea is needed less often. Care should be taken not to decrease the $PaCO_2$ below a patient's baseline outpatient $PaCO_2$ (known or estimated), as without mechanical ventilation this $PaCO_2$ cannot be sustained. The patient is assessed for liberation from mechanical ventilation when bronchospasm has improved, sedation needs are minimal, secretions are minimized, and respiratory muscle strength is adequate. If mechanical ventilation is prolonged, a tracheostomy may be of benefit.

12. Miscellaneous agents—Mucolytic agents (guaifenesin, *N*-acetylcysteine) are of unproven benefit as testing in clinical trials has been minimal. Although there is an appealing rationale for its use, *N*-acetylcysteine may cause bronchospasm and must be given with caution, if at all.

F. Chest Wall Disorders That Increase the Work of Breathing

Patients with kyphoscoliosis or other chest wall abnormalities who develop acute ventilatory failure will often respond to noninvasive ventilation, oxygen, and measures to increase sputum clearance and treat respiratory infections. Some patients who do not improve will opt for tracheostomy and long-term mechanical ventilation. Large pleural effusions (often malignant) are usually drained with intermittent thoracentesis or a chest tube. Pleurodesis can be performed chemically and/or surgically to prevent recurrence of effusion. Large pneumothoraces are evacuated by a chest tube and usually do not require surgical intervention. Rib fractures that impair ventilation are usually treated by fixation and/or intercostal nerve blocks.

G. Neuromuscular Coupling Defects and Respiratory Muscle Failure

Neuromuscular respiratory failure is easy to treat acutely. Disease-specific treatment considerations are outlined below and in Table 25–6.

1. Guillain-Barré Syndrome (GBS)—Plasmapheresis or intravenous immunoglobulin hasten recovery in GBS and may prevent respiratory failure. In refractory cases, both are often used. Steroids are of unproven benefit.

2. Myasthenia gravis—Plasmapheresis hastens recovery in acute myasthenia gravis. Thymectomy is rarely used acutely. Steroids and other immunosuppressants are of less proven benefit but are frequently employed.

3. Organophosphate (insecticide) overdose—Pralidoxime and atropine are effective anticholinergic agents that improve muscle function and decrease secretions in organophosphate overdose. Secretion clearance is often a major problem.

4. Antitoxins—Antitoxins are available for botulism and most toxins associated with neuromuscular blocking defects (snake bites, etc). The use of botulinum antitoxin may not shorten the duration of mechanical ventilation if respiratory failure develops but improves other organ dysfunctions.

5. Chest physiotherapy, IPPB, and other measures—Atelectasis and ineffective clearance of sputum and saliva are common in neuromuscular processes. Good oral care, careful observation, positioning, and frequent suctioning are key measures. IPPB with a bedside device may be helpful in treating and preventing atelectasis, whereas chest physiotherapy may aid established lobar atelectasis and improve sputum clearance. Bronchodilators may improve mucociliary function and improve sputum clearance. Rotating inflation beds may decrease atelectasis and improve sputum clearance in neurologically impaired patients.

6. Noninvasive positive pressure ventilation—NPPV may be a useful therapy in neuromuscular coupling defects if the patient is alert and able to protect the airway. It is less useful in GBS and botulism due to the slow improvement in respiratory dysfunction in these two illnesses. The chronic use of NPPV has been demonstrated to decrease mortality in decompensated ALS, and to be of benefit in other motor neuron diseases and myopathies.

7. Mechanical ventilation—If needed, mechanical ventilation is usually straightforward in patients with myopathies and neuromuscular coupling defects. A tracheostomy will decrease upper airway complications and improve comfort if intubation is needed for more than 2 weeks. Atelectasis may be difficult to prevent even with PEEP or large VTs due to diaphragm weakness.

Prognosis

A. Failure of Central Drive

Opiate and other substance overdoses are usually not lethal if caught early, brain hypoxia is avoided, and abstinence occurs. Aspiration pneumonias during obtundation can be associated with acute lung injury and a mortality rate of 30–40%. Obesity hypoventilation usually has a poor prognosis if recurrent respiratory failure occurs and patients are unable to lose weight or comply with medical therapy. Brain stem injury to the respiratory center from stroke, trauma, or tumor has a poor prognosis for recovery. Brain stem compression due to mass occupying lesions or increased intracranial pressure may be relieved with surgical therapy. Meningitis and encephalitis are usually treatable without chronic impairment in respiratory function if the patient survives with a return to consciousness. Poliomyelitis was once a frequent cause of chronic ventilatory failure in the United States, but is now rare. In developing countries polio remains associated with a poor prognosis for recovery when respiratory failure develops.

B. NEUROMUSCULAR COUPLING DEFECTS

When mechanical ventilation is required, ventilator dependence in GBS and botulism often lasts for months. Ventilatory failure is < 10% in myasthenia gravis and only transient mechanical ventilation is usually required. In all of these conditions, prognosis for recovery is excellent and mortality is low. Respiratory failure is uncommon in Eaton–Lambert syndrome, but carries a poor prognosis if present. Patients with ALS have a variable prognosis after an episode of ventilatory failure. Home-based NPPV improves survival in ALS if patients accept it. Many patients also benefit from home mechanical ventilation through a tracheostomy, which appears to be the safest ventilatory strategy; their prognosis is thereafter dependent on the frequency of pneumonia and progression to dementia. ALS patients who develop acute ventilatory failure and who thereafter refuse any ventilatory assistance have a poor prognosis and usually die of respiratory failure in the subsequent year. Critical illness polyneuropathy may take months to resolve and can lead to extended rehabilitation stays, but overall prognosis for recovery is good.

C. INCREASED WORK OF BREATHING DUE TO LUNG AND CHEST WALL DISEASE

Acute ventilatory failure from asthma has a good prognosis with supportive care, although patients may die in the prehospital setting during subsequent exacerbations due to rapid worsening of bronchospasm. Patients with severe COPD and their first episode of respiratory failure can generally be weaned off mechanical ventilation, but their long-term prognosis is poor if they develop recurrent episodes of ventilatory failure and are not candidates for lung transplant. Patients with kyphoscoliosis without cor pulmonale have an average survival of 9 years after their first episode of ventilatory failure, although patients with cor pulmonale have an average survival of only 1 year without chronic home ventilation.

D. FAILURE OF RESPIRATORY MUSCLES

The rare cases of acute myositis that lead to ventilatory failure have a good prognosis. Neuromuscular blockade-associated myopathy may take weeks to months to resolve, but the overall prognosis is good. Patients with muscular dystrophies with acute ventilatory failure usually have chronic ventilatory failure, and will need chronic home ventilation through a tracheostomy if that is consistent with their wishes. They may live for many years on home ventilation, although quality of life is generally poor.

Behrendt CE: Acute respiratory failure in the United States: incidence and 31-day survival. Chest 2000;118:1100. [PMID: 11035684]. (A good epidemiological picture based on 61,000 patients.)

Brochard L: Noninvasive ventilation for acute respiratory failure. JAMA 2002;288:932. [PMID: 12190351]. (A review of this evolving treatment and its impact to decrease ICU infections, lower length of stay, and improve survival.)

Huh M, Davis W: Intravenous immune globulin versus plasma exchange in Guillain-Barré syndrome. N Engl J Med 1992;327:817. [PMID: 1501670]. (Comparison of these treatments for Guillain-Barré syndrome.)

Levy BD, Kitch B, Fanta CH: Medical and ventilatory management of status asthmaticus. Intensive Care Med 1998;24:105. [PMID: 9539066]. (Treatment options for acute asthma are discussed in detail.)

Madison JM, Irwin RS: Chronic obstructive pulmonary disease. Lancet 1998;352:467. [PMID: 9708769]. (Treatment for acute COPD exacerbation and its controversies are highlighted.)

Martin TJ et al: A randomized, prospective evaluation of noninvasive ventilation for acute respiratory failure. Am J Respir Crit Care Med 2000;161:807. [PMID: 10712326]. (An important study where noninvasive ventilation lowered the need for intubation.)

Niewoehner DE et al: Effect of systemic glucocorticoids on exacerbations of chronic obstructive pulmonary disease. Department of Veterans Affairs Cooperative Study Group. N Engl J Med 1999;340:1941. [PMID: 10379017]. (A careful study showing a benefit for short courses of systemic glucocorticoids for COPD exacerbations.)

Provencio JJ, Bleck TP, Connors AF Jr: Critical care neurology. Am J Respir Crit Care Med 2001;164:341. [PMID: 11500331]. (Important aspects of neurology in ICU patients.)

Sivak ED, Shefner JM, Sexton J: Neuromuscular disease and hypoventilation. Curr Opin Pulmon Med 1999;5:355. [PMID: 10570736]. (Disease entities, clinical presentations, and treatment are presented.)

Stoller JK: Clinical practice. Acute exacerbations of chronic obstructive pulmonary disease. N Engl J Med 2002;346:988. [PMID: 11919309]. (Recent treatment updates for COPD.)

Chronic Ventilatory Failure

Enrique Fernandez, MD

ESSENTIALS OF DIAGNOSIS

- *Insidious nonspecific symptoms include headache and memory impairment.*
- *Elevated P_{CO_2} on blood gas analysis is a late finding and is necessary for diagnosis.*
- *Vital capacity and maximal inspiratory pressure may help with etiology and severity.*
- *Important causes include neuromuscular disease, chronic obstructive pulmonary disease (COPD), and central hypoventilation.*

General Considerations

The term **respiratory failure** specifies the failure of the entire integrated respiratory system, including the lungs, chest wall, and brain, to maintain adequate oxygenation of arterial blood and proper elimination of carbon dioxide (Figure 26–1). Ultimately, respiratory failure interferes with respiration at the cellular level. Somewhat arbitrary values for arterial oxygen tension (PaO_2) and arterial carbon dioxide tension ($PaCO_2$) define respiratory failure, as gas exchange at the tissue level cannot be easily measured. These values are influenced by altitude of residence, age, and metabolic processes as well as by breathing itself. At altitude, oxygenation and $PaCO_2$ are both lower than at sea level. With advanced age, oxygenation worsens and P_{CO_2} may rise slightly. Respiratory failure for a patient at rest at sea level is defined by a PaO_2 or $PaCO_2$ far outside the normal range: usually below 60 mm Hg for PaO_2 or above 45–50 mm Hg for $PaCO_2$.

Ventilatory failure is generally diagnosed by the presence of an arterial P_{CO_2} above 45 mm Hg. This may result from a decreased central nervous system respiratory drive to breathe or be secondary to impaired function of the respiratory muscles and/or mechanical abnormalities of the chest wall. Most often, however, ventilatory failure is caused by diseases affecting the lung mechanics, such as chronic obstructive lung disease (Figure 26–1). Hypoxemia in the setting of ventilatory failure results from low alveolar oxygen tension (PaO_2) and worsens with increasing arterial carbon dioxide tension ($PaCO_2$). Progressive worsening of ventilation (progressive hypoventilation), even in the absence of intrinsic lung disease, will not only increase arterial $PaCO_2$ but also decrease alveolar (PaO_2) and arterial (PaO_2) oxygen tension.

The **alveolar gas equation** relates ventilatory failure to hypoxemia, as an increased $PaCO_2$ has a reciprocal relation to PaO_2 [Appendix, Eq. (1)]. A derivative of this equation, the **alveolar–arterial oxygen difference** [Appendix, Eq. (2)], should be used at the bedside to distinguish ventilatory failure from hypoxemic respiratory failure in which ventilation is preserved but oxygen levels are low. **Hypoxemic respiratory failure** is usually acute and is caused by conditions such as pneumonia, acute respiratory distress syndrome (ARDS), or pulmonary embolism (see Chapter 15).

Ventilatory respiratory failure, the inability to excrete adequate carbon dioxide, may be acute, chronic, or both. In chronic ventilatory failure, carbon dioxide (CO_2) retention is slow and progresses over months or years, allowing the body to use compensatory mechanisms to diminish harmful effects. Metabolic compensation (HCO_3 retention through the kidneys) restores the pH of the blood toward normal. For example, the patient with chronic ventilatory failure may have a $PaCO_2$ of 60 mm Hg or more, and live comfortably at home for years, whereas a rapid rise to a $PaCO_2$ of 60 mm Hg is associated with changes in mental status and the need for prompt medical evaluation.

Pathogenesis

Hypoxemia may be caused by a shunt, ventilation–perfusion ($\dot{V}/\dot{Q}$) mismatching, or hypoventilation.

A. SHUNT

A shunt can be thought of as blood flowing past a nonventilated collection of alveoli, defined as the acinus or gas exchange unit. With a shunt, the blood is not oxygenated and CO_2 is not removed. A total shunt is defined as perfusion maintained without any ventilation, such as seen in an intracardiac defect or arteriovenous malformation.

B. VENTILATION–PERFUSION MISMATCHING

Abnormalities in oxygenation often characterize ventilation–perfusion mismatching (low $\dot{V}/\dot{Q}$). With lung

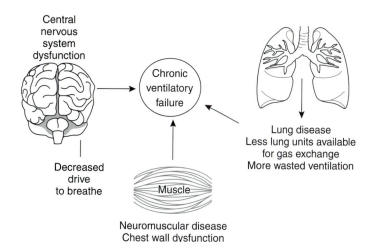

Figure 26–1. Mechanisms of chronic ventilatory failure.

disease, regional variations in ventilation and perfusion are substantial. Lung diseases such as interstitial lung diseases and pneumonia all have areas of $\dot{V}/\dot{Q}$ mismatching with low $\dot{V}/\dot{Q}$ and hypoxemia. Totally matched ventilation–perfusion means that each **acinus** (gas exchange unit) receives exactly the right amount of ventilation to oxygenate the hemoglobin and remove carbon dioxide. Each ideal alveolus would receive equal portions of alveolar ventilation ($\dot{V}A$), estimated at 4.5 L/min, and alveolar perfusion, which averages 5 L/min. The ideal lung would therefore have a $\dot{V}A/\dot{Q}$ of 4.5/5 or 0.9, and each acinar unit would have a $\dot{V}A/\dot{Q}$ 0.9 as well.

Due to ventilation–perfusion ($\dot{V}/\dot{Q}$) mismatching and shunting of blood through bronchial arteries, however, the PaO_2 is always lower than the ideal PAO_2. A normal difference between alveolar and arterial oxygen tension, the **[P(A–a)O$_2$] difference or gradient** [Appendix, Eq. (2)], is about 10 mm Hg in a normal young individual and widens with age, up to 30 mm Hg, in a 70-year-old healthy subject. Use of this calculation is an excellent bedside tool to help formulate a differential diagnosis [Appendix, Eq. (2)] to separate diseases causing hypoxemia due to alveolar dysfunction (such as pulmonary embolism, pneumonia, or ARDS) from those of hypoventilation.

C. HYPOVENTILATION

Carbon dioxide (CO_2) is continuously produced by tissues and excreted by the lungs. Three factors determine the level of CO_2 in the blood, or $PaCO_2$: (1) **carbon dioxide production** by the tissues, (2) **minute ventilation** [breaths per minute times tidal volume (VT)], which is the volume of each breath, and (3) the amount of **dead space,** VD/VT.

Carbon dioxide production depends on metabolic rate, which is approximately 200 mL/min for a healthy individual. Metabolic rate increases from muscular activity, and rises 7% for each °F rise in body temperature (13% for each °C rise in body temperature). When the brain's respiratory center control is normal, $PaCO_2$ is maintained close to 40 mm Hg by increasing the breathing rate or VT as needed (autoregulation), despite wide fluctuations in production of CO_2. However, increased production of CO_2 from fever or seizures can cause a large increase in arterial $PaCO_2$ for patients with minute ventilation limited by neuromuscular or obstructive lung disease.

For each breath, the gas that does not contact the circulation is the **dead space**. Dead space units (high $\dot{V}/\dot{Q}$) do not primarily cause hypoxemia but may lead to increased $PaCO_2$ [Appendix, Eq. (3)]. **Anatomic dead space** refers to the gas that remains in the large airways and is part of normal ventilation. **Physiological dead space** (VD/VT) includes anatomic dead space plus overventilated lung units that lack blood flow. Although people with normal lungs can increase respiratory effort to compensate for any VD or "wasted" ventilation, patients with limited lung function cannot. Physiological VD is often high for persons with severe lung disease such as chronic obstructive lung disease. Normal VD is < 30% of a breath; ventilation is > 70% efficient. In the patient with severe lung disease the VD may be increased to 60–70% of each breath and ventilation is only 40% efficient or less. Under these conditions, ventilation is grossly inefficient and retention of CO_2 may ensue. Conditions causing this type of ventilatory failure (hypoventilation) are shown in Table 26–1.

Table 26–1. Causes of ventilatory failure (hypoventilation).

Impaired ventilatory control	Landry–Guillain–Barré syndrome[1,2]
Idiopathic	Polyneuropathies associated with lupus or polyarteritis
Primary alveolar hypoventilation (Ondine's curse)	Toxins (lead, thallium, triorthocresyl phosphate)
Structural	Saxitoxin
Brain stem infarction or neoplasm	Infectious, diabetes mellitus, chronic alcoholism,
Functional	idiopathic
Obesity–hypoventilation syndrome	Neuromuscular junction
Myxedema	Myasthenia gravis[2]
Drugs (narcotics, sedatives, metabolic abnor-	Botulism[1]
malities, metabolic alkalosis)	Eaton–Lambert syndrome[1]
Chest wall abnormalities	Tick paralysis
Kyphoscoliosis (> 100°)	Black widow spider bite
Thoracoplasty	Organophosphate poisoning[1]
Fibrothorax	Antibiotic toxicity
Neuromuscular disease	Muscle
Upper motor neuron (any lesion in the cortex, brain	Progressive/dystrophies
stem, spinal cord)	Muscular dystrophies[2]
Trauma[1]	Myotonic dystrophy[2]
Space-occupying lesions	Myopathy
Tumor[2]	Polymyositis/dermatomyositis[2]
Syringomyelia[2]	Other collagen vascular diseases[2]
Multiple sclerosis[2]	Malnutrition[2]
Quadriplegia	Acid maltase deficiency
Lower motor neuron	Carnitine palmityltransferase deficiency
Anterior horn lesions	Endocrine[2] (exogenous steroids, hypoactivity or
Poliomyelitis[2]	hyperactivity of the thyroid, adrenal, and pituitary
Amyotrophic lateral sclerosis[2]	glands)
Werdig-Hoffman disease	Metabolic (electrolyte and acid–base disturbances, hypoxemia)
Spinal muscular atrophies	**Airway obstruction**
Postpolio syndrome	Upper airway
Peripheral nerves	Tracheal stenosis[2]
Trauma	Laryngeal or nasal polyps[2]
Diaphragmatic paralysis[2]	Obstructive sleep apnea[2]
Nutritional polyneuropathy[2] (beriberi)	Tonsillar hypertrophy[2]
Critical illness polyneuropathy[2]	Lower airway
Lyme disease	Chronic obstructive pulmonary disease[1,2]

[1]Leads to acute respiratory failure.
[2]Leads to chronic respiratory failure and superimposed acute exacerbations.

Rossi A, Poggi R, Roca J: Physiologic factors predisposing to chronic respiratory failure. Respir Care Clin North Am 2002;8:379. [PMID: 12481963]. (The concepts of lung and chest wall/muscle physiology are discussed in further detail.)

D. RESPIRATORY MUSCLE FUNCTION AND RESPIRATORY FAILURE

Neuromuscular diseases are accompanied by a variable degree of involvement of the inspiratory and expiratory muscles of respiration. Respiratory muscle weakness is a well-recognized cause of respiratory failure.

Weakness of inspiratory muscles affects the ability to increase minute ventilation in response to increased ventilatory demands from conditions such as fever or infection. The normal response to high ventilatory demands is tachypnea (increased respiratory rate), which enhances the work of breathing by increasing dead space ventilation. With inspiratory muscle weakness, there are also reductions in VT and in vital capacity (VC), which predispose to atelectasis and to further increases in ventilatory demand and work of breathing.

Weakness of expiratory muscles impairs cough effectiveness and clearance of secretions. There is less impact on respiratory mechanics and ventilatory function, because the elastic recoil of the stretched chest wall and lung tissue provides the principal driving force for expiratory flow. Complications arise with weakness of the upper airways and bulbar musculature. These include paresis of laryngeal and glottic muscles, which diminish effective swallowing and coughing. Weakness of the tongue and retropharyngeal structures causes positional airway obstruction, which leads to a higher risk of aspiration, atelectasis, and respiratory failure. If the process continues, the increased work of breathing accelerates CO_2 retention.

In addition to its primary role in neuromuscular disease, respiratory muscle dysfunction contributes to ventilatory failure in other diseases that predispose to hypercapnic respiratory failure. These include obstructive airway diseases such as COPD and chest wall deformities such as kyphoscoliosis. An alternate way to classify respiratory muscle dysfunction is by the mechanism of muscle fatigue. Muscle fatigue is defined as the loss of muscle capacity to develop force or shortening, reversible by rest. Muscle fatigue can involve problems with inadequate supply, compromised reserve, or increased demand. These are outlined in Table 26–2. Understanding these mechanisms promotes selection of clinical interventions to improve fatigue.

Macklem PT: Respiratory muscles: The vital pump. Chest 1980; 78:753. [PMID: 7428459]. (This is a detailed overview of respiratory muscle function.)

Rossi A, Poggi R, Roca J: Physiologic factors predisposing to chronic respiratory failure. Respir Care Clin North Am 2002; 8:379. [PMID: 12481963]. (The concepts of lung and chest wall/muscle physiology are discussed.)

Table 26–2. Reasons for muscle fatigue.

Excessive energy demand
  Sepsis
  Fever
  COPD
  Hyperthyroidism
Inadequate energy supply
  Diminished blood flow
  Anemia
  Lack of energy stores
  Increased work of breathing
    Increased resistance
    Decreased compliance
    Hyperventilation
    Suboptimal pattern of breathing
Diminished respiratory muscle strength
  Neuromuscular diseases
  Disuse (chronic mechanical ventilation)
  Malnutrition
  Hypomagnesemia
  Hypothyroid
  Hypokalemia
  Endotoxemia
  Aminoglycosides
  Paralytic drugs

Clinical Findings

A. SYMPTOMS AND SIGNS

Diagnosis is approached by first recognizing the presence of a condition predisposing to respiratory failure and then seeking clinical evidence of hypoxemia and/or hypercapnia. Because it is impossible to accurately assess PaO_2 or $PaCO_2$ by clinical means alone, it is critical for patients at risk for respiratory failure to move quickly and to check oxygen saturation and arterial blood gas. Although correlation between the severity of the underlying lung or muscular disease and the development of respiratory failure is not exact, it is important to elicit as much information as possible concerning the patient's history and current clinical status. Symptoms of CO_2 retention are extremely variable and correlate poorly with $PaCO_2$ level. If $PaCO_2$ increases rapidly, there is easily discernible impairment of consciousness; however, with chronic slowly progressive CO_2 retention, compensatory mechanisms make symptoms subtle. Morning headaches, memory impairment, and peripheral vasodilation with bounding pulses are common symptoms and signs. Tremor and asterixis are seen with severely elevated CO_2 levels.

Central cyanosis is the primary physical sign of hypoxemia. It can be detected when the level of hypoxemia is close to the level causing tissue damage (SaO_2 <70% and PaO_2 <40 mm Hg). Hypoxia produces a range of neurological manifestations, from mild confusion to coma, but because the differential diagnosis of confusion is broad, its clinical recognition is difficult. Signs of cor pulmonale including jugular venous distention and dependent edema that is not due to venous stasis, cirrhosis, or cardiomyopathy may be the primary clues to diagnosis. Finally, only the **arterial blood gases** will determine the diagnosis and degree of ventilatory failure.

Bedside observations provide important information about respiratory muscle fatigue (Table 26–3). The first clinical sign is an **increase in respiratory frequency,** with shallow V_{Ts}. Normal contraction of the diaphragm produces descent with displacement of the abdomen anteriorly. In contrast, if the diaphragm does not contract normally and the pleural pressure becomes negative via contraction of intercostals and thoracic accessory muscles, the diaphragm moves toward the head (cranially) and the abdomen moves inward with inspiration. This **"paradoxical" movement of the diaphragm** is an excellent clinical indicator that the diaphragm is working against a fatiguing load. **Respiratory alternans,** in which respiratory movements are abdominal for a few breaths, followed by a series of

Table 26–3. Physical findings of respiratory failure/inspiratory muscle fatigue.

Finding[1]	Clinical Correlate	Severity
Increase in respiratory rate with shallow tidal volume	Exercise intolerance ± sensation dyspnea	Mild
Drop in maximal inspiratory pressure (PI$_{max}$, NIF)		Moderate
Decrease in vital capacity		
Paradoxical movement of the diaphragm		
Respiratory alternans	Increase in PaCO$_2$	
Terminal fall in respiratory rate	Respiratory arrest	Severe

[1]Findings are ranked in order of increasing severity. Note that the changes of muscle dysfunction on examination occur early and the blood gas changes late, with more severe compromise.

breaths in which the respiratory movements take place predominantly by rib cage movements, is also a sign of fatigue. An increase in PaCO$_2$ follows abdominal paradox and respiratory alternans, but the development of severe acidemia (a low pH) is a late manifestation. Respiratory rate and minute ventilation fall only when respiratory arrest and death are imminent.

In many types of chronic respiratory failure, there are disease-specific clues on physical examination. For neuromuscular disorders, muscular atrophy and an ability to breathe deeply should be assessed. In amyotrophic lateral sclerosis (ALS), muscle fasciculations are characteristic. Severe kyphoscoliosis that can lead to respiratory failure is discernible from clinical observation alone. Severe COPD has accompanying weight loss, muscle wasting, hyperexpansion of the thorax, and prolonged expiration. The disorders causing loss of central drive lack associated physical examination clues and the patients generally appear surprisingly comfortable with their respiratory failure.

Cohen CA et al: Clinical manifestations of inspiratory muscle fatigue. Am J Med 1982;73:308. [PMID: 6812417]. (A focus on symptoms and signs of muscle fatigue.)

Rochester DF, Esau SA: Assessment of ventilatory function in patients with neuromuscular disease. Clin Chest Med 1994;15:751. [PMID: 7867289]. (Physical examination and laboratory parameters used in diagnosis of respiratory muscle dysfunction in neuromuscular disease.)

B. Diagnostic Studies

The two diagnostic tests that best correlate with imminent ventilatory failure are maximal inspiratory pressure and vital capacity. Measurement of **maximal inspiratory pressure** (PI$_{max}$) at the mouth is sometimes called the negative inspiratory force or NIF. A maximal inspiratory pressure of 90 cm H$_2$O is normal, and 30–50 cm H$_2$O is indicative of emerging respiratory failure. Values < 25 cm H$_2$O correlate well with hypercapnia. Measurement of **vital capacity** (VC) is less sensitive than PI$_{max}$ but is technically easier, and estimates the ventilatory reserve of the patient. As a rule of thumb for neuromuscular disease, a VC of 30–40 mL/kg indicates emerging respiratory failure. When VC is < 30 mL/kg, respiratory failure is established. In patients with ventilatory failure, a VC < 10–15 mL/kg (of ideal body weight) fails to allow adequate spontaneous ventilation. For a patient with progressive neuromuscular ventilatory failure, serial measurements of VC may anticipate the change in arterial blood gases and herald the need for respiratory support.

Other diagnostic techniques are less useful (Table 26–4). The **maximal voluntary ventilation** (MVV), the amount of air moved per minute at maximum patient effort, is quite effort dependent and therefore often overestimates the severity of muscle impairment. In ventilatory failure due to primary pulmonary disease the **physiological dead space** (VD/VT) has historically been a useful measurement [Appendix, Eq. (3)]. Because this requires measurements of expired gas that are not routinely performed, its use is now usually reserved for patients on long-term mechanical ventilation to ascertain if they are candidates for weaning. From a retrospective review of patients in respiratory failure, spontaneous respiration cannot be supported long term when the VD/VT ratio is > 0.6.

Diaphragm fluoroscopy can be used to evaluate diaphragm function looking for unilateral movement of a diaphragm upward with inspiration (paradox). It is insensitive in assessing weakness, especially when there is bilateral dysfunction.

Table 26–4. Diagnostic studies for chronic ventilatory failure.

Maximal inspiratory pressure (MIP or PI$_{max}$)
Vital capacity (VC)
Maximal voluntary ventilation (MVV), which is effort dependent
Dead space ventilation (VD/VT)
Diaphragm fluoroscopy
EMG accompanied by an EMG power spectral shift
Tension time index (TTI)
Arterial blood gases (ABG)
Electrolytes
Other: PO$_4$, Mg^{2+}, TSH, HCO$_3$, hematocrit

Other laboratory methods to detect muscle fatigue include the use of the electromyogram (EMG) and the tension time index (TTI). The EMG is made up of a spectrum of frequencies. With fatigue, the EMG power spectrum shifts with a characteristic increase in low-frequency power and a decrease in high-frequency power. Also, the relaxation rate of the inspiratory muscles falls, and the time constant of relaxation increases. Accessory muscles of respiration are recruited to respond to the increased load. The level of activation of inspiratory muscle groups leads to asynchronous movement of chest and abdomen. Although a powerful tool, this is rarely used clinically. The TTI is the product of inspiratory time divided by the total breathing cycle time and the transdiaphragmatic pressure per breath divided by maximal transdiaphragmatic pressure. Fatigue is indicated as this TTI increases, showing longer time needed to inspire and lower transdiaphragmatic pressures. Muscle endurance longer than 30 min is achieved with a TTI of 0.30 or shorter.

The **arterial blood gases** will determine the diagnosis and degree of the ventilatory failure with an elevated P_{CO_2} the hallmark of diagnosis. Oximetry is insensitive in detecting ventilatory failure as recruitment of muscles of respiration will occur to preserve oxygenation until the chronic ventilatory failure process is advanced. Because electrolyte and hormone abnormalities lead to muscle dysfunction, other laboratory tests that aid in the assessment of fatigue include potassium, phosphorus, magnesium, and thyroid-stimulating hormone (TSH) to check for hypothyroidism. Bicarbonate is elevated as renal compensation for hypercarbia. The hematocrit is sometimes elevated in the 50–60% range as a response to the hypoxemia.

Flaminiano LR, Celli BR: Respiratory muscle testing. Clin Chest Med 2001;22:661. [PMID: 11787658]. (Further detail on diagnostic testing is provided.)

Rochester DF, Esau SA: Assessment of ventilatory function in patients with neuromuscular disease. Clin Chest Med 1994; 15:751. [PMID: 7867289]. (Physical examination and laboratory parameters used in diagnosis of respiratory muscle dysfunction in neuromuscular disease.)

Roussos C: Function and fatigue of respiratory muscles. Chest 1985;88(Suppl):124S. [PMID: 3160552]. (Discussion of muscle physiology and interaction of muscle function and central nervous system.)

Vollestad NK, Sejersted OM: Biochemical correlates of fatigue. A Brief Review. Eur J Appl Physiol 1988;57:336. [PMID: 3286252]. (This paper discusses the pathophysiology of muscle biochemistry and fatigue.)

Differential Diagnosis

There are numerous diseases causing chronic respiratory failure. In general, these are categorized as restrictive, including both neuromuscular and chest wall disorders, intrinsic lung disease, or chronic problems with central drive to breathe (Figure 26–1).

If an obtunded mental status is not the result of respiratory failure or hypoxemia, other causes should be sought. These include stroke, dementia, depression, sleep deprivation, metabolic abnormalities such as hyponatremia, hypoglycemia, vitamin B_{12} deficiency, severe hypothyroidism, drug overdosing, meningitis from infection or carcinoma, or systemic infection. Table 26–1 is a comprehensive list of causes of chronic respiratory failure from abnormal drive, chest wall deformities, neuromuscular disease, and airway obstruction. The differential diagnosis of acute respiratory failure is discussed in Chapter 25.

Treatment

A. OVERVIEW

The first step in the treatment of chronic ventilatory failure is to treat the cause. Unfortunately, reversible processes in chronic ventilatory failure are uncommon. This contrasts with acute respiratory failure in which treatment can induce dramatic reversal in respiratory failure. Most of the time, hypoxemia is treated with supplemental oxygen, bronchospasm by the use of bronchodilators, and increases in metabolic rate by treatment of infection. When appropriate, maneuvers to improve cough or mobilize secretions are used. On rare occasions, patients may benefit from electrical pacing of the diaphragm. The ultimate treatment for most patients, however, is supplemental ventilation. Support can be from either negative-pressure or positive-pressure ventilators. Negative-pressure ventilators include the cuirass, pulmowrap, and iron lung. They expand the lung by creating a negative pressure surrounding the thorax leading to passive inflation of the lungs. Unfortunately, these devices are often cumbersome and impede patient mobility. Noninvasive positive-pressure ventilation (NIPPV) is the successful support of patients with chronic respiratory insufficiency using intermittent mechanical ventilation to the lungs without an artificial airway. The noninvasive positive-pressure ventilators are connected to the patient's airway through a facemask that covers the nose or nose and mouth. These have a prominent role in treating chronic respiratory failure.

NIPPV has many advantages and fewer complications compared to mechanical ventilation via a tracheostomy. The complications that are specific for ventilation through an endotracheal tube or a tracheostomy are shown in Table 26–5. In mechanical ventilation for acute respiratory failure, the higher rates of infection from endotracheal intubation are accompanied by longer intensive care unit (ICU) stays and higher mor-

Table 26–5. Complications of invasive
mechanical ventilation.

Related to the placement of the endotracheal tube
  Aspiration of gastric contents, gastric distention
  Hypotension
  Trauma of the teeth, pharynx, larynx, trachea
  Hypotension, decreased cardiac output, cardiac arrest
  Generalized seizures
  Ulceration, edema, hemorrhage, stenosis
  Barotrauma
Loss of airway defense mechanisms
  Inflammation
  Chronic bacterial colonization
  Impairment of clearance mechanisms
  Sinusitis (5–25% with nasal intubation)
  Nosocomial pneumonia (21%)
After removal of the endotracheal tube
  Sore throat, hoarseness
  Cough, sputum production, hemoptysis
  Upper airway obstruction caused by vocal cord dysfunction
    or laryngeal swelling
Complications due to tracheotomy
  Stomal infection, hemorrhage
  Intubation of a false lumen
  Mediastinitis
  Acute injury of trachea and surrounding structures:
    esophagus, blood vessels
Other complications
  Respiratory muscle dysfunction
  Respiratory muscle atrophy
  Increased work of breathing

tality compared to noninvasive ventilation; these same benefits are hypothesized for chronic use. Additional benefits of noninvasive ventilation include patient comfort and the ability to eat, speak, and communicate. Potential problems include gas delivery through an interface that allows air leak around the mask or through the mouth that diminishes the effectiveness of the system. The treatment goal is to provide adequate comfort while minimizing the occurrence of an air leak from the mask.

B. NONINVASIVE POSITIVE-PRESSURE VENTILATION

1. Mechanism—Ventilatory support benefits patients by reversing respiratory muscle fatigue. Respiratory muscle fatigue can be overt but is often "incipient," with the respiratory muscles working against a load that they can initially handle but are unable to sustain for a long period of time. It is thought that incipient fatigue induces only mild depletion of energy substrates, and the muscles' metabolic processes rapidly recover with "rest." However, for muscles subjected to a heavy work load, or under conditions of malnutrition or low cardiac output plus neuromuscular disease, recovery, which includes the restoration of glycogen stores, takes longer. Muscle fiber damage after prolonged exercise has been well demonstrated in humans and may contribute to chronic respiratory failure. Patients who need prolonged ventilatory support may need to regenerate severely damaged respiratory muscle fibers, which may explain why it takes a long time for respiratory "rest" on mechanical ventilation to achieve clinical improvement. The increased acidity in chronic respiratory failure inhibits ATP utilization, which further impairs muscle contraction. Other reversible factors that impair diaphragmatic contractility and facilitate fatigue include metabolic acidosis in addition to respiratory acidosis, hypophosphatemia, and hypomagnesemia.

How overnight noninvasive ventilation stabilizes and improves daytime gas exchange is somewhat controversial. First, in acute respiratory failure, resting (unloading) respiratory muscles seems to be the most important factor in patient improvement. In chronic ventilatory failure, however, respiratory center resetting seems to be the prime mechanism of improvement. Evidence for the resting theory of chronically fatigued respiratory muscles is provided by recording of the diaphragmatic EMG during assisted noninvasive ventilation showing a clear decrease of the electrical signal compared to the electrical activity recorded during spontaneous ventilation. Second, indices of respiratory strength and endurance improve following varying periods of noninvasive ventilation. Importantly, as few as 4–6 h of intermittent ventilation gradually decreases the $PaCO_2$ with improvement of symptoms such as headaches, hypersomnolence, and memory loss.

Noninvasive ventilation may also improve pulmonary mechanics by resetting the respiratory center to a lower $PaCO_2$. Patients with chronic respiratory insufficiency have decreased neural output from the brain's respiratory center to the respiratory muscles. The muscle work will adapt to a level that protects them from muscle fatigue, a phenomenon called "central fatigue." Resetting the respiratory center to a lower $PaCO_2$ level is likely the primary mechanism of improvement for patients with chronic ventilatory failure.

Chronic hypoventilation is highly exaggerated at night, especially during the deep stages of sleep. Increasing accumulation of bicarbonate, with respiratory center desensitization to CO_2 and worsening hypoventilation during the day compensate for this. Use of nocturnal ventilation improves nighttime hypoventilation, the body excretes the bicarbonate in the urine, and the respiratory center resets itself to a lower CO_2, with improvement of daytime hypercapnia. This is frequently seen, for example, in patients with sleep apnea presenting with cor pulmonale. Daytime assisted ventilation is as effective as nocturnal ventilation in reversing hypoventilation. Discontinuation of nocturnal ventilation produces slow deterioration of daytime gas exchange and return of symptoms, which again improve when nocturnal ventilation is reinstated. The improvement in gas exchange and symptoms with therapy does not necessarily mean there are parallel changes in respiratory muscle strength or endurance, changes in pulmonary mechanics, or improvement of microatelectasis.

Bellemare F, Bigland-Ritchie B: Central components of diaphragmatic fatigue assessed by phrenic nerves stimulation. J Appl Physiol 1987;62:1307. [PMID: 3571083]. (Central fatigue as a mechanism of chronic respiratory muscle dysfunction.)

Belman MJ et al: Efficacy of positive vs. negative pressure ventilation in unloading the respiratory muscles. Chest 1990;98:850. [PMID: 2119950]. (Comparison of positive- and negative-pressure ventilation for chronic ventilatory failure.)

Schonhofer B et al: Daytime mechanical ventilation in chronic respiratory insufficiency. Eur Respir J 1997;10:2840. [PMID: 9493671]. (The effects of noninvasive positive-pressure ventilation are not specific to nighttime sleep.)

2. Restrictive disorders—Assisted noninvasive ventilation is most effective in patients with restrictive chest wall diseases, in whom the primary abnormality is in the respiratory muscle pump, with the lungs being normal (Figure 26–1). The ventilator simply takes over the function of the failing respiratory muscle pump. Restrictive disorders that lead to chronic ventilatory failure include neuromuscular diseases and diseases of the chest wall (Table 26–1). Prevention of these underlying conditions is important and feasible. The number of patients with severe chest disorders decreases yearly, as survivors of polio epidemics gradually die and the mutilating thoracoplasties for tuberculosis treatment are no longer needed. Due to vaccination against poliomyelitis, curative treatment for tuberculosis, and better surgical procedures to correct and stabilize the vertebral spine, new patients with thorax deformities are now rare in the United States.

The progression of neuromuscular and chest wall diseases due to respiratory failure is usually slow. In general, it takes years before ventilatory failure is manifest. Amyotrophic lateral sclerosis is an exception, as this disease progresses to respiratory failure over months or a few years. Worsening dyspnea, orthopnea, a decrease in the ability to perform activities of daily living, or signs of cor pulmonale should prompt an in-depth evaluation for ventilation need. Advanced restrictive patients merit yearly evaluation for progression of chronic respiratory failure. The two diagnostic tests that correlate best with imminent ventilatory failure are vital capacity and maximal inspiratory pressure and these should be serially assessed.

Patients with restrictive diseases should be evaluated for hypoxemia and hypercapnia during sleep with the goal of starting nocturnal ventilation. Dysfunction will first manifest during rapid eye movement (REM) sleep, where the normal hypotonia of upper airways and chest wall muscles is enhanced, leading to increased airway resistance and further hypoventilation. Oxygen therapy alone can produce a significant rise in $PaCO_2$ with marked worsening of respiratory acidosis. Because of this, oxygen should be avoided as the sole treatment for patients with hypercapnic respiratory failure unless its use is carefully assessed during sleep with parameters of hypercapnia such as arterial PCO_2, endotracheal CO_2, or transcutaneous CO_2.

When patients with restrictive thoracic disease develop respiratory failure, the use of NIPPV should aim to achieve the following five goals: (1) improve and stabilize gas exchange, (2) improve sleep quality, (3) ameliorate daytime symptoms, (4) eliminate or improve cor pulmonale, and (5) extend survival.

The effects of nocturnal ventilation on daytime gas exchange are substantial in a variety of restrictive chest wall processes and neuromuscular diseases. Daytime PaO_2 has improved from 10 to 20 mm Hg and daytime $PaCO_2$ has improved from 7 to 15 mm Hg after 1 year of nocturnal positive pressure ventilation. The improvement in daytime $PaCO_2$ occurs in a period of a day to a few weeks, with slow reduction of the baseline $PaCO_2$. Once a plateau has been reached, $PaCO_2$ tends to remain stable, with further worsening depending on the natural history of the underlying disease.

Quality of life is improved in patients with restrictive disorders using NPPV. After a few nights of assisted ventilation, patients feel better; hypersomnolence and morning headache are the first symptoms to disappear. Comparison of the number of hospital days before and after initiation of nasal ventilation has shown a decrease from 34 days to 5 days for patients with scoliosis, from 31 days to 5 days for patients with sequelae of tuberculosis, and from 18 days to 7 days for patients with Duchenne's muscular dystrophy.

If ventilatory failure and its complications are untreated, life expectancy of patients with restrictive thoracic disorders is low. Scoliotic patients with chronic hypoventilation complicated by right heart failure have a 50% 1-year mortality with 80% dead at 2 years. Similarly, 50% of patients with ALS are dead 3 years after diagnosis, and only 10% are alive at 10 years. Use of nocturnal NIPPV has improved survival. The 5-year survival of postpolio patients on NIPPV is 94–100% and the 5-year survival of patients with kyphoscoliosis is 60–80%. Survival for Duchenne's muscular dystrophy has been 85% at 1 year and 73% at 5 years. Similar excellent results are seen with other thoracic restrictive diseases. In ALS, NPPV is less effective than ventilation through a tracheostomy: 5-year survival with NIPPV was only 32% (8 of 25 patients), whereas survival for those who received tracheal ventilation was 54% (27 of 50 patients). For ALS, NPPV may be less effective because patients have abnormal bulbar function, difficulty with secretions, and aspiration.

Temporary withdrawal of NIPPV in regular users shows that the earliest regression is the reappearance of nocturnal hypoventilation, mainly during REM sleep, followed by the reappearance of fatigue, frequent arousals, daytime hypersomnolence, or morning headache. Reinstallation of ventilation resolves symptoms and gas exchange abnormalities. These findings support the effectiveness of NPPV in improving chronic hypoventilation and symptoms in patients with restrictive thoracic disorders. Although NIPPV is clearly beneficial for these patients, the question of when to start assisted ventilation is less certain. There is no evidence that prophylactic use of NPPV prior to ventilatory failure is useful. Therefore timing is driven by symptoms and arterial blood gas (ABG) assessment.

A consensus conference has reviewed the rationale for NPPV in restrictive thoracic disorders and agreed to the following clinical indicators:

1. **Symptoms:** Fatigue, dyspnea, morning headache, hypersomnolence, nightmares, enuresis.
2. **Physiological criteria (one of the following):**
   a. $PaCO_2 \geq 45$ mm Hg (daytime).
   b. Nocturnal oximetry demonstrating oxygen saturation ≤88% for 5 consecutive minutes.
   c. For progressive neuromuscular disease, maximal inspiratory pressure ≤60 cm H_2O or FVC ≤50% predicted.

For symptomatic patients without daytime blood gas abnormalities, nocturnal monitoring of gas exchange is indicated, which includes continuous SpO_2 and ABGs early in the morning to detect nocturnal hypoventilation. Other probable but less clear-cut indicators for nocturnal ventilation include cor pulmonale, nocturnal oxygen desaturation for ≥10% of total monitoring time, repeated hospitalizations with bouts of acute respiratory failure, and failure to respond to continuous positive airway pressure (CPAP) alone when there is concomitant obstructive sleep apnea.

Baydur A et al: Long term non-invasive ventilation in the community for patients with musculoskeletal disorders: 46-year experience and review. Thorax 2000;55:4. [PMID:10607795]. (Long-term patient outcomes in chronic ventilatory failure from musculoskeletal disease.)

Bourke SC, Gibson GJ: Sleep and breathing in neuromuscular disease. Eur Respir J 2002;19:1194. [PMID:12108875]. (This is a recent review of pathophysiology and management.)

Cazzolli PA, Oppenheimer EA: Home mechanical ventilation for amyotrophic lateral sclerosis: nasal compared to tracheostomy intermittent positive pressure ventilation. J Neurol Sci 1996;139(Suppl):123. [PMID: 8899671]. (Case series with one patient out at 14 years including a discussion of bulbar involvement and invasive ventilation.)

Consensus Conference: Clinical indications for noninvasive positive pressure ventilation in chronic respiratory failure due to restrictive lung disease, COPD, and nocturnal hypoventilation: a consensus conference report. Chest 1999;116:521. [PMID: 10453883]. ("Expert" derived guidelines for treatment of chronic respiratory failure.)

Leger P et al: Nasal IPPV: long-term follow up in patients with severe respiratory insufficiency. Chest 1994;105:100. [PMID: 8275718]. (Another long-term follow-up series.)

Piper AT, Sullivan CE: Effects of long-term nocturnal nasal ventilation on spontaneous breathing during sleep in neuromuscular and chest wall disorders. Eur Respir J 1996;9:1515. [PMID: 8836668]. (Nocturnal positive-pressure ventilation induces improvements in respiratory drive during sleep and while awake.)

3. Chronic obstructive pulmonary disease—The effectiveness of noninvasive ventilation in patients with COPD is controversial. Unfortunately, for these patients treatment is mainly aimed at improving symptoms and at improving airway obstruction. In the Nocturnal Oxygen Therapy Trial (NOTT) and the Medical Research Council (MRC) trial, long-term oxygen therapy improved survival and is the only therapy proven to do this for patients with COPD. The benefit of oxygen is not immediate, however, and takes months to be noticeable (500 days in the MRC). During this early period, mortality was highly related to hypercapnia. It has thus been suggested that reducing the high $PaCO_2$ further improves survival.

Reviewing the pathophysiology of ventilatory failure in patients with severe COPD will help explain why noninvasive ventilation might benefit these patients. COPD is the most common cause of respiratory failure; its primary abnormality is in the lungs, but the respiratory muscle pump is also severely affected because of the **increase in the work of breathing** and the decreased capacity of the respiratory muscles to cope with the **increased ventilatory load**. Noninvasive ventilation might improve patients with COPD by aiding the work of the respiratory muscle pump. Complete abolition of electrical activity of the diaphragm is often more difficult to obtain in patients with COPD than in patients with restrictive syndromes.

The work of breathing is markedly elevated in patients with COPD due to increased airway resistance and hyperinflation, which may cause high intrinsic positive end expiratory pressure ($PEEP_i$). The O_2 cost of breathing in patients with COPD may be enormous, increasing from about 2.5 mL/min in healthy individuals up to 30 mL/min in patients with COPD (from 2% to 15% of total body oxygen consumption). Ventilatory reserve is markedly decreased; resting ventilation is about 40–50% of the patient's maximal ventilatory capacity whereas it is 5% in healthy subjects. Hyperinflation affects the inspiratory muscles, making them operate in an abnormal position of the length–tension curve. With progressive hyperinflation, the inspiratory muscles shorten and cannot produce maximal force. The higher the hyperinflation, the greater the decrease in PI_{max}. Hyperinflation also affects the geometry of respiratory muscles, especially the diaphragm. A flattened diaphragm with an infinite radius of curvature cannot generate any inspiratory force. Hyperinflation decreases the expansion of the lower rib cage and negatively affects elastic recoil of the thoracic cage.

Hypoxemia is a common finding in COPD due to wasted ventilation (dead space) and ventilation–perfusion mismatching. Gas exchange abnormalities are further enhanced during sleep in patients with severe COPD. In normal subjects, there is some degree of hypoventilation during sleep, due to blunting of the drive to breathe; there is a normal rise of $PaCO_2$ of up to 5–7 mm Hg. This is augmented in patients with COPD, with production of acidosis and secondary retention of bicarbonate and decreased chemosensitivity to CO_2. Hypoxic and hypercapnic drives to breathe are diminished in REM sleep. This alveolar hypoventilation and hypoxemia are particularly accentuated during REM sleep. In addition to gas exchange abnormalities, patients with COPD have impaired sleep quality, with shortened total sleep time and frequent arousals. Sleep-deprived normal subjects have blunted ventilatory response to both hypoxia and hypercapnia. Impaired sleep quality in patients with COPD may further reduce chemosensitivity to hypoxia and hypercapnia.

Potential beneficial effects of NPPV in patients with COPD include the following: (1) improvement in nocturnal hypoventilation, (2) lowered work of breathing by providing inspiratory assistance, (3) improvement in hypoxemia and acidosis with subsequent improvement in right heart failure, and (4) decreased stimulus for arousals and improvement in quality of sleep. Although all the pathophysiological abnormalities described related to impairment of inspiratory muscles and gas exchange defects during sleep have provided investigators with a rationale for using NIPPV in patients with COPD, there are conflicting results.

Patients with marked CO_2 retention benefit most from NIPPV. The degree of airway obstruction is not a criterion for ventilation unless there is a concomitant high $PaCO_2$. The NOTT study showed that supplemental oxygen alone improves sleep quality. Therefore, before initiating NPPV, patients with COPD should fail a trial of O_2 supplementation alone. Although the evidence is far from definitive, the Consensus statement has selected the following guidelines.

1. **Disease documentation:** Establish and document an appropriate diagnosis through history, physical examination, and diagnostic tests; ensure optimal management of the primary disorder and also optimal management of any underlying disorder.

2. **Indications for use of NIPPV:**
    a. Symptoms: fatigue, dyspnea, hypersomnolence, and morning headache
    b. Physiological criteria:
        i. $PaCO_2 \geq 55$ mm Hg
        ii. $PaCO_2$ 50–54 mm Hg and nocturnal desaturation $\leq 88\%$ for 5 continuous minutes while receiving oxygen therapy ≥ 2 L/min
        iii. $PaCO_2$ 50–54 mm Hg and two or more hospitalizations in a 12-month period related to recurrent episodes of hypercapnic respiratory failure

Other indications may include failure to respond to optimal medical therapy such as maximal bronchodilator therapy and/or steroids, O_2 supplementation if indicated, and failure to respond to CPAP when moderate-to-severe obstructive sleep apnea is present. It is important to reassess the patient after 2 months of therapy and continue only if compliance is adequate (>4 h/24 h) and the therapeutic response is favorable.

Consensus Conference: Clinical indications for noninvasive positive pressure ventilation in chronic respiratory failure due to restrictive lung disease, COPD, and nocturnal hypoventilation: a consensus conference report. Chest 1999;116:521. PMID: 10453883]. ("Expert"-derived guidelines for treatment of chronic respiratory failure.)

Medical Research Council Working Party Report: Long-term domiciliary oxygen therapy in chronic hypoxic cor pulmonale complicating chronic bronchitis and emphysema. Lancet 1981;1:681. [PMID: 6110912] (A landmark article on oxygen use and improved survival.)

Nocturnal Oxygen Therapy Trial Group: Continuous O_2 nocturnal oxygen therapy in hypoxemic chronic obstructive lung disease; a clinical trial. Ann Intern Med 1980;93:391. [PMID: 6776858]. (The other landmark article on oxygen use and improved survival.)

Sharp JT et al: Respiratory muscle function in patients with chronic obstructive pulmonary disease in relationship to disability and to respiratory therapy. Am Rev Respir Dis 1974;110:154. [PMID: 4613221]. (Pathophysiology of muscle function in patients with COPD.)

4. Hypoventilation disorders or obstructive sleep apnea—Respiratory failure from central hypoventilation is incompletely understood and poorly characterized. The hypoxic drive and the ventilatory response to CO_2 are decreased during sleep, especially during REM

Table 26–6. Disorders primarily associated
with nocturnal hypoventilation.

Central alveolar hypoventilation
Idiopathic central sleep apnea
Obesity–hypoventilation syndrome
Obstructive sleep apnea combined with COPD and pul-
monary hypertension or congestive heart failure, the over-
lap syndrome

---

sleep, in healthy subjects. This response is greatly exaggerated in patients, leading to nocturnal hypoventilation. COPD, chest wall deformities, or chronic restrictive lung diseases all predispose patients to hypoventilate
at night. In addition, several disorders are considered
primary disorders of hypoventilation (Table 26–6).

These conditions all exhibit alveolar hypoventilation
unexplained by primary lung or muscle disease and are
exacerbated during sleep. Diagnostic workup should
start with history, examination, and blood gases.
Chronic alveolar hypoventilation is only rarely of adult
onset and almost always requires ventilation. Persons
with central sleep apnea, obesity–hypoventilation syndrome, or the overlap syndrome present with sleepiness
as the central symptom and thus their diagnostic algorithm usually includes a sleep study after the ABG. In
treating these conditions, supplemental oxygen, respiratory center stimulants, CPAP, and assisted ventilation
have all been used. For the majority (~60%) of these,
treatment targeted at the sleep disorder with oxygen
(for central sleep apnea) or CPAP (for obstructive or
central sleep apnea) is adequate, as confirmed by repeat
ABG showing improvement in daytime P_{CO_2}.

The role of NPPV in treating these disorders is still
poorly defined. Compliance with NPPV requires patient motivation, but this has improved with newer
mask and machine technology. CPAP is often the treatment of choice for obstructive sleep apnea. If in spite of
CPAP use the patient progresses to respiratory failure,
initiation of NPPV can be considered to improve
symptoms and hypoventilation. Only a minority of patients (those with obesity–hypoventilation syndrome or
obstructive or central sleep apnea unresponsive to
CPAP alone) require NIPPV. NPPV is therefore indicated in patients who have failed to respond to other
specific treatments, including respiratory center stimulants, weight loss, and supplemental oxygen.

Berger KI et al: Obesity hypoventilation syndrome as a spectrum of
respiratory disturbances during sleep. Chest 2001;120:1231.
[PMID: 11591566]. (An important and interesting classification of this confusing topic.)

Consensus Conference: Clinical indications for noninvasive positive pressure ventilation in chronic respiratory failure due to
restrictive lung disease, COPD, and nocturnal hypoventilation: a consensus conference report. Chest 1999;116:521.
PMID: 10453883]. ("Expert"-derived guidelines for treatment of chronic respiratory failure.)

Martin TJ, Sanders MH: Chronic alveolar hypoventilation: a review for the clinician. Sleep 1995;18:617. [PMID: 8560127].
(A comprehensive view of the clinical presentation associated
with sleep-disordered breathing and other pulmonary disorders.)

Mehta S, Hill NS: Noninvasive ventilation, state of the art. Am J
Respir Crit Care Med 2001;163:540. [PMID: 11179136]. (A
comprehensive discussion of indications for noninvasive ventilation, types of devices, application procedures, and personnel time.)

Prognosis

Prognosis in chronic respiratory failure depends on the
underlying disease. Prognosis is particularly poor for
ALS compared to other neuromuscular diseases. Prognosis for COPD is worst when COPD is accompanied
by cor pulmonale. Little is known about prognosis
from central hypoventilation disorders as these have not
been systematically investigated. With treatment, patients with many of the disorders that cause chronic respiratory failure can live for decades.

Appendix: Equations

A. EQUATION 1: ALVEOLAR GAS EQUATION

$$P_{AO_2} = P_{IO_2} - \frac{P_{aCO_2}}{RQ} \tag{1}$$

or

$$P_{AO_2} = [F_{IO_2} \times (P_B - P_{H_2O})] - \frac{P_{aCO_2}}{RQ} \tag{2}$$

Assuming barometric pressure (P_B) = 747 mm Hg,
water vapor pressure (P_{H_2O}) = 47 mm Hg (at 37°C),
and respiratory quotient (RQ) = 0.8, then for a subject
breathing room air (F_{IO_2} = 0.21) at sea level, Eq. (2) becomes

$$P_{AO_2} = 147 - \frac{P_{aCO_2}}{0.8} \tag{3}$$

B. EQUATION 2: THE ALVEOLAR–ARTERIAL [(A–a)O₂] DIFFERENCE (GRADIENT)

(A–a)O_2 is $P_{AO_2} - P_{aO_2}$, with P_{aO_2} the arterial oxygen
measured on alveolar blood gas and P_{AO_2} the gas reaching the alveolus.

For example, a sleepy 18-year old comes to the
emergency room with a history of "trying" a new drug

but can't recall the name. If $PaCO_2$ is 50 and PaO_2 is 75, the A–a oxygen gradient is

$$PAO_2 - PaO_2 = 84.7 - 75$$
$$= 9.7$$

which is normal. Even though the oxygen level appears low, this hypoxemia is from hypoventilation, not ventilation–perfusion mismatching from pneumonia or pulmonary embolism.

C. EQUATION 3. PHYSIOLOGICAL DEAD SPACE VENTILATION

A normal range is 0.20–0.40:

$$VD/VT = [PaCO_2 - PECO_2]/PaCO_2$$

where $PaCO_2$ is arterial gas measurement of CO_2 and $PECO_2$ is expired gas measurement of CO_2.

For example, if $PECO_2 = 40$ mm Hg and $PECO_2 = 18$ mm Hg

$$VD/VT = (40 - 18)/40$$
$$= 22/40$$
$$= 0.55$$

which is elevated to a range that makes independent breathing difficult.

Mechanical Ventilation: Invasive and Noninvasive

27

Michael B. Fessler, MD, & Carolyn H. Welsh, MD

ESSENTIALS OF DIAGNOSIS

- Positive pressure mechanical ventilation is used to treat acute and chronic respiratory failure.
- It is important to be alert for complications of mechanical ventilation including barotrauma, ventilator-induced lung injury, and hemodynamic compromise.
- Early assessment of readiness to wean reduces duration of ventilation.
- Use of noninvasive ventilation lessens infection and duration of time in intensive care and improves mortality.

General Considerations

Mechanical ventilation has resulted in profoundly improved survival from acute and chronic respiratory failure. Nevertheless, growing awareness of the potential for ventilators to worsen patient outcomes has increased the necessity to understand subtle points of patient/ventilator interactions. In this chapter the central issues of mechanical ventilation including indications, modes, settings, complications, patient monitoring, weaning, and noninvasive ventilation will be discussed.

Mechanical ventilation in the intensive care unit (ICU) is delivered under positive pressure in contrast to normal human breathing in which inspiration induces negative pressure in the thorax. This makes the complications of barotrauma and hypotension predictable. To achieve ventilation, rate, tidal volume (V_T), fraction of inspired oxygen (F_{IO_2}), and positive end-expiratory pressure (PEEP) are selected, as discussed in the section on ventilator setting below. It is useful to track the product of V_T and rate, the minute ventilation ($\dot{V}_E$), to assess for complications and readiness to wean. A normal $\dot{V}_E$ is less then 10 L/min.

Indications for Mechanical Ventilation

With the exception of apnea, there are no absolute clinical indicators for mechanical ventilation, so decisions must be individualized. In acute respiratory failure associated with disorders such as chronic obstructive pulmonary disease (COPD), a proven intermediary role for noninvasive positive-pressure ventilation (NIPPV) has clarified the indications for intubation to ventilate (invasive positive-pressure ventilation, IPPV). Importantly, mechanical ventilation does not mandate endotracheal intubation, nor does intubation require mechanical ventilation. For example, endotracheal tube placement may be life saving in a case of impending upper airway obstruction or high risk for aspiration, without need for a ventilator.

General indications for IPPV are listed in Table 27–1. With the availability of both high-flow oxygen sources and NIPPV, isolated oxygenation failure as a reason for IPPV is rare. Intubation for hypoxia is indicated when NIPPV has failed or is contraindicated. Contraindications include inability to protect the airway, patient intolerance, and hemodynamic instability/cardiac arrest. For hypercapnic ventilatory failure, the absolute value of arterial carbon dioxide (CO_2) tension/pressure (Pa_{CO_2}) is less important than either the corresponding arterial pH (indicating acid/base compensation) or the trend in Pa_{CO_2} (indicating clinical trajectory). Both the inability to "protect" the airway from aspiration and the need for pulmonary toilet for excess secretions are indications for intubation but not ventilation, and are not listed in Table 27–1.

Pierson DJ: Indications for mechanical ventilation in adults with acute respiratory failure. Respir Care 2002;47:249. [PMID: 11874605]. (Comprehensive discussion of the evolving indications for mechanical ventilation in specific respiratory disorders.)

Modes of Mechanical Ventilation

A "mode" of mechanical ventilation refers to the program by which the ventilator interacts with the patient,

Table 27–1. Indications for mechanical ventilation.

Apnea
Oxygenation deficit refractory to other interventions
Acute/impending ventilatory ("hypercapnic") failure

---

the relationship between the possible types of breaths allowed by the ventilator, and the variables that define inspiration. Inspiration is defined by three variables: trigger, limit, and cycle. *Trigger* is the change detected by the ventilator that causes inspiration to begin; *limit* is the value that cannot be exceeded during inspiration (volume, pressure, or flow); and *cycle* is the value that when reached, terminates inspiration. Using these definitions, three breath types are possible: full ventilator control (mandatory), partial ventilator control (assisted), and full patient control (spontaneous).

Using these variables, the modes of mechanical ventilation are easily understood. The most commonly used modes in adults are volume limited. In *controlled mechanical ventilation* (CMV), there is no patient triggering; rather, all breaths are ventilator triggered, limited, and cycled. CMV is used in patients who make no respiratory effort, such as those with neuromuscular paralysis. In *assist/control ventilation* (ACV), by contrast, the clinician sets a minimum rate and tidal volume. The patient can trigger the ventilator at a more rapid rate, and will receive the set volume each time. In *intermittent mandatory ventilation* (IMV), ventilator-limited (ie, volume or pressure) breaths are similarly delivered at a set (minimum) rate, but the patient can breathe spontaneously by triggering a demand valve between machine-limited breaths. In current ventilators IMV is modified to *synchronized IMV* (SIMV), in which the ventilator synchronizes machine breaths with patient effort.

In the patient who does not trigger the ventilator, CMV, ACV, and SIMV are qualitatively identical. In assist control, there is a greater potential for respiratory alkalosis and intrinsic PEEP (PEEP$_i$), or "autoPEEP," persistent positive alveolar pressure at end expiration, often with associated hyperinflation, due to delivery of full machine breaths for all patient efforts. The hyperinflation results from insufficient time for the lungs to empty. Although SIMV has been associated with less alkalosis than the ACV mode in two trials, it may involve increased patient work of breathing. ACV and SIMV are about equal in popularity nationwide, with use dependent on institutional preference.

In principle, machine breaths in the assist/control or IMV modes can be defined by a set volume or pressure. If volume control is selected, the tidal volume is fixed, and airway pressure varies with the resistance and compliance of the patient's lungs and chest wall (see *Respiratory Mechanics* below). If pressure control is selected, a fixed inspiratory pressure level is maintained for a set inspiratory time or inspiration:expiration (I:E) ratio, and tidal volume and flow vary with patient effort and mechanics.

No well-designed prospective trial has shown an important clinical difference in outcome between pressure- and volume-controlled ventilation. Supporters of volume-controlled ventilation point out that a minimal minute ventilation is ensured, whereas supporters of pressure-controlled ventilation point out that airway pressure is fixed below a protective ceiling despite changes in respiratory mechanics and flow varies with patient demand. A third important difference is that in volume ventilation, sudden decreases in compliance (eg, pneumothorax) present as dramatic elevations in airway pressure, whereas in pressure ventilation, such events present more subtly, with hypoventilation. For the same reason, PEEP$_i$, by decreasing the pressure gradient driving inspiratory airflow, may present as hypoventilation in pressure modes. Consequently, in pressure-controlled ventilation, measures to increase alveolar ventilation, such as increasing respiratory rate, may paradoxically worsen ventilation by aggravating PEEP$_i$ and directly increasing dead space ventilation.

Two additional common modes of ventilation are *continuous positive airway pressure* (CPAP) and *pressure support ventilation* (PSV). CPAP is spontaneous breathing with no mandatory or assisted breaths; a constant level of pressure is applied to the airway throughout the respiratory cycle. Of note, the mode CPAP is similar to PEEP, which is not a mode but is the addition of baseline positive pressure during mechanical ventilation. In PSV, breaths are patient triggered, pressure limited, and flow cycled. That is, with no machine backup rate, the ventilator assists the patient's inspiratory effort with a preset pressure. Patients determine their own respiratory rate, inspiratory time, and tidal volume. PSV can be combined with other modes, such as SIMV, to assist patient efforts between the set machine breaths.

Although the ventilator performs the full work of breathing in CMV and the patient performs the full work of breathing in CPAP, two important points should be emphasized. First, the ideal work of breathing for the mechanically ventilated patient remains unclear (ie, the ideal amount that prevents muscle atrophy, yet permits rest). Second, patient work of breathing is not necessarily less in ACV or SIMV than in PSV, particularly if patient–ventilator synchrony is optimized in PSV (see *Features of Patient–Ventilator Interaction* below).

Several newer "alternative" ventilatory modes have been developed in recent years in an attempt to combine attractive features of pressure and volume ventilation into a single mode that will deliver the minimum necessary ventilator pressure for a tidal volume goal. Modes including mandatory minute ventilation (MMV) "automatically" titrate the amount of ventilator assistance to changing patient mechanics and breathing drive. These modes have not yet been shown to improve clinical end points in prospective trials, but are increasingly encountered in general practice.

Campbell RS et al: Pressure-controlled versus volume controlled ventilation: does it matter? Respir Care 2002;47:416. [PMID: 11929615]. (Theoretical discussion of differences between the two, pointing out that the differences may be smaller than commonly perceived.)

Ventilator Settings

The major variables to set for the volume-controlled modes, ACV and SIMV, are respiratory rate, tidal volume, flow rate and pattern, FIO_2, and PEEP level.

A. RESPIRATORY RATE

Although a rate of 10–20 breaths/min is generally appropriate for most patients with respiratory failure, patients with airflow limitation who are at risk for developing $PEEP_i$ may benefit from lower rates and patients with a need for high minute ventilation due to metabolic acidosis need higher rates. In SIMV, it is best to initially deliver at least 80% of minute ventilation with machine breaths. In ACV, setting the rate about 4 breaths/min below the patient rate ensures that the patient and not the machine is dictating minute ventilation, and yet provides adequate backup if the patient becomes apneic.

B. TIDAL VOLUME

Although tidal volumes as high as 10 mL/kg (and perhaps higher) may be appropriate for patients without lung disease, lower volumes are otherwise indicated. In acute respiratory distress syndrome (ARDS), the use of a tidal volume of 6 mL/kg (ideal body weight) was associated with improved mortality compared with 12 mL/kg, and should be considered the standard of care. A tidal volume of 6–8 mL/kg is often used in obstructive lung disease (asthma, COPD) to avoid high airway pressures and development of $PEEP_i$. In fact, studies of asthma and ARDS suggest that a lung protective ventilatory strategy, termed "permissive hypercapnia," may lead to improved outcomes. This strategy reduces tidal volumes and/or rate and allows a respiratory acidosis to a pH as low as 7.15–7.20. Generally, when increased ventilation is needed, it is more effective to adjust minute ventilation by changes in rate rather than tidal volume, because increases in tidal volume occasionally have the paradoxical effect of slowing respiratory rate.

Frequent arterial blood sampling to check CO_2 tension in the stable patient can be avoided by noting the minute ventilation needed to achieve a given level of $PaCO_2$.

C. FLOW RATE AND PATTERN

The peak flow rate determines the maximal inspiratory flow delivered by the ventilator during inspiration. Although 60 L/min is a common initial peak flow setting, higher flows, with subsequent higher peak inspiratory pressure (see *Monitoring the Ventilated Patient* below), are commonly needed for high ventilatory demand or underlying airway obstruction. Flow is delivered during the inspiratory period via one of three waveforms: constant (square wave), decelerating (ramp wave), or sinusoidal. Although important differences in clinical outcome have not been demonstrated for particular flow patterns, decelerating flow is most commonly used because it may achieve better gas exchange (ie, lower alveolar–arterial oxygen gradient and lower dead space) as well as lower peak inspiratory pressure, despite higher mean airway pressure. To improve oxygenation in ARDS, mean airway pressure is increased. To do this in volume-controlled modes, the peak inspiratory flow rate is decreased. In pressure control ventilation, inspiratory time is increased (pressure control) to reach an I:E ratio greater than 1, a practice termed *inverse ratio ventilation* (IRV). As IRV is uncomfortable for the patient, often requiring deep sedation or even paralysis, and carries the risk of gas trapping, it should be used selectively and by experienced clinicians.

D. FRACTION OF INSPIRED OXYGEN

The FIO_2 is typically started at 1.0 (100% oxygen). Although the literature does not stipulate a cutoff for a safe level of inspired oxygen in humans, concerns over oxygen radical-mediated lung injury have led to the common practice of decreasing the FIO_2 below 0.5–0.6 as soon as feasible. Pulse oximetry may be used to titrate FIO_2, with one study suggesting that a threshold of 92% in light-skinned patients and 95% in darker-skinned patients ensures adequate oxygenation. Measurement of partial pressure of arterial oxygen by arterial blood gas (PaO_2 >55–60 mm Hg is typically acceptable) is recommended at the start of ventilation to verify accuracy of pulse oximetry for each patient.

F. PEEP

PEEP is selected to improve oxygenation. It can also be used to improve work of breathing and inspiratory triggering in patients with $PEEP_i$. Potential adverse effects of PEEP include elevation of intracranial pressure and hemodynamic compromise/hypotension.

PEEP improves oxygenation mostly by "recruiting" lung units. Paradoxically, PEEP may sometimes worsen oxygenation by (1) decreasing cardiac output and thereby the oxygen saturation of mixed venous blood returning to the lungs, (2) directing pulmonary blood flow to more consolidated airspaces by compressing alveolar capillaries in nondiseased, more compliant airspaces, or (3) promoting right-to-left interatrial shunting. Because high levels of PEEP reduce cardiac output and impair oxygen delivery to tissues, measurement of the effect of PEEP on oxygen delivery, termed a "best PEEP trial," may be helpful.

In patients with airflow limitation (eg, COPD), $PEEP_i$ increases the work of breathing by increasing the inspiratory effort needed to initiate ventilator flow. In such patients with dynamic airflow limitation and expiratory airway collapse, addition of ventilator PEEP up to ~85% of the $PEEP_i$ level may improve inspiratory triggering and work of breathing. However, given the potential for worsening of hyperinflation, particularly for patients with asthma, PEEP for this purpose should be used cautiously. A stable inspiratory plateau pressure (Pplat) after addition of ventilator PEEP suggests absence of worsened hyperinflation (see *Monitoring the Ventilated Patient* below).

Complications of Mechanical Ventilation

Multiple direct complications of mechanical ventilation have been described (see Table 27–2). Other indirectly associated complications of mechanical ventilation include critical illness polyneuropathy, acalculous cholecystitis, and venous thromboembolism. Three of these,

Table 27–2. Complications of mechanical ventilation.

Pulmonary
   Barotrauma (eg, pneumothorax, pneumomediastinum, systemic gas embolism, etc)
   Ventilator-induced lung injury (ie, volutrauma, atelectrauma, biotrauma)
   Oxygen toxicity
   Ventilator-associated pneumonia
   Tracheal stenosis
Cardiac
   Reduced cardiac output/hypotension
   Right ventricular ischemia
   Propagation of right-to-left interatrial shunt
Gastrointestinal
   Ileus
   Gastrointestinal hemorrhage
Renal
   Fluid retention
   Hyponatremia
Cerebrovascular
   Increased intracranial pressure

barotrauma, ventilator-induced lung injury, and altered hemodynamics, will be discussed below, as both direct and indirect complications have important practical implications.

A. BAROTRAUMA

Barotrauma is the term for the specific complications of extraalveolar air such as pneumothorax or pneumomediastinum thought to occur from alveolar rupture into the adjacent bronchovascular interstitium. It is less common than in earlier days of positive pressure ventilation, likely because of attention to patient ventilator synchrony and high peak airway pressures. In rare instances the air extravasates into blood vessels with resultant air emboli in the brain, heart, or skin causing changes in mental status, cardiac arrhythmias, and livedo reticularis.

B. VENTILATOR-INDUCED LUNG INJURY (VILI)

Intriguingly, although VILI is synergistic with preexistent lung injury, positive-pressure ventilation of even the *normal* lung can produce pathological hyaline membrane changes indistinguishable from ARDS. Studies in the early 1970s introduced the concept of "barotrauma," or pressure-induced lung injury, demonstrating that high inflation pressures injured the lung. Subsequent studies showed that the injurious variable was the *transpulmonary* pressure distending the lung rather than peak alveolar pressure (ie, alveolar pressure minus pleural pressure), or, more simply, end-inspiratory *volume*. This, in turn, led to the current VILI concept of volume-induced lung injury, or "volutrauma," with its implication that patients with decreased chest wall compliance from abdominal distention or other restrictive causes may be relatively "protected" from high airway pressures on the ventilator. A multicenter NIH-sponsored ARDS trial, which demonstrated improved mortality using a low (6 mL/kg ideal body weight) compared to a high tidal volume strategy (12 mL/kg ideal body weight), supports this volutrauma idea.

The lung in patients with ARDS is heterogeneously affected, with the dependent, consolidated lung not participating in gas exchange. Only the relatively nondiseased, compliant portion of the lung is vulnerable to overdistention by the delivered tidal volume. This has led practitioners to theorize that pressure ventilation, with a uniform pressure ceiling in all lung units, is less injurious to the relatively normal lung than volume ventilation, which directs volume along the path of least resistance primarily to the nondiseased lung. Despite these claims, however, no well-designed, randomized, controlled trial has shown a difference in outcome between pressure- and volume-targeted ventilation in patients with ARDS.

Finally, perhaps the most interesting recent concept of VILI is that of "biotrauma," the idea that VILI may lead to multiple organ dysfunction syndrome by "leakage" of both stretch-induced injurious lung cytokines and bacteria into the systemic circulation. Lower tidal volumes have been shown to generate fewer cytokines, and are associated with less extrapulmonary organ dysfunction. This phenomenon may explain why most patients with ARDS die of extrapulmonary complications rather than from respiratory failure itself.

C. ALTERED HEMODYNAMICS

Positive-pressure ventilation and PEEP both cause hypotension by reducing cardiac output, with a blood pressure drop that is most dramatic immediately following endotracheal intubation. PEEP decreases venous return, and thus cardiac output, primarily by compressing the inferior vena cava. By increasing pulmonary vascular resistance and right ventricular afterload, high levels of PEEP may also: (1) decrease right ventricular systolic function, particularly for patients with underlying right ventricular dysfunction or right coronary artery disease, (2) aggravate right ventricular ischemia, and (3) propagate right-to-left interatrial shunting through a patent foramen ovale. PEEP *reduces* left ventricular afterload, and thereby may occasionally lead to *improved* left ventricular function and cardiac output in patients with dilated cardiomyopathy. Because of this therapeutic effect of the ventilator, both occult left ventricular ischemia and left ventricular systolic dysfunction may occasionally complicate ventilator weaning.

Hurford WE: Cardiopulmonary interactions during mechanical ventilation. Int Anesthesiol Clin 1999;37:35. [PMID: 10445172]. (Concise description of the physiological mechanisms by which positive-pressure ventilation affects different aspects of cardiac function.)

Kacmarek RM: Ventilator-associated lung injury. Int Anesthesiol Clin 1999;37:47. [PMID: 10445173]. (Review of the primary literature detailing the mechanisms by which mechanical ventilation injures the lung.)

Monitoring the Ventilated Patient

Managing a patient on the mechanical ventilator necessitates monitoring respiratory physiological variables. These variables track progression and resolution of disease, complications of mechanical ventilation, patient comfort, work of breathing, and likelihood of successful patient liberation from the ventilator. Although a number of sophisticated monitoring variables have been developed in recent years, only those most useful and readily available are within the scope of this chapter. Discussed below are: (1) clinically practical respiratory mechanical variables, (2) an algorithm for approaching the mechanically ventilated patient in acute distress, and (3) features of patient–ventilator interaction.

A. RESPIRATORY MECHANICS

Variables indicated on all mechanical ventilators include exhaled tidal volume and airway pressure. For the patient on volume-cycled ventilation for whom breath-to-breath volume is constant, airway pressure at any moment depends on: (1) the *impedance* of the *respiratory system* to air delivery (ie, respiratory system *compliance* and airflow *resistance*), (2) patient effort, and (3) patient synchrony with the ventilator. The latter two points will be discussed in the section *Features of Patient–Ventilator Interaction. Respiratory system* refers to the lung (parenchyma and airways) and its surrounding chest wall (pleura and thoracoabdominal cage). Although lung and chest wall mechanics may be distinguished with the use of invasive tools such as the esophageal balloon, this is rarely needed. Specifically, it is important to remember that pressures caused by changes in compliance of the chest wall, such as pneumothorax or even abdominal distention, are transmitted to the lung.

A simplified schema for understanding respiratory mechanics on the ventilator is that of the two-compartment model of the respiratory system, depicted in Figure 27–1. In this model, the respiratory system is thought of as a pipe, or airways compartment in which airflow occurs, in series with a balloon, or alveolar compartment, in which inflation occurs. As volume is delivered by the ventilator through the airway opening, pressure builds up in the inflating balloon, or alveolar compartment, as a function of its *compliance* (pressure = volume/compliance), and along the pipe, or airway, as a function of its resistance to airflow (pressure = flow × resistance). This occurs in addition to any baseline pressure exceeding atmospheric maintained in the system during the respiratory cycle (ie, PEEP and/or PEEP$_i$).

Pressure at the airway opening (Pao) will increase with any increase in PEEP, PEEP$_i$, flow, resistance (eg, bronchospasm), or tidal volume, and with any decrease in compliance (eg, pneumothorax). Pao increases progressively during inspiration with volume delivery by the ventilator until it reaches its peak, the *peak inspiratory pressure* (PIP), at the moment the full tidal volume is delivered. Pao likewise normally decreases to atmospheric (or to PEEP, if PEEP is programmed into the ventilator) at the end of exhalation, as the respiratory system empties. The downstream pressure in the alveolar compartment (which includes PEEP and PEEP$_i$), reflecting respiratory system compliance, can be measured at the airway opening in isolation from the additional pressure generated in the airways by stopping flow (ie, making flow zero), and thereby making pressure generated by flow through the airways zero. This principle is identical to the measurement of pulmonary capillary wedge pressure with a pulmonary artery catheter balloon inflation stopping flow and re-

Figure 27–1. Two-compartment (airway, alveolus) model of the respiratory system. During inspiration, pressure at the airway opening (Pao) equals the sum of the downstream component pressures (Paw—the pressure generated by resistive losses along the airway and Pplat—the elastic pressure acting to distend the alveolus). Alv, alveolus; ao, airway opening; aw, airway; C, compliance; R, resistance; V, volume; V̇, flow.

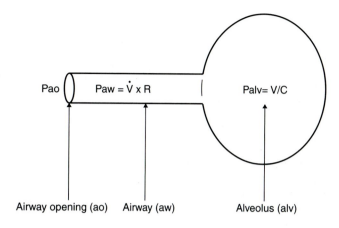

vealing static pressure in the left atrium. In practice, the maximum pressure of the alveolar compartment reached at completion of the tidal volume, or *plateau pressure* (Pplat), can be monitored by programming a 1.0-s end-inspiratory pause of zero flow (see Figure 27–2). The PIP − Pplat difference equals the flow-resistive pressure (ie, the pressure generated by flow along the airways).

These measurements apply best to volume-controlled ventilation, in which flow and tidal volume are programmed. By contrast, in pressure-controlled ventilation in which a constant pressure is applied to the airway opening for a prescribed inspiratory time, PIP is often equal to Pplat, as can be demonstrated by observing an end-inspiratory period of zero flow on the ventilator flow-time graph.

The monitoring variables of static compliance (Cstat), resistance to airflow (R), and intrinsic PEEP (PEEP$_i$) can be easily derived at the bedside. These variables are used to adjust the ventilator, follow disease progression, and monitor response to therapy. Cstat, reflecting the compliance or distensibility of the alveo-

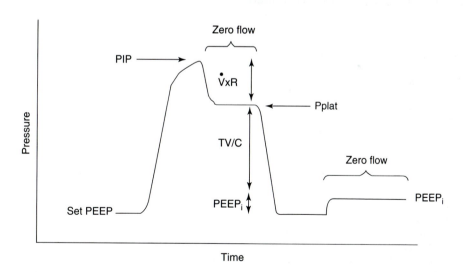

Figure 27–2. Schematic pressure waveform during volume ventilation. A pause of zero flow removes the pressure generated by flow in the airways, revealing the static downstream alveolar pressure at end inspiration (Pplat) and end expiration (PEEP$_i$, intrinsic PEEP, or "autoPEEP"). The variables comprising Pplat and PIP are indicated in the middle of the figure. C, compliance; PEEP$_i$, intrinsic PEEP; PIP, peak inspiratory pressure; Pplat, plateau pressure; R, resistance; TV, tidal volume; V̇, flow.

lar compartment, is calculated by dividing the volume change of the alveolar compartment during inspiration by the corresponding pressure change in isolation from airways pressure:

$$Cstat \ (mL / cm \ H_2O) = tidal \ volume \ / (Pplat - PEEP) \quad (1)$$

It is useful to monitor Cstat daily in patients with alveolar diseases, such as ARDS, as it reflects both evolving disease status and the associated increase in work of breathing. However, because $PEEP_i$ increases end-inspiratory alveolar pressure (Pplat), failure to recognize $PEEP_i$ and to subtract it from Pplat will lead to a falsely low value of Cstat.

R can be derived by dividing the change in pressure associated with airflow by the airflow generating this pressure.

$$R \ (cm \ H_2O / L / s) = (PIP - Pplat) / flow \quad (2)$$

It is useful to monitor R daily in patients with airways disease, such as status asthmaticus or COPD exacerbation. Although airflow resistance in these disorders is most important during exhalation, Eq. (2) is actually a measure of *inspiratory* resistance. To easily apply Eq. (2), which requires a value for flow, constant ("square wave") flow should be programmed on the ventilator. A useful bedside trick is to set the square wave flow value to 60 L/min (or 1 L/s), in which case the denominator becomes 1, and the PIP–Pplat difference easily measurable on the ventilator becomes equal to R in the standard units of cm H_2O/L/s. It is also useful to follow $PEEP_i$, or "*autoPEEP*," in patients with airways disease exacerbation. Normally, at end exhalation (before the next delivered breath), the tidal volume in the alveolar compartment fully empties, and both expiratory airflow and alveolar pressure fall to zero. However, if elevated airflow resistance slows alveolar emptying beyond the

available expiratory period, particularly in settings of decreased expiratory time (eg, elevated respiratory rate) and/or decreased alveolar driving pressure (eg, emphysema), positive alveolar pressure, or $PEEP_i$, may persist at end exhalation. $PEEP_i$ is often initially detected by observing the flow graphic on the ventilator for persistent flow at end-expiration. $PEEP_i$ is measured by programming a 1.0-s *end-expiratory pause* of zero flow into the ventilator. $PEEP_i$ may cause hypoventilation, hypotension, or a false elevation in pulmonary capillary wedge pressure. Strategies to minimize $PEEP_i$ include decreasing the respiratory rate, use of bronchodilators, or addition of PEEP.

B. THE MECHANICALLY VENTILATED PATIENT IN ACUTE RESPIRATORY DISTRESS

A useful approach to the ventilated patient who develops acute hypoxemia is depicted in Figure 27–3. By observing PIP and measuring Pplat, the problem can often be localized either to the alveolar or the airways compartment, and an immediate differential diagnosis can be generated. Specifically, elevation of PIP with an unchanged Pplat (ie, PIP–Pplat increased) may indicate mucus plugging or bronchospasm. Elevation of both PIP and Pplat in parallel (ie, PIP–Pplat unchanged) may indicate pneumothorax, pulmonary edema, or pneumonia. Alternatively, if neither is elevated, the possibility of a vascular event altering gas exchange should be considered (ie, pulmonary embolism).

C. FEATURES OF PATIENT–VENTILATOR INTERACTION

Evaluating the interaction between patient and ventilator can be a difficult process, but is essential because reflex action to sedate the distressed patient prolongs time on the ventilator. Some of the common causes of dyssynchrony can be detected by monitoring the flow-time graphic on the ventilator as discussed below.

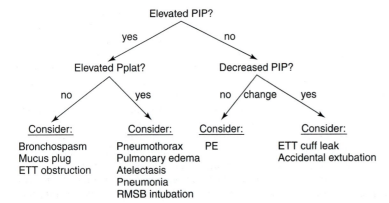

Figure 27–3. Approach to the mechanically ventilated patient with acute hypoxemia or respiratory distress. ETT, endotracheal tube; PE, pulmonary embolism; PIP, peak inspiratory pressure; Pplat, plateau pressure; RMSB, right mainstream bronchus.

D. EFFECT OF INSPIRATORY FLOW

A common cause of patient–ventilator dyssynchrony is inappropriate inspiratory flow. Many critically ill patients have an elevated respiratory drive with a demand for inspiratory flow that exceeds that delivered by the ventilator, thereby creating distress and increasing the work of breathing. The patient creates abnormally large negative pressure inspiratory attempts, detected by observing a scooped (concave up) shape in the inspiratory pressure graphic. Although increasing inspiratory flow may occasionally solve the problem, increasing flow or decreasing inspiratory time have both, somewhat paradoxically, been shown to increase respiratory rate in ventilated patients. Hence, increasing inspiratory flow to reduce $PEEP_i$ may paradoxically worsen $PEEP_i$ by causing tachypnea, thereby *decreasing* expiratory time. Perhaps the best choice for the distressed patient is to make an empiric flow change and observe the result. Alternatively, if no ideal flow can be achieved, switching to a pressure mode (in which inspiratory flow is variable and determined by the patient), such as pressure support or pressure control, may solve the problem.

E. INEFFECTIVE TRIGGERING

A second common cause of dyssynchrony is ineffective triggering of inspiratory flow. In pressure triggering, the ventilator delivers a tidal breath whenever the patient's inspiratory effort decreases pressure in the ventilator circuit to the *set sensitivity,* commonly −1 to −2 cm H_2O. However, a patient who has $PEEP_i$, or persistent positive alveolar pressure at the onset of inspiration, instead needs to pull a negative pressure equal to set sensitivity *plus* the value of $PEEP_i$ to start ventilator flow, and may not be strong enough to do this. Such failed inspiratory attempts can be perceived on physical examination as gulps without associated tidal breaths delivered by the ventilator. Alternatively, double triggering or double efforts for a single tidal breath are seen. If these are noted, both the patient and the ventilator should be looked at carefully for $PEEP_i$.

F. PREMATURE EXPIRATORY CYCLING

PSV, although typically thought to be a comfortable mode, can be a problem for patients with airflow limitation. PSV uses a fall in inspiratory flow (eg, to 25% of peak flow) to switch from inspiration to expiration. However, for patients with long time constants for filling and emptying of the respiratory system, as in emphysema, this can cause mechanical inflation to persist well into neural expiration. Consequently, the patient "bucks" the ventilator by recruiting expiratory muscles although the ventilator is still delivering inspiratory flow. This phenomenon can be perceived on the venti-

lator pressure-time graphic as a distortion of the typical PSV square wave inspiratory pressure pattern by an end-inspiratory upward pressure spike, and can often be avoided by limiting inspiratory time, using a mode such as pressure control ventilation, in which inspiratory time is set.

G. MISCELLANEOUS CAUSES OF DYSSYNCHRONY

Other possible causes of dyssynchrony include patient discomfort with low tidal volume "protective" ventilation, poor trigger sensitivity, auto-triggering of the ventilator by water in the circuit, and insufficient pain control. As stated, monitoring of the flow-time and pressure-time graphic can be diagnostic. $PEEP_i$ can be easily detected by noting persistent end-expiratory flow on the flow-time graphic (ie, expiratory flow does not return to zero). Excessive secretions in need of suctioning often appear as a "saw tooth" pattern on the graphic screen.

Hess DR et al: Pulmonary mechanics and graphics during positive pressure ventilation. Int Anesthesiol Clin 1999;37:15. [PMID: 10445171]. (Concise explanation of the method of monitoring respiratory mechanics in ventilated patients, including theoretical underpinnings and practical features.)

Jubran A: Advances in respiratory monitoring during mechanical ventilation. Chest 1999;116:1416. [PMID: 10559107]. (Scholarly review of several aspects of monitoring of gas exchange, mechanics, and work of breathing in ventilated patients, including practical clinical points.)

Tobin MJ et al: Patient-ventilator interaction. Am J Respir Crit Care Med 2001;163:1059. [PMID: 11316635]. (Describes important aspects of ventilator triggering, flow, and inspiration–expiration switching.)

Weaning

A. WEANING STRATEGY

Although a number of trials have investigated the best way to "liberate" patients from mechanical ventilation, no method is clearly superior. A few important points can be made. First, most patients (~75%) do not need to be "weaned" from the ventilator; a graduated reduction of support is unnecessary, particularly for postoperative patients. The majority can simply be extubated after their first successful attempt at spontaneous breathing. For patients who fail their initial attempts at spontaneous breathing, synchronized intermittent mandatory ventilation (SIMV) weaning appears to be inferior and may even prolong the duration of mechanical ventilation. Next, most of the long list of classic "weaning parameters" (eg, maximum inspiratory pressure, respiratory rate, vital capacity) are poorly predictive of successful liberation. The clinical *gestalt* of even experienced practitioners is often poorly predictive of successful liberation. Lastly, the duration of ventilation can be reduced by using validated clinical parameters, such as the rapid-shallow breathing index (RSBI), in a protocol-directed approach.

Most experts agree that the process of liberation should involve an initial achievement of clinical criteria of readiness (eg, $SaO_2 \geq 90\%$ with $FIO_2 \leq 0.5$ and PEEP ≤ 5 cm H_2O, no or low-dose vasopressors, mental status at least easily arousable, some indication of improvement in the initial cause of respiratory failure, minute ventilation ideally <12–15 L/min), followed by some form of initial spontaneous breathing trial (SBT). The initial trial may be by a T-piece (breathing without any assistance through the endotracheal tube with a flowing gas source), PSV, or CPAP (ie, PEEP without inspiratory pressure assistance). Initial SBT failure (for failure criteria, see Table 27–3) should be followed by reassessment and a more gradual weaning mode, as discussed below. Nevertheless, even these basic clinical criteria of readiness can be misleading; for example, a study of brain-injured patients on mechanical ventilation demonstrated that a low Glasgow Coma Scale score had poor predictive power for extubation success. Because of this, multiple studies have attempted to validate more sophisticated physiological variables assessing readiness for liberation from ventilation.

Perhaps the best-validated and easiest index to assess readiness to wean is the RSBI, which is the respiratory rate divided by tidal volume in liters. When the RSBI is less than 100, *as measured for 1 min on T-piece*, the patient is likely to achieve successful extubation. Some experts emphasize the importance of carefully judging the timing of weans to avoid muscle fatigue caused by a failed SBT, whereas others contend that no physiological variable should prevent an attempt at an SBT. Regarding the appropriate length of the initial SBT, a large randomized controlled trial demonstrated that 30 and 120 min were equivalent at predicting success.

Table 27–3. Criteria for assessing tolerance of a spontaneous breathing trial.

Acceptable oxygenation: $SaO_2 \geq 90\%$ or $PaO_2 \geq 60$ mm Hg on $FIO_2 \leq 0.5$

Acceptable ventilation: increase in $PaCO_2 \leq 10$ mm Hg or pH decrease ≤ 0.10

Acceptable respiratory rate: respiratory rate ≤ 35 breaths/min or < 50% increase in rate

Acceptable hemodynamics: heart rate ≤ 140 beats/min or an increase $\leq 20\%$ of baseline; systolic blood pressure ≥ 80 mm Hg and ≤ 160 mm Hg, or change of < 20% from baseline

RSBI (rate/tidal volume) < 100 breaths/min/L

No signs of elevated work of breathing, such as thoracoabdominal paradox or excessive use of accessory muscles

No signs of distress, such as diaphoresis or agitation

Commonly accepted parameters for judging "success" of an SBT are listed in Table 27–3.

For those patients who fail the initial SBT, three different methods for subsequent weaning are generally used: SIMV, PSV, and T-piece. The latter two have gained predominant support in the literature as effective weaning modes, and the former should be abandoned as a primary weaning strategy.

SIMV involves a stepwise reduction of the mandatory respiratory rate (eg, a decrease by two breaths/min twice daily) until the patient can tolerate a minimal rate (~4 breaths/min), with the remainder of breaths unassisted. Although the initial theory was for SIMV mode to permit "rest" during assisted breaths and progressive "exercise" during unassisted breaths, the respiratory center cannot rapidly alter its output in time to "respond" to these different breath types. Consequently, the work of breathing is comparable between assisted and unassisted breaths, progressively increasing for both breath types as the set respiratory rate is reduced. The overall concept of trading ventilator work for patient work appears to have been incorrect. Furthermore, in addition to SIMV inducing fatigue, an overly regimented protocol of graduated reduction of respiratory rate needlessly prolongs ventilator time.

PSV typically involves the stepwise reduction in PS level (eg, by 2 cm H_2O twice daily) until a minimal PS level is reached (eg, 5 cm H_2O). This low pressure is thought to approximate the work of breathing off the ventilator by "overcoming" the additional work of breathing imposed by the endotracheal tube. PSV was the most effective mode when compared to SIMV and T-piece in a large randomized trial, and is used in many centers. Two potential problems of uncertain clinical importance can be encountered with PSV weaning. First, the postextubation work of breathing may actually be better approximated by unassisted breathing through the endotracheal tube (ie, T-piece), and PSV may underestimate the amount of work that a patient will have to perform after extubation, thereby leading to more frequent reintubation. Second, as discussed above, patients with marked airflow limitation (eg, COPD) may "buck" the PS mode by initiating expiration before mechanical inflation is completed.

T-piece involves unassisted spontaneous breathing by disconnection of the endotracheal tube from the ventilator circuit and reconnection to a flowing, oxygen-enriched source of gas. It was the most effective weaning mode in a second large randomized controlled trial. Although progressive increases in T-piece trial duration and daily number (eg, increasing from a few minutes twice a day to two or more hours several times daily) are commonly used, and, in fact, may be necessary in chronically ventilator-dependent patients, once-daily T-piece trials have been shown to be as effective as multiple daily trials for patients without complications. Whereas a large randomized trial demonstrated that for an *initial* SBT, a 30-min T-piece trial was as effective as a 120-min T-piece SBT in predicting extubation success, tolerance of a 120-min SBT may constitute a better test of readiness for extubation for those patients undergoing a subsequent weaning T-piece SBT after a failed initial trial. Large randomized controlled trials have indicated that the *mean* time to SBT failure is 40–50 min. Furthermore, patients who have undergone longer courses of mechanical ventilation may benefit from even longer SBTs. A study of patients with COPD ventilated for ≥15 days found the majority failed a T-piece trial after a *median* of 120 min. Because prolonging T-piece trials much beyond 120 min may produce fatigue, this decision needs to be cautiously individualized. In addition to the SBT tolerance parameters listed in Table 27–3, some practitioners advise that the RSBI be measured again at the end of the SBT. The predictive value of the RSBI has been better when measured after 30 min of spontaneous breathing than after 1 min. Although checking an arterial blood gas at the end of the SBT is not always necessary, it may help in situations in which the patient appears marginal for extubation, has been ventilated long term, or has an elevated minute ventilation. Ensuring an adequate cough and absence of secretions requiring frequent suctioning is also reassuring.

In sum, for the patient who fails an initial attempt at spontaneous breathing, several strategies, all using SBTs, are available for progressive withdrawal from the ventilator: daily SBTs (T-piece, CPAP, or PS); T-piece, CPAP, or PS trials of increasing duration; or gradual decreases in PS level. In certain cases an argument can be made for the superiority of one of these methods. For example, patients with COPD may occasionally have difficulty tolerating PSV. Second, because patients with congestive heart failure (CHF) may derive enough assistance in cardiac performance from positive pressure ventilation (see *Altered Hemodynamics* above), it is arguably most predictive to perform their SBTs on T-piece.

B. THE DIFFICULT-TO-WEAN PATIENT

Failure to wean commonly reflects an imbalance of excessive respiratory workload and insufficient respiratory muscle strength or endurance, with a typical pattern of tachypnea and shallow tidal volumes. A long list of etiological considerations in the difficult-to-wean patient is given in Table 27–4. Depending on the clinical scenario, occult coronary ischemia, occult left ventricular dysfunction/pulmonary edema, PEEP$_i$, concretions narrowing the endotracheal tube, and critical illness myopathy/polyneuropathy should be considered. Most patients, particularly those with diaphragmatic dysfunction, congestive heart failure, emphysema, morbid obe-

Table 27–4. Causes of failure to wean from mechanical ventilation.

Respiratory muscle weakness
 Electrolyte depletion (eg, hypokalemia, hypomagnesemia), malnutrition
 Critical illness polyneuropathy
 Inadequate rest
 Prolonged paralysis or myopathy (eg, neuromuscular agents, corticosteroids, aminoglycosides)
Decreased ventilatory drive
 Hypothyroidism
 Excessive administration of sedatives or opiates
Increased ventilatory load
 Increased resistance: bronchospasm, secretions, plugged endotracheal tube
 Decreased lung compliance: pulmonary edema, ARDS
 Decreased chest wall compliance: pleural effusions, abdominal distention, and obesity
 Increased minute ventilation: elevated dead space ventilation, fever, and overfeeding
 Intrinsic PEEP
Cardiac problems
 Left ventricular dysfunction
 Coronary ischemia

---

sity, or abdominal distention, should be positioned upright during weaning. Electrolytes affecting muscle function, including potassium, magnesium, and phosphate, should be repleted, and correction of metabolic acidosis should be considered, particularly if excessive minute ventilation persists. Lastly, in patients with COPD exacerbation who fail SBTs, extubation straight to noninvasive positive pressure ventilation [ie, bilevel positive airway pressure (BiPAP)] can be tried. In such patients, studies show improved weaning rates, less nosocomial pneumonia, and decreased mortality.

Epstein SK: Weaning from mechanical ventilation. Respir Care 2002;47:454. [PMID: 11929617]. (Description of the pathophysiology of weaning failure as well as the various phases of weaning of the patient, including references to important studies in the literature.)

Manthous CA et al: Liberation from mechanical ventilation—a decade of progress. Chest 1998;114:886. [PMID: 9743181]. (Refreshing review of recent advances in our understanding of weaning of the mechanically ventilated patient.)

Tobin MJ: Advances is mechanical ventilation. N Engl J Med 2001;345:1133. [PMID: 11430329].

Noninvasive Ventilation

Noninvasive ventilation (ie, ventilatory assistance without the use of an endotracheal tube) can be delivered with the use of either (1) negative-pressure ventilators that apply subatmospheric pressure to the chest wall (eg, the iron lung), or (2) NIPPV that delivers positive-pressure assistance to the airway by mask. Although negative-pressure ventilation has been shown in uncontrolled trials to benefit patients with chronic respiratory failure due to chest wall, neuromuscular, and central hypoventilation disorders, poor patient acceptance, ineffectiveness for many patients, and barriers imposed on patient care have limited its application in acute respiratory failure.

By contrast, NIPPV is preferred in the acute setting. NIPPV can be delivered by several appliances, each available in several sizes, including face masks that cover both the nose and mouth, nasal masks, "nasal pillows" that fit into the nostrils, and cushion devices that fit across the nostrils. Selecting the correct mask size, in particular avoiding the mistake of an oversized mask, as well as proper preparation of the patient (ie, bedside coaching, slow upward titration of the pressure level), are critical. Full-face masks may be most effective for dyspneic patients. Compared to full face masks, nasal masks likely lessen aspiration risk from regurgitation, allow easier secretion clearance, lower the risk of asphyxiation with ventilator malfunction, decrease facial pressure sores, and improve speech, oral care, and feeding. One disadvantage of nasal masks is that most patients in acute respiratory failure are mouth breathers, and a leak through the mouth prevents efficient ventilation. This is sometimes improved by a chin strap. Fortunately, small leaks do not generally compromise the effectiveness of NIPPV. Because gastric distention is unlikely in conscious patients with pressure support levels lower than 25 cm H_2O, placement of a nasogastric tube is not routinely needed. Patient comfort and avoidance of facial skin necrosis may be aided by periodic removal of the mask, or cycling between two types of masks.

Several modes of pressure delivery are available for NIPPV, including volume-targeted ventilation, pressure-controlled ventilation, BiPAP ventilation, and CPAP. Pressure-targeted ventilation tends to be best tolerated by patients. BiPAP is a term that refers to a specific brand of bilevel PAP ventilator. Bilevel PAP, which cycles between a high-pressure level (inspiratory) and a low-pressure level (expiratory), is similar in concept to PSV used with PEEP. An important difference between the two, however, is that with bilevel PAP the expiratory pressure is equivalent to PEEP, but the inspiratory pressure level is equal to the pressure support level plus PEEP. Thus, a pressure of 15/5 set on bilevel pressure is equivalent to 10/5 with the pressure support mode. CPAP alone (continuous positive pressure without added inspiratory support) improves work of breathing in patients with both airflow limitation and pulmonary edema, and may occasionally be adequate treatment for acute respiratory failure.

Success of NIPPV in acute respiratory failure depends upon both proper patient selection and proper patient monitoring. Selection and exclusion criteria for NIPPV candidates are listed in Table 27–5. Careful monitoring of the acute respiratory failure patient undergoing NIPPV is of paramount importance to ensure successful treatment and to avoid postponing invasive mechanical ventilation if it becomes necessary. Useful parameters to monitor include respiratory rate, use of accessory muscles, abdominal paradox, mental status, and gas exchange. It is important to avoid relying blindly on the initial settings, but rather to adjust them empirically (eg, stepwise increases in inspiratory pres-

Table 27–5. Selection and exclusion criteria for candidates for NIPPV.

Selection Criteria (At Least Two Should Be Present)	Exclusion Criteria (Any May Be Present)
Respiratory distress with moderate-to-severe dyspnea, use of accessory muscles, abdominal paradox	Respiratory arrest
	Cardiorespiratory instability (eg, hypotension with impaired perfusion, serious dysrhythmia, and myocardial infarction with pulmonary edema)
pH < 7.35 and $Paco_2$ > 45 mm Hg	Uncooperative patient
Respiratory rate ≥ 25/min (adults)	Recent facial, esophageal, or gastric surgery
	Craniofacial trauma or burns
	High aspiration risk (inability to manage secretions)
	Inability to protect airway
	Fixed anatomic abnormalities of the nasopharynx (eg, choanal atresia, severe laryngomalacia)
	Impending upper airway obstruction

sure), always carefully observing the result. Improvements in pH and $PaCO_2$ within 30–120 min are predictive of the eventual success of NIPPV. Significant worsening of gas exchange during this time likely indicates the need for endotracheal intubation.

NIPPV has improved patient outcomes in acute respiratory failure. A meta-analysis found both reduced need for endotracheal intubation and decreased mortality with the use of NIPPV. Two recent prospective, randomized trials have documented that NIPPV—in the form of bilevel PAP or isolated PS (ie, with expiratory pressure of zero), respectively—improves outcomes in *severe exacerbations of COPD*. Improved outcomes have included decreased need for intubation (number of patients who need to be treated to prevent one intubation is about two or three), lower rates of complications, shorter hospital stays, and reduced mortality. The number of patients who need to be treated to prevent one death from COPD by using NIPPV instead of conventional therapy was only about 5–15. It should be noted, however, that the selection criteria in these trials imposed high rates of patient exclusion, and other trials have failed to document improved outcomes in *mild* exacerbations of COPD (eg, pH >7.35). Placing the inclusion and exclusion criteria in these trials side by side, it appears that a COPD severity "window" between no need for ventilatory assistance and need for invasive assistance is appropriate for NIPPV (ie, moderate-to-severe dyspnea associated with pH ~7.25–7.35 and respiratory rate of ~25–35 breaths/min, in the absence of the contraindications listed in Table 27–5). By contrast, although two retrospective reviews suggest that use of NIPPV may avoid intubation in status asthmaticus, NIPPV in acute respiratory failure related to *asthma* has not been rigorously examined in a prospective manner.

Noninvasive CPAP has proven to be an effective adjunct for *acute pulmonary edema* in randomized, controlled trials. In contrast, bilevel PAP cannot, at this time, be recommended for pulmonary edema because, curiously, it was associated with a higher rate of my-

ocardial infarction in a small trial. The use of NIPPV has also been examined in several subsets of patients suffering from *acute hypoxemic respiratory failure*. In acute hypoxemic respiratory failure *unrelated to COPD*, bilevel PAP has led to shorter duration of mechanical ventilation, reduced length of ICU stay, and fewer serious complications, such as nosocomial pneumonia and sinusitis. However, in one trial, of the patients initially treated with NIPPV, 31% required intubation subsequently, and of these, 9 of 10 died, raising the concern that inappropriate delay of endotracheal intubation in this patient subset may reduce survival. In acute hypoxemic respiratory failure following *solid organ transplantation*, or in *neutropenic patients*, NIPPV was associated with fewer intubations, fewer serious complications, and perhaps lower mortality. Overall, the emerging picture for NIPPV in the ICU is one of benefit in lessening nosocomial infections and in improving survival. As discussed above (see *Weaning*), another interesting application for NIPPV is facilitation of extubation in patients with COPD who fail an initial spontaneous breathing trial.

Lastly, NIPPV has a role in treating chronic conditions. In chronic respiratory failure, NIPPV is useful in long-term management of neuromuscular disease and severe kyphoscoliosis, and may have a role in patients with COPD with marked hypercapnia, as judged by gas exchange, quality of life, and sleep efficiency. Similarly, long-term use of nocturnal CPAP in patients with chronic CHF and sleep-related central apneas improves symptoms of heart failure, increases left ventricular ejection fraction, and may improve survival.

Hess DR: Noninvasive positive pressure ventilation for acute respiratory failure. Int Anesthesiol Clin 1999;37:85. [PMID: 10445175]. (Review of the evidence for clinical application of noninvasive ventilation with a focus on more practical issues of its use.)

Hillberg RE et al: Noninvasive ventilation. N Engl J Med 1997; 337:1746. [PMID: 9392701]. (Concise review of the available forms of noninvasive ventilation and evidence for their clinical efficacy.)

Sleep Apnea & the Upper Airway Resistance Syndrome

John R. Ruddy, MD

ESSENTIALS OF DIAGNOSIS

- *Snoring, or otherwise noisy respiration in sleep.*
- *Periods of respiratory pauses (apneas) witnessed by bed partner or parents.*
- *Fragmented sleep or complaints of insomnia.*
- *Daytime sleepiness and/or fatigue.*
- *Personality changes, intellectual deterioration.*
- *Depression.*

General Considerations

Although the sleep-related breathing disorders (SRBD) have been recognized only recently, they are among the most common of all the respiratory disorders. These conditions occur in all age groups but are seen most frequently in middle-aged men.

Estimates from epidemiological studies suggest that 1–5% of the general adult population has obstructive sleep apnea syndrome (OSAS) as defined by evidence of abnormal breathing during sleep combined with symptoms of daytime sleepiness. Other studies have demonstrated that 24% of men and 9% of women aged 30–60 years have an elevated apnea–hypopnea index (AHI) without symptoms.

The impact of mild asymptomatic and often unrecognized obstructive sleep apnea (OSA) on other conditions such as hypertension and cardiovascular disease is an area of extensive research. Population studies indicate a prevalence of sleep-disordered breathing (SDB) in men that is two to three times greater than in women. The prevalence increases throughout the adult years at least until about age 65.

Young T et al: Epidemiology of obstructive sleep apnea. Am J Respir Crit Care Med 2002;165:1217. [PIMD:11991871]. (State-of-the-art review.)

Pathogenesis

The obstructive sleep-related breathing disorders can be viewed as manifestations of ever-increasing resistance to airflow in the upper airway. At one end of the continuum is an airway that is always patent in all stages of sleep, positions, and airway inflammation. On the other end is an airway that frequently collapses (obstructive apnea) whenever the patient sleeps. These events can lead to cortical and autonomic nervous system arousals and oxygen desaturations, producing cardiovascular effects. Between these extreme end points a patient may exhibit primary snoring (without evidence of sleep disruption or airway obstruction), sleep fragmentation associated with airflow limitation (and usually snoring) and excessive daytime sleepiness (EDS) but without overt hypopneas or apneas [known as the upper airway resistance syndrome (UARS)], and sleep-related hypopneas associated with arousals and desaturations.

Ventilation occurs when air flows down a gradient of pressure created when the muscles of respiration contract to create negative intrapleural pressure. The muscles dilating the upper airway are activated in a phasic manner allowing the airway to remain open during inspiration. Most patients with sleep apnea appear to have an anatomically narrowed airway, whose patency is maintained during wakefulness due to increased upper airway tone. With sleep onset a normal reduction in airway tone occurs that leaves the upper airway vulnerable to collapse during inspiration. The episodes can be associated with oxygen desaturations and cortical and autonomic arousals. Systemic and pulmonary artery pressures acutely rise and the heart rate increases. These events lead to sleep fragmentation and patients with OSA tend to have increased amounts of light Stage 1 sleep and reduced amounts to Stages 3 and 4 and rapid eye movement (REM) sleep.

Central apneas occur when the respiratory effort of the diaphragm and intercostal muscles ceases, producing a momentary pause in breathing. The causes of central sleep apnea (CSA) are varied, but appear to relate to conditions or circumstances that affect the repiratory control system (eg, neurological disorders of the brain stem, congestive heart failure, and breathing at high elevation). In some of these conditions (eg, hypoxia at altitude) the drive to breathe during wakefulness leads to an excessive reduction in carbon dioxide (CO_2) levels, which results in a respiratory pause after sleep onset. The pause that follows typically allows CO_2 levels to "overshoot" and an electroencephalographic (EEG) arousal is triggered. Respiration is resumed and another period of "hyperventilation" occurs setting up a pattern of cyclic central apneas and repetitive arousal from sleep. For further discussion of ventilatory disorders see Chapters 25 and 26.

Clinical Findings

A. Symptoms and Signs

The typical patient with OSAS has a long history of loud snoring and daytime sleepiness. The degree of snoring varies greatly, ranging from being intermittent or occasional with less severe presentations to a persistent and intense occurrence with more significant disease. Respiratory pauses (ie, witnessed apnea), often following crescendo snoring and preceding inspiratory snorts at the resumption of airflow, are highly suggestive of obstructive apnea. Repetitive awakenings and frank insomnia often occur. Patients will frequently avoid sleeping in the supine position as this potentiates airway occlusion. Awakening with a dry mouth, sore throat, heartburn, or a headache is common. Nocturnal polyuria, enuresis, and impotence can accompany OSAS.

Changes in daytime alertness and function are also typically reported, although the severity of these symptoms ranges from subtle decrements in performance on the job or at school to dramatic and potentially life-threatening episodes of sleepiness that occur while driving or operating machinery. Because daytime function can deteriorate very gradually, the patient may have little awareness of the degree of the impairment. Therefore, obtaining patient history from family members or co-workers can be helpful. Depression, irritability, and personality changes are all commonly reported.

Patients with CSA often complain of disrupted sleep without significant snoring and minimal daytime sleepiness. Awakening with a breathless sensation is common. When CSA accompanies other medical conditions, such as congestive heart failure (CHF), neurological disorders, or alveolar hypoventilation, the symptoms may primarily relate to those conditions (eg, exercise intolerance, dyspnea with exertion, peripheral edema, muscle weakness, and postural dizziness).

Individuals with SDB tend to be overweight, with at least 60% having a body mass index of greater than 28 kg/m². A neck circumference greater than 43 cm in men is predictive of OSA. Abnormalities of the upper airway on examination are common, typically with evidence of an elongated uvula, low-lying soft palate, and crowding from the lateral pharyngeal walls. The mucosa of the uvula and soft palate often appears erythematous and swollen. Nasal obstruction (such as from polyps or a deviated nasal septum), macroglossia, retrognathia, and micrognathia can all potentiate airway obstruction. Adenotonsilar hypertrophy is a common cause of aiway obstruction in children. The general medical examination may be notable for hypertension (HTN), which occurs in at least 40% of patients with OSAS.

Diagnostic classifications of various SRBDs are given in Table 28–1.

B. Laboratory Findings

Chemistry and hematology studies are usually normal, unless apnea-related hypoxemia is severe or associated with waking hypoxia, in which case polycythemia may be present.

C. Special Examinations

Assessment of respiration and sleep quality during a typical sleep period is necessary to correctly diagnose and estimate the severity of an SRBD. A formal nocturnal polysomnogram (PSG) assesses sleep quality by recording electroencephalograms (EEGs), electrooculograms (EOGs), and electromyograms (EMGs) to determine the sleep–wake state. This is combined with assessments of respiratory effort (eg, monitoring movement of the thorax and abdomen or intrathoracic pressure changes via an esophageal pressure monitor), airflow, and oxygen saturation. Additionally, body position, leg movement, electrocardiogram, and snoring sounds are typically monitored. These assessments are combined to produce a graphic representation of the entire sleep–wake state, known as a hypnagram (Figure 28–1).

Along with this type of graphic summary other important measures are calculated, such as the apnea–hypopnea index (AHI), respiratory disturbance index (RDI), arousal index, and mean and lowest oxygen saturation (Table 28–2). The effect of body position (especially the supine position) and sleep stage on the occurrence of respiratory events and snoring can be assessed. Cardiac rhythm and rate can be monitored.

Apneas are defined as the total absence of airflow for at least 10 s. They are classified as being a central apnea if there is neither respiratory effort nor airflow, obstructive apnea if there is persistent effort without airflow, or mixed apnea if they begin as a central event but then demonstrate effort without airflow (see Figures 28–2 and 28–3). Most patients exhibit a combination of all three types during a recording, but the predominant pattern is most commonly obstructive.

Table 28–1. Diagnostic classification.

Condition	Apnea–Hypopnea Index (Respiratory Events/h)	Arousals/h	Snoring	Daytime Alertness
Simple snoring	< 5	< 10	+	Normal
Upper airway resistance syndrome	< 10	Often > 15	+/–	Impaired
Obstructive sleep apnea syndrome				
Mild	5–15	5–20	+	Mild impairment
Moderate	15–30	10–30	+	Moderate impairment
Severe	> 30	> 20	++	Severe impairment
Central sleep apnea syndrome	> 5 central apnea/h	> 10	+/–	Variable

Hypopneas are defined as a decrease in airflow for at least 10 s usually followed by either an arousal or a change in oxygen saturation. The definition of what constitutes a hypopnea is less standardized and varies among sleep laboratories. The definition given by the American Academy of Sleep Medicine is a 30% reduction in airflow or thoracoabdominal effort lasting for at least 10 s associated with a 4% fall in oxygen saturation.

A respiratory effort-related arousal (RERA) is an arousal that follows a measured increase in respiratory effort that abruptly decreases at the time of the arousal.

Although nocturnal polysomnograms are usually done in a laboratory dedicated to sleep recordings, they can be performed in the home setting using portable equipment. If home studies are utilized for patient care, it is important to ensure that the technology has been validated to accurately assess respiratory disturbances and sleep state, if desired. Home recordings of oxygen saturation alone are not sufficient to rule out an SRBD.

That SRBDs represent a continuum of disease must be kept in mind when interpreting the result of a PSG. Most clinicians agree that an AHI greater than 10/h is abnormal and an AHI less than 5/h is in the normal range for adults when diagnosing OSAS. An AHI between 5 and 10/h is in a gray zone and decisions for treatment rely more heavily on the presence and severity of daytime symptoms. The UARS by definition occurs in patients who have a normal AHI but who are

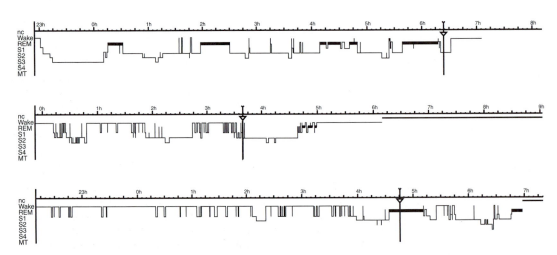

Figure 28–1. Hypnagrams in three separate patients. *Top:* Relatively normal hypnagram. Note sleep onset at 23:00 and a prolonged period of Stage 4 sleep from 23:15 to about 00:10. Periods of REM sleep (thick black lines) get longer as the night progresses. The final awakening was 6:35 AM. *Middle:* Very fragmented sleep with frequent shifts from wakefulness to Stage 1 sleep. Very little REM sleep occurred. This patient had OSAS. *Bottom:* Prolonged latency to consolidated sleep at aproximately 3:50 AM. This was a split night study with CPAP initated at 3:30 AM. Wakefulness; REM sleep; S1, Stage 1; S2, Stage 2; S3, Stage 3; S4, Stage 4; MT, patient movement time.

Table 28–2. Frequent abbreviations and definitions.

Abbreviation	Definition
AHI	Apnea–hypopnea index = $\dfrac{\text{Total number of apneas + hypopneas}}{\text{Total sleep time (min)}} \times 60$
AI	Arousal index = $\dfrac{\text{Total number of arousals}}{\text{Total sleep time (min)}} \times 60$
CPAP	Continuous positive airway pressure
CSA	Central sleep apnea
EDS	Excessive daytime sleepiness
MSL	Mean sleep latency
MSLT	Multiple Sleep Latency Test
MWT	Maintenance of Wakefulness Test
OSA	Obstructive sleep apnea
OSAS	Obstructive sleep apnea syndrome
PSG	Polysomnogram
RDI	Respiratory disturbance index = $\dfrac{\text{Total number of apneas + hypopneas + RERA}}{\text{Total sleep time (min)}} \times 60$
RERA	Respiratory effort-related arousal
SDB	Sleep-disordered breathing
SRBD	Sleep-related breathing disorder
UARS	Upper airway resistance syndrome

excessively sleepy. This diagnosis is suggested in patients with frequent arousals (usually more than 10/h) that typically, but not always, follow evidence of snoring.

The diagnosis can be confirmed with the demonstration of repetitive episodes of increasing respiratory effort prior to arousals. Usually this is done with an intrathoracic pressure measurement via an esophageal balloon. Additionally, a successful empiric trial of continuous positive airway pressure (CPAP), titrated to eliminate snoring and decrease sleep fragmentation, can support the diagnosis of UARS if daytime symptoms improve.

The diagnosis of a clinical sleep disorder requires a combination of abnormal findings on a sleep recording with clinical symptoms of daytime dysfunction, usually daytime sleepiness or fatigue. Daytime alertness can be quantified by utilizing surveys of self-reported sleepiness such as the Epworth sleepiness scale or with daytime sleep laboratory studies. The Epworth sleepiness scale is a point score obtained when patients answer eight questions concerning everyday situations in which sleepiness may occur. Patients rank the likelihood of dozing off from none (0 point) to high (3 points). Normal controls score in the range of 6–8 points. Patients with untreated OSAS typically have mean scores of approximately 12–14 points. Most clinicians feel a score of 11 or more suggests EDS.

Sleep laboratory studies assessing daytime alertness include the Multiple Sleep Latency Test (MSLT) and Maintenance of Wakefulness Test (MWT). In these tests, patients are given four or five opportunities to sleep at 2-h intervals during a day in the sleep laboratory. The tests last 20 min and the time from the start of each test until sleep occurs (as defined by EEG) is defined as the sleep latency. The tests differ in that patients are lying in bed and instructed to close their eyes in the MSLT whereas they are dressed, sitting, and told to try to stay awake in the MWT. Normative data have been published suggesting that in the MSLT, a mean sleep latency (MSL) on all five naps of less than 5 min demonstrates severe sleepiness and an MSL greater than 10 min is normal. In the MWT an MSL above 11 min is considered normal.

Doghramji K et al: A normative study of the Maintenance of Wakefulness Test (MWT). Electroencephalogr Clin Neurophysiol 1997;103:554. [PMID: 9402886]. (An MSL of 10.9 min was the limit of normal in 64 normal controls.)

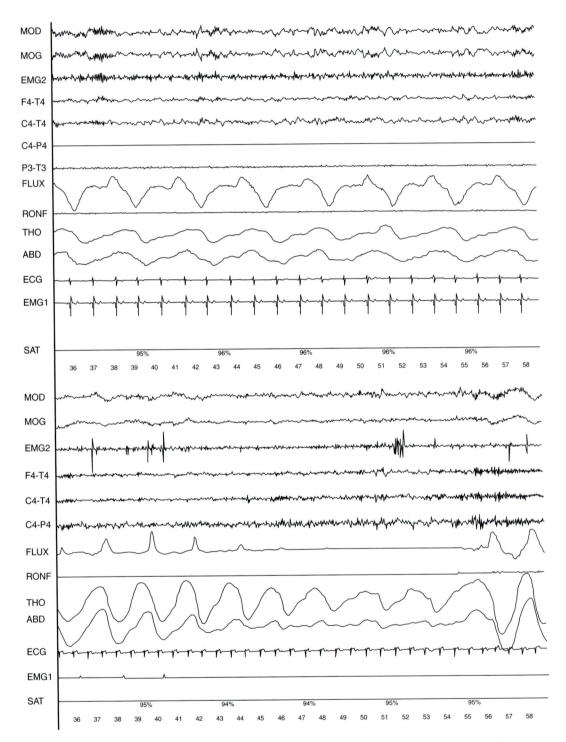

Figure 28–2. ***Top:*** Relatively normal respiration in non-REM sleep. ***Bottom:*** Obstructive apnea lasting 12 s. Note the flat airflow tracing with persistent respiratory effort. There is an EEG arousal. MOG and MOD, electrooculograms; F4–T4, C4 –T4, C4–P4, P3–T3, electroencephalograms; FLUX, nasal–oral airflow; RONF, snoring sounds; THO thoracic effort; ABD, abdominal effort; EMG1, anterior tibialis electromyogram; EMG2, submental electromyogram; SAT, oxygen saturation.

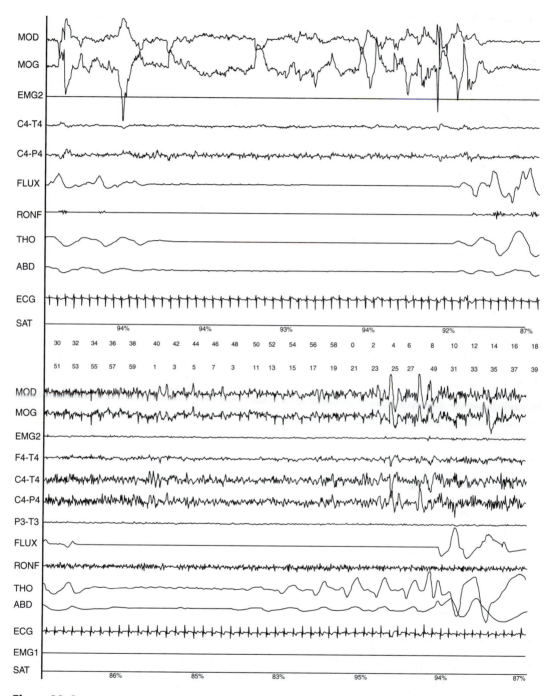

Figure 28–3. ***Top:*** Central apnea, duration 31 s, in REM sleep. The desaturation lags behind the apnea. Note the phasic eye movements and absence of respiratory effort. ***Bottom:*** Mixed apnea lasting 36 s. Essentially no respiratory effort is seen for 15 s, followed by 21 s of effort without airflow. An EEG arousal occurred. MOG and MOD, electroocculograms; F4–T4, C4–T4, C4–P4, P3–T3, electroencephalograms; FLUX, nasal–oral airflow; RONF, snoring sounds; THO thoracic effort; ABD, abdominal effort; EMG1, anterior tibialis electromyogram; EMG2, submental electromyogram; SAT, oxygen saturation.

Differential Diagnosis

The SRBDs must be differentiated from other causes of EDS. Patients with narcolepsy typically have a history indicating an earlier age of onset of sleep attacks, the occurrence of cataplexy, and the absence of snoring. Narcoleptic patients demonstrate EDS on the daytime MSLT. They often have an MSL of less than 5 min with evidence of sleep onset REM on at least two naps (see Chapter 29).

A sleep log from individuals with EDS secondary to insufficient sleep will show shortened total sleep times. A successful trial of sleep extension is diagnostic and therapeutic. Depression can also present with EDS and may be diagnosed based on the usual constellation of symptoms and a successful trial of antidepressant medications. The periodic limb movement disorder caused by frequent limb movements (usually leg jerks) can cause disrupted sleep and daytime sleepiness similar to OSAS (see Chapter 29).

Primary hypersomnia [also known as idiopathic central nervous system (CNS) hypersomnia] is an uncommon condition in which EDS is chronic and is not associated with snoring or other aspects of an SRBD. Sleep laboratory studies in these patients demonstrate essentially normal sleep for prolonged periods followed by an MSLT showing EDS without evidence of REM activity.

Daytime sleepiness accompanying difficulty sleeping at night occurs with disturbances in circadian rhythm. Other disorders, such as sleep-related panic attacks, the worsening of reactive airways disease, and chronic obstructive pulmonary disease (COPD) should be considered and may require evaluation in a sleep laboratory for diagnosis.

Complications

The effects of the SRBD can be classified as those relating to an individual's state of alertness and those relating to overall health.

Patients with OSAS have daytime sleepiness by definition and some studies demonstrate increasing levels of self-reported sleepiness with increasing AHI. Snoring by itself, in patients with a normal AHI, is associated with increased sleepiness. Cognitive dysfunction is often reported by patients and decreased psychomotor efficiency has been demonstrated to be related to increased AHI. These symptoms may impair performance on the job or in school. Although patients with OSAS treated with CPAP (see Treatment section) exhibit improved levels of alertness, they may not completely normalize their performance on daytime tests, which suggests an irreversible effect on brain function in certain patients.

Vehicular accidents are more likely to occur in patients with OSAS or snoring than in normal subjects. The increased rate of accidents is seen even in patients who deny daytime sleepiness, indicating that the impact of these disorders is likely unrecognized by the patients.

Depression, irritability, and personality changes are frequently reported by patients and their family members. Some studies assessing the quality of life in patients with OSA indicate changes in multiple scales consistent with other moderately severe chronic conditions.

The effect of OSA on other aspects of individuals' health status has been an area of active research and vigorous debate. Systemic hypertension is felt to be present in at least 40% of patients with OSAS. Approximately 30% of asymptomatic patients in hypertension clinics may have undiagnosed OSA. The prevalence of OSA is even higher in patients with resistant or difficult-to-control hypertension. Although obesity may contribute to hypertension in many patients with OSA, OSA itself is felt to be an independent risk factor for elevated blood pressure. The risk of hypertension increases in a dose–response fashion with increasing AHI. Additionally, OSA may obliterate the nocturnal sleep-related drop in blood pressure (BP) that is seen in normal subjects and in hypertensive patients without OSA. Treatment of OSA can lead to improvements in BP control.

The Sleep Heart Health Study demonstrated increased prevalence of cardiovascular disease in patients with an AHI greater than 11/h. Other case-controlled studies have documented increased prevalence of OSA in patients who suffered a myocardial infarction. The risk of having a cerebral vascular event is also greater in individuals with an elevated AHI. Taken together, these findings suggest that SDB is an important independent contributor to cardiovascular disease.

Lavie P et al: Sleep apnea syndrome: a possible contributing factor to resistant hypertension. Sleep 2001;24:721. [PMID: 11560187]. (Patients with resistant hypertension have higher levels of SDB.)

Leung RS et al: Sleep apnea and cardiovascular disease. Am J Respir Crit Care Med 2001;164:2147. [PMID: 11751180]. (State-of-the-art review.)

Peppard PE et al: Prospective study of the association between sleep disordered breathing and hypertension. N Engl J Med 2000;342:1378. [PMID: 10805822]. (Dose–response relationship between SDB at baseline and the presence of elevated BP 4 years later.)

Treatment

A. Obstructive Sleep-Disordered Breathing

The goal of treatment of SDB is to reduce or eliminate the abnormal breathing episodes during sleep allowing sleep quality to improve. Hopefully, this leads to better daytime function and a reduction in risk of cardiovascular disease. The degree of disease severity that warrants treatment appears to be variable as some patients with an apparently mild disorder (eg, those with UARS) on PSG may have a significant impairment of daytime function and hence will benefit from therapy. For relatively asymptomatic patients, the level of breathing disorders benefiting from intervention is uncertain and currently under debate. Most clinicians suggest starting therapy if the AHI is in the range of 20–30/h even if the patient denies symptoms, and many suggest treatment at AHI levels as low as 5/h if there is evidence of HTN or cardiovascular disease.

There are three general categories of treatment: behavorial, medical, and surgical. Each treatment should be appropriately tailored to the severity and needs of the patient. Often combining elements of multiple forms of treatment are necessary to yield success in a given patient.

1. Behavorial therapy—Weight loss, if maintained, has been associated with improved breathing during sleep. A 10% weight loss in obese patients has been associated with approximately a 25% decrease in AHI.

The patient should be encouraged to avoid sleep deprivation and respiratory depressants, including alcohol, which can worsen existing OSA. Exposure to smoke and other airway irritants should be eliminated as these can increase airway inflammation and OSA. The supine position should be avoided if PSG evidence indicates that in this position SDB is worse. This can be accomplished by having the patient wear a sleep shirt with a pocket in the center of the back containing uncomfortable objects such as a tennis ball. Sleeping with the head elevated approximately 30–60° can be helpful. The patient should also be counselled about the potential of accidents due to daytime sleepiness and encouraged to avoid driving or operating dangerous machinery until daytime alertness improves.

2. Medical therapy—Treatment of nasal congestion due to allergies and irritants is encouraged; saline nasal washes and topical nasal steroids are typically used for this purpose.

CPAP is currently the most reliable medical treatment for SDB. CPAP is essentially a technique in which patients sleep wearing a mask (either nasal or oral–nasal) that is connected to a small portable bedside blower unit. Air delivered to the patient acts as a "pneumatic splint" to keep the airway open. Typically CPAP therapy is initiated during an in-laboratory sleep study when the air pressure is titrated to overcome the sleep-related airway obstruction. For any given patient, the pressure needed may vary depending on the stage of sleep and the body position. Many sleep laboratories perform "split night" studies that combine an initial baseline section for diagnostic purposes followed by a CPAP titration section. Some patients will require additional studies to define effective pressure settings.

Autotitrating CPAP devices are commercially available and are currently in use. These devices vary in the manner in which they assess airway obstruction (eg, the detection of snoring or changes in airflow) and mask leaks. In general, autotitrating CPAP devices can lead to improvements in sleep quality and daytime performance similar to fixed CPAP therapy in patients with uncomplicated OSAS. Auto-CPAP therapy is currently recommended only after the diagnosis of OSA has been made by conventional techniques. This therapy is not recommended in patients with congestive heart failure (CHF), COPD, daytime hypoxemia, and sleep-related hypoxemia unrelated to OSA. Additionally, patients who have had previous upper airway surgery [such as uvulopalatopharyngoplasty (UPPP)] or who do not snore should not be treated with an autotitrating CPAP device that utilizes the detection of snoring as a trigger for changes in pressure.

Regardless of the method of initiating therapy, the patient must have a properly fitting and comfortable mask to avoid air leaks. Adding humidification to the system and treating nasal congestion may be helpful and improve compliance. CPAP therapy has been demonstrated to improve oxygen saturation, sleep quality, daytime alertness, and cardiac function. However, patients can have difficulty tolerating this therapy over time leading to published compliance rates of approximately 50–80%. Closely following the patient's progress with a special CPAP support team may improve compliance.

A variation on this technique is bilevel pressure therapy. This employs a similar type of device that allows the selection of different inspiratory and expiratory pressures. Although patients often find this more comfortable, its use has not been shown to increase compliance.

Oral appliances are intraoral devices that are worn during sleep with the intention of maintaining a patent airway, generally by advancing the mandible. A variety of devices are currently in clinical use and vary in their composition, design (eg, either fixed or adjustable), and overall tolerability. Because the distance the mandible is advanced may be a crucial factor in defining the device's efficacy and appears to be dependent on the clinician fitting the device, its effectiveness is unpredictable. Therefore follow-up PSGs are suggested. Although most of the studies evaluating the effectiveness of oral appliances have been in patients with mild to moderate OSA, these devices can also be used successfully in patients with severe disease or those who have failed CPAP or surgical treatment.

Supplemented oxygen can be used to lessen the severity of apnea-related desaturations. Although sleep continuity may not improve, this therapy might be considered in patients who do not tolerate other therapies. Oxygen may need to be added to CPAP therapy in patients with coexistent pulmonary disease such as COPD.

3. Surgical therapy—A variety of surgical proceedures have been used in attempts to treat OSAS and snoring. The understanding that airway obstruction often occurs at multiple sites in the airway is critical when recommending or planning surgical intervention. UPPP is the most frequently performed procedure and is designed to reduce airway obstruction at the level of the soft palate. The reported success rates for UPPP in OSAS is often in the range of 40–50%.

Laser-assisted uvuloplasty (LAUP) has been used, particularly as treatment for snoring. Although there may be short-term improvement in the majority of cases, the effectiveness decreases with time. Additionally, numerous patients have developed scarring and stenosis that lead to worsening of symptoms and even the development of overt OSA in patients who were previously nonapnic snorers. The maxillomandibular advancement procedure is associated with better success rates, often 90%. This procedure is often done in a staged fashion, used only after patients have failed initial procedures such as UPPP. Tracheotomy is an option that bypasses the upper airway obstruction. It is used for patients with severe life-threatening OSAS who can not be otherwise treated. Bariatric surgery, if leading to persistent weight loss, may be helpful in morbidly obese patients.

Regardless of which surgical procedure is selected, a follow-up PSG is recommended to assess the effectiveness of the therapy.

B. Central Sleep Apnea (CSA)

Treatment of patients with CSA begins with subcategorization of these patients into three groups: those with evidence of coexistent obstructive sleep apneas, those with evidence of waking or daytime alveolar hypoventilation, and those without either waking hypoventilation or OSA.

Patients who have CSA in conjunction with OSAS or any evidence of airflow limitation should be treated initially like a "pure OSA patient." Often the central events resolve (either acutely or over time) once the airway obstruction has been eliminated. Follow-up PSGs are recommended to determine if further treatment is needed.

Patients with waking hypoventilation (eg, Ondine's curse) but no evidence of airflow limitation often exhibit CSA as the sleep-related reduction in ventilatory drive results in central events. These patients can benefit from nocturnal ventilation, usually administered via a nasal mask. Sometimes tracheostomy will be necessary to deliver this therapy.

Patients without evidence of waking hypoventilation should be carefully evaluated for evidence of nasal obstruction, CHF, or neurological disease. If found, these conditions should be treated thoroughly and the patient reevaluated. If CSA persists, an in-laboratory titration of CPAP and/or oxygen is recommended. Acetazolamide has been used with moderate success in short-term studies involving few patients. For further discussion of the treatment of Cheyne– Stokes respiration–central sleep apnea associated with CHF (see Chapter 30).

Berger G et al: Laser-assisted uvuloplasty for snoring: medium to long-term subjective and objective analysis. Arch Otolaryngol Head Neck Surg 2001;127:412. [PMID: 11296050]. (LAUP results deteriorate over time.)

Bettega G et al: Fifty-one consecutive patients treated by maxillofacial surgery. Am J Respir Crit Care Med 2000;162:641. [PMID: 10934100]. (AHI decreased from 59 to 11/h in patients treated with extensive maxillomandibular surgery.)

Scheller M et al: Bariatric surgery for treatment of sleep apnea syndrome in 15 morbidly obese patients: long-term results. Otolarygol Head Neck Surg 2001;125:299. [PMID: 11593162]. (Average RDI decreased from 96 to 11/h with bariatric surgery.)

Sin D et al: Long-term compliance rates to CPAP in obstructive sleep apnea. Chest 2002;121:430. [PMID: 11834653]. (Intensive follow-up leads to CPAP compliance of 88% at 6 months.)

Walker-Engström M et al: 4-year follow-up of treatment with dental appliance or uvulopalatopharyngoplasty in patients with obstructive sleep apnea. Chest 2002;121:739. [PMID: 11888954]. (Normalization of AHI to less than 10/h in 63% of patients treated with mandibular devices and 33% of patients treated with UPPP at 4 years.)

Evaluation of Sleepiness & Sleep Disorders Other Than Sleep Apnea: Narcolepsy, Restless Leg Syndrome, & Periodic Limb Movements

29

Carolyn H. Welsh, MD

ESSENTIALS OF DIAGNOSIS

- *Sleepiness results from habits leading to inadequate time asleep, alterations in daily sleep patterns, primary sleep disorders, medications, or medical diseases; not all sleepiness is from sleep apnea.*
- *Taking a good history is critical to treatment of disease and appropriate sleep laboratory referral.*

General Considerations

Hypersomnolence is defined as sleepiness or drowsiness during the day, sometimes even after a full night's sleep. Sleepiness can lead to irritability, depression, or lack of vigilance, with resultant falling asleep when driving. Sleepiness can also impair cognitive function and lead to poor job performance. The impact of sleepiness on health and daytime functioning is underestimated and often ignored by physicians as well as the public. Accidents on the road are increasingly associated with sleepiness and are expensive. In the United States, the indirect costs of sleep-related accidents are estimated to be one hundred billion dollars per year.

Sleepiness is common, and can be caused by poor general sleep habits as well as sleep disorders (Table 29–1). Sleepiness from inadequate hours of sleep is widespread in our society, with fewer hours of sleep time today compared to 100 years ago for the average adult. Changes in circadian rhythm in sleep, such as advanced or delayed sleep phase, may lead to enhanced sleepiness. For example, getting to bed at 4:00 AM and arising at 7:00 AM for school may be the most comfortable schedule for an adolescent, but results in daytime sleepiness (delayed sleep phase). There are large num-

bers of people doing shift work, and others with poor quality sleep or inadequate sleep due to insomnia. Daytime sleepiness is frequently a hallmark of obstructive sleep apnea, as discussed in Chapter 28. Sleepiness may also result from underlying medical conditions as well as primary sleep disorders such as sleep apnea, narcolepsy, or restless leg syndrome. Often, patients with sleepiness from insomnia, defined as the inability to get to sleep or stay asleep, or those with poor sleep habits are referred for sleep apnea evaluation without having had a sleep history taken by the referring physician. To evaluate sleep apnea appropriately and distinguish it from other conditions, it is important to take a good sleep history, know how common systemic diseases impact sleep, and learn how to refer appropriate patients to a sleep laboratory for diagnostic sleep apnea testing.

Clinical Findings

A good sleep history is important in assessing sleepiness. A recent survey in an ambulatory care setting indicated that physicians and nurses rarely inquired about sleep. Patients are often reluctant to address sleep problems during an office visit even when they experience sleep difficulties; asking about sleep can provide physicians with insight into disease and efficacy of treatments. Particular questions about sleep include the time a patient goes to bed, the time of actual getting to sleep, whether there are nocturnal awakenings, and if so when and for what reason. It is also important to determine how long it takes a person to return to sleep if they have awakenings. Other important parts of the history include timing of morning awakening and arising and a detailed history of naps in the daytime. Bed partner observations are often critical in assessing sleep and should include inquiries about restlessness, snoring, breathing cessation, and impact of sleeplessness on daily functioning.

Table 29–1. Diagnoses and conditions causing sleepiness.

Diagnosis	Prevalence	Finding
Insomnia	Very common	Trouble initiating or maintaining sleep
Lack of sufficient sleep	Very common	Sleeps in on weekends
Poor sleep hygiene	Very common	Sleepiness or insomnia
Circadian rhythm problem	Common	Pattern of advanced or delayed time of sleep
Obstructive sleep apnea	Common	Cessation of breathing at night
Central sleep apnea	Moderate	Congestive heart failure or neurological disease
Periodic limb movements disorders	Common, 20% over age 65	Leg jerking, unrefreshed sleep
Parasomnias	Rare, childhood predominant	Sleepwalking, sleep terrors; no recall of events; sleepiness rare
Narcolepsy	Rare	Very, very sleepy
Restless leg syndrome	Common	Legs symptoms worse in the evening and relieved by activity
Depression	Common	Usually insomnia, 10% with sleepiness
Idiopathic hypersomnia	5–10% of patients in sleep clinics	Similar to narcolepsy

A full medication history often reveals use of medications that affect sleep in symptomatic patients. Medications used to treat anxiety disorders and psychosis can cause either insomnia or excess sleepiness. Medications that prevent patients from getting to sleep or maintaining sleep may lead to daytime sleepiness. The selective serotonin reuptake inhibitors (SSRIs), for example, often cause insomnia whereas many of the antipsychotic medications and several of the tricyclic antidepressants frequently increase symptoms of sleepiness. Common medications that induce sleepiness are listed in Table 29–2.

Physical examination generally does not provide major clues for sleepiness, aside from the observation that a patient is falling asleep during an interview. Excessive leg movements of restless leg syndrome are rarely noticeable.

Special Studies

A. Sleep Diary

Often an unexpectedly short time allotted for sleep may explain daytime sleepiness. A patient who goes to bed at 11:00 PM, gets to sleep at 11:30 PM, and is up at 5 AM to prepare for work gets only 5.5 h of sleep. This is probably insufficient, as the average adult requires 7–8 h of sleep nightly. A sleep log or diary may help gather information on sleep habits that a patient is not able to articulate during an interview. To compile a useful diary, patients are asked to track for 2–4 weeks the time

they go to sleep, when they awaken, sleep interruptions, and napping. They are also asked to include times of meals, medications, and reasons they awoke during sleep, as well as related events in their lives such as family crises or other stressful events and conditions. As an example, a 3:00 AM onset of sleep time with awakening at 7:30 AM daily for work may not be mentioned during a brief conversation in the office, but will be obvious from a sleep log. It is also possible that the sleep onset at 3:00 AM may be from a circadian alteration in the sleep–wake cycle, such as a delayed sleep phase. Not all delayed sleep is problematic, but it can lead to chronic sleep deprivation for those needing to arise early in the morning for work or school. See Table 29–3 for other tests used to assess sleepiness.

B. Subjective Sleep Scores

Assessment of subjective scores of sleepiness may improve focus on when to refer a patient to a sleep laboratory for assessment or provide insight on ongoing treatments. The Epworth Sleepiness Scale score evaluates whether eight common situations induce sleep and scores each situation on a scale of zero to three. A score of 6–7 is normal, 11 is common for people with sleep apnea, and 18 is characteristic of people with narcolepsy. The Stanford Sleepiness Scale estimates current level of sleepiness. The Functional Outcomes of Sleep Questionnaire (FOSQ) is a well-validated questionnaire that determines how disorders of excessive sleepiness affect patients' abilities to conduct normal activities. Re-

Table 29–2. Medications that increase sleepiness.

Benzodiazepines
  Chlordiazepoxide
  Flurazepam
  Diazepam
  Temazepam
  Lorazepam
  Triazolam
Seizure medications
  Phenobarbital
  Diphenylhydantoin, phenytoin
  Primidone
  Gabapentin
  Carbamazepine
  Valproic acid
Tricyclic antidepressant medications
  Amitriptyline
  Doxepin
Neuroleptic medications
  Chlorpromazine
  Thioridazine
  Clozapine
  Mirtazapine
Trazodone
Nefazodone
Clonidine
α-Methyldopa
Antihistamines, especially first generation

peating the assessment helps determine whether function is improved by treatment. Use of one or more of these scores can quantify a baseline level of sleepiness and ascertain response to treatment.

C. PHYSIOLOGICAL TESTING

Polysomnography is the diagnostic gold standard for sleep apnea, but is not uniformly needed for complaints of excessive sleepiness. A sleep history is of primary importance in identifying insufficient sleep as the cause of symptoms. Details of polysomnography and multiple sleep latency testing, the latter used to assess the time needed to fall sleep, are included in Chapter 28 and under the discussion of narcolepsy below.

Oximetry detects oxygen desaturation and pulse rate with a finger or ear probe. Although nocturnal oximetry is widely used as a screen for sleep apnea, its use for this purpose is not validated and other abnormalities of breathing may be missed. Nocturnal oximetry at present should be limited to patients with conditions such as chronic obstructive or interstitial lung disease where nocturnal hypoxemia is suspected and the likely treatment is supplemental oxygen.

Differential Diagnosis

Causes of daytime sleepiness are diverse and include alterations in circadian rhythm, insufficient sleep, insomnia, obstructive and central sleep apnea, and upper airway resistance syndrome. Apneas cause sleepiness in part by greater frequency of arousals, leading to increased sleep fragmentation, decreased total sleep time, increased Stage 1 sleep, and diminished slow wave and rapid eye movement (REM) sleep. Narcolepsy, restless leg syndrome, and periodic limb movements cause daytime hypersomnolence and often masquerade as obstructive sleep apnea. Psychiatric disorders impact sleep

Table 29–3. Tests for sleepiness assessment.

Test	Finding
History	Reason for sleepiness
Subjective scores to assess sleepiness	
Epworth Sleepiness Scale score	Rough quantification of overall sleepiness
Stanford Sleepiness Scale	Sleepiness at the time of questioning
Functional Outcomes of Sleep Questionnaire (FOSQ)	Impact of sleepiness on life
Vigilance testing	Slowed reflexes/possibility of danger in driving
Actigraphy	Records movements while awake, inactivity in sleep; used over 24 h
Polysomnography	Sleep latency (short if sleepy, long if insomnia)
	Arousals
	Sleep apnea events
	Periodic limb movements (normal up to 5/h)
Multiple sleep latency test (MSLT)	Short sleep latency (less than 5 min in daytime)
Maintenance of wakefulness test (MWT)	Propensity to sleep or stay awake in a quiet environment

and can cause either insomnia or daytime sleepiness. Up to 90% of patients with major depressive disorders have sleep disturbances. Medical diseases that cause sleepiness include congestive heart failure (CHF), chronic obstructive lung disease, asthma, seizures, and Parkinson's disease. Sleepiness due to these latter diseases is discussed in Chapter 30. Common causes of daytime sleepiness are listed in Table 29–1.

Treatment

A good history often pinpoints the reason for sleep problems. Solutions start with treatment of medical conditions that may be inducing sleepiness, such as heart failure, chronic obstructive pulmonary disease (COPD) or seizures. Improvement in sleep habits, termed sleep hygiene, is sometimes the most important treatment for persons with sleep complaints. Sleep hygiene should be reviewed with the patient to improve sleep. Hygiene advice includes avoidance of tobacco, alcohol, and caffeine, improvement of the sleep environment, relaxation techniques before bedtime, and sleep restriction for insomniacs. A synopsis of these recommendations is included in Table 29–4.

A detailed discussion of insomnia is not possible here. The American Academy of Sleep Medicine provides practice parameters for behavioral treatment of insomnia. Drug therapies can be used on occasion to improve sleep. Adjustments in medications or the time of

day when they are delivered can markedly improve sleepiness. For example, a dose of furosemide at 10:00 PM often causes multiple awakenings for trips to the bathroom at night. The awakenings that lead to sleep deprivation can be avoided if the diuretic is given earlier in the day. Many antidepressant medications, including the SSRIs used for depression, lead to insomnia and are better dosed early in the day.

Chesson AL Jr et al: Practice parameters for the nonpharmacologic treatment of chronic insomnia. An American Academy of Sleep Medicine report. Standards of Practice Committee of the American Academy of Sleep Medicine. Sleep 1999; 22:1128. [PMID: 10617175]. (Detailed recommendations for insomnia treatment are outlined here.)

Douglas NJ: "Why am I sleepy?" Sorting the somnolent. Am J Respir Crit Care Med 2001;163:1310. [PMID: 11371393]. (The author discusses narcolepsy, periodic limb movement disorder, delayed sleep phase syndrome, and shift work.)

Johns MW: A new method for measuring daytime sleepiness: the Epworth Sleepiness Scale. Sleep 1991;14:540. [PMID: 1798888]. (This includes information on how to use the Epworth scale.)

Namen AM et al: Performance of sleep histories in an ambulatory medicine clinic. Chest 1999;116:1558. [PMID: 10593776]. (Obtaining a history of sleep habits is underused but quick to perform with excellent insights.)

NARCOLEPSY

 ESSENTIALS OF DIAGNOSIS

- Narcolepsy patients present with daytime sleepiness, cataplexy, hallucinations, sleep paralysis, and nocturnal sleep fragmentation.
- Cataplexy is the hallmark symptom, but may lag for years behind other symptoms or never appear.
- Diagnosis is based on a history of extreme sleepiness during the day with demonstration of short sleep latency and sleep onset REM periods by multiple sleep latency testing (MSLT).
- Biochemical diagnostic testing for HLA DQB1* 0602 or low or absent cerebral spinal fluid hypocretin can be useful.

General Considerations

Narcolepsy is an uncommon but dramatic disorder with an incidence in the North American population of

Table 29–4. Sleep hygiene recommendations.

Optimize sleep scheduling and sleep environment
    Get a regular sleep–wake schedule
    Consider avoiding naps
    Remain active and exposed to bright light during the day
    Perform regular exercise in late afternoon, not just before bedtime
    Consider a hot tub bath 1–2 h before bedtime
    Avoid extreme heat or cold in bedroom
Avoid sleep-altering foods and supplements
    Coffee
    Tobacco
    Alcohol
    Have only a light bedtime snack, avoid heavy evening meals
Stimulus control strategy
    Go to bed when you feel sleepy
    Restrict bedroom to sleep and sex; avoid use for TV, paperwork, eating, or challenging activities
    If sleep is unsuccessful within 30 min, get up and engage in quiet activity until sleepy again
    Stay in bed as long as sleep is needed but no longer

approximately 0.05%. Risk of narcolepsy for first-degree relatives of narcolepsy patients is 0.9–2.3%, which is 10–40 times higher than in the general population. It presents with profound sleepiness, drop attacks (cataplexy) that are induced by emotion, sleep-associated paralysis, and hallucinations. Although rare, its impact on life is severe and therefore appropriate diagnosis and treatment are important. The usual age of onset of symptoms is during teen or young adult years, between ages 15 and 30. Six percent of patients, however, manifest symptoms before age 10. Other sleep disorders including periodic limb movements and sleep apnea may coexist with narcolepsy, making diagnosis difficult. Lack of awareness of this disorder by physicians has led to underdiagnosis in the community, with diagnosis lagging onset of symptoms by as much as 10 years.

Pathogenesis

Narcolepsy is characterized by loss of sleep regulation, with appearance of REM sleep manifestations during wakefulness. Hypocretin has recently been described as a molecule that is lacking or dysfunctional in both animal models of narcolepsy and patients with narcolepsy. Hypocretin, considered an organizing transmitter regulating sleep state, is primarily located in the prefornical area of the hypothalamus with neuronal projections to sleep centers of the brain. It stimulates monoaminergic tone and is thought to integrate the monoaminergic and cholinergic brain pathways of sleep and wakefulness, and thereby regulate sleep.

A better understanding of the mechanisms of narcolepsy has developed from animal models of the disease. A genetic defect in canine narcolepsy that results in a nonfunctional hypocretin (orexin) receptor has been identified. A preprohypocretin knockout mouse model also shows narcolepsy-like symptoms. In humans, low or reduced hypocretin levels are seen in the cerebrospinal fluid of narcoleptic patients, presumed to result from functional hypocretin depletion in the hypothalamus. The low hypocretin activity is thought to lead to sleepiness and inappropriate appearance of REM sleep by activating or overstimulating cholinergic nerves or by depleting adrenergic nerves.

Prior to discovery of hypocretin as a unifying biochemical abnormality in the pathogenesis of narcolepsy, pathogenic investigation focused on an autoimmune nature of narcolepsy. There is an association of narcolepsy with HLA class II antigens DR15 (DR2), especially DQB1*0602. Although most narcoleptic patients have this HLA type, the majority of people with DQB1*0602 never develop narcolepsy. An autoimmune etiology still remains of interest, due to the uncommon nature of the disease in at-risk individuals and the discrepancy of the disease in monozygotic twins. Ongoing assessment of autoimmune mechanisms leading to depletion of hypocretin continues.

Clinical Findings

Symptoms of narcolepsy include the traditional tetrad of sleepiness, cataplexy, hallucinations, and sleep paralysis. Three symptoms, cataplexy, hallucinations, and paralysis, are characterized as REM phenomena occurring inappropriately during wakefulness. In narcolepsy, sleepiness is profound and usually more debilitating than in other disorders causing sleepiness, including sleep apnea. There are often actual microsleeps or sleep attacks as well as episodes of falling asleep at inopportune moments. All patients with narcolepsy have daytime sleepiness as reflected in their history and by Epworth Sleepiness Scale scores in the high teens and above. Sleep at night may be fragmented. On awakening in the mornings, patients with narcolepsy claim that their sleepiness is improved but 1–2 h later it recurs. Napping often relieves symptoms for several hours, but sleepiness recurs on average several times each day.

The presence of cataplexy is pathognomonic for narcolepsy. Cataplexy is the sudden loss of muscle tone triggered by emotion, especially anger, laughter, excitement, surprise, or even a joke. Cataplexy can vary from dramatic to subtle with findings such as falling down, stumbling, sagging jaw, head nod, slurred speech, or muscle twitching. When this symptom is present in a sleepy patient, diagnostic testing with a multiple sleep latency test may not be needed to confirm the diagnosis, although it is generally recommended.

Hallucinations are present in the majority of patients. Visual hallucinations are most common, but auditory symptoms are somewhat more specific for narcolepsy. Hallucination content is often frightening or gloomy. Paralysis either at sleep onset (hypnogogic) or awakening (hypnopompic) can be frightening. Patients are aware of an inability to move, lasting from seconds to minutes. The cataplexy, hallucinations, and paralysis all suggest a disordered control of REM sleep with intrusion into times of wakefulness. In narcolepsy, there is also early development of REM sleep shortly after the onset of sleep, rather than after the average 90-min lag in adults.

The most common symptom in narcolepsy is sleepiness, which occurs in all patients. Sleep fragmentation or frequent awakening at night is the second most common symptom, occurring in almost 90% of patients. It is often overlooked for the more dramatic REM manifestations of paralysis and hallucinations, which occur in 70–80% of patients.

There are no characteristic findings on physical examination for narcolepsy. Narcolepsy patients have been found to be on average 1 kg heavier than age-matched controls. Patients with narcolepsy may appear drowsy and nod off during conversations in the office, experiencing short episodes of sleep called microsleeps.

Polysomnography (PSG) is routinely performed for people with suspected narcolepsy to look for sleep-disordered breathing such as obstructive sleep apnea and periodic limb movements. These are more common in patients with narcolepsy than in the general population. Findings on sleep study include a short sleep latency of < 10 min, REM sleep starting < 60 min after sleep onset, frequent awakenings, and often an increased amount of light (Stage I) sleep.

Multiple sleep latency testing (MSLT) is the diagnostic test of choice for narcolepsy. This test is performed the night after a full sleep study that shows an absence of sleep apneas or adequate treatment by nasal continuous positive airway pressure (CPAP) therapy. After a night in the sleep laboratory, five nap studies are recorded at 2-h intervals. Patients are instructed to try to fall asleep. Each attempt at a nap is stopped at 20 min if there is no sleep or after 15 min of sleep. Because use of medications such as antidepressants, stimulants, or narcotics may induce sleepiness or facilitate sleep-onset REM periods, MSLT should be performed after medications have been removed for 14–15 days. In most laboratories, patients undergo a urine toxicology screen for opiates, phencyclidine, cannabinoids, benzodiazepines, cocaine, barbiturates, and amphetamines to exclude these drugs as a cause of their sleepiness. The two characteristic MSLT findings in narcolepsy are short sleep latency (time needed to get to sleep) and sleep-onset REM periods. Normal sleep latency is 10–20 min. Less than 5 min is pathological and is characteristic of narcolepsy. Sleep-onset REM periods do not normally occur; two periods of REM sleep during an MSLT plus short sleep latency are considered diagnostic of narcolepsy.

If the MSLT study is diagnostic of narcolepsy, appropriate treatment for daytime sleepiness can be initiated. If sleepiness and cataplexy are both present, the diagnosis is straightforward. There are, however, patients whose diagnosis remains perplexing. Some of these are diagnosed with idiopathic hypersomnia. Patients with idiopathic hypersomnia are similarly sleepy, but generally have slightly longer sleep latencies during the nap studies and lack sleep-onset REM periods. Cataplexy is not associated with idiopathic hypersomnia.

Multiple wake testing (MWT) is an alternate nap study format. Patients in a quiet environment are instructed to stay awake rather than fall asleep. It is less well standardized than the MSLT and therefore more difficult to interpret. It is currently used less frequently, although it may be a better way to assess ability to stay awake.

Differential Diagnosis

Several conditions, including obstructive sleep apnea, present with daytime sleepiness. Obstructive sleep apnea is a common problem in middle-aged adults with sleepiness (see Chapter 28). Table 29–1 lists conditions causing sleepiness and highlights distinguishing features. Idiopathic hypersomnia is a diagnosis of exclusion. Patients have symptoms similar to narcolepsy but without cataplexy or sleep-onset REM on diagnostic testing. Lack of a sufficient amount of sleep or insomnia can cause daytime sleepiness. A history of late bedtimes, lengthy time needed to get to sleep, awakening(s) at night, and awakening time in morning suggest insufficient sleep. Sleeping in on weekends further suggests lack of sufficient sleep during the week. Circadian rhythm disorders can present with increased sleepiness. These include delayed sleep phase (common in adolescents) or advanced sleep phase (more common in older adults). Sleepiness may be associated with shift work and frequently changing schedules. Taking a history and obtaining a sleep diary can usually pinpoint the altered times of sleepiness in these latter conditions.

Restless leg syndrome and periodic limb movements can present with sleepiness and are discussed below. Although sleepiness is an important symptom in these conditions, they do not often cause the profound degree of sleepiness seen with narcolepsy. Cardiac and respiratory disorders including CHF, asthma, and chronic obstructive lung disease may present with a primary complaint of sleepiness. In addition, neurological and psychiatric conditions such as dementia, seizures, or mood disorders can present with sleepiness as a chief complaint. Chapter 30 highlights several of these conditions.

Complications

Narcoleptic patients have sleepiness that is more profound than seen with any of the sleep disorders. This can lead to poor work performance and ultimately job loss or marital and family strife. A great concern is the risk of falling asleep while driving, which endangers the life of the patient and other drivers on the road. Patients must be counseled to avoid driving until their sleepiness is treated.

Prevention

There is no known prevention of narcolepsy.

Treatment

The goal of treatment of narcolepsy is to improve alertness by improving sleep hygiene and by developing effective medication strategies that have minimal side effects. Medications are also used to treat the symptoms of cataplexy.

Nonpharmacological treatments include several behavioral interventions that complement drug therapy. Regular sleep and wake times are more important for persons with narcolepsy than for most people. Prevention of sleep deprivation is important to avoid worsening sleepiness. Counseling a patient to avoid shift work is useful, as the sleep–wake pattern imposed by this work schedule adds to sleep deprivation. Work in a stimulating environment that helps the patient stay awake during the day may be beneficial. Scheduling short naps during the daytime is a particularly useful strategy for most patients. Discussion of the diagnosis of narcolepsy with supervisors should be strongly considered, as patients with narcolepsy are frequently erroneously labeled as lazy and suboptimal employees. The Americans with Disabilities Act should be discussed with the employer to facilitate appropriate accommodation in the workplace. Driving poses risks related to falling asleep at the wheel if narcolepsy is undertreated and safety while driving or even a ban on driving should be discussed. When symptoms of sleepiness worsen, it is important to consider repeating a sleep study to see if sleep apnea or periodic limb movements have newly developed. Because these are more common in people with narcolepsy, they, rather than a progression of narcolepsy itself, may worsen sleepiness.

Medications to treat sleepiness in patients with narcolepsy are outlined in Table 29–5. Modafinil is considered a first-line drug. It promotes wakefulness through mechanisms different from amphetamine stimulants. It also may improve cognitive performance during sleep deprivation in normal adults. Side effects include headache, nervousness, nausea, and rhinitis. There appears to be less potential for addiction than for amphetamines. Methylphenidate (ritalin), commonly prescribed for attention deficit hyperactivity disorder, is a stimulant that has been used with great success in treating narcolepsy. Side effects include nervousness, anorexia, dizziness, palpitations, and tachycardia. It is thought to be a reasonably safe treatment for children with narcolepsy.

Amphetamines such as dextroamphetamine and methamphetamine are stimulants currently used to treat the daytime sleepiness associated with narcolepsy. These may have a somewhat greater impact on sleepiness than modafinil, but also have more side effects. There is potential for abuse, although patients with narcolepsy are less likely than other people to abuse amphetamines. The recommendation is to start dosing low and increase slowly, titrating to sleepiness. Toxicity of amphetamines includes anxiety, irritability, palpitations, tremor, anorexia, headache, and insomnia. Pemoline, another effective medication for sleepiness, was transiently withdrawn from the U.S. market because of a 4- to 17-fold increase in risk of acute hepatic failure. It is currently available, but frequent monitoring of liver function enzymes is mandatory. Experience with selegiline, a monoamine oxidase inhibitor, is limited, but presents the possibility of treating both sleepiness and cataplexy with a single compound.

γ-Hydroxybutyrate (sodium oxybate) is a hypnotic agent with a short half-life that is used to treat cataplexy. Side effects include rebound insomnia and respiratory depression. It is recreationally abused as the "date rape" drug. Sodium oxybate is currently available only in one central pharmacy in the United States due to its potential for abuse and must be monitored closely. It is dosed at bedtime and repeated 4 h later. Its putative advantage is based on four studies that show it diminishes episodes of cataplexy and improves quality of nighttime sleep, leading to improvements in daytime sleepiness.

Table 29–5. Treatment of daytime sleepiness in narcolepsy.

Drug	Estimated Daily Dose	Side Effects
Modafinil	200–400 mg	Headache, nausea
Methylphenidate	20–100 mg	Nervousness, insomnia
Dextroamphetamine	30–100 mg	Tachycardia, constipation, restlessness, insomnia
Methamphetamine	40–80 mg	Longer duration of action, same side effects
Selegiline	20–40 mg	Nausea, orthostatic hypotension
Pemoline	75–150 mg	Acute liver failure
Sodium oxybate	3–9 in divided doses at bedtime and 4 h later	Nausea, weight loss, drowsiness, enuresis, risk of recreational use

Table 29–6. Drug treatment of cataplexy in narcolepsy.

Medication	Estimated Starting Dose
Imipramine	10 mg
Clomipramine	10 mg
Protriptyline	10 mg
Fluoxetine	20 mg
Venlafaxine	37.5 mg
Selegiline	20 mg (also treats daytime sleepiness)
Sodium oxybate	3–9 g, divided dose

Medications used specifically to treat the symptoms of cataplexy are outlined in Table 29–6. The SSRI drugs are now more commonly prescribed because the tricyclic antidepressant medications have more anticholinergic side effects.

Prognosis

Prognosis for persons with narcolepsy is good with a normal life expectancy. Unfortunately, none of the treatments achieves a cure; it is a lifelong condition. There is continued daytime sleepiness for most patients despite therapy with stimulants or modafinil.

Hungs M, Mignot E: Hypocretin/orexin, sleep and narcolepsy. Bioessays 2001;23:397. [PMID: 11340621]. (This is a review of the role of hypocretin in narcolepsy.)

Littner M et al for the Standards of Practice Committee: Practice parameters for the treatment of narcolepsy: an update for 2000. Sleep 2001;24:451. [PMID: 11403530]. (These are guidelines for use of medications.)

Narcolepsy web site http://www.Narcolepsynetwork.org. (Web site of a national nonprofit organization of patients and professionals involved with narcolepsy with frequently updated scientific and medical information.)

RESTLESS LEG SYNDROME

 ESSENTIALS OF DIAGNOSIS

- Restless leg syndrome is a common cause of impaired sleep, either sleepiness or insomnia, that often presents in early adulthood.
- There is a familial association for two-thirds of patients with an autosomal dominant pattern.
- Sensations of creeping or crawling in legs are characteristic.
- There is an urge to move the legs and sometimes the arms, with the motor restlessness worsening with rest and improving with movement.
- Circadian variability in symptoms is seen, with the worst symptoms in the evening and early night.

General Considerations

Restless leg syndrome (RLS) can impair quality of sleep and lead to frequent arousals and sleepiness during the daytime. RLS is defined as an urge to move the legs, worst in the evening, and an associated disagreeable sensation sometimes called creeping or crawling that is heightened by inactivity. Exact prevalence is not known. There are estimates that it occurs in 1.2–15% of the population, which makes it one of the most common and treatable causes of sleep problems. Eighty percent of persons with RLS will have periodic leg movements of sleep, although the converse is not true.

About 50% of patients with idiopathic or primary RLS have symptom onset before age 20. People with a secondary form of the disorder have onset later, concurrent with their medical disorder. Primary RLS is an autosomal dominant condition, distinct from secondary RLS, in which other medical conditions such as iron deficiency, a postgastrectomy state, neurological cord lesions, pregnancy (19% of pregnant patients), uremia (50% of patients undergoing hemodialysis), rheumatoid arthritis, amyloid, and folate or B_{12} deficiency are associated with onset of symptoms. Uremia is the second most common reason for RLS after primary RLS and is an underappreciated predisposing condition. Women with idiopathic or primary RLS frequently have worsening of symptoms during pregnancy.

Pathogenesis

Primary RLS is an inherited disorder, probably with an autosomal dominant pattern. The dopaminergic nervous system may be important in the pathogenesis of RLS. Women with high activity of the monoamine oxidase A (MAO-A) gene and correspondingly low synaptic dopamine levels have a greater risk for RLS than women with a lower activity allele. Low doses of levodopa relieve RLS symptoms in many patients. Linkage analysis with a family pedigree suggests that the gene(s) for RLS are on chromosome 12q, although this has yet to be confirmed.

It is estimated that 20–50% of renal failure patients on dialysis have symptoms of restless legs. Approximately 20% of pregnant women also experience RLS. It is hypothesized that iron deficiency may disrupt functioning of the brain's dopaminergic system as iron is a critical cofactor for tyrosine hydroxylase, a rate-limiting enzyme in dopamine synthesis. Studies using single-photon emission computed tomography or positron emission tomography (SPECT, PET) scanning show that there is a small decrease in dopamine measures in the striatum of the brain in patients with secondary RLS compared to control subjects.

Clinical Findings

A. SYMPTOMS AND SIGNS

Obtaining a good sleep history for patients with RLS is critical as treatment differs markedly from therapy for sleep apnea or narcolepsy. Diagnosis is based mostly on history without reliance on laboratory testing. Patients often present with sleepiness, although the degree of sleepiness is less than occurs with narcolepsy. Classic symptoms include painful sensations and leg jerking prior to sleep that often interfere with the ability to initiate sleep. The sensations can be tingling, burning, painful, or aching. Patients describe a strong urge to move their legs. The movements are often flexion of the hip, knee, or ankle. Motor restlessness is worsened by rest and temporarily improved with activity. Symptoms are generally most apparent in the evening and night and less irksome earlier in the day.

Symptoms can be triggered or exacerbated by stress or alcohol ingestion.

Findings on physical examination are those of observed restlessness. Patients may have stiff legs and flexion of legs and arms. There are no focal neurological findings.

B. LABORATORY TESTING

There are no specific diagnostic tests for RLS, although recent understanding of the genetic associations may lead to better understanding of specific laboratory abnormalities and subsequent development of laboratory tests.

Serum ferritin levels are inversely proportional to restless leg symptoms; iron deficiency exacerbates symptoms. Ferritin levels in the low or low-normal range (45–50 μg/L) are associated with worsening of symptoms, even in patients without anemia. Evaluation for folate, magnesium, and B_{12} deficiencies as well as creatinine and blood urea nitrogen is recommended.

Because 80% of patients have periodic limb movements (PLMs), a polysomnogram or overnight sleep study frequently shows flexor leg movements as defined further in the section on PLMs below (Figure 29–1).

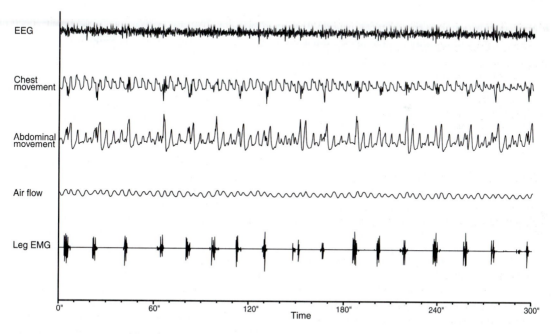

Figure 29–1. The polysomnographic appearance of the leg movements of periodic limb movement disorder is seen in the leg electromyogram (EMG) channel. They are repetitive, last 0.5–5 s (1 s on this tracing), and are 5–90 s apart (20–30 s in this tracing). There are often arousals at the end of the leg movements, although these are not demonstrated here; the associated deflections in the electroencephalogram (EEG), chest, and abdominal channels are motion artifacts.

PLMs are more common in the first half of the night. Sleep latency is often prolonged as leg/arm movements and symptoms interfere with sleep initiation.

Differential Diagnosis

The diagnosis should be considered in sleepy patients or those with unrefreshing sleep and in patients in whom an appropriate history has been elicited. Other diagnostic considerations in patients with sleep-related movements include fleeting myoclonic jerks that occur upon falling asleep. They are described as jolting movements at the onset of sleep, occur in 50–60% of normal persons, and are quicker and less sustained than RLS movements. Other conditions in which jerking leg movements are common include narcolepsy, fibromyalgia, PLMs without RLS, REM sleep behavior disorder, postpolio syndrome, lumbar spine radiculopathy, and nocturnal seizures.

Complications

Complications of RLS include insomnia for the patient and disturbed sleep for both the patient and bed partner. Daytime sleepiness is variable but can be severe.

Prevention

There is no known prevention for idiopathic RLS. Avoidance of some drugs, alcohol, and caffeine can alleviate symptoms, although this is not uniformly helpful.

Treatment

Treatment starts with activities that improve symptoms. Moderate physical activity is useful in some patients. Fatigue and stress may be exacerbants and avoidance of these help minimize symptoms. Some patients try hot baths prior to bedtime. Transcutaneous electrical nerve stimulation is of potential benefit, although there is little evidence to show efficacy at the present time. Avoidance of certain foods and drugs can be helpful including caffeine, alcohol, antihistamines, neuroleptics, antidepressants, or drugs that have dopamine antagonist activity such as calcium channel blocking agents, prochlorperazine, and metoclopramide. Specific medications such as SSRIs, tricyclic antidepressants, and lithium may worsen RLS. Bupropion reduces leg movements and may be a better antidepressant for people with RLS that the SSRIs or tricyclic antidepressant agents.

Recently published guidelines for treatment of RLS include recommendations for use of dopamine precursors, dopamine-receptor agonists, opioids, and benzodiazepines (Table 29–7). Dopamine agonists such as pergolide and pramipexole are used successfully for many

Table 29–7. Treatment of restless leg syndrome.

Dopamine precursors
  Levodopa ± carbidopa
Dopamine agonists
  Pergolide
  Pramipexole
  Ropinirole
  Bromocriptine
Opioids
  Propoxyphene
  Narcotics
    Codeine
    Oxycodone
    Methadone
    Tramadol
Benzodiazepine
  Clonazepam
Anticonvulsants
  Carbamazepine
  Gabapentin
Clonidine

patients. Side effects of pergolide include nausea, dizziness, insomnia, and nasal congestion. Most people tolerate pramipexole better, but occasionally daytime sleepiness is associated with pramipexole, which can be dangerous when driving or performing activities requiring vigilance. The dopamine precursor levodopa alleviates symptoms for a large number of patients. Levodopa/carbidopa is often a first-line drug for RLS due to its low cost. Small studies have suggested that benzodiazepines or certain anticonvulsants may be beneficial in treating RLS.

Treatment is not uniformly effective, especially with the benzodiazepines and anticonvulsant medications. Combinations of low doses of several medications or alternating drugs may help ameliorate loss of efficacy that occasionally occurs with some medications. Up to 80% of patients using levodopa may have augmentation, defined as RLS symptoms that begin appearing earlier during the day or involve new parts of the body with increasing severity. Dopaminergic agents appear to have less risk of augmentation than levodopa and can be substituted if augmentation occurs. Brief periods off levodopa may decrease augmentation, but this has not been substantiated. Other less common problems with levodopa include tolerance, need for increased doses of medication to treat symptoms, and rebound. Rebound is worsening of symptoms at the end of the action period of the drug, such as in the early morning for a nighttime dose of levodopa/carbidopa. Effective strategies for rebound include use of sustained release preparations of levodopa/carbidopa or switching to a dopaminergic agonist.

Treatment of iron deficiency or anemia can improve symptoms of secondary RLS and should be considered prior to use of the medications discussed above.

Prognosis

Lifespan for patients with primary RLS is typically normal. Although symptoms are bothersome, they rarely preclude daily activities. Idiopathic RLS begins at any age, with a peak in late childhood, and is only slowly progressive over years. Secondary RLS progresses more rapidly. When periodic limb movements are associated with Parkinson's disease or REM sleep behavior disorder, prognosis is that of the underlying disease.

Information site for the Restless Leg Syndrome Foundation at http://www.rls.org/frames/home_frame.htm. (Physician and patient information, updated every 2 years.)

National Heart Lung and Blood Institute working group on restless leg syndrome: Restless leg syndrome. Detection and management in primary care. Am Fam Physician 2000;62:108. [PMID: 10905782]. (This is a practical overview of diagnosis and treatment.)

Silber MH: Sleep disorders. Neurol Clin 2001;19:173. [PMID: 11471763]. (This is an overview of treatment for narcolepsy and restless leg syndrome.)

Winkelmann J et al: Clinical characteristics and frequency of the hereditary restless leg syndrome in a population of 300 patients. Sleep 2000;23:597. [PMID: 10947127]. (This is a good clinical description of restless leg syndrome.)

PERIODIC LIMB MOVEMENTS

 ESSENTIALS OF DIAGNOSIS

- *Periodic limb movements are a physiological finding on sleep studies characterized by dorsiflexion of the big toe with flexor movements of legs and/or arms.*
- *The impact of periodic limb movements on sleep quality is controversial; they can be associated with insomnia, sleepiness, or a normal degree of sleepiness.*
- *There is increased frequency with aging, iron deficiency, and renal disease.*

General Considerations

Periodic limb movements (PLMs) are defined as repetitive stereotyped leg and arm movements resulting in fragmented sleep. They are primarily a polysomnographic finding, but may result in daytime sleepiness by causing frequent awakenings at night. Their impact on sleep symptoms has recently been questioned.

The characteristic movements are large toe dorsiflexion with anterior tibialis leg muscle contractions lasting 0.5–5 s in duration (Figure 29–1). They occur by definition in clusters of at least four and are separated by 5–90 s. These are frequently followed by an arousal by electroencephalogram (EEG) or an awakening. The normal index of these limb movements is 0–5/h.

PLMs are considered to cause excessive sleepiness by leading to sleep interruptions and thereby sleep deprivation, although there is some debate about their importance. They can occur without an underlying disorder but are common in several sleep disorders such as RLS, Parkinson's disease, and sleep apnea syndromes. PLMs increase with age, with a prevalence of 5–6% in young adults and 25–58% in elderly, community-dwelling adults. A recent large epidemiological study of 18,980 Europeans aged 15–100 years found an incidence of 3.9%. Other associated conditions include renal disease, fibromyalgia, and folate and B_{12} deficiency. In the European survey, associated features for PLMs included snoring, daily coffee intake, use of hypnotics, stress, and shift work or work on a night shift.

Pathogenesis

The pathogenesis of PLMs is poorly understood. They are associated with sleep-disordered breathing, RLS, dopamine function, and iron deficiency. In one study 14 of 20 patients with PLMs of sleep had upper airway resistance syndrome; the apneic events were considered to cause an associated limb movement. A population study in the elderly found PLMs correlated with sleep-disordered breathing in women. There is an association and overlap with RLS in some patients.

The dopaminergic system appears to be important in the pathogenesis of PLMs. Iron is a cofactor for tyrosine hydroxylase in synthesizing dopamine and is hypothesized to be instrumental in manifestations of PLMs.

Clinical Findings

A. SYMPTOMS AND SIGNS

Patients with PLMs may present with sleepiness during the day or a complaint of interrupted sleep at night with the characteristic repetitive limb movements. The bedclothes are found in disarray, there are awakenings from sleep, and sleep is often unrefreshing. There may be comments about leg jerking at night by a bed partner. Alternatively, there may be insomnia or no symptoms. The uncertain clinical significance makes treatment decisions difficult. An additional confusing feature is that there may be variability in the number of movements from night to night. Patients who are sleepy or have insomnia from PLMs are considered to have periodic limb movement disorder.

Laboratory Testing

The number of limb movements per hour is counted on sleep study or polysomnography and more than five per hour is defined as high. There should be at least four limb movements clustered together to classify them as PLMs; single jerks are not counted. The number of movements is generally highest at the beginning of the night and drops during the second half of the night. There is some variability in the index from night to night.

For symptomatic limb movements, the same diagnostic testing used for RLS needs to be considered. Specifically, an assessment for renal disease, iron deficiency, and ferritin level may reveal definable causes for the movements. A ferritin level < 50 ng/mL (50 μg/L) may worsen the condition. Folate, B_{12}, and magnesium deficiencies may occasionally contribute to periodic limb movement disorder.

Differential Diagnosis

Conditions causing nocturnal limb movements are listed under the differential diagnosis section for RLS above. Leg cramps and RLS are most commonly considered in the differential diagnosis. Although a majority of patients (80%) with RLS have PLMs, the converse is not true. RLS is a more specific diagnosis than PLMs, with distinctive leg sensations more noticeable in the evening and often relieved by movement.

Treatment

Because iron is considered a cofactor for tyrosine hydroxylase in processing dopamine, treatment with iron is considered for patients with low ferritin even when they are not anemic. Treatment with medications targeted at diminishing movements is recommended for those symptomatic from the leg movements; exactly which patients to treat is uncertain, but probably should include those who are sleepy, those with arousals after leg movements by polysomnography, and those who awaken with movements. The medications are the same as for RLS and are listed in Table 29–7.

Prognosis

There is great variability in the estimated prognosis for periodic limb movement disorder. Some experts are unconvinced that PLMs are associated with poor quality sleep or daytime sleepiness and think that they are manifestations of the upper airway resistance seen in sleep apnea. These patients should, accordingly, be treated for sleep apnea. A recent long-term follow-up of a cohort of adults showed no consistent change in severity of PLMs in the elderly over an 18-year follow-up period. A large number of PLMs in patients with renal failure was shown to correlate with higher mortality. Use of erythropoietin in one tantalizing study of patients undergoing dialysis reduced the number of PLMs in sleep.

Benz RL et al: Potential novel predictors of mortality in end-stage renal disease patients with sleep disorders. Am J Kidney Dis 2000;35:1052. [PMID: 10845816]. (Periodic limb movements are a poor prognostic sign in renal disease.)

Chervin RD: Periodic leg movements and sleepiness in patients evaluated for sleep-disordered breathing. Am J Respir Crit Care Med 2001;164:1454. [PMID: 11704595]. (The rate of leg movements shows no correlation with daytime sleepiness.)

Exar EN, Collop NA: The association of upper airway resistance with periodic limb movements. Sleep 2001;24:188. [PMID: 11247055]. (Subtle upper airway obstruction leads to periodic limb movements.)

Gehrman P et al: Long-term follow-up of periodic limb movements in sleep in older adults. Sleep 2002;25:340. [PMID: 12003165]. (The prevalence of PLMs is high in the elderly, but the severity of the disorder does not progressively worsen with increasing age.)

Ohayon MM, Roth T: Prevalence of restless leg syndrome and periodic limb movement disorder in the general population. J Psychosom Res 2002;53:547. [PMID: 12127170]. (Prevalence and risk factors for RLS and PLMD are distinguished.)

Medical Conditions That Often Cause Daytime Sleepiness

Carolyn H. Welsh, MD

ESSENTIALS OF DIAGNOSIS

- *Sleepiness in the day or wakefulness at night (insomnia) can be caused by medical disorders other than sleep apnea.*
- *Conditions such as heart failure, chronic obstructive lung disease, asthma, gastroesophageal reflux, fibromyalgia, Parkinson's disease, and seizures are associated with sleepiness and manifestations during sleep.*
- *Treatment directed at the underlying medical condition often decreases sleepiness and improves patient function.*

General Considerations

Many respiratory diseases have manifestations during sleep. Medical, neurological, and psychiatric conditions may present as primary sleep problems or generate sleep complaints, in particular, sleepiness during the daytime. Insomnia, especially awakening from sleep (sleep maintenance insomnia), is common in patients with sleep apnea and narcolepsy but also in patients with chronic obstructive pulmonary disease (COPD), asthma, gastroesophageal reflux, and fibromyalgia. It may be difficult when patients first present to separate symptoms due to pulmonary diseases from those caused by sleep-disordered breathing. This can be especially challenging for the physician, because sleep apnea, heart failure, and COPD are all common in middle-aged and older adults and may all be present in the same patient. It is important to identify patients with impaired sleep resulting from medical conditions other than sleep apnea as treatment differs. This chapter highlights common medical diagnoses associated with daytime sleepiness or sleep symptoms that may masquerade as sleep apnea. For details on a general approach to sleepiness and the sleep disorders that come to the attention of an internist, specifically sleep apnea, narcolepsy, restless leg

syndrome, and periodic limb movements, see Chapters 28 and 29.

Common medical conditions with sleep manifestations are listed in Table 30–1. The conditions highlighted in this chapter include cardiac, pulmonary, musculoskeletal, and neurological disorders. Both sleepiness and difficulty staying asleep with frequent nocturnal awakenings are particularly problematic for some patients with congestive heart failure, COPD, asthma, gastroesophageal reflux disease, Parkinson's disease, and fibromyalgia. Seizures may present with daytime sleepiness even without documented nocturnal awakenings.

CONGESTIVE HEART FAILURE

ESSENTIALS OF DIAGNOSIS

- *Obstructive sleep apnea and central sleep apnea (Cheyne–Stokes respirations) are common in heart failure and disrupt sleep.*
- *Treatment of central sleep apnea in patients with heart failure improves survival.*

General Considerations

Congestive heart failure (CHF) is a common problem, often presenting with shortness of breath or fatigue as its primary symptoms. It increases in frequency with age. There are 40,000 deaths and close to one million hospitalizations annually in the United States from heart failure. Smoking is a shared risk factor for both ischemic heart disease, which leads to heart failure, and COPD. It may be difficult to distinguish which of these disorders is causing problems with sleep when the diseases coexist. Many patients with advanced CHF describe fatigue, lack of energy, tiredness, or weakness with exercise. A smaller number complain of sleepiness and drowsiness. Cheyne–Stokes respiration, a type of

Table 30–1. Conditions that impair sleep and lead to daytime sleepiness.

Medical conditions
 Congestive heart failure
 Chronic obstructive pulmonary disease
 Asthma
 Gastroesophageal reflux
 Fibromyalgia
 Parkinson's disease
 Seizures
 Liver failure
 Uremia
 Hypothyroidism
 Nonketotic hyperosmolar coma
 Hypoglycemia
 Central nervous system infection
 Stroke
 Chronic fatigue syndrome
 Dementia
Psychiatric conditions
 Psychoses
 Mood disorders, especially depression
 Anxiety disorders
 Panic disorders
 Alcoholism
 Dementia

central sleep apnea characterized by an absent ventilatory effort with a waxing and waning breathing pattern, is associated with excess mortality in CHF. As many as 40–45% of people with heart failure from systolic dysfunction may have the Cheyne–Stokes form of central sleep apnea. Management of central sleep apnea in these patients is an important component of their heart failure therapy, and improves outcome.

Pathogenesis

Central apneas are defined as cessation of breathing without any respiratory muscle effort. They appear to result from loss of ventilatory drive. Carbon dioxide retention is rare. Hyperventilation leads to hypocapnia and subsequent hypopnea or apnea until the arterial carbon dioxide pressure ($PaCO_2$) rises. Arousals from sleep are common during the hyperventilation phase after a central apnea. These arousals lead to fragmented sleep and subsequent daytime sleepiness. A hyperadrenergic state, common in heart failure and sleep apnea, appears to worsen heart failure itself. When lying in the supine position edema fluid that has pooled in the legs during the day returns to the circulation and predisposes patients with heart failure to pulmonary edema at night.

Clinical Findings

General symptoms of heart failure include shortness of breath with exertion, fatigue, and often daytime sleepiness. Dyspnea may worsen at night either as orthopnea or paroxysmal nocturnal dyspnea (PND). Symptoms that awaken patients with heart failure exacerbation are often nonspecific and may be difficult to distinguish from a COPD exacerbation, a primary sleep disorder such as sleep apnea, or a response to medications that interrupt sleep. A common presentation of Cheyne–Stokes breathing in CHF is trouble staying asleep, termed sleep maintenance insomnia. This is often characterized as gasping, grunting, or choking during sleep, accompanied by frequent body movements. After a sleepless night, daytime sleepiness ensues. Frequent Cheyne–Stokes respirations are noted in up to 45% of patients with a low ejection fraction. Obstructive sleep apnea is also seen in patients with heart failure.

Physical findings associated with a diagnosis of heart failure include tachycardia, a diffuse point of maximal impact on cardiac palpation, an S3 gallop, distant heart sounds, crackles in the lung bases, jugular venous distention, hepatojugular reflux, tricuspid regurgitation, ascites, and dependent edema. Although hypoxemia is often present during sleep, many patients with severe central sleep apnea and Cheyne–Stokes respiration do not desaturate below 90% oxygenation.

Techniques that quantify cardiac ejection fraction can confirm left ventricular heart failure but are nonspecific with regard to whether Cheyne–Stokes breathing is the cause of sleepiness. These techniques include echocardiogram, nuclear medicine-gated blood pool scan, and cardiac catheterization.

Oximetry at night is frequently used to identify oxyhemoglobin desaturation. However, even with severe central apneas, oxygen saturation may be preserved. This technique will not detect many patients with central sleep apnea, and therefore is not recommended as a screening tool for this condition. Polysomnography, an 18-channel sleep study, is the recommended procedure if central sleep apnea is suspected. Both central and obstructive sleep apnea can be diagnosed in patients with heart failure with these studies. Other sleep study findings in heart failure include light sleep and frequent arousals.

Differential Diagnosis

Diagnostic considerations for sleep problems in people with CHF include obstructive sleep apnea, asthma, or COPD exacerbations. Nocturnal ischemia can be difficult to distinguish from heart failure. Additionally, medications used to treat CHF, hypertension, or hyperlipidemia occasionally lead to insomnia. These include β-blockers and statin medications used to treat hyperlipidemia. Cheyne–Stokes respiration/central sleep apnea may be from causes other than a low ejection fraction including cerebral disorders, uremia, and dwelling at high altitude.

Treatment

Treatment of heart failure with medications including β-blockers, angiotensin-converting enzyme inhibitors, or angiotensin receptor blockers may lessen the central apneic episodes and improve sleep complaints. Some patients with CHF require diuretics such as furosemide. Treatment of nocturnal ischemia, if present, with nitrates or calcium channel blockers is also beneficial.

Oxygen therapy or continuous positive airway pressure (CPAP) is a therapeutic option specific for central apnea once treatment of heart failure has been optimized. Oxygen has been a mainstay of treatment but is not universally successful. CPAP can be difficult to implement but is often recommended as the treatment of choice, improving the prognosis of CHF with central apnea. Clinical trials are currently underway to further assess its efficacy. Bilevel mask therapy (BiPAP, VPAP, and others) differs from CPAP in that there is both a set inspiratory and expiratory pressure. It is sometimes advocated in patients with CHF, but clinical trials of efficacy are lacking. Another treatment option is theophylline. Alternatively, benzodiazepines or other short acting hypnotic drugs such as zolpidem have been tried to diminish the degree of hypocapnia and rebound hypercapnia, prevent arousals, and promote sleep, but good clinical data for this approach are lacking. If obstructive apnea coexists with heart failure, assessment and treatment of this with weight loss and CPAP therapy can lessen nocturnal hypoxemia.

Prognosis

The overall prognosis of CHF has improved with the use of after-load-reducing (hydralazine/nitrates, angiotensin-converting enzyme inhibitors, angiotensin receptor blockers) and β-blocking drugs. Preservation of cardiac function and survival are both improved with these treatments. Persons with Cheyne–Stokes breathing and heart failure have a higher mortality than patients with heart failure without central sleep apnea, however, this poor prognosis can be improved with CPAP treatment. Specific improvements include a lower mortality and decreased need for transplantation in patients with Class III and IV heart failure and Cheyne–Stokes respiration.

Javaheri S: Treatment of central sleep apnea in heart failure. Sleep 2000;23(Suppl 4):S224. [PMID:10893108]. (The authors report a more detailed discussion of central sleep apnea in heart failure and include methods of treatment.)

Sin DD et al: Effects of continuous positive airway pressure on cardiovascular outcomes in heart failure patients with and without Cheyne-Stokes respiration. Circulation 2000;102:61. [PMID:10880416]. (This article indicates improved cardiac function and a trend to improved mortality and transplantation rates for patients with heart failure treated with continuous positive airway pressure.)

Yamashiro Y, Kryger MH: Review: sleep in heart failure. Sleep 1992;16:513. [PMID: 8235235]. (Clinical points of sleep and heart failure are discussed.)

CHRONIC OBSTRUCTIVE PULMONARY DISEASE (COPD)

 ESSENTIALS OF DIAGNOSIS

- *Cough, wheezing, and shortness of breath impair sleep in patients with COPD.*
- *Hypoxemia worsens during sleep, from hypoventilation and ventilation–perfusion mismatching, leading to nocturnal awakening and daytime sleepiness.*
- *Hypoxemia and awakenings are most severe during rapid eye movement (REM) sleep.*

General Considerations

COPD is common, especially in men and increasingly in women of middle to older age. It is the fourth leading cause of death in the United States affecting more than 14 million people. Although it primarily affects the lungs, it is a systemic disease with a profound impact on physical function. Many patients with COPD are quite sleepy during the day. Their sleep symptoms include both daytime sleepiness and insomnia and they experience both difficulty getting to sleep and frequent awakenings at night from symptoms of cough and shortness of breath or hypoxemia. Sleep is characterized by more light stages, decreased amounts of the restorative slow wave sleep and REM sleep, and frequent arousals. Oxygen desaturations are common at night even for persons whose oxygen saturation during the daytime is normal.

Pathogenesis

Chronic bronchitis leads to nighttime cough and wheeze, which can disrupt sleep. Shortness of breath predominates with emphysema. Nocturnal hypoxemia is thought to contribute to nighttime awakenings and poor sleep in patients with COPD by four mechanisms:

hypoventilation from lower lung volumes during sleep, hypoventilation from a lower respiratory rate during sleep, worsening of ventilation–perfusion matching in the supine position, and the steep slope of the oxyhemoglobin desaturation curve causing precipitous drops in saturation. Hypoxemia in humans is more common in the supine position due to loss of diaphragm use. It is more common in sleep than during wakefulness, especially REM sleep in which the decreased muscle tone of REM prevents lung hyperexpansion. Hyperexpansion is particularly important for patients with COPD to preserve lung function and oxygenation; when hyperexpansion is lost during sleep there is brisk oxygen desaturation.

Although cough and hypoxemia are the most important reasons for sleep problems in patients with COPD, medications used to treat COPD may also worsen the ability to sustain sleep. Theophylline may increase periodic limb movements or induce insomnia, both of which worsen sleep efficiency. β-agonists can also induce insomnia. Systemic corticosteroids, especially when used in the afternoon or evening, alter circadian cortisol rhythm and may disrupt nocturnal sleep.

Clinical Findings

A clinical diagnosis of COPD severe enough to cause sleep problems is generally obvious, but recognition of altered sleep as a problem in patients with COPD is often ignored. Respiratory symptoms of cough, phlegm, and dyspnea on exertion occur. Physical examination shows a prolonged expiratory phase, diminished breath sounds, wheezes, and findings of right-sided heart failure (manifestations of COPD on physical examination are discussed in further detail in Chapter 7). Spirometry in COPD usually shows an obstructive pattern. Sleep symptoms early in the course of disease are mostly due to cough from bronchitis or may be related to the medications used to treat bronchospasm and inflammation. Symptoms late in the course of disease can be due to hypoxemia. It is estimated that 10% of patients with COPD have concomitant COPD and sleep apnea. This "overlap syndrome" with both diseases coexisting appears to worsen nocturnal pulmonary hypertension and sleep complaints. Therefore, a person with well-treated COPD who remains sleepy should be evaluated for sleep apnea if the history suggests obesity, nocturnal snoring, and awakening.

A polysomnography or formal sleep study is indicated only when sleep apnea is also suspected. Nocturnal oximetry alone can detect patients who are hypoxemic at night despite good daytime oxygenation; this is the preferred initial diagnostic test in COPD. Of patients with COPD who have an acceptable arterial oxygen tension (>60 mm Hg) on awakening, 25% will show at least a 5% decrease in oxygen saturation during REM sleep, making oximetry a useful test at pinpointing those who need oxygen treatment.

Differential Diagnosis

Sleep disruption and daytime sleepiness may be due to many conditions, but sleep disruption in patients with COPD is most often confused or complicated by insomnia, anxiety, depression, CHF, and asthma. Combinations of sleep apnea and COPD, the overlap syndrome, may be difficult to assess and treat.

Treatment for Nocturnal Worsening of COPD

Adequate control of cough and bronchospasm is important. Treatment may include use of nocturnal anticholinergic drugs such as an ipratropium bromide inhaler, which improves sleep quality. Alternatively, theophylline or a long acting β-agonist may be beneficial, although evaluation of sleep quality shows mixed results. Use of a long-acting bronchodilator at bedtime (salmeterol or formoterol) rather than shorter acting agents can prevent sleep interruptions. Treatment of accompanying sinus drainage that induces cough improves sleep. Good sleep hygiene should be reviewed with particular stress placed on smoking cessation as nicotine disturbs sleep.

The best treatment for many patients is detecting and treating nocturnal hypoxemia. This can be accomplished with provision of home oxygen therapy after nocturnal oximetry monitoring. Most patients with COPD with nocturnal desaturation also have exercise desaturation, and an exercise oximetry test may suffice to detect those at risk for nocturnal desaturations. Other interventions include assessment for concomitant sleep apnea if symptoms are present and sleepiness remains after bronchodilator drugs, sleep hygiene recommendations, and oxygen have been used. Anxiety or depression may contribute to insomnia, but need to be treated cautiously with sleep depressant medications to avoid oversedation and a drop in ventilatory drive.

Noninvasive bilevel ventilation using a nasal or facemask is an excellent treatment for acute COPD exacerbations. There is, however, an equivocal role for chronic nocturnal ventilation in COPD. Whether home nocturnal ventilation should be provided chronically in selected patients with COPD is uncertain and is under investigation (for further discussion, see Chapters 26 and 27).

Prognosis

Patients with COPD have decreased survival, especially if they are hypoxic and have cor pulmonale. Use of oxygen improves survival. Poor oxygenation during sleep likely contributes to pulmonary hypertension and cor pulmonale, but sleep quality itself is not known to prognosticate survival.

Brown LK: Sleep-related disorders and chronic obstructive pulmonary disease. Respir Care Clin North Am 1998;4:493. [PMID: 9770263]. (Details about the overlap syndrome of sleep apnea and COPD are discussed.)

Flenley DC: Sleep in chronic obstructive lung disease. Clin Chest Med 1985;6:651. [PMID: 2935359]. (Pathophysiology of sleep hypoxemia in COPD.)

McNicholas WT: Impact of sleep in COPD. Chest 2000;117:48s. [PMID: 10673475]. (Multiple strategies are useful in improving sleep for patients with COPD.)

ASTHMA

 ESSENTIALS OF DIAGNOSIS

- *The majority of patients with asthma have sleep complaints at least once a week.*
- *Symptoms are described as shortness of breath, wheezing, chest tightness, coughing, and air hunger.*
- *Nocturnal symptoms peak in the early morning hours (3–4 AM).*
- *Nocturnal asthma symptoms lead to insufficient sleep and present as either insomnia or sleepiness during the day.*

General Considerations

Asthma is defined as variable airflow obstruction and hyperreactivity of airways. It is a disease of children and adolescents as well as adults. Sleep-related asthma is defined as asthma attacks that occur during sleep with accompanying symptoms of shortness of breath, wheezing, coughing, air hunger, and chest tightness. Insomnia, excessive sleepiness, or both may result. Sleep deprivation from frequent arousals or awakenings leads to daytime sleepiness. The frequency of nocturnal wheezing is surprisingly high with two-thirds of patients with asthma in Great Britain reporting wheezing three nights per week. The majority, 61–74% of patients with asthma, report nocturnal awakenings. It is thought that worsening of asthma at night is an indication of disease severity; patients with nocturnal flares tend to have more severe disease. There is an association of nocturnal wheezing with asthma mortality and death rates from asthma are highest in the early morning.

Pathogenesis

Reasons for nocturnal exacerbations of asthma are multiple. The most important mechanisms include circadian changes in hormone levels and inflammation. Circadian variability in cortisol hormone levels contributes to nighttime worsening of symptoms. Cortisol peaks at 6 AM after a nadir at midnight; as a result bronchospasm and awakenings occur more frequently in the early morning hours. These circadian changes are associated with increases in eosinophils, increased airway obstruction, and heightened airway reactivity in the early morning hours. Inflammation likely contributes to nocturnal worsening of asthma. There are more granulocytes in lung bronchoalveolar lavage fluid and more inflammatory markers in the early morning hours including CD4 lymphocytes, superoxide generation, and CD51 production. Higher levels of leukotriene E4 are associated with the morning dipping pattern of asthma.

Other hypotheses have been raised to explain nocturnal flares of asthma. Nocturnal allergen exposure to agents such as bed mites may be important. Alternatively, there may be a late asthmatic response to allergen exposure early in the day.

Gastroesophageal reflux (GER) and sinus drainage can worsen asthma and may be more important at night than during the day due to lying in a supine position. A recumbent position and sleep itself may worsen obstruction. Enhanced vagal tone may be important in nocturnal asthma, in part by facilitating reflux of gastric acid into the esophagus.

There may also be an association between sleep-disordered breathing and asthma. One condition may worsen the other. For example, sleep-disordered breathing may exacerbate asthma by increased vagal stimulation, or asthma may increase sleep-disordered breathing through heightened airflow rate. Alternatively, inflammation of the nose, mouth, and pharynx as well as the airways may be caused by common mechanisms such as allergies.

Clinical Findings

Asthma symptoms include shortness of breath, wheezing, coughing, air hunger, and chest tightness; these characterize nighttime asthma symptoms, too. Symptoms typically improve with bronchodilator medications. When asked, Do you awaken from sleep? What awakens you? How many hours do you sleep? Are you sleepy during the daytime?, a large number of patients with asthma describe nocturnal awakenings. Although many patients with asthma have awakenings at night, a smaller number have life-threatening bronchoconstriction.

Patients with asthma at night have a higher amplitude in the day–night variation in peak expiratory flow rates. Those with nocturnal asthma may have an even higher variation between day and night flows than patients without nocturnal symptoms. Sleep studies are rarely indicated for these patients unless obstructive sleep apnea is a complicating problem.

Differential Diagnosis

Asthma is usually easy to distinguish from COPD by lack of prior or current tobacco smoking and onset of symptoms at a younger age. Sometimes early morning awakenings are characteristic of angina or CHF; these should be considered for persons in the appropriate age, sex, and risk categories.

Treatment

Treatment of nocturnal asthma in general is the same as for asthma, with a stepwise approach for increasing levels of asthma severity as outlined in Chapter 6. There are, however, several specific treatments for asthma with nocturnal worsening (Table 30–2). These include ridding the sleeping area and home of pets that can induce a late asthmatic response. A reduction in household mites can be achieved by low humidity. Also, avoidance of carpeting lowers allergen exposure and may decrease asthma severity. If GER has been identified, treatment can start with head of bed elevation and a bedtime histamine 2 (H2) blocker. Use of long-acting β-agonists such as salmeterol or formoterol at bedtime results in a sustained level of bronchodilation and may avoid some of the nocturnal awakenings. Some advocate use of longer acting β-agonists rather than theo-

Table 30–2. Treatment of nocturnal asthma.

Environmental strategies
    Pet removal
    Low humidity
    Avoidance of carpeting
Treatment of gastroesophageal reflux
    Head of bed elevation
    Bedtime histamine 2 blocker
Long-acting medications
    β-agonists
    Salmeterol
    Formoterol
Chronotherapy
    Evening use of sustained release theophylline
    Afternoon dosing of corticosteroids

phylline to minimize sleep complaints for patients with milder asthma.

Chronotherapy involves timing medication regimens based specifically on nocturnal asthma exacerbations. It is defined as use of treatment targeted at circadian events and involves several strategies anticipating nocturnal flares. First, sustained dose theophylline before bedtime improves symptoms compared to conventional dosing. Additionally, steroids delivered in the early afternoon increase the peak expiratory flow rate more than the same doses delivered in the morning or at bedtime.

Bohadana AB, Hannhart B, Teculescu DB: Nocturnal worsening of asthma and sleep-disordered breathing. Review article. J Asthma 2000;39:85. [PMID: 11990234]. (Discussion of the hypotheses of nocturnal worsening of asthma.)

Kraft M: Corticosteroids and leukotrienes: chronobiology and chronotherapy. Chronobiol Int 1999;16:683. [PMID: 10513889]. (A more detailed discussion of the fascinating circadian rhythms of cortisol and its impact on asthma symptoms and treatment.)

Turner-Warwick M: Epidemiology of nocturnal asthma. Am J Med 1988;85:6. [PMID: 3400687]. (Study showing a high frequency of nocturnal symptoms in an unselected asthma population.)

SLEEP-RELATED GASTROESOPHAGEAL REFLUX DISEASE (GERD)

 ESSENTIALS OF DIAGNOSIS

- *Gastroesophageal reflux (GER) often presents as a sour taste, cough, or heartburn.*
- *GER is common in patients with asthma, sleep apnea, and in patients who are obese.*
- *Treatment of these underlying conditions often improves GER.*
- *Although it is a common problem, the impact of GER in disturbing sleep is uncertain.*

General Considerations

Heartburn is the classic symptom of GER. Of the general population 7–10% complain of daily heartburn, and 30% experience it at least weekly. It is more common after age 40, in obese people, and in those with asthma. A relationship of GER symptoms to sleep apnea has recently been described with many patients having both disorders. In a Gallup survey almost 50% of participants with GER responded that their reflux led to daytime sleepiness. The real clinical impact of reflux on sleep, however, is uncertain.

Pathogenesis

Reflux of stomach contents into the esophagus, mouth, and lungs leads to symptoms or even tissue injury. The usual barrier to reflux is the lower esophageal sphincter (LES). Relaxation of LES pressure to below 10 mm Hg, which is seen with obesity or pregnancy, facilitates reflux of contents into the esophagus. The markedly negative thoracic pressures in asthma exacerbations may also facilitate reflux. Although a causal role for GER in asthma has been sought, the contribution of GER to asthma is unclear. Increased vagal tone at night is thought to mediate the lowering of esophageal sphincter tone. There is a circadian pattern to acid secretion that may be important, with acid secretion peaking between 9 PM and midnight.

Clinical Findings

Patients may be asymptomatic or have difficulty elucidating symptoms. They may have a sour or bitter taste in the mouth, cough or choking, and heartburn. Less typical symptoms include dysphagia, belching, chest pain, hoarseness, bad breath, and aspiration. Patients may awaken from sleep with GER; it is sometimes difficult to determine if they awaken from the symptoms of asthma or reflux when the two problems coexist.

Differential Diagnosis

Peptic ulcer disease awakens people from sleep with pain or abdominal discomfort and may be described as epigastric burning, heartburn, or an unpleasant taste in the mouth. Pain may radiate to the chest or back. Myocardial ischemia pain may mimic gastrointestinal pain. Patients may have asthma or reflux and asthma together.

Treatment

Treatment includes elevation of the head of the bed and avoidance of foods that precipitate reflux. Substances that reduce lower esophageal pressure including caffeine, cigarettes, and alcohol should also be reduced or avoided. Weight loss is important in treatment. Treatment of sleep apnea if present with CPAP can improve reflux symptoms by as much as 50%. Medications that improve GERD include antacids, H2 receptor antagonists, prokinetic agents, and proton pump inhibitors. Surgery is reserved for severe GERD and can be an open or laparoscopic fundoplication. A transoral suturing technique via flexible endoscopy and radio frequency treatment to the gastroesophageal junction are not yet standard of care but are undergoing evaluation as alternative surgical procedures.

Gislason T et al: Respiratory symptoms and nocturnal gastroesophageal reflux. A population-based study of young adults in three European countries. Chest 2002;121:158. (GER in young adults in Northern Europe is associated with asthma and obstructive sleep apnea syndrome.)

Harding SM: Nocturnal asthma: role of nocturnal gastroesophageal reflux. Chronobiol Int 1999;16:641. [PMID: 10513887]. (Nocturnal reflux was noted by pH probe in 82% of patients with asthma with 77% claiming symptoms of reflux.)

Katz PO: Gastroesophageal reflux disease: new treatments. Rev Gastroenterol Disord 2002;2:66. [PMID: 12122962]. (Newer surgical strategies to treat gastroesophageal reflux.)

FIBROMYALGIA

 ESSENTIALS OF DIAGNOSIS

- *Nonrestorative sleep, daytime sleepiness, and accompanying pain are characteristic.*
- *There is an absence of other rheumatological disease.*
- *There is α wave intrusion into sleep.*

General Considerations

Fibromyalgia is common, occurring in 3–10% of the adult population. Sleep complaints and sleep disturbances are prominent in this condition. Fibromyalgia is characterized by diffuse musculoskeletal pain, chronic fatigue, and unrefreshing sleep. Patients have increased tenderness in specific localized anatomic areas without laboratory evidence of contributing articular or metabolic disease. There is a frequent complaint of light sleep and patients are generally more symptomatic during nocturnal hours. There may be associated periodic limb movements. When the sleep problems of fibromyalgia are addressed, pain improves. Relationships between sleep complaints and pain may be bidirectional; it is often difficult to ascertain if the sleep problem predates or follows the musculoskeletal pain. Symptoms are often, unfortunately, dismissed as unimportant.

Pathogenesis

The mechanisms that cause fibromyalgia are not clear. There may be a vigilant state hyperarousal state that leads to worsening pain. Some experts think sleep is probably the primary problem and the musculoskeletal symptoms are secondary, whereas others believe that the musculoskeletal symptoms induce the sleep problem. Still others suggest that the primary process is a low threshold of pain. The absence of an elevated erythrocyte sedimentation rate (ESR) suggests this is not an inflammatory disease.

Clinical Findings

Clinical findings of fibromyalgia are nonspecific. Patients frequently complain of unrefreshing sleep and tiredness during the daytime. They also describe light sleep with easy awakening, awakening with stiffness and myalgias, and fatigue. After a good night's sleep, stiffness is less prominent. Fibromyalgia is defined by the presence of tender zones within the muscles. The presence of 11 of these 18 tender zones supports a diagnosis. By definition, there is no identifiable rheumatological disease.

Laboratory Findings

A hallmark of fibromyalgia is the presence of α waves on electroencephalogram (EEG) during non-REM sleep. α-wave activity has a frequency of 8–13 Hz and generally occurs during an awake drowsy state. In one trial, the amount of α activity during non-REM sleep tracked with greater subjective sensation of pain. In contrast to the collagen vascular diseases, in fibromyalgia there is no elevation of the ESR or other inflammatory mediators.

Differential Diagnosis

The differential diagnosis is broad and includes chronic fatigue syndrome, insufficient sleep, depression, and other rheumatological diseases such as rheumatoid arthritis.

Treatment

Patient education about the disorder is important. Attention is directed to the precepts of sleep hygiene including regular sleep and wake times, exercise, and avoidance of stimulants at bedtime. There is no role for corticosteroids. Opiate drugs should be minimized. There is some treatment efficacy for sleep symptoms with low dose amitriptyline, selective serotonin reuptake inhibitors (SSRIs) such as paroxetine, or more sedating antidepressants such as trazodone. Use of exercise programs has been moderately effective in improving sleep symptoms.

Prognosis

Prognosis is good.

Harding SM: Sleep in fibromyalgia patients: subjective and objective findings. Am J Med Sci 1998;315:367. [PMID: 9638893]. (This article includes details of sleep architecture in fibromyalgia and treatment suggestions.)

Moldofsky H, Lue FA: The relationship of alpha delta EEG frequencies to pain and mood in 'fibrositis' patients treated with chlorpromazine and L-tryptophan. Electroencephalogr Clin Neurophysiol 1980:50:179. [PMID: 6159193]. (Tracking of α waves in deep sleep correlated with pain and hostility.)

PARKINSON'S DISEASE

 ESSENTIALS OF DIAGNOSIS

- Of people with Parkinson's disease 75% have sleep disturbances.
- Insomnia and daytime sleepiness are common and multifactorial.
- A major diagnostic concern is to decide whether there is too much versus too little disease-treating medication.

General Considerations

Parkinson's disease is a disease of the elderly with a prevalence of 5% in persons 80–84 years old. It is estimated that Parkinson's disease and Parkinson's syndrome affect 347 of 100,000 people older than age 40. Sleep problems are common, including insomnia and difficulty initiating and maintaining sleep. There are sleep disturbances specific to the neurological disorder such as cough and aspiration, periodic limb movement disorder/restless leg syndrome, and REM sleep behavior disorder. Daytime drowsiness is a frequent result. Sleep complaints plague 75% of persons with Parkinson's disease during the course of their illness, with worsening as the disease progresses.

Pathogenesis

The underlying physiological problem in Parkinson's disease is ascribed to reduced dopamine content in the basal ganglia of the brain with loss of needed dopaminergic input from the substantia nigra. It is likely that dysregulation of the serotonergic, noradrenergic, and cholinergic neuronal systems throughout the brain also contribute to the sleep problems in patients with Parkinson's disease.

Clinical Findings

General features of Parkinson's disease include resting tremor, truncal rigidity with stiffness and inability to relax muscles (including cog wheeling rigidity), brady-kinesia (slow initiation of movement), and loss of postural reflexes that leads to gait instability. Two of these four features are required for diagnosis. Parkinson's syndrome has a clinical presentation similar to Parkinson's disease. The latter is an idiopathic process whereas the syndrome has an identifiable etiology, such as drug-induced (phenothiazine), toxin-induced (carbon monoxide), or postinfection (encephalitis).

Sleep difficulties are a major clinical problem for patients with Parkinson's disease and are multifactorial. Sleep fragmentation is characteristic with a large number of awakenings. There is often prolonged sleep latency with difficulty falling asleep. Some of the sleep interruption may be from physical discomfort and inability to move caused by bradykinesia. Either insomnia or daytime sleepiness may result from treatment medications or the schedule of medications. Dopamine agonists that are dosed in the evening may lead to insomnia, whereas other medications such as levodopa, amantadine, or anticholinergic agents can cause hallucinations. Other problems include bradykinesia and discomfort related to waning drug effects in the middle of the night. If doses are too low, patients may have nocturnal rigidity and excessive limb movements. Swallowing difficulties with cough and aspiration occur late in the course of the disease.

Periodic limb movements have been noted in at least one-third of patients with Parkinson's disease. Flexor movements starting in the great toe and extending into the leg characterize these. Periodic limb movements become more common as the effect of L-dopa wears off in the early morning hours. Parkinson's syndrome is also associated with another disruptive condition, the REM sleep behavior disorder, which is defined as the uncharacteristic presence of motor activity during REM sleep. This condition may antedate other Parkinson's symptoms by many years. Dementia is a late finding in Parkinson's disease and is associated with poor quality sleep. Circadian rhythm problems are also more common than in the general population, leading to advanced sleep phase and early morning awakenings.

Findings on physical examination are characteristic of Parkinson's disease. These include tremor, bradykinesia, truncal rigidity, and difficulty walking. The pill-rolling tremor may lessen with sleep, although it does not usually disappear.

Specific laboratory studies are not often helpful in determining a cause for sleep problems in patients with Parkinson's disease. Diagnostic imaging of the brain can identify evidence of other neurological disorders that are in the differential diagnosis. Polysomnography or full sleep study is indicated in selected cases, to identify concomitant apneas or periodic limb movements of sleep.

Differential Diagnosis

Other neurodegenerative disorders including progressive supranuclear palsy, olivopontocerebellar degeneration, and Shy-Drager syndrome are similar to Parkinson's disease and are often classified as causing a Parkinson's syndrome. Parkinson's disease may be misdiagnosed as dementia or stroke.

Complications

Complications germane to sleep in patients with Parkinson's disease include nocturnal aspiration, depression, and hallucinations. Aspiration of secretions with subsequent cough, stridor, and even pneumonia is common and induces poor quality sleep. Several of the medications used to treat Parkinson's disease cause insomnia. There is a high rate of depression in patients with Parkinson's disease, which can lead to further insomnia with daytime sleepiness. One-third of patients are thought to experience hallucinations from either the disease or treatment medications.

Treatment

General treatment for Parkinson's disease involves use of medications that increase dopamine levels. Five classes of agents do this: dopaminergic agonists, dopamine precursors, dopamine releasers, catechol-O-methyltransferase inhibitors, and monoamine oxidase B inhibitors (Table 30–3). Anticholinergic drugs, antidepressant medications, and benzodiazepines are often used and can affect sleep. Dopaminergic medications, although generally beneficial to sleep, can interrupt sleep or cause insomnia. Low doses of levodopa or dopaminergic agents in the evening promote sleep but high doses can disrupt sleep. Because of the complex nature of treatment, late disease is fraught with the difficulty of determining whether the drug or the disease is causing the sleep symptoms.

Prognosis

Death generally occurs 10–25 years after onset of disease. Improving quality of life through adjustment of medications and addressing sleep problems needs constant attention. This may be best accomplished by referral to a specialist in Parkinson's disease.

Askenasy JJM: Sleep in Parkinson's disease. Acta Neurol Scand 1993;87:167. [PMID: 8475684]. (Sleep is a major quality of life issue for patients with Parkinson's disease.)

Trenkwalder C: Sleep dysfunction in Parkinson's disease. Clin Neurosci 1998;5:107. [PMID: 10785836]. (High frequency of sleep symptoms and discussion of the multiple causes of sleep problems.)

Table 30–3. Treatment for Parkinson's disease.

Dopaminergic treatment for Parkinson's disease
  Dopamine precursors
    Levodopa/carbidopa (carbidopa inhibits decarboxyla-
      tion of peripheral levodopa)
  Dopaminergic agonists
    Pergolide
    Pramipexole
    Ropinirole
    Bromocriptine
  Monoamine oxidase inhibitor
    Selegiline
  Dopamine releaser
    Amantadine
  Catechol-*O*-methyltransferase inhibitor (prevent
      dopamine breakdown)
    Entacapone
    Tolcapone
Nondopaminergic treatment
  Anticholinergic drugs
    Benztropine
    Trihexyphenidyl hydrochloride
  Vitamin E

NOCTURNAL SEIZURES

 ESSENTIALS OF DIAGNOSIS

- *Of seizures 25% are nocturnal with 10% being only nocturnal.*
- *Sleepiness or hypersomnia may be the manifestation of a seizure or the result of a postictal state, an accompanying primary sleep disorder such as sleep apnea, or the use of seizure medications.*
- *Seizures may be confused with parasomnias, such as sleep terrors, or with narcolepsy.*

General Considerations

Seizures are the third most common neurological disorder in the United States, trailing only stroke and Alzheimer's disease. Nocturnal seizures cause sleepiness during the daytime. It is estimated that 25% of patients with seizures have nocturnal seizures and 8–10% have only nocturnal seizures. Ongoing seizures are important to consider in the patient with daytime sleepiness, although they are less common than sleep apnea or insufficient sleep due to poor sleep habits. Frontal and tem-

poral lobe seizures are more likely to induce sleepiness than other seizure types.

The relationship between seizures and sleep is complex. There are several ways in which seizures may cause daytime sleepiness. First, seizures may trigger sleep-disordered breathing or parasomnias. Conversely, obstructive sleep apnea may trigger seizures by inducing hypoxemia. The somnolence of a postictal state after seizures may mimic sleep disorders, but sleep apnea and parasomnias may mimic seizures, making diagnosis difficult. Concomitant sleep apnea, periodic limb movements, or other sleep disorders may be the reason for sleepiness, even in a patient with seizures. Perhaps most commonly, however, seizure medications contribute to daytime sleepiness in a third of patients. These symptoms occasionally improve with continued use.

Pathogenesis

Epilepsy is a paroxysmal disorder of nerve signal propagation in the cerebral cortex, and seizures are manifestations of epilepsy. Seizures are more common during non-REM sleep, especially stage 2 sleep.

Clinical Findings

Tonic–clonic generalized seizures are characterized by generalized movements and altered consciousness. Not all seizures are generalized. Partial complex seizures occur frequently during sleep. These seizures are characterized by alteration in consciousness and automatisms. Sleep seizures are often associated with a temporal lobe focus. A postictal confusional state or sleepiness is common in partial complex seizures, and there may be retrograde amnesia. Enuresis is reported with nocturnal seizures. Some patients with seizures have them only during sleep, making diagnosis difficult. There are no characteristic findings on physical examination for seizures, although there may be transient localized neurological findings of weakness or aphasia.

Laboratory Studies

The EEG is the diagnostic test of choice for evaluation of seizures. A usual work-up includes use of 12–16 EEG channels. The EEG may need to be repeated, as a seizure may not occur in every 24-h period. Use of simultaneous video recording to detect stereotypic activity can be useful in nocturnal seizures. Findings with tonic–clonic seizures include bilateral synchronous spike and slow wave complexes. Partial complex seizures have spikes or spikes and waves in a more localized distribution, especially during non-REM sleep.

For new-onset seizures in an adult, a computed tomography (CT) scan or other imaging for brain tumors should be undertaken. Biochemical assessment for hypoxemia, low glucose, hyponatremia, and low calcium may help assess reasons for new onset seizures.

Differential Diagnosis

There are numerous sleep conditions that are mistaken for seizures. These include sleep starts, parasomnias, REM sleep behavior disorder, and narcolepsy. Sleep starts (hypnic or myoclonic jerks) are jerking movements at sleep onset. They often involve the legs, but can include arm and head movements too. Two-thirds of the population experience these jerks in the transition from wake to sleep; they are not only common but have no associated medical implications. Parasomnias are sleep problems of stereotypic behavior such as confusional arousals, sleepwalking, head banging, and sleep terrors. The events are never remembered and often occur in the first half of the night. In contrast to seizures, daytime sleepiness is very uncommon with parasomnias. Onset is usually in childhood.

REM sleep behavior disorder is defined as motor activity during REM sleep when it should not occur. Often combative behavior and kicking or thrashing are noted. Daytime sleepiness may or may not be seen. Nightmares and posttraumatic stress disorder (PTSD) are occasionally confused with seizures.

The cataplexy associated with narcolepsy is sometimes mistaken for seizures. Narcolepsy is a disorder in which organizational boundaries between REM sleep and wakefulness are lost. Narcolepsy presents with both the drop attacks of cataplexy and severe daytime sleepiness. Characteristic symptoms and findings of narcolepsy are discussed in Chapter 29.

Complications

Seizure medications may worsen sleep apnea by blunting respiratory drive and by facilitating weight gain.

Treatment

Seizure medications are a common cause of sleepiness for patients with epilepsy. Patients on several medications are more likely to be sleepy than those on only one drug. The highest degree of sleepiness results from use of phenobarbital, with carbamazepine and valproate each causing sleepiness in approximately 40% of users. Phenytoin is associated with sleepiness in 15–20% of those using it. Thus, not only the seizure itself but also the medication may cause daytime sleepiness or hypersomnia.

The recommendation is to treat nocturnal seizures with seizure medications and assess serially for treatment-related sleepiness versus an ongoing seizure problem. Sleep deprivation should be avoided as it can pre-

cipitate seizures. If clinically appropriate, patients should be assessed for sleep apnea.

Prognosis

Prognosis depends on etiology and type of seizure. Seizures from brain tumors, for example, have a worse prognosis than idiopathic seizures. The benign focal epilepsy of childhood has a greater than 90% remission rate by age 18. Idiopathic tonic–clonic seizures have a good prognosis. Patients with partial seizures frequently will continue to have seizures (35%).

Chokroverty S: Diagnosis and treatment of sleep disorders caused by co-morbid disease. Neurology 2000;54:S8. [PMID: 10718679]. (This includes a nice discussion of seizures and sleep.)

Manni R, Tartara A: Evaluation of sleepiness in epilepsy. Clin Neurophysiol 2000;111(Suppl 2):s111. [PMID: 10996563]. (Excellent discussion of the interaction of sleep and epilepsy.)

Minecan D et al: Relationship of epileptic seizures to sleep stage and sleep depth. Sleep 2002;25:899. [PMID: 12489898]. (The article compiles sleep EEG information tabulated by sleep stage and hypothesizes reasons for seizures during stage 2 sleep.)

STROKE

Stroke or cerebrovascular accident can induce acute or chronic problems with sleep. Patients often aspirate and/or choke on saliva or secretions, which may awaken them from sleep. In bulbar stroke, an infarct of the respiratory control centers in the medulla may cause central sleep apnea. Problems with oral musculature after a stroke may induce obstructive apneas. Patients with diffuse cerebral disease can have associated central sleep apnea. There is an interesting epidemiological association between habitual snoring and an increased risk of stroke, although a causative role is unclear.

Partinen M: Ischaemic stroke, snoring and obstructive sleep apnea. J Sleep Res 1995;4:156. [PMID: 10607193]. (This presents in detail the current understanding of the relationship between stroke and sleep apnea.)

PSYCHIATRIC DISORDERS & DEMENTIA

Psychiatric disorders impact sleep and lead to daytime sleepiness. Patients with medical diseases frequently have coexisting psychiatric disorders. Alternatively, their medical disease can lead to depression or anxiety, both of which impair nocturnal sleep and cause daytime sleepiness or insomnia. Depression generally is associated with early morning arousals, although atypical depression leads to increased sleepiness. Psychiatric disorders impact sleep causing both insomnia and daytime sleepiness. It has been estimated that 90% of patients with major depressive disorder have sleep disturbances. Depression, anxiety, schizophrenia, or mood disorders are conditions that need to be considered for patients presenting with increased sleepiness. Schizophrenic psychoses may present as sleep disorders but more commonly present as disorganized sleep and an inability to sleep at night with concomitant daytime sleepiness. Alcoholism and recovery from drinking even after up to a year of abstinence are underappreciated reasons for poor quality sleep and sleepiness.

Dementia impacts sleep in many ways. Insomnia and sleep fragmentation are common symptoms and concomitant depression is frequently seen. One hypothesis suggests there is a loss of normal circadian rhythms as disease advances. As clinical disease worsens, patients can become agitated and combative with wandering and shouting in the early evening or night. Roughly 12% experience this sundowning syndrome.

SECTION IX

Occupational & Environmental Lung Diseases

Pneumoconiosis

Delos D. Carrier, MD, MSPH, & Lee S. Newman, MD, MA

Pneumoconiosis refers to any nonmalignant chronic lung disease resulting from inhalation and deposition of mineral, metallic, or dust particles in the pulmonary interstitium. The most common agents responsible for pneumoconioses are asbestos, silica, and coal. The effect of these agents is dependent on the intensity and duration of exposure as well as their clearance after deposition in the lung parenchyma.

ASBESTOSIS & ASBESTOS-RELATED PLEURAL DISEASE

 ESSENTIALS OF DIAGNOSIS

- A careful occupational and environmental history of past inhalational exposures.
- Evidence of pleural disease and/or interstitial lung disease (especially bilateral reticular infiltrates).

General Considerations

Asbestos is a group of naturally occurring fibrous magnesium silicates that are ubiquitous throughout the world. There are six types of asbestos; one is serpentine (chrysotile) and five are fibrous amphiboles (amosite, crocidolite, anthophyllite, tremolite, and actinolite). Most disease results from direct or indirect exposure to asbestos-containing materials during mining, milling, manufacturing, installation, or removal of asbestos-containing products. Increased risk among workers is not

generally observed until at least 20 years following initial exposure. However, patients with particularly high levels of exposure may develop clinically evident disease within 10 years. The three major categories of asbestos-related disease are asbestosis, asbestos-induced pleural disease, and cancer. Asbestosis is parenchymal lung fibrosis that results from asbestos exposure. As with coal workers' pneumoconiosis and silicosis, the degree of fibrosis is related to the amount and duration of exposure.

Pathogenesis

Typical asbestos fibers found in the lungs are 20–50 μm in length. They deposit initially at bifurcations of conducting airways and in alveoli. Fibers greater than 3 μm in diameter generally do not penetrate the distal lung, but those with diameters less than 3 μm readily translocate into the interstitium and pleural space. Fibers greater than 5 μm in length tend to be incompletely phagocytosed and are retained in tissues where they initiate and sustain cellular and molecular events that result in fibrogenesis. Asbestos triggers a chronic inflammatory process promoted by oxidative injury and profibrotic growth factors and cytokines. The principal determinants of the rate of disease progression are cumulative dose, fiber type, and individual susceptibility.

Prevention

The most significant preventive intervention in patients with asbestosis is smoking cessation. Cigarette smoking in asbestos workers increases the prevalence of radiographic pleuroparenchymal changes and markedly increases the incidence of lung carcinoma.

Additional preventive measures include limiting exposure to asbestos. The Occupational Safety and Health Administration (OSHA) has developed regulations to control exposure in the workplace. Similar regulations have also been developed by the Mine Safety and Health Administration (MSHA) regarding exposure of miners. These regulations require use of approved protective equipment, such as respirators, and recommended work practices and safety procedures to limit exposure. Respiratory protection requires that workers be issued the proper size and type of mask, based on respirator fit testing procedures, and that they be trained to recognize the hazards of asbestos.

Clinical Findings

The clinical, physiological, and radiographic findings of asbestosis also occur in other diseases associated with diffuse pulmonary fibrosis, particularly the interstitial pneumonias. A key distinguishing radiographic feature of asbestosis is the presence of bilateral pleural plaques associated with linear interstitial opacities. Patients with asbestosis usually have a history of occupational asbestos exposure.

A. SYMPTOMS AND SIGNS

Symptoms of asbestosis are similar to those that occur in other interstitial lung diseases. Patients experience gradual onset of exertional dyspnea and a dry, nonproductive cough 20–40 years after initial exposure. Other symptoms may include chest tightness, chest pain, malaise, and loss of appetite. Hemoptysis is not characteristic and when present should prompt an investigation for lung cancer. Physical examination reveals dry bilateral basilar rales, especially during inspiration, that are unaffected by coughing. Wheezing does not usually occur. Although other physical abnormalities are unusual in early stages of disease, patients may develop digital clubbing, cyanosis, and signs of cor pulmonale as pulmonary fibrosis becomes more severe. Severe digital clubbing or clubbing in radiographically mild disease suggests coexistent lung cancer.

B. LABORATORY FINDINGS AND DIAGNOSIS

The earliest physiological changes in asbestosis include evidence of small airway dysfunction. Lung volumes decline in a pattern consistent with pulmonary restriction as disease progresses. The diffusion capacity of the lung for carbon monoxide (DL_{co}) may be reduced and arterial blood gases typically demonstrate hypoxia at rest or with exercise. Physiological limitation and symptoms may precede radiographic changes. Isolated severe obstructive disease is usually not solely attributable to asbestos exposure. However, asbestosis does produce airflow obstruction due to inflammation and fibrosis of

terminal and respiratory bronchioles, even in nonsmokers.

Definitive diagnosis is based on demonstration of diffuse interstitial fibrosis with asbestos (ferruginous) bodies on histological examination of lung tissue. However, biopsy is rarely performed because the diagnosis can usually be made on the basis of history and chest imaging.

C. IMAGING STUDIES

Chest radiographs in asbestosis typically show linear/reticular interstitial markings in lower and mid lung fields, usually associated with calcified or noncalcified pleural thickening along the mid chest wall bilaterally and/or along the dome of the diaphragm. Approximately 10% of patients with asbestosis have normal chest radiographs. Bilateral calcified plaques are relatively specific markers for asbestos exposure. They may be well circumscribed or diffuse. Pleural disease can occur in the absence of coexisting parenchymal disease.

Some asbestos-exposed patients develop pleural effusions, resulting in diffuse pleural scarring and obliteration of the costophrenic angle on radiographs and computed tomography (CT). Benign asbestos-related pleural effusions may be asymptomatic, but more commonly are associated with pleuritic chest pain. They are often the first manifestation of asbestos-related lung disease, occurring as early as 10 years after exposure.

Rounded atelectasis, which occurs when visceral pleural plaques invaginate and fold upon the pulmonary parenchyma to form a cicatricial rounded mass, is common in asbestos-related pleural disease. Although these lesions may be confused with a neoplastic process on routine radiographs, high-resolution CT (HRCT) is helpful in identifying their benign nature. The typical appearance on HRCT is a pleura-based mass associated with focal pleural thickening and curvilinear displacement of vessels and bronchi into the mass.

HRCT is also more sensitive than chest radiographs for diagnosing asbestosis and other asbestos-related pleural abnormalities. HRCT may show curvilinear subpleural septal lines, parenchymal fibrous bands, bronchiolar thickening, and honeycombing. CT images taken with the patient lying prone can distinguish early asbestosis from dependent interstitial fluid. Although 85% of parietal pleural plaques are calcified by histology, calcification is only recognized in 15% of cases by chest radiograph. The proportion is significantly higher with HRCT. Similarly, it can be difficult to distinguish noncalcified plaques from fat, muscle, diaphragmatic undulation, previous rib fractures, or postinflammatory change on chest radiographs. Of lesions thought to be pleural plaques on radiograph, 10–20% are actually localized areas of fat deposition on the inner surface of the chest wall. HRCT is superior to chest radiograph in correctly identifying pleural thickening and pleural plaques and in differentiating pleural changes from chest wall fat and other artifacts. Although the combination of pulmonary fibrosis and pleural changes on CT boosts the accuracy of diagnosis, asbestosis does occasionally occur in the absence of pleural abnormalities. Thus, a fibrotic-appearing HRCT scan that lacks evidence of pleural disease does not exclude asbestosis.

Differential Diagnosis

Clinical diagnosis hinges on an exposure history, compatible imaging and/or histological findings, appropriate latency and clinical course, and exclusion of other known causes of pulmonary fibrosis. Lung biopsy is not necessary for diagnosis in most cases of asbestosis. Other disorders in the differential diagnosis include various forms of pneumoconiosis (eg, mixed dust pneumoconiosis, silicosis), chronic beryllium disease, idiopathic forms of interstitial lung disease, and chronic hypersensitivity pneumonitis.

Complications

Complications of asbestosis include episodes of acute respiratory failure related to an increased incidence of pulmonary infections (bronchitis and pneumonia) as well as chronic respiratory failure and cor pulmonale from progressive hypoxia.

Treatment

The fibrotic process in asbestosis cannot be modified by any currently available medication once it is established. Management includes control of respiratory infections, supplemental oxygen for hypoxemia, and symptomatic relief from right heart failure. There is no documented benefit of corticosteroid or other immunosuppressive therapy. The natural progression of the disease includes gradual worsening of lung function and gas exchange, eventually leading to permanent disability. Lung cancer and mesothelioma are significant concerns. Most importantly, the interaction between cigarette smoking and asbestosis as co-risk factors for lung cancer is profound. Age standardized rates reveal a 6- to 10-fold increase in the incidence of lung cancer in individuals with both types of exposure compared to those exposed only to asbestos. Smoking prevention and cessation are integral parts of the counseling of asbestos-exposed patients. Regular surveillance with HRCT may be justified in current and past smokers to identify lung cancer at an early, resectable stage. However, studies proving efficacy of such screening in high-risk populations are still lacking.

Prognosis

Regression of asbestosis is rare. It is generally slowly progressive due to accumulating inflammation and fibrotic damage caused by retained asbestos fibers. Rapid progression after onset of symptoms is unusual. However, progression of disease eventually interferes with activities of daily living and requires supplemental oxygenation. The end result of disease progression is commonly pulmonary and cardiac failure.

Cohort studies have shown an increase in lung cancer with all major forms of asbestos exposure. The amphiboles are considered to be more carcinogenic than chrysotile for development of mesothelioma and are more prone to produce pleural fibrosis. The risk of asbestosis is similar for both chrysotile and amphibole fibers.

Malignant mesothelioma, a rare tumor of the pleura and peritoneum, is caused by prior asbestos exposure. All types of asbestos fibers are associated with development of mesothelioma. Tobacco smoking does not elevate this risk.

SILICOSIS

 ESSENTIALS OF DIAGNOSIS

- *A careful occupational and environmental history of past inhalational exposure.*
- *Evidence of interstitial lung disease, especially bilateral, nodular, upper lung zone disease.*

General Considerations

Silicosis refers to diffuse interstitial fibronodular lung disease caused by inhalation of crystalline silica. It is the most prevalent chronic occupational lung disease in the world. Despite efforts to regulate dust exposures in the United States the disease continues to be a problem. Silicosis results most commonly from exposure to quartz, cristobalite, or tridymite silica polymorphs. Amorphous silica, which is noncrystalline (eg, vitreous silica glass), is relatively less toxic. Exposure commonly occurs in workers involved in hard-rock mining, silica milling, quarrying and stone work, foundry work (quartz sand is used to make molds), sand blasting, pottery making, glass making, and cleaning boilers. Silicosis presents in acute and chronic forms. Acute silicosis develops within months of exposure, usually after intensive inhalation of fine particles. Accelerated silicosis develops over 5–10 years and is generally associated with exposure to higher dust levels than chronic silicosis. Chronic silicosis may be either simple or complicated and typically develops 15 or more years after initial exposure. Complicated silicosis is characterized by coalescence of individual silicotic nodules that ultimately form large conglomerate masses called progressive massive fibrosis (PMF).

Prevention

Efforts to prevent silicosis center on limiting exposure to the dust. Eliminating exposure is critical in preventing new cases. In addition, further exposure to high levels of airborne silica in patients with established silicosis is associated with progressive pulmonary disease. Regional public health authorities should be contacted in this regard when new cases of silicosis are discovered. Additional measures designed to preserve lung function in patients with established disease include screening for tuberculosis (see below) and management of hypoxia.

Clinical Findings

Most diagnoses are presumptive and based on the combination of typical radiographic features of nodular silicosis and an occupational history of silica exposure followed by a suitable latency period. The diagnosis is usually made without invasive testing, as histological examination of lung tissue is not needed. When biopsies are performed they are usually done to exclude malignancy, rheumatoid nodules, or infection.

A. SYMPTOMS AND SIGNS

Most forms of silicosis are insidious in onset; signs and symptoms develop after a 10- to 30-year latency period following first exposure. Symptoms may be due to silica-induced chronic bronchitis as well as to silicosis. Patients may complain of cough, sputum production, and dyspnea. Although many remain minimally symptomatic, others over time experience progressive loss of energy as well as signs and symptoms of cor pulmonale. Most workers with simple silicosis do not progress to complicated disease. Symptoms of PMF include fatigue, dyspnea, and cough. Typical physical signs in silicosis include fine, bilateral crackles and tracheal deviation in advanced disease due to PMF-induced upper lung volume loss.

B. LABORATORY FINDINGS

Blood tests are nonspecific and usually not helpful. Elevation of serum immunoglobins, circulating immune complexes, rheumatoid factor, and antinuclear antibodies occurs. Tuberculin skin tests may be positive in patients with silicotuberculosis.

Lung function abnormalities are uncommon in simple silicosis. When abnormal, pulmonary function tests demonstrate a restrictive defect, often with concurrent airflow obstruction. PMF produces severe restriction, loss of pulmonary compliance, and hypoxemia.

The histopathology of silicosis typically consists of nodular masses with surrounding fibrosis and emphysema. Silicotic nodules are made of centrally located whorls of collagen and reticulin with surrounding macrophages, fibroblasts, mast cells, and lymphocytes. Early silicotic nodules are more cellular with less fibrosis. Nodules can be diffuse but usually cluster near upper lung zone respiratory bronchioles. In acute silicosis, air spaces fill with a periodic acid–Schiff (PAS) stain-positive proteinaceous exudate often indistinguishable from that present in idiopathic pulmonary alveolar proteinosis. Features of desquamative interstitial pneumonitis and diffuse alveolar damage may be found in such cases as well.

C. IMAGING STUDIES

Chest radiographs in simple silicosis typically feature rounded opacities ranging in size from 1 to 10 mm and occurring in the upper lung zones bilaterally. As nodules coalesce the upper lung zones become fibrotic with volume loss and apical retraction of the hila. Presence of coalesced nodules is diagnostic of complicated silicosis; larger masses suggest a diagnosis of PMF. Areas of emphysema and bullae appear with more advanced disease. There is frequently mild enlargement of hilar and mediastinal lymph nodes. Eggshell calcifications in hilar lymph nodes occur in 10% of cases. Accelerated silicosis has many of the same radiographic features as simple silicosis but develops after a shorter latency period. Bilateral ground-glass opacifications occur with acute silicosis (also called silicoproteinosis) and may mimic pulmonary edema or alveolar hemorrhage.

Plain chest radiography is less sensitive than HRCT in detecting silicosis. HRCT improves detection of early nodules, coalescence, and silica-induced emphysema.

Differential Diagnosis

Diagnosis of silicosis relies upon an occupational history of silica dust exposure, presence of silicotic nodules on chest radiography or CT, and exclusion of other illnesses that may mimic silicosis. These include mycobacterial and fungal infections as well as other granulomatous diseases such as sarcoidosis, chronic beryllium disease, and hypersensitivity pneumonitis. Silicosis and coal workers' pneumoconiosis are radiographically very similar. In fact, many coal miners have been exposed to both coal dust and silica. Diagnosis of acute silicosis is based on a history of excessive silica exposure, usually occurring recurrently over fewer than 1–3 years, coupled with imaging studies showing ground-glass opacification. Examination of lung tissue is occasionally necessary to distinguish this condition from pneumonia, alveolar hemorrhage, or noncardiogenic pulmonary edema.

Complications

Complications of silicosis include concomitant lung infections, lung cancer, spontaneous pneumothorax, and broncholithiasis. Of particular concern is concurrent infection with tuberculosis. Although the incidence of tuberculosis is increased in all forms of the disease, the highest rates of infection occur in patients with acute and accelerated silicosis. Presence of a positive tuberculin skin test should prompt a thorough evaluation for silicotuberculosis; some authorities recommend treatment for active tuberculosis in this setting regardless of microbiology results.

Other illnesses associated with silica exposure include connective tissue diseases such as systemic sclerosis, rheumatoid arthritis, and systemic lupus erythematosus.

The risk of lung cancer is increased among workers with silicosis. Less information on cancer is available for workers exposed to silica who do not have silicosis.

Patients with PMF may develop chronic respiratory failure and cor pulmonale.

Treatment

There is no specific treatment for silicosis. Treatment is geared toward prevention of complications, eliminating continued exposure to silica dust, and managing the consequences of chronic respiratory failure. Because of the strong association between silicosis and tuberculosis, concurrent mycobacterial infection should be considered in any patient with silicosis, especially those with relatively rapid clinical deterioration. Conversion of the tuberculin skin test without clinical evidence of active tuberculosis warrants isoniazid prophylactic therapy. A number of drug regimens have been proposed for treatment of active silicotuberculosis. Recent evidence suggests that a 4.5- to 6-month regimen consisting of rifampin, pyrazinamide, isoniazid, and streptomycin is effective with a relapse rate of less than 4%. Some three-drug regimens that include isoniazid and rifampin with either ethambutol, pyrazinamide, or streptomycin for 9–24 months are associated with relapse rates between zero and 5%.

Hypoxemia and cor pulmonale are managed with supplemental oxygen and supportive care. Anecdotally, corticosteroids may be helpful when silicosis is associated with autoimmune disease. In patients with acute or accelerated silicosis, corticosteroids may produce transient improvement in pulmonary function.

Patients with silicosis should avoid additional silica exposure. Silicosis and silica exposure are associated with increased risk of lung cancer.

Prognosis

Generally, patients with simple silicosis have a normal lifespan and many have no physical impairment. Mild respiratory symptoms develop in others. Complicated silicosis, however, may progress to severe respiratory disability with premature mortality. The likelihood of impairment and death is increased if tuberculosis develops and is inadequately treated. Development of rheumatoid arthritis or an elevated rheumatoid factor may also herald progression of lung disease. Silica-related air flow obstruction, with bronchitis or emphysema, produces significant impairment and is often associated with progressive abnormalities in diffusion capacity, gas exchange, and exercise tolerance. Conglomerate silicotic masses are harbingers of severe impairment, cor pulmonale, and premature death from respiratory failure. When silicosis develops at an early age, the prognosis is poor, usually reflecting previous intense exposures and a correspondingly high risk of progression. Favorable prognostic factors include lower average exposures, advanced age at time of diagnosis, simple silicosis, and an observed slow rate of progression.

COAL WORKERS' PNEUMOCONIOSES

 ESSENTIALS OF DIAGNOSIS

- *A careful occupational and environmental history of past inhalational exposures.*
- *Evidence of interstitial lung disease (especially bilateral rounded opacities with upper lobe predominance).*

General Considerations

Coal workers' pneumoconiosis (CWP) results from inhalation of coal dust. Coal workers are at risk for other respiratory conditions including silicosis, anthrasilicosis, or mixed-dust pneumoconiosis from combined exposure to both coal and hard-rock dust. There is significant clinical overlap among these conditions. Miners who work at the leading edge of the unmined coal seam are exposed to the highest concentrations of airborne coal and silica dust when the hard rock adjacent to coal seams is cut. By comparison, surface workers who maintain equipment or who clean, process, and load coal are exposed to lower levels of respirable coal dust, although they are still at some risk. A recent study showed that CWP continues to occur in the United States at rates ranging from 1.4% to 14%.

Prevention

Preventive strategies require regular workplace monitoring of respirable coal dust levels and medical surveillance of the workforce. Proper ventilation and dust suppression allow employers to meet compliance and regulatory dust exposure standards. Physicians should not assume that their patients who work in coal mines have been adequately protected or that use of a respirator is adequate to protect workers from coal dust. All coal miners should be offered periodic tests of lung function and chest imaging.

Clinical Findings

The coal macule is the main pathological lesion in CWP. Macules are focal accumulations of coal dust, dust-laden macrophages, and fibroblasts. They are located around respiratory bronchioles and associated with varying degrees of fibrosis and focal emphysema. This emphysema occurs in both smoking and nonsmoking coal miners. Macules increase in size and number with increasing dust deposition and time. They are typically found in mid and upper portions of the lungs. Complicated CWP occurs when individual macules grow into masses or coalesce with other macules. Large opacities are defined as being greater than 1.0 cm in diameter on chest imaging. Coalesced nodules look radiographically like PMF that occurs in patients with silicosis. Masses can grow to consume the space occupied by the upper lobes. Latency is approximately 20–40 years.

A. SYMPTOMS AND SIGNS

Simple CWP is usually an asymptomatic condition without evidence of pulmonary impairment on lung function tests. Patients, however, often report bronchitis from coal dust exposure regardless of whether they have pneumoconiosis detected on chest radiograph. As simple CWP advances into complicated CWP, patients develop cough, sputum production (sometimes with expectoration of black sputa), and dyspnea. Coal dust, like silica dust, commonly causes chronic bronchitis in exposed workers. Physical signs include bilateral dry

rales, rhonchae, tracheal deviation due to PMF, and signs of right heart failure. PMF is associated with dyspnea at rest or with exertion, symptoms of chronic bronchitis, recurrent chest infections, right ventricular hypertrophy, and episodes of right heart failure.

B. LABORATORY FINDINGS

The radiographic appearance of simple CWP is not necessarily associated with abnormal pulmonary function tests. However, miners with the heaviest exposures to coal dust have lower mean forced expiratory volume (FEV_1) than those exposed to lower levels. This suggests a dose–response relationship between airflow obstruction and dust exposure. Declines in forced vital capacity (FVC) and FEV_1/FVC ratio are also related to the degree of exposure. The relationship between exposure and lung function abnormalities persists even after adjusting for tobacco use by miners. Coal dust and tobacco smoke produce similar decrements in lung function. The greatest reduction in FEV_1 occurs in patients with the most severe CWP. PMF is associated with a mixed obstructive/restrictive pattern, frequently with reduction in DL_{CO} and oxygen desaturation at rest and during exercise.

C. IMAGING STUDIES

Radiographs in simple CWP are characterized by the presence of small rounded opacities in the lung parenchyma. The upper lobes are involved more than the lower lobes early in the disease process. There may also be minor enlargement of hilar lymph nodes. The radiographic appearance of CWP is very similar to that for silicosis. These diseases are principally distinguishable by exposure history or occasionally by histology. Simple CWP is usually detected on chest radiograph before symptoms or signs develop. As disease progresses to complicated CWP, the nodules increase in size and coalesce. PMF is associated with significant numbers of nodules greater than 1.0 cm in diameter. The size cutoff distinguishing PMF from complicated CWP is arbitrary. The two conditions represent points along a continuum of disease severity as opposed to distinct clinical entities. As with silicosis, HRCT is more sensitive than simple radiographs in detecting coal macules, emphysema, and coalescing masses.

Differential Diagnosis

In most cases CWP is diagnosed presumptively, based on appropriate chest radiograph or CT appearance coupled with a history of exposure. Most miners have worked in coal mines at least 10 years at the time of diagnosis. The differential diagnosis of CWP consists of other disorders that produce upper lung zone nodules and includes silicosis, mycobacterial and fungal infections, and other granulomatous diseases such as sarcoidosis, chronic beryllium disease, and hypersensitivity pneumonitis. Miners with simple CWP are at increased risk of developing complicated CWP. The differential diagnosis of CWP complicated by PMF includes cancer and infection.

Complications

CWP is associated with an increased incidence of mycobacterial infections, although they are less common than in silicosis. Coal workers may also develop Caplan's syndrome, which presents radiographically as multiple peripheral nodules (0.5–5 cm in diameter) superimposed on simple, nodular CWP. CWP patients with Caplan's syndrome either have rheumatoid arthritis or will develop it within the next decade.

The incidence of chronic respiratory failure and cor pulmonale is increased in CWP complicated by PMF.

Treatment

There is no specific therapy for CWP. Treatment focuses on avoiding or reducing ongoing dust exposure, symptom control, and management of cor pulmonale/chronic respiratory failure. Change in occupation is commonly required to lower dust exposure. However, disease progression can occur despite this intervention. Periodic spirometry and radiography are useful to monitor disease progression. Symptomatic patients require evaluation of gas exchange and supplemental oxygen for hypoxia. Patients with cough and dyspnea associated with airflow limitation benefit from treatment with inhaled bronchodilators. Patients with hyperresponsive airways may benefit from inhaled corticosteroids. Pulmonary rehabilitation may help improve cardiovascular conditioning and maintain activity levels in patients with PMF complicated by chronic respiratory failure.

Prognosis

All forms of CWP may progress, even in the absence of further dust exposure. The prognosis of simple CWP, however, is controversial, in part due to difficulty in eliminating the confounding effects of tobacco use. Although life expectancy of coal workers is similar to that of people in other professions, coal workers have increased mortality from lung disease, tuberculosis, and stomach cancer. Conversely, mortality from cardiovascular disease and lung cancer is lower. Complicated

CWP and coal-related PMF are associated with chronic respiratory failure and cor pulmonale, resulting in significant pulmonary disability and premature death. Approximately 4% of deaths in coal miners are attributable to CWP, primarily from PMF. Risk factors for development of PMF include magnitude of dust exposure, rank of the coal mined (anthracite carries the most risk, followed by bituminous and lignite), and silica content of the coal dust. Active tuberculosis may also be a risk factor for PMF, although this relationship is controversial.

OTHER PNEUMOCONIOSES

Pneumoconioses have been described after exposure to numerous other dusts, however, the incidence of these diseases is much lower than that for asbestosis, silicosis, or CWP. Some of these conditions and the associated dust exposures are listed in Table 31–1. As in all pneumoconioses, obtaining a history of exposure and recognizing an appropriate constellation of signs, symptoms, pulmonary function tests, and radiographic abnormalities are critical to diagnosis. Referral to a pulmonary occupational medicine specialist should be obtained if the history suggests one of these disorders.

Beckett WS: Occupational respiratory diseases. N Engl J Med 2000;342:406. [PMID: 10666432]. (General review of pathophysiology and pathogenesis of various forms of occupational lung disease.)

Newman LS: Occupational illness. N Engl J Med 1995;333:1128. [PMID: 7565952]. (General review of evaluation and clinical manifestations of categories of occupational illness.)

Table 31–1. Dust exposure associated with selected pneumoconioses.

Disease	Dust
Asbesosis	Asbestos
Silicosis	Silica
Coal workers' pneumoconiosis	Coal dust
Talcosis	Hydrated magnesium silicate
Mixed dust pneumoconiosis	Coal dust, smoke from fires, and silicates
Kaolin-induced pneumoconiosis	Hydrous aluminum silicate
Aluminum-induced pneumoconiosis	Bauxite (Al_2O_3)
Hard-metal disease (giant cell pneumonitis)	Cobalt
Berylliosis	Beryllium
Silicosiderosis	Silica and iron

Hypersensitivity Pneumonitis

Cecile Rose, MD, MPH

ESSENTIALS OF DIAGNOSIS

- *Known repeated exposure to an immunologically sensitizing organic or chemical antigen.*
- *Symptoms and signs frequently include dyspnea on exertion and inspiratory rales.*
- *Pulmonary physiology typically demonstrates a restrictive or mixed pattern with reduced diffusion capacity of the lung for carbon monoxide ($D_{L_{CO}}$).*
- *Abnormalities on chest imaging most commonly include infiltrates on radiograph and centrilobular nodules on high-resolution computed tomography (HRCT).*
- *Lung histopathology demonstrates cellular bronchiolitis and interstitial granulomas.*

General Considerations

Hypersensitivity pneumonitis (HP), also known as extrinsic allergic alveolitis, refers to a constellation of inflammatory lung diseases caused by repeated exposure and immunological sensitization to a variety of organic and chemical antigens. Diagnosis relies on a combination of findings including a history of repeated antigen exposure; characteristic signs and symptoms, most commonly including exertional dyspnea and inspiratory crackles on examination; pulmonary function abnormalities often including decreased diffusion capacity and restrictive changes; radiological abnormalities, classically with infiltrates on chest radiograph or centrilobular nodules on HRCT; and characteristic histological findings of cellular bronchiolitis and interstitial granulomas.

The three general categories of antigens that cause HP are microbial agents, animal proteins, and low-molecular-weight chemicals. Microbial agents include bacteria and fungi. Multiple species of thermophilic bacteria frequently contaminate decaying vegetable matter and are causally associated with farmer's lung, the prototypical example of HP. Thermophiles as well as other bacterial species may also contaminate ventilation systems and humidifiers and cause HP from exposure to indoor aerosols. Nontuberculous mycobacteria contaminating hot tubs and metal working fluids are also thought to cause HP. Many fungi, including *Rhizopus, Penicillium, Aspergillus*, and *Alternaria*, are causative antigens in various occupational settings such as woodworking, agriculture, and lumber milling, and as contaminants of air-handling systems or water-damaged indoor settings. Avian antigens are the most common animal proteins associated with HP. Environmental and occupational history taking should always examine the possible presence of birds in the home and participation in bird hobbies. Cases of HP have been associated with apparently trivial exposures such as feather duvets and decorations, down comforters, and dusty laundry from bird hobbyists. A few low-molecular-weight chemicals are known to cause HP, including isocyanates, the pesticide pyrethrum, Pauli's reagent (sodium diazobenzenesulfate), and copper sulfate.

The epidemiology of HP is problematic due to variable clinical case definitions and underrecognition of disease. Most epidemiological studies have focused on farmer's lung; estimates of incidence and prevalence vary significantly by region. HP prevalence among dairy and cattle ranchers in Wyoming was found to be 3%, whereas prevalence rates in Wisconsin dairy farmers are as high as 12%. Prevalence of HP among bird hobbyists ranges from 0.5% to 21%. Among isocyanate workers, the prevalence is approximately 1%. Attack rates in outbreaks of HP may be quite high. HP occurred in 52% of office workers exposed to a contaminated humidification system. Attack rates of 27% and 65% in sequential HP outbreaks occurred among lifeguards exposed to microbial-contaminated aerosols at an indoor swimming pool.

Grammer LC: Occupational allergic alveolitis. Ann Allergy Asthma Immunol 1999;83:602. [PMID: 10619329]. (Review of epidemiology, pathogenesis, and clinical presentation of HP.)

Rose CS et al: "Lifeguard lung": endemic granulomatous pneumonitis in an indoor swimming pool. Am J Public Health 1998;88:1795. [PMID: 9842376]. (Epidemiological investigation of an outbreak of HP among lifeguards at an indoor pool.)

Pathogenesis

Both environmental and host factors appear to play a role in risk for HP. A number of studies have shown that HP occurs more frequently in nonsmokers. However, smokers who develop farmer's lung have a poorer prognosis, with lower vital capacities, more frequent clinical recurrences, and worse 10-year survival than nonsmokers with farmer's lung. Exposure factors such as antigen concentration, duration of exposure before symptom onset, frequency and intermittency of exposure, particle size, antigen solubility, use of respiratory protection, and variability in work practices influence disease prevalence, latency, and severity. Farmer's lung disease is most common in regions with heavy rainfall where feed is likely to become damp and in harsh winter conditions where contaminated hay is used to feed cattle in indoor barns with minimal ventilation. Pigeon breeder's lung is most common during the summer sporting season when exposure is highest.

HP is characterized by the presence of activated T-lymphocytes in bronchoalveolar lavage (BAL) and an interstitial mononuclear cell infiltrate on lung biopsy. Pathogenesis involves repeated antigen exposure leading to immunological sensitization and subsequent immune-mediated lung inflammation. The mechanisms underlying this series of events appear primarily to involve cell-mediated immunity, with interleukin (IL)-12 and interferon-γ playing essential immunomodulatory roles.

Prevention

Recognition of an index case of HP may have considerable public health importance, as others exposed to the same environment are also at risk for disease. Each case represents a sentinel health event, indicating the need for further investigation of the implicated environment to identify risk to others and opportunities for prevention. Potential intervention includes control of moisture problems by preventing leaks and eliminating aerosol humidifiers or hot tubs. Prevention of bird breeder's HP includes removal of birds from the home as well as careful clean-up to remove fleecy furnishings such as carpets that may be sources of on-going dust exposure and wet-wiping of surfaces. Changes in work practices to reduce the prevalence of farmer's lung include efficient drying of hay and cereals before storage, use of mechanical feeding systems, and better ventilation of farm buildings.

Zejda JE, McDuffie HH, Dosman JA: Epidemiology of health and safety risks in agriculture and related industries. Practical applications for rural physicians. West J Med 1993;158:56. [PMID: 8470386]. (Review of preventive measures employed by the agricultural sector to decrease the risk of farmer's lung.)

Clinical Findings

A. SYMPTOMS AND SIGNS

There is often considerable overlap in clinical presentation of HP among acute, subacute, and chronic forms.

Respiratory symptoms such as cough and dyspnea and systemic symptoms of fever, chills, and myalgias typically occur 4–12 h after antigen exposure in acute HP. Physical findings include fever and inspiratory crackles. Subacute and chronic forms of HP present with insidious onset of dyspnea and cough accompanied by nonspecific systemic symptoms such as malaise, fatigue, myalgias, low grade fever, and weight loss. Physical examination may be normal or remarkable for basilar crackles. Cyanosis and right-sided heart failure occur in more advanced disease.

B. LABORATORY FINDINGS

Finding specific immunoglobulin G (IgG) precipitating antibodies (precipitins) in serum of patients with suspected HP is a helpful diagnostic clue but is not sensitive, specific, or required for diagnosis. Serum precipitins are markers of antigen exposure and are detectable in 3% to 30% of asymptomatic farmers and 50% of asymptomatic pigeon breeders. False negative results are common. Of patients with farmer's lung disease, 30–40% in one study had no detectable precipitins.

Peripheral leukocytosis is common in acute forms of HP. Mild elevations in erythrocyte sedimentation rate, C-reactive protein, and immunoglobulins of IgG, IgM, or IgA isotype may occur in all presentations of HP, reflecting acute or chronic inflammation.

C. PHYSIOLOGY

Patients with HP may exhibit obstructive, restrictive, or mixed patterns on pulmonary function testing. Normal values of spirometry and lung volumes are not uncommon in early disease. Abnormalities of gas exchange, particularly during exercise, are the most sensitive physiological indicators of early HP. Restrictive changes and a decreased diffusion capacity ($D_{L_{CO}}$) are common in acute HP. Mixed restrictive and obstructive impairments along with decreased $D_{L_{CO}}$ occur in subacute and chronic HP. Up to 10% of patients with farmer's lung may have obstruction alone and tests of nonspecific bronchial hyperreactivity such as methacholine challenge may be positive.

D. IMAGING STUDIES

Chest radiographs are often normal when disease is detected early. Typical radiographic changes in acute HP include diffuse ground-glass opacification and fine reticulonodular infiltrates, often with lower lung field predominance. Reticulonodular infiltrates are more prominent in subacute HP. Fibrosis with upper lobe retraction, reticular opacities, volume loss, and honeycombing occur with chronic disease.

High-resolution computed tomography (HRCT) is more sensitive than plain radiography for diagnosing

HP. A number of HRCT abnormalities have been described. Ground-glass hazy opacities that likely represent active alveolitis or fine fibrosis are most common in acute illness but also occur in subacute and chronic HP, especially if there is ongoing exposure (Figure 32–1). Centrilobular nodules are also quite common. These nodules may represent cellular bronchiolitis and are typically round, poorly defined, and less than 5 mm in diameter. They often occur with ground glass opacification; this combination is highly suggestive of HP. Both nodules and ground-glass opacification may regress with removal from exposure. HRCT also frequently reveals irregular linear opacities, traction bronchiectasis, and honeycombing in subacute or chronic HP. These changes likely reflect fibrosis. Unfortunately, the presence and location of fibrotic changes are nonspecific and HRCT cannot reliably distinguish chronic HP from idiopathic pulmonary fibrosis. HRCT also occasionally demonstrates emphysematous changes in chronic HP. These changes probably result from underlying bronchiolar inflammation and obstruction. In chronic farmer's lung, radiological emphysema may be more common than fibrosis, even after accounting for effects of tobacco smoking. In one study of farmer's lung 13 of the 20 patients with evidence of emphysema on HRCT had never smoked.

E. HISTOPATHOLOGY

Lung histopathological changes in patients with HP typically include the triad of cellular bronchiolitis, lymphoplasmocytic interstitial infiltrates, and poorly formed nonnecrotizing granulomas. The complete triad is not always present and pathological features vary with disease stage. Granulomas are described in 60–70% of acute cases of HP but in less than 50% of patients with chronic HP. Giant cells, airspace foam cells, and bronchiolitis obliterans with organizing pneumonia (BOOP) may also occur. A fibrotic pattern similar to usual interstitial pneumonitis (UIP) is common in chronic HP.

Colby TV, Coleman A: The histologic diagnosis of extrinsic allergic alveolitis and its differential diagnosis. Prog Surg Pathol 1989;10:11. (Discussion of typical histopathological changes that are present in HP.)

Krasnick J et al: Hypersensitivity pneumonitis: problems in diagnosis. J Allergy Clin Immunol 1996;97:1027. [PMID: 8655880]. (Case report of pigeon breeder's HP with a discussion of value of serum precipitins in diagnosis.)

Lynch DA et al: Hypersensitivity pneumonitis: sensitivity of high-resolution CT in a population-based study. AJR Am J Roentgenol 1992;159:469. [PMID: 1503007]. (Comparison of sensitivity of chest radiographs and HRCT in detection of HP.)

Lynch DA et al: Can CT distinguish hypersensitivity pneumonitis from idiopathic pulmonary fibrosis? AJR Am J Roentgenol 1995;165:807. [PMID: 7676971]. (Efficacy of HRCT in differentiating HP from idiopathic pulmonary fibrosis and desquamative interstitial pneumonia.)

Matar LD, McAdams HP, Sporn TA: Hypersensitivity pneumonitis. AJR Am J Roentgenol 2000;174:1061. [PMID: 10749251]. (Discussion of the HRCT patterns in HP.)

Patel RA et al: Hypersensitivity pneumonitis: patterns on high-resolution CT. J Comput Assist Tomogr 2000;24:965. [PMID: 11105719]. (Pictorial essay demonstrating HRCT patterns of HP.)

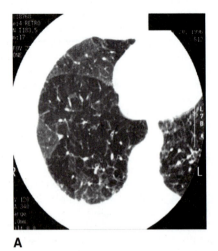
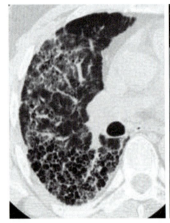
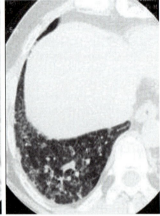

A   **B**

Figure 32–1. A: HRCT features of acute or subacute HP often include profuse centrilobular nodules, air trapping, and ground-glass attenuation. ***B:*** HRCT features of chronic HP may include reticular opacities, ground-glass, air trapping, and honeycombing.

Differential Diagnosis

The clinical presentation of HP mimics that of a number of other interstitial lung diseases (ILD), and a strong clinical index of suspicion combined with careful history-taking skills are essential in establishing the diagnosis. Clinical signs and symptoms do not readily distinguish HP from sarcoidosis, chronic beryllium disease (CBD), rheumatological lung diseases, or idiopathic interstitial lung diseases. Unlike sarcoidosis, CBD, and connective tissue-related ILD, extrapulmonary manifestations do not occur in HP. Although the classic histopathological triad of HP is helpful in the differential diagnosis of granulomatous lung diseases, the histological findings of HP are nonspecific and do not replace careful history taking for antigen exposure when granulomatous lung disease is diagnosed. HP may be mistaken for asthma in cases characterized by physiological obstruction and bronchial hyperreactivity. Failure to respond to conventional asthma therapy should prompt consideration of the possibility of HP. HP should also be included in the differential diagnosis of emphysema, particularly in nonsmokers.

Diagnosis

Evaluation of all patients with suspected HP should include a detailed clinical history, physical examination, chest HRCT (unless the plain film is clearly abnormal), complete pulmonary function tests (including lung volumes, pre- and postbronchodilator spirometry, and $D_{L_{CO}}$), and fiberoptic bronchoscopy with BAL and transbronchial biopsy. The cornerstone of diagnosis is a detailed history of symptoms in conjunction with occupational and environmental exposures. A clinical history suggesting a temporal relationship between symptoms and certain activities provides important clues to the diagnosis of HP, although such a pattern is not always apparent in subacute or chronic forms of the disease. Work history should include a chronology of current and previous occupations, with descriptions of specific work processes and exposures. The work history should also include a list of specific chemical, particulate, and other aerosol exposures, presence of persistent respiratory or constitutional symptoms in exposed co-workers, and use of respiratory protection. Review of Material Safety Data Sheets (MSDS) for specific chemicals such as isocyanates may supplement the work history. The environmental history should explore exposure to pets and other domestic animals (especially birds); hobbies such as gardening and lawn care that may involve sensitizing chemical exposures; recreational activities such as use of hot tubs and indoor swimming pools that may generate microbial bioaerosols; use of humidifiers, cool mist vaporizers, and humidified air conditioners that may be sources of microbial bioaerosols; moisture indicators such as leaking, flooding, or previous water damage to carpets and furnishings; and visible mold or mildew contamination in indoor environments.

Treatment

The cornerstone of therapy of HP is preventing continued exposure to the offending antigen. Elimination of the antigen is the preferred approach and has the added benefit of preventing disease in other exposed individuals. Removal of the contaminated source is straightforward in cases of home humidifier and hot tub-related HP. On-site investigation of the work and home environments by an experienced industrial hygienist may be helpful in cases in which the causative exposure is uncertain, particularly when disease is progressive. Unfortunately, antigen abatement is not always feasible, and removal of the patient from the implicated environment may be necessary. The role of respirators in preventing HP is unclear. Respirators have been used when removal from exposure was impossible. Although respirators may provide protection in circumstances with limited duration of exposure, verification of their efficacy in preventing new onset or recurrent HP requires further investigation. Moreover, respirators are difficult to wear for extended periods and require adequate fit testing and maintenance; noncompliance with their use is common.

Oral corticosteroids are frequently used to supplement antigen avoidance in severe or progressive HP. Corticosteroids are probably unnecessary in cases in which pulmonary function abnormalities are minor and spontaneous recovery is likely with removal from exposure. In more severe cases initial therapy with 40–60 mg/day of oral prednisone should be started and continued for at least 4–6 weeks. Pulmonary function tests should be monitored in the first 4–6 weeks following initiation of treatment. A gradual taper to a minimum sustaining dose should follow if there is objective improvement in physiology. Corticosteroids should be tapered and discontinued if no improvement occurs.

Additional therapy includes supplemental oxygen and other supportive measures in hypoxemic patients. Inhaled corticosteroids and β-agonists may be helpful in patients with airflow limitation. Cytotoxic agents such as cyclophosphamide and azathioprine have been used in cases refractory to corticosteroids. Regular monitoring for side effects and adverse reactions from immunosuppressive agents is essential. Cytotoxic therapy should be continued for at least 6–9 months to assess functional improvement and efficacy in preventing disease progression. Prophylaxis for pneumocystis pneumonia, appropriate vaccination, and prompt treatment of intercurrent infection are recommended for patients receiving corticosteroids and/or cytotoxic therapy.

Craig TJ et al: Bird antigen persistence in the home environment after removal of the bird. Ann Allergy 1992;69:510. [PMID: 1471783]. (Demonstrates the persistence of bird antigen for up to 18 months after both removal of the offending bird and environmental cleaning, suggesting adequate therapy may actually require removal of the patient from the environment.)

Kusaka H et al: Two-year follow up on the protective value of dust masks against farmer's lung disease. Intern Med 1993;32:106. [PMID: 8507920]. (Evaluates the practicality and efficacy of dust masks in preventing farmer's lung HP.)

Natural History & Prognosis

The clinical course of HP is variable. Permanent sequelae include persistent bronchial hyperresponsiveness, emphysema, and progressive interstitial fibrosis. An accelerated decline in lung function with continued antigen exposure has been demonstrated for most forms of HP, underscoring the importance of cessation of exposure. However, the clinical course of HP is variable even with antigen avoidance. Acute HP generally resolves without sequelae. However, progressive impairment may occur with recurrent attacks or following a single severe attack. The subacute and chronic forms of HP, characterized by insidious symptoms and more subtle clinical abnormalities, are frequently recognized later in the disease course. These patients often have a worse prognosis for this reason than do patients with acute disease. Disease progression occurs in some patients with subacute and chronic HP despite cessation of exposure.

Long-term mortality rates for patients with chronic HP range from 1% to 10%. Prognostic factors include age, duration of exposure after onset of symptoms, time of exposure prior to diagnosis, and presence of scarring. The prognosis for bird breeder's lung may be worse than for farmer's lung, with 5-year mortality rates approaching that of idiopathic pulmonary fibrosis.

Kokkarinen J, Tukiainen H, Terho EO: Mortality due to farmer's lung in Finland. Chest 1994;106:5092. [PMID: 7774328]. (Retrospective review of mortality and causes of death in patients with farmer's lung HP.)

Yoshizawa Y et al: A follow-up study of pulmonary function tests, bronchoalveolar lavage cells, and humoral and cellular immunity in bird fancier's lung. J Allergy Clin Immunol 1995;96:122. [PMID: 7622754]. (Demonstration of persistent presence of sensitized inflammatory cells and increased antibody production in bronchoalveolar lavage fluid after removal of antigen.)

Drug-Induced Lung Disease

33

Stephen K. Frankel, MD

 ESSENTIALS OF DIAGNOSIS

- *Drug-induced lung disease has a number of different and distinct clinical manifestations.*
- *Drug-induced lung disease is a diagnosis of exclusion.*
- *Diagnosis depends upon identifying the exposure and requires a thorough drug history.*
- *Lung biopsy may be supportive by demonstrating an appropriate pattern of lung injury but is not diagnostic*

General Considerations

Drug-induced lung disease may present with a variety of manifestations and has been associated with over 100 separate agents. However, if the agents to which a patient has been exposed and the interval since exposure are known, the potential pulmonary complications from that exposure will be fairly limited. In addition, there are stereotypical patterns of injury that suggest the possibility of drug-induced lung injury.

The diagnosis of drug-induced lung disease is usually one of exclusion as there is no single test that can confirm or refute this diagnosis. Depending upon the clinical manifestation of toxicity, signs and symptoms will vary and may mimic common entities such as pneumonia, heart failure, collagen-vascular disease, or cancer. Likewise, chest imaging rarely specifically suggests drug toxicity. Diagnosis usually requires ruling out other causes of the patient's disease and identifying an appropriate exposure, appropriate time interval between exposure and disease, and appropriate clinical manifestation for a suspect drug.

Establishing exposure requires a thorough medication history that reviews not only current medications but all drugs that the patient has ever taken, including over-the-counter agents. This history should also include herbal and alternative medications, nutritional supplements, and illicit drug use. Drug-induced lung disease may occur within minutes of taking a medication or many years after taking a drug. Specific prompts

and questioning are frequently necessary to clarify issues such as trade names, medications received during hospitalizations, and nondrug therapies such as radiation or supplemental oxygen. A specific search for the use of more common offenders such as amiodarone, nitrofurantoin, or methotrexate is useful when patients present with a clinical picture suggestive of drug-induced lung disease.

Clinical Findings (Table 33–1)

A. Bronchospasm

Bronchospasm is most frequently associated with β-blockers, cocaine, intravenous contrast, nonsteroidal antiinflammatory drugs (NSAIDs), aspirin, and propellants, including those used in metered dose inhalers. Reactions occur within minutes to hours of taking the medication, but with less severe reactions, patients may continue taking the offending medication for weeks, months, or years. Clinically, patients report shortness of breath and chest tightness, and physical examination reveals wheezing and a prolonged expiratory phase. Chest radiographs are often normal but may reveal increased lung volumes or hyperlucency. Pulmonary function tests (PFTs) demonstrate obstructive physiology with a positive bronchodilator response. Differential diagnosis includes common entities such as asthma and chronic obstructive pulmonary disease (COPD), such that drug-induced bronchospasm is often overlooked. Treatment includes administration of inhaled bronchodilators and discontinuation of the offending medication.

B. Acute or Subacute Pneumonitis

Although this category of drug reaction is often subdivided by mechanism between hypersensitivity reactions and nonimmunologically mediated interstitial pneumonitis, they are grouped together for the purposes of this discussion as there is uncertainty and overlap in the mechanism of injury for a number of agents. Moreover, the clinical presentation of these entities is similar. Patients present several days to months after the initiation of therapy with dyspnea and nonproductive cough. Additional symptoms may include fever, chills, fatigue, malaise, chest discomfort, rash, arthralgias, or myalgias. Extrapulmonary symptoms are more common in but not exclusive to hypersensitivity reactions. Examination

Table 33–1. Clinical presentations of drug-induced lung disease.

Barotrauma
  Amphetamines
  Cocaine
  Marijuana

Bronchiolitis obliterans
  Gold
  Penicillamine

Bronchiolitis obliterans with organizing pneumonia
  Amiodarone
  Bleomycin
  Cocaine
  Cytosine arabinoside
  Gold
  Methotrexate
  Mitomycin C
  Penicillamine
  Radiation

Bronchospasm
  Acetylcysteine
  Amphetamines
  Aspirin
  β-Blockers
  Cocaine
  Cytosine arabinoside
  Dipyridamole
  Intravenous contrast
  Methacholine
  Nonsteroidal antiinflammatory drugs
  Pentamidine (inhaled)
  Paclitaxel
  Propellants
  Protamine

Drug-induced lupus
  Chlorpromazine
  Hydralazine
  Isoniazid
  Penicillamine
  Phenytoin
  Procainamide

Eosinophilic lung disease
  β-Lactam antibiotics
  Carbamazepine
  Diphenylhydantoin
  Isoniazid
  L-Tryptophan
  Minocycline
  Nitrofurantoin
  NSAIDs
  Pentamidine (inhaled)
  Sulfa agents
  Sulfonamides
  Tetracycline

Pleural effusion
  Amiodarone
  Bromocriptine
  Drugs associated with drug-induced lupus
  Interleukin-2
  Methysergide
  Nitrofurantoin
  Sclerotherapy
  Tocolytics

Pulmonary edema
  Aspirin
  Amphetamines
  Chlordiazepoxide
  Cocaine
  Cytosine arabinoside
  Hydrochlorothiazide (HCTZ)
  Intereukin-2
  Opiates
  Protamine
  Tocolytics
  Tricyclic antidepressant overdose

Pulmonary fibrosis
  Amiodarone
  Azathioprine
  Bleomycin
  Busulfan

  Chlorambucil
  Combination chemotherapy
  Cyclosphosphamide
  Melphalan
  Mercaptopurine
  Mitomycin C
  Nitrofurantoin
  Nitrosoureas (BCNU, CCNU, methyl--CCNU)
  Procarbazine
  Radiation

Pulmonary hemorrhage
  Anticoagulants
  Cocaine
  High-dose combination chemo-therapy
  Mitomycin C
  Penicillamine
  Platelet IIb/IIIa inhibitors

Pulmonary hypertension
  Anorectic agents
  Cocaine

Pneumonitis
  Amiodarone
  Azathioprine
  Bleomycin
  Cocaine
  Cyclohosphamide
  Gold
  Methotrexate
  Nitrofurantoin
  Penicillamine
  Paclitaxel
  Radiation

Talc granulomatosis
  Amphetamines
  Cocaine
  Opiates

may reveal tachypnea, rales, decreased breath sounds, or evidence of consolidation. Hypoxemia and hypocapnia are the most common arterial blood gas findings and chest radiographs typically demonstrate interstitial, alveolar, or mixed infiltrates. These changes are generally bilateral. Chest computed tomography (CT) imaging characterizes these areas as patchy, heterogeneous ground glass abnormalities, reticular infiltrates with alveolar septal wall thickening, and/or airspace consoli-

dation. The most common pulmonary function abnormality is a reduced diffusion capacity of the lung for carbon monoxide (DL_{CO}). Restrictive findings may also be seen. Pneumonitis characterized as a hypersensitivity reaction often but not necessarily always has lymphocytosis or eosinophilia in bronchoalveolar lavage fluid and occasionally demonstrates peripheral eosinophilia. Treatment usually consists of removal of the drug and a trial of corticosteroids.

C. Pulmonary Fibrosis/Late Fibrosing Pneumonitis

Pulmonary fibrosis is a late complication of multiple chemotherapeutic and immunosuppressive agents, radiation, nitrofurantoin, and amiodarone. Patients present months to years after therapy with insidious, progressive dyspnea on exertion, decreasing exercise tolerance, vague chest discomfort or pleuritic chest pain, nonproductive cough, fatigue, malaise, and/or weight loss. Examination reveals basilar predominant, mid to late inspiratory rales similar to those found in idiopathic pulmonary fibrosis. Other findings may include tachypnea, decreased breath sounds, or bronchial breath sounds. Pulmonary hypertension, cor pulmonale, or chronic respiratory failure may complicate end-stage disease. Chest imaging typically demonstrates bilateral reticular infiltrates with volume loss. Other findings include traction bronchiectasis, honeycombing, pleural fibrosis, and atelectasis. PFTs commonly show a reduced $D_{L_{CO}}$ and restrictive physiology. Arterial blood gases demonstrate hypoxemia and hypocapnia. The differential diagnosis in these patients includes idiopathic pulmonary fibrosis, connective tissue disease-associated interstitial lung disease, asbestosis, drug-induced pulmonary fibrosis, radiation fibrosis, familial interstitial lung disease, idiopathic nonspecific interstitial pneumonitis (NSIP), and fibrosing hypersensitivity pneumonitis. A careful drug history is important in all patients who present with pulmonary fibrosis as the exposure may have taken place years before onset of disease. Treatment includes discontinuation of the drug and supportive therapy such as supplemental oxygen. A trial of corticosteroids may also be indicated in some cases, but prognosis is generally poor once patients develop clinically apparent pulmonary fibrosis.

D. Noncardiogenic Pulmonary Edema

The alveolar endothelial–epithelial barrier, which determines the permeability of the lung to water and osmotically active particles, is sensitive to injury by a variety of agents such that pulmonary edema is a fairly common manifestation of drug toxicity. Patients generally present within hours or days of drug exposure and report dyspnea, frothy sputum, and cough. Examination reveals tachypnea, dependent rales, and hypoxemia. Chest radiographs show interstitial and/or alveolar infiltrates consistent with pulmonary edema. Differential diagnosis includes cardiogenic and noncardiogenic pulmonary edema, atypical infections, noninfectious pneumonitis, and lymphangitic spread of cancer. Treatment is discontinuation of the drug, supportive care, and diuresis.

E. Acute Respiratory Distress Syndrome (ARDS)/Diffuse Alveolar Damage (DAD)

Clinically, it may be difficult to distinguish among noncardiogenic pulmonary edema, acute pneumonitis, and ARDS/diffuse alveolar damage, as there is considerable overlap among these presentations. Generally, drugs that cause ARDS result in more severe injury (severe hypoxemia or respiratory failure), a more protracted course, and poorer response to therapy. Histopathology demonstrates not only edema, type II pneumocyte hyperplasia with atypia, and inflammatory cell infiltrates but also epithelial necrosis and formation of hyaline membranes. Examples of agents that cause ARDS/DAD are gemcitabine and cytosine arabinoside.

F. Drug-Induced Lupus

Procainamide, hydralazine, penicillamine, and isoniazid are the agents most commonly associated with drug-induced lupus. Patients generally present with pleuritis, pleural effusion, pneumonitis, arthralgias, myalgias, skin disease, serositis, and constitutional symptoms. Severe complications such as cerebritis or nephritis are exceedingly rare. Serologies frequently demonstrate antinuclear antibody (ANA) seropositivity and, rarely, more specific double-stranded DNA antibodies. Drug-induced lupus almost always responds to withdrawal of the offending agent with resolution of symptoms over weeks to months.

G. Pulmonary Hemorrhage

Diffuse alveolar hemorrhage is a rare manifestation of drug-induced injury, largely limited to cocaine, high-dose combination chemotherapy, penicillamine, and anticoagulants/antiplatelet agents. The most common presentation includes dyspnea, hemoptysis, hypoxemia, and alveolar infiltrates on chest radiograph. However, up to one-third of patients with alveolar hemorrhage do not present with hemoptysis, frequently resulting in misdiagnosis as pneumonia. Diagnosis is made when bronchoscopy yields a bloody return on bronchoalveolar lavage that does not clear with serial lavage.

H. Barotrauma

Pneumothorax, pneumomediastinum, and pneumopericardium may occur with inhalational drug use. These are not complications of the drugs per se as much as the method of delivery of the drug. The proposed mechanism of injury is that deep inhalation followed by a Valsalva maneuver along with coughing raises intraalveolar pressure. This increased pressure results in tears in the parenchyma and tracking of air back along bronchovascular sheaths into the pleural space and mediastinum. Barotrauma has been reported most commonly with crack cocaine use, but may also occur with methamphetamines and marijuana. A careful search must be undertaken to rule out other causes of barotrauma such as perforated esophagus, chest trauma, and "pocket shots" (direct injection by the user into a central vein.) Treatment consists of supportive care, including chest tube thoracostomy for clinically significant pneumothoraces.

I. BRONCHIOLITIS OBLITERANS

Bronchiolitis obliterans (BO) is a rare manifestation of drug-induced lung disease resulting in progressive small airway scarring. It occurs with both penicillamine and gold therapy. "Mid-inspiratory squeaks" are the classic finding suggestive of BO. Other findings on examination include tachypnea, wheeze, hyperinflation, and decreased breath sounds. Imaging generally reveals only air trapping and hyperinflation. PFTs demonstrate hyperinflation and airflow limitation. Prognosis for these patients is poor and treatment with corticosteroids or immunosuppressive agents is generally unrewarding.

J. BRONCHIOLITIS OBLITERANS WITH ORGANIZING PNEUMONIA

Bronchiolitis obliterans with organizing pneumonia (BOOP) is a pathological diagnosis characterized by the appearance of granulation tissue in airspaces and small airways. Although occasionally idiopathic, BOOP generally occurs as a complication of another disease such as infection, connective tissue disease, drug-induced injury, or inhalation exposures. Patients commonly report progressive dyspnea on exertion and nonproductive cough. Chest imaging reveals patchy, focal airspace disease. BOOP is generally responsive to corticosteroids.

K. TALC GRANULOMATOSIS

Talc granulomatosis is an immunological response to the deposition of foreign material in the pulmonary parenchyma or vasculature. Drug-induced talc granulomatosis occurs when patients inject or inhale filler materials such as talc, methylcellulose, or baking soda with illicit drugs. Patients present with progressive dyspnea on exertion, decreasing exercise tolerance, chest discomfort, cough, or pulmonary hypertension. Chest imaging may be normal or may reveal diffuse interstitial infiltrates or micronodular/nodular disease. Differential diagnosis includes infections such as *Pneumocystis carinii* pneumonia and tuberculosis [this population is at increased risk for human immunodeficiency virus/acquired immunodeficiency syndrome (HIV/AIDS)] and noninfectious entities such as sarcoidosis. Diagnosis requires biopsy demonstrating granulomatous disease and birefringent crystals seen with polarized light. Talc granulomatosis is often poorly responsive to therapy,

but some patients will improve following a course of corticosteroids.

L. PULMONARY INFILTRATES WITH EOSINOPHILIA

Many drugs have been associated with the development of eosinophilic pulmonary infiltrates. In developed countries, drug reaction is probably the leading cause of Löffler's syndrome. Patients are often asymptomatic, but may complain of nonproductive cough, dyspnea, wheezing, rash, arthralgias, or fevers. Prior to the identification of eosinophilia, the differential diagnosis includes pneumonia, drug-induced pneumonitis, heart failure, cancer, and connective tissue disease. Identification of peripheral eosinophilia or eosinophilia in bronchoalveolar lavage fluid narrows the differential to drug reaction, parasitic infection, eosinophilic pneumonia, Churg–Strauss vasculitis, allergic bronchopulmonary aspergillosis, and idiopathic hypereosinophilic syndrome. The interval between initiation of the drug and development of clinically apparent disease is highly variable due to the often mild symptoms associated with this condition. Nonetheless, most patients are usually still taking or have only recently stopped taking the drug at time of diagnosis. A subset of these reactions may also be classified as acute hypersensitivity responses. Patients generally respond within days to drug withdrawal, but in severe cases a course of corticosteroids is beneficial.

M. PULMONARY HYPERTENSION

Although rare, patients who have taken the anorectic agents dexfenfluramine, phenteramine, fenfluramine, or aminorex have greatly increased risk for development of primary pulmonary hypertension. Acute and chronic cocaine use has also been associated with development of pulmonary hypertension. See Chapter 18 for a further discussion of this condition.

N. PLEURAL DISEASE

Pleural effusion is a common finding in drug-induced lung disease. Drugs listed in Table 33–1 under drug-induced lupus, noncardiogenic pulmonary edema, and pleural disease are all associated with development of pleural effusions. Pleural fibrosis is a rare complication of drug therapy, most commonly associated with methysergide, bromocriptine, ergotamines, amiodarone, bleomycin, and mitomycin C use.

Ben-Noun L: Drug-induced respiratory disorders: incidence, prevention and management. Drug Saf 2000;23:143. [PMID: 10945376]. (Good general review of drug-induced lung disease.)

Erasmus JJ, McAdams HP, Rossi SE: High-resolution CT of drug-induced lung disease. Radiol Clin North Am 2002;40:61. [PMID: 11813820]. (Review of radiological manifestations of drug-induced lung disease.)

Specific Drug Reactions

A. ANTINEOPLASTIC AGENTS

1. General considerations—Many individual chemo-therapeutic agents and combinations of agents have well-described pulmonary toxicity (Table 33–2). The majority of pulmonary complications are either acute/subacute pneumonitis or pulmonary fibrosis. Additional complications also include pulmonary edema, ARDS, pulmonary hemorrhage, bronchospasm, respiratory failure, BOOP, and pulmonary infiltrates with eosinophilia. The differential diagnosis of cancer patients with pulmonary symptoms and infiltrates days to weeks following chemotherapy includes infection, drug- or radiation-induced lung injury, and neoplasm. Physical examination and imaging studies are often nonspecific and diagnosis commonly requires broncho-scopic evaluation to distinguish between these possibilities. Empiric therapy for one or more conditions is often necessary. Therapy commonly includes cortico-steroids for both interstitial pneumonitis and pulmonary fibrosis. Early-onset interstitial disease is significantly more responsive to therapy than late-onset fibrosis.

Risk factors for development of pulmonary toxicity depend upon the agent(s) used. However, factors that are important include treatment with agents with a high incidence of pulmonary toxicity, cumulative dose of an agent, previous or concurrent radiation therapy, use of multiple cytotoxic agents, underlying pulmonary disease, oxygen therapy, and decreased drug clearance.

2. Bleomycin—Bleomycin is used in the treatment of germ cell tumors and lymphoma. Toxicity occurs in 10% of patients and is more common with cumulative doses >450 U and advanced age (especially >70 years). Radiation therapy and oxygen administration may also be risk factors, although these interactions are controversial. Respiratory symptoms such as cough and dyspnea are more common during and immediately following combination therapy with bleomycin and radiation compared to chemotherapy alone. However, the incidence of pulmonary symptoms between these two groups of patients is similar 2–3 years after therapy, suggesting no long-term sequelae. Mortality is increased in animals treated with both oxygen and bleomycin, implying a synergistic effect of these agents. However, human data indicating an increased risk of pneumonitis does not exist. Nevertheless, because of concerns raised by animal data, oxygen supplementation should be used cautiously during and after bleomycin therapy.

Table 33–2. Pulmonary toxicity associated with chemotherapy

Agent	Pulmonary Toxicity
Ara-C (cytosine arabinoside)	Noncardiogenic pulmonary edema, BOOP
ATRA (all-*trans*-retinoic acid)	Retinoic acid syndrome (see text)
Bleomycin	Pneumonitis, pulmonary fibrosis, pulmonary nodules
Busulfan	Pulmonary fibrosis
BCNU (bischloroethyl nitrosourea, carmustine)	Pulmonary fibrosis
Chlorambucil	Pulmonary fibrosis
Cyclophosphamide	Pulmonary fibrosis
Gemcytabine	ARDS/diffuse alveolar damage
High-dose combination chemotherapy	Pneumonitis, pulmonary fibrosis, diffuse alveolar hemorrhage
Interleukin-2	Noncardiogenic pulmonary edema, pleural effusion
Melphalan	Pulmonary fibrosis
Methotrexate	Pneumonitis
Mitomycin C	Pulmonary fibrosis, alveolar hemorrhage (HUS), acute hypersensitivity reaction (see text)
Procarbazine	Pulmonary infiltrates with eosinophilia, pneumonitis
Paclitaxel	Bronchospasm, angioedema, pneumonitis
Radiation therapy	Pneumonitis, pulmonary fibrosis

Pulmonary toxicity associated with bleomycin includes pulmonary nodules, acute pneumonitis, and pulmonary fibrosis. Pulmonary fibrosis is the most common complication. Therapy with corticosteroids is recommended, although results are variable. Mortality is approximately 20–30%.

3. Mitomycin C—Mitomycin C toxicity may present with pulmonary fibrosis similar to bleomycin-induced lung disease; however, mitomycin C also has three other unusual pulmonary manifestations: acute hypersensitivity reactions, BOOP, and hemolytic–uremic syndrome (HUS). Acute reactions occur when mitomycin C is given together with a vinca alkaloid and is characterized by cough, dyspnea, bronchospasm, chest pain, hypoxemia, infiltrates, and occasionally acute respiratory failure. This complication has a good prognosis when treated with supportive care and corticosteroids. Hemolytic–uremic syndrome presents with diffuse alveolar hemorrhage associated with renal failure, thrombocytopenia, and microangiopathic hemolytic anemia. It is rare but has a dismal prognosis with mortality rates approaching 70%.

4. Nitrosoureas—Carmustine (BCNU), the prototypic nitrosourea, is associated with pulmonary fibrosis. Patients present months to years following therapy with dyspnea on exertion, constitutional symptoms, hypoxemia, rales, and infiltrates on chest radiograph. Up to 20% of patients receiving carmustine develop lung disease. Risk factors include higher cumulative doses and preexisting lung disease. Other nitrosoureas, such as lomustine (CCNU) and semustine, produce similar pulmonary toxicity albeit with lesser frequency.

5. Busulfan—Busulfan is an alkylating agent that is associated with development of clinically significant pulmonary fibrosis in approximately 5% of patients. Toxicity appears to be related to duration of therapy.

6. Cyclophosphamide—Cyclophosphamide is a cytotoxic alkylating agent that is used to treat cancer and also an immunosuppressive agent used to treat diseases such as rheumatoid arthritis and idiopathic pulmonary fibrosis. Cyclophosphamide toxicity may present either as subacute pneumonitis weeks after exposure or pulmonary fibrosis months to years following exposure. Radiation and multidrug regimens increase the risk for toxicity in cancer patients. As an immunosuppressive agent, low-dose cyclophosphamide is associated with a <1% incidence of pulmonary complications. Corticosteroids improve the acute pneumonitis but are of lesser benefit in patients with fibrosis.

7. Cytosine arabinoside—Cytosine arabinoside is associated with noncardiogenic pulmonary edema and ARDS. Symptoms occur within days of drug administration. Patients present with relatively acute onset shortness of breath, hypoxemia, and infiltrates. Treatment with corticosteroids is recommended in conjunction with supportive care.

8. Interleukin-2—Interleukin-2 (IL-2) is used in immunotherapy or biochemotherapy of melanoma and renal cell carcinoma. IL-2 administration occasionally causes a "sepsis syndrome" with fever, chills, hypotension, and noncardiogenic pulmonary edema. Patients present with dyspnea, hypoxemia, and infiltrates. When patients develop this complication it must be differentiated from an infectious complication.

9. Retinoic acid—Retinoic acid promotes differentiation of acute promyelocytic leukemia (APL) cells into mature granulocytes. With initiation of therapy for APL, patients can sequester large numbers of these newly differentiated cells in their pulmonary vasculature, resulting in dyspnea, hypoxemia, and occasionally respiratory failure. Chest radiographs demonstrate bilateral airspace disease. Treatment includes supportive care and corticosteroids. Leukopheresis may be indicated in particularly severe cases.

10. High-dose chemotherapy/bone marrow transplantation—High-dose combination chemotherapy, such as that used in bone marrow transplantation or with stem cell rescue, has been associated with acute pneumonitis, pulmonary fibrosis, and diffuse alveolar hemorrhage. The prognosis for patients with diffuse alveolar hemorrhage is extremely poor in spite of aggressive supportive care and high-dose corticosteroids.

11. Radiation therapy—Radiation therapy is a common and effective tool used for the treatment of cancer. Although great care is taken to minimize the biological impact of radiation on normal lung tissue, the pulmonary parenchyma and vasculature are inevitably exposed to clinically significant doses of radiation that may result in radiation pneumonitis or radiation fibrosis.

Radiation pneumonitis may occur as early as 2 weeks or as late as 6 months after therapy. Most cases appear within 1–3 months. Patients present with dyspnea, nonproductive cough, chest discomfort, fever, hemoptysis, rales, evidence of consolidation, or a friction rub. Chest radiographs are generally abnormal with interstitial and/or alveolar infiltrates in the involved lung. Infiltrates develop within the radiation ports as opposed to having an anatomic distribution, thereby assisting in the diagnosis. However, radiation-induced lung injury may also present with lung involvement outside the irradiated region and even in the contralateral lung. Approximately 80% of patients with radiation pneumonitis respond to a course of treatment with corticosteroids. Dose and duration are generally determined by the severity of pneumonitis and responsiveness in the individual case, but a starting dose of 60 mg of prednisone or equivalent with a gradual taper over several weeks is usually employed.

Radiation fibrosis occurs between 6 months and 3 years after therapy and is irreversible. Patients commonly present with either an abnormal chest radiograph during follow-up or with insidious progression of dyspnea on exertion and decreasing exercise tolerance. Patients may or may not have an antecedent history of radiation pneumonitis. Fibrosis is more common in patients who had preexisting disease, larger doses of radiation, and less fractionation of a given radiation dose. Radiation fibrosis may be distinguished from other forms of pulmonary fibrosis via an asymmetric, nonanatomic distribution, but unfortunately, radiation fibrosis is not always limited to the irradiated lung. Radiation fibrosis is not responsive to corticosteroid or cytotoxic therapy. Recommendations for therapy focus on preventing additional fibrosis by avoiding additional chest irradiation or chemotherapeutic agents with synergistic toxicity.

Preventive strategies should be undertaken by the radiation oncologist to minimize the potential for pulmonary toxicity prior to the initiation of treatment. Such measures may include dose fractionation, shielding, and three-dimensional conformal radiotherapy.

Abid SH, Malhotra V, Perry MC: Radiation-induced and chemotherapy-induced pulmonary injury. Curr Opin Oncol 2001;13:242. [PMID: 11429481]. (Discussion of patterns of lung injury that typically result from chemotherapeutic drugs and radiation therapy.)

Movsas B et al: Pulmonary radiation injury. Chest 1997;111:1061. [PMID: 9106589]. (Thorough review of clinical syndromes, risk factors, pathogenesis, and treatment of radiation-induced lung injury.)

Sleiffer S: Bleomycin-induced pneumonitis. Chest 2001;120:617. [PMID: 11502668]. (Concise review of clinical presentation, risk factors, and management of bleomycin lung disease.)

B. CARDIOVASCULAR DRUGS (TABLE 33–3)

1. Amiodarone—Amiodarone is widely used in the treatment of ventricular and supraventricular arrhythmias. Lung disease remains the most serious complication of therapy with an incidence of about 5% (1–10%). Initially believed to be limited to patients on higher daily and cumulative doses, pulmonary toxicity is now known to occur regardless of dose or duration. Amiodarone-induced pulmonary toxicity presents with either a subacute pneumonitis/hypersensitivity reaction or chronic alveolitis with fibrosis. Bronchospasm, noncardiogenic pulmonary edema, ARDS, and pulmonary nodules/masses have also been reported but are exceedingly rare.

Early amiodarone toxicity presents with fever, cough, shortness of breath, chest discomfort, tachyp-

Table 33–3. Pulmonary toxicity associated with cardiovascular agents.

Agent	Pulmonary Toxicity
Amiodarone	Early pneumonitis, late pneumonitis with fibrosis
ACE inhibitors	Cough, angioedema, bronchospasm
β-Blockers	Bronchospasm
Dipyridamole	Bronchospasm
Flecainide	Pneumonitis/ARDS
Hydralazine	Drug-induced lupus
Mexilitine	Pulmonary fibrosis
Tocainide	Pneumonitis/ARDS
Platelet glycoprotein IIb/IIIa inhibitors	Alveolar hemorrhage
Protamine	Bronchospasm, noncardiogenic pulmonary edema
Procainamide	Drug-induced lupus

nea, rales, rhonchi, and/or evidence of consolidation. Laboratory studies reveal leukocytosis, an increased sedimentation rate, and occasionally peripheral eosinophilia. Chest radiographs demonstrate bilateral, symmetric, or asymmetric alveolar or, less commonly, interstitial infiltrates. Heart failure and pneumonia are often included in the differential diagnosis. Amiodarone toxicity remains a diagnosis of exclusion.

Late amiodarone toxicity occurs more commonly than early toxicity and has a more indolent course. Patients complain of low-grade fevers, fatigue, malaise, weight loss, decreased exercise tolerance, dyspnea on exertion, nonproductive cough, and chest discomfort. Examination is nonspecific with tachypnea, tachycardia, rales, decreased breath sounds, and/or evidence of consolidation. Imaging studies most commonly show diffuse interstitial infiltrates, although other patterns have been noted. CT of the chest sometimes suggests the diagnosis of amiodarone toxicity when high attenuation infiltrates are present (iodinated amiodarone is more radioopaque than inflammation or edema). The most common PFT finding is a reduced $D_{L_{CO}}$ (>15–20% of predicted values). Restrictive abnormalities may also occur. Bronchoalveolar lavage fluid was initially thought to be useful in diagnosis when either foamy alveolar macrophages or lymphocytosis with a $CD8^+$ predominant population were noted. However, the presence of foamy macrophages signifies only amiodarone exposure, not amiodarone-induced pulmonary toxicity and is of no diagnostic utility. Lymphocytosis/CD8[+] cells in bronchoalveolar lavage fluid occurs only in a minority of cases and is neither sensitive nor specific for amiodarone toxicity.

Treatment for amiodarone-induced lung toxicity includes discontinuation of the drug as well as corticosteroid therapy. The extremely long half-life of the drug (30–45 days) and the need for alternative antiarrhythmic therapy for life-threatening ventricular arrhythmias complicate discontinuation of amiodarone. The latter concern has been somewhat alleviated by the availability and efficacy of implantable defibrillators. Corticosteroid dose and duration must be tailored to individual patients based upon the severity of disease and response to therapy. An initial dose of 40–60 mg per day of prednisone or equivalent tapered over 2–6 months is appropriate for most patients. Patients started on amiodarone therapy should have baseline PFTs and chest radiographs performed. Serial monitoring of PFTs to screen for toxicity is controversial as an isolated reduction in D_{LCO} does not necessarily correspond with amiodarone-induced lung toxicity. However, a reduced D_{LCO} is highly sensitive when patients have appropriate symptoms and an abnormal chest radiograph.

2. β-Blockers—β-Blockers provoke bronchospasm in sensitive patients and must be given with caution to patients with reactive airways disease. Cardioselective agents cause less bronchoprovocation than less selective agents, as do agents with partial agonist activity. Although dose may be important, β-blocker-induced bronchospasm has also been observed with topical ophthalmological preparations in patients with glaucoma. Treatment consists of avoidance of β-blockade in β-blocker-sensitive patients and the use of inhaled β-agonists, supplemental oxygen, and, if severe, corticosteroids.

3. Angiotensin-converting enzyme (ACE) inhibitors—Of patients treated with an ACE inhibitor 10% develop cough that is believed to be caused by increased production of bradykinin. Some patients tolerate this annoying side effect, however, others have to discontinue the medication. A minority of patients develop angioedema from ACE inhibitors with potentially serious complications. The drug must be discontinued in these patients.

4: IIB/IIIA inhibitors—There are multiple case reports of alveolar hemorrhage following administration of platelet glycoprotein IIb/IIIa inhibitors.

Jessurun GA, Boersma WG, Crijns HJ: Amiodarone-induced pulmonary toxicity. Predisposing factors, clinical symptoms and treatment. Drug Saf 1998;18:339. [PMID: 9589845]. (Good review of clinical presentation, risk factors, and treatment of amiodarone- induced lung disease.)

C. Antiinflammatory Agents/ Immunosuppressive Agents

Antiinflammatory/immunosuppressive agents are frequently used in autoimmune disorders such as rheumatoid arthritis, systemic lupus erythematosus (SLE), scleroderma, and idiopathic interstitial pneumonias and in transplantation (Table 33–4). Determining the etiology of new pulmonary disease can be complex as it may represent worsening of the underlying disease, opportunistic infection, or drug toxicity. Diagnosis of drug-induced lung disease in this setting relies on exclusion of other etiologies.

1. Methotrexate—Methotrexate is an inhibitor of folate metabolism and is used in the treatment of autoimmune disease and cancer. Methotrexate pneumonitis is a common complication that occurs in 5–10% of patients. Patients present weeks to months after starting therapy with nonproductive cough, dyspnea, fatigue, fever, tachypnea, rales, and hypoxemia. Chest radiographs may demonstrate mixed, alveolar, or interstitial infiltrates or be normal. Up to one-third of patients demonstrate peripheral eosinophilia. Treatment includes discontinuation of the drug and a trial of corticosteroids. Pulmonary manifestations reported with high-dose methotrexate treatment for cancer include noncardiogenic pulmonary edema, pleuritis, and pleural effusion.

2. Penicillamine—Penicillamine is clinically beneficial in a number of diseases including rheumatoid

Table 33–4. Pulmonary toxicity associated with antiinflammatory agents/immunosuppressive agents.

Agent	Pulmonary Toxicity
Acetylsalicyclic acid (aspirin)	Bronchospasm, noncardiogenic pulmonary edema
Azathioprine	Pulmonary fibrosis
Cyclophosphamide	Pneumonitis, pulmonary fibrosis
Gold	Acute pneumonitis, bronchiolitis obliterans
Leukotriene antagonists	Churg–Strauss syndrome
Methotrexate	Pneumonitis
NSAIDs	Bronchospasm
Penicillamine	Pulmonary–renal syndrome, bronchiolitis obliterans, pneumonitis, pulmonary fibrosis, drug-induced lupus

arthritis, scleroderma, primary biliary cirrhosis, heavy metal chelation, and Wilson's disease. Pulmonary complications from penicillamine are very rare but include pulmonary–renal syndrome, bronchiolitis obliterans, acute hypersensitivity pneumonitis, chronic alveolitis with fibrosis, and drug-induced lupus.

Penicillamine-induced pulmonary–renal syndrome closely resembles Goodpasture's syndrome. Patients present with pulmonary hemorrhage and rapidly progressive glomerulonephritis. Unlike Goodpasture's syndrome, anti-glomerular basement membrane (GBM) antibodies are usually not seen, although ANA titers are frequently elevated. Respiratory failure and renal failure are common. The prognosis of this disorder is poor. Treatment includes plasmapheresis and immunosuppression with cyclophosphamide or azathioprine.

3. Gold—Gold therapy is used primarily in the treatment of rheumatoid arthritis. It is often difficult to distinguish between pulmonary complications related to rheumatoid arthritis and complications from the gold therapy. Gold-induced pulmonary complications are rare, occurring in <1% of patients, and present as either acute pneumonitis or, rarely, as bronchiolitis obliterans. The acute pneumonitis is a hypersensitivity phenomenon. Patients present with fever, rash, and constitutional symptoms as well as dyspnea and cough. Although up to 50% of afflicted patients have peripheral eosinophilia, lymphocytes usually predominate in bronchoalveolar lavage fluid. Treatment consists of withdrawal of the drug and a trial of corticosteroids.

4. Aspirin and NSAIDs—Aspirin and other nonsteroidal antiinflammatory drugs are associated with bronchospasm. The mechanism of disease involves increased generation of leukotrienes LTC4, LTD4, and LTE4 via inhibition of cyclooxygenase. Aspirin-sensitive patients with asthma are particularly responsive to leukotriene inhibitors. Aspirin overdose may be associated with noncardiogenic pulmonary edema, respiratory alkalosis due to increased central drive, and respiratory failure.

5. Leukotriene antagonists—An association between leukotriene antagonists and Churg–Strauss syndrome has been suggested in several case reports and series. It is not clear whether this association is causal or due to unmasking of occult Churg–Strauss by reductions in corticosteroid dose following initiation of antileukotriene therapy.

Imokawa S et al: Methotrexate pneumonitis: review of the literature and histopathological findings in nine patients. Eur Respir J 2000;15:373. [PMID: 10706507]. (Review of clinical presentation, physiology, radiology, and pathology of methotrexate pneumonitis.)

Tomioka R, King TE: Gold-induced pulmonary disease: clinical features, outcome and differentiation from rheumatoid lung disease. Am J Respir Crit Care Med 1997;155:1011. [PMID: 9116980]. (Clinical review focusing on differentiation of gold-induced lung disease from rheumatoid lung disease.)

D. ANTIMICROBIALS

1. Nitrofurantoin—Nitrofurantoin is an antibiotic that is commonly used for treatment of urinary tract infections. Two distinct pulmonary syndromes are associated with nitrofurantoin, acute hypersensitivity pneumonitis and chronic alveolitis with pulmonary fibrosis. Fever, chills, cough, dyspnea, chest discomfort, wheezing/bronchospasm, arthralgias, myalgias, and/or rash characterize the former. Examination is nonspecific with tachypnea, tachycardia, wheeze, rales, rhonchi, or decreased breath sounds. Chest radiographs usually reveal interstitial and/or alveolar infiltrates. Laboratory studies demonstrate peripheral eosinophilia in 80–90% of patients. Treatment includes discontinuation of the drug with or without a brief course of corticosteroids.

Chronic alveolitis with fibrosis occurs with long-term suppressive doses of nitrofurantoin and is much less common than the acute reaction. Patients present with fatigue, weight loss, nonproductive cough, and dyspnea on exertion. Tachypnea and rales are commonly heard on chest examination, and chest radiographs reveal reticular infiltrates and honeycombing consistent with pulmonary fibrosis. Treatment includes withdrawal of the drug and a trial of corticosteroids.

2. Other antimicrobial agents—Many antimicrobial agents have been associated with pulmonary infiltrates and peripheral eosinophilia. Signs and symptoms are similar to those described for acute hypersensitivity pneumonitis from nitrofurantoin. Reactions occur extremely rarely given the widespread use of many of these drugs, but have been reported with penicillins, cephalosporins, tetracycline, minocycline, sulfa drugs, isoniazid, ethambutol, and rifampin.

E. ILLICIT DRUGS

1. Cocaine—Cocaine is either inhaled or injected as cocaine hydrochloride or smoked and inhaled in its free base form, which is better known as "crack" cocaine. The inhaled form may lead to sinus symptoms, epistaxis, and ulceration of the nasal septum, whereas complications of intravenous use include septic emboli and talc granulomatosis. However, inhaled crack cocaine produces the most significant and varied pulmonary complications. These are summarized in Table 33–5.

Most pulmonary complications of crack cocaine occur within 1–2 h of use, although patients may present up to 48–72 h after using the drug. Typical symptoms include cough, wheezing, shortness of breath, hemoptysis, chest pain, and carbonaceous sputum. Findings from physical examination correlate with the

Table 33–5. Pulmonary complications of crack cocaine.

Pulmonary Manifestation	Comments
Upper airway injury/burns	The preparation of free base cocaine requires the use of ether or other solvents. Residual solvent may be highly volatile and cause upper airway burns.
Bronchospasm/asthma	Wheezing and asthma exacerbations are common. Treatment includes bronchodilators, steroids, and oxygen.
Barotrauma	Pneumothorax, pneumomediastinum, and pneumopericardium have all been reported.
Pulmonary edema	Both cardiogenic and noncardiogenic.
Hemoptysis and pulmonary hemorrhage	Hemoptysis is a common presenting complaint and may occur incidentally or along with crack lung, pulmonary hemorrhage, barotrauma, or cardiovascular complications.
"Crack lung"	A clinical syndrome characterized by chest symptoms and pulmonary infiltrates occurring within 48–72 hours of crack use. Patients frequently complain of shortness of breath along with chest pain +/– cough. Hypoxemia is common. Patients improved within 1–5 days with supportive care. Patients who have undergone biopsy have demonstrated a constellation of histopathologic findings including diffuse alveolar damage with hyaline membranes, edema, hemorrhage, type II cell hyperplasia, and inflammatory infiltrates (lymphocytes, eosinophils and monocytes/macrophages).
Bronchiolitis obliterans with organizing pneumonia	There are case reports of cocaine use leading to BOOP, although this is a rare complication.
Eosinophilic lung disease	Presents a pulmonary infiltrates associated with wheezing and peripheral eosinophilia and eosinophilia on brochoalveolar lavage. Responsive to corticosteroids.
Cough and sputum	Up to 50% of chronic crack cocaine users report having a cough often productive of carbonaceous sputum.

specific pulmonary complication (eg, rales with pulmonary edema and crepitus/subcutaneous emphysema with barotrauma). Electrocardiograms and chest radiographs are important in the evaluation of complications of cocaine abuse. Chest pain may be due to either cardiac complications such as ischemia, infarct, or dissection, pulmonary complications, or both. Similarly, pulmonary edema associated with cocaine use may be either cardiogenic (secondary to a cardiomyopathy or malignant hypertension) or noncardiogenic (due to direct toxic effects of the drug on the pulmonary epithelium).

Long-term sequelae of cocaine use have been difficult to study but include a mild reduction in DL_{CO}, chronic pulmonary hemorrhage, pulmonary hypertension, and mild interstitial fibrosis.

2. Amphetamines—Methamphetamine is the most commonly abused amphetamine. It is known by a variety of street names including "ice," "crystal," and "crank." Pulmonary complications occur less frequently than with cocaine, but include bronchospasm, barotrauma, airway burns, pulmonary hypertension, granulomatosis, and noncardiogenic pulmonary edema.

3. Opiates—In addition to respiratory depression and septic emboli, opiates are associated with noncardiogenic pulmonary edema and talc granulomatosis. Noncardiogenic pulmonary edema occurs with morphine, fentanyl, and naloxone as well as heroine. Patients present with dyspnea, cough, and/or chest fullness. Chest radiographs reveal interstitial or, less commonly, alveolar edema. Treatment includes discontinuation of the drug and supportive measures.

Haim DY et al: The pulmonary complications of crack cocaine. A comprehensive review. Chest 1995;107:233. [PMID: 7813284]. (Comprehensive review of the pharmacology of cocaine and pulmonary syndromes associated with crack cocaine.)

F. OTHER AGENTS

1. Tocolytics—Tocolytic agents (terbutaline, salbutamol, ritodrine) are used to inhibit preterm labor and are associated with noncardiogenic pulmonary edema. The differential diagnosis of gravid patients presenting with shortness of breath includes tocolytic-induced pulmonary edema, pulmonary embolism, amniotic fluid embolism, bronchospasm, peripartum cardiomyopathy, aspiration, or ARDS. Treatment includes discontinuation of the drug, diuresis, supplemental oxygen, and supportive care.

2. Anorectic agents—Anorectic agents that were previously available by prescription (fenfluramine and dexfenfluramine) but have since been removed from the market are associated with a greater than 20-fold increase in the risk for primary pulmonary hypertension. Patients presenting with pulmonary hypertension should be asked about their use of these drugs. Patients who are known to have taken these drugs should be screened for pulmonary hypertension and valvular heart disease.

Occupational Asthma

E. Rand Sutherland, MD, MPH

ESSENTIALS OF DIAGNOSIS

- *Typical symptoms of asthma, bronchodilator reversible expiratory airflow limitation, and airway hyperresponsiveness.*
- *Symptoms due to asthma rather than an alternative diagnosis.*
- *Onset after entering the workplace.*
- *Directly attributable to exposures in the workplace.*
- *Specific immunoglobulin E (IgE) formation or positive skin testing may only represent allergic sensitization.*
- *Specific inhalational challenge may confirm the diagnosis.*

General Considerations

Occupational asthma can be defined as new-onset asthma that is directly attributable to one or more exposures in the workplace and not to exposures encountered outside the workplace. A diagnosis of occupational asthma can be made only after a diagnosis of asthma has been established and after the onset of asthma has been clearly related to the workplace. In addition to providing an environment in which asthma may be induced, the workplace can provide a number of exposures that exacerbate preexisting asthma and it is important to distinguish between preexisting asthma that is exacerbated by work and true occupational asthma.

Occupational asthma is the most prevalent occupational lung disease in the industrialized world. Studies in Canada and the United Kingdom indicate that occupational asthma accounts for up to approximately 50% of all cases of work-related lung disease, and a significant proportion of patients who are disabled due to asthma relate their disability to occupational asthma. United States Social Security Administration disability data indicate that approximately 15–20% of those individuals who are disabled due to asthma have occupational asthma.

Over 200 agents have been identified as causes of occupational asthma. Isocyanates are commonly implicated, as are wood dusts, anhydrides, dyes, metals, cereals, and latex. Common causes of occupational asthma in at-risk workers are listed in Table 34–1. Risk for occupational asthma appears to be directly related to the type of workplace exposures that an individual sustains, although traditional risk factors for asthma such as atopy are also considered to be risk factors for the development of occupational asthma.

Pathogenesis

The pathogenesis of occupational asthma is complex and multifactorial, involving both environmental and host factors. The majority of patients with occupational asthma develop the disease within the first 1–2 years of exposure, although there are differences in the time to development of occupational asthma based on the molecular weight of the inciting antigen.

Occupational asthma can be classified as one of two types: immunological or nonimmunological (Table 34–2). The immunological type of occupational asthma can occur through either IgE-dependent or IgE-independent mechanisms, depending in part on the molecular weight of the causative agent. The nonimmunological type of asthma, also known as irritant-induced asthma or reactive airway dysfunction syndrome (RADS), develops through poorly understood mechanisms as a result of airway inflammation induced by inhalational injury and usually presents without a latency period. These differences in pathogenesis lead to differences in clinical presentation and timing of the signs and symptoms of airflow limitation.

Immunological occupational asthma may occur through IgE-dependent or IgE-independent mechanisms. Induction of specific IgE antibodies may occur in response to exposure to high-molecular-weight antigens ($\geq$5000 Da) such as animal or vegetable proteins, which can act as complete antigens. Furthermore, some low-molecular-weight agents (eg, platinum salts) can also induce specific IgE antibody production, but only after interacting with proteins and acting as haptens to form functional antigens. Once these specific IgE antibodies have been formed, they bind to antigens present on the surface of inflammatory cells and initiate a sequence of proinflammatory events. In all cases, the in-

Table 34–1. Selected causes of occupational asthma in at-risk workers.

Agent	Workers at Risk
Chemicals	
Acid anhydrides	Epoxy resin, plastic workers
Complex amines	Painters, photographers
Diisocyanates	Plastic and varnish workers
Methacrylates	Health care workers, histologists
Enzymes	
Proteases	Detergent industry workers
Metals	
Cobalt	Hard-metal grinders
Chromium, nickel	Metal platers
Platinum salts	Platinum refiners
Plant proteins	
Latex	Health care workers
Wheat	Bakers, millers
Psyllium	Pharmacists, nurses
Wood dusts	
Western Red Cedar	Carpenters, sawmill operators

teraction between the antigen and IgE results in an inflammatory cascade mediated by histamine, leukotrienes, and other cytokines and ultimately orchestrated by a cellular immune response consisting of eosinophils, mast cells, neutrophils, and airway epithelial cells. Exposure to the causative agent in occupational asthma caused by IgE-dependent mechanisms often leads to either an isolated "early" response, with bronchoconstric-

Table 34–2. Pathogenesis of occupational asthma.

Immunological	Nonimmunological
Onset months to years after exposure	Irritant-induced, RADS
IgE-mediated or IgE-independent mechanisms	Symptom onset acute after a toxic inhalational exposure
IgE mediated	Direct damage to airway epithelium implicated
Primarily high-molecular-weight antigens (eg, animal, plant proteins)	Constitutes approximately 15% of occupational asthma cases
Early or biphasic asthmatic response	
IgE independent	
Primarily low-molecular-weight antigens (eg, isocyanates)	
T-lymphocyte (CD8+) the primary effector cell	
Late or biphasic asthmatic response	

tion that begins a few minutes after exposure, peaks at about 30 min after exposure, and then tapers over the next 30–60 min; or a biphasic reaction, in which an additional "late" asthmatic reaction occurs 4–6 h after exposure, peaks 8–10 h after exposure, and then tapers over the next 12–36 h.

A number of low-molecular-weight agents (eg, isocyanates) cause immunological occupational asthma but do so through IgE-independent mechanisms. Biopsy specimens from patients with immunological non-IgE-mediated occupational asthma demonstrate that activated CD8+ T-lymphocytes are the primary inflammatory cell type found in this form of occupational asthma. The appropriate low-molecular-weight antigens can also induce a proliferative response in peripheral blood lymphocytes of patients with occupational asthma without inducing specific IgE formation, further supporting the role of these cells in the airway inflammatory process. Although up to 20% of patients with occupational asthma caused by agents such as plicatic acid (the causative antigen in Western Red Cedar asthma) or isocyanates may have IgE antibodies specific to these agents, the presence of these specific antibodies can be an indication of prior sensitization only and not an indication of IgE-mediated airway inflammation in response to the antigen. Therefore, the presence of specific IgE antibodies alone cannot be used as a diagnostic criterion for occupational asthma. In IgE-independent occupational asthma, inhalational challenge may produce either an isolated late asthmatic reaction or a biphasic response.

The mechanisms of irritant-induced occupational asthma are incompletely understood. This type of occupational asthma appears not to be immunologically mediated, but rather caused by direct airway inflammation as a result of a toxic inhalational exposure. Airway epithelial cell damage has been hypothesized to lead to the onset of neurogenic inflammation and nonspecific activation of inflammatory cells in the airway. Proinflammatory mediators secreted directly by the airway epithelium may additionally lead to altered epithelial and endothelial permeability, resulting in airway hyperresponsiveness and airway obstruction. These patients may not demonstrate an asthmatic response to an inhaled antigen, although airway hyperresponsiveness to nonspecific agents such as methacholine will usually be present.

Prevention

Because occupational asthma is a disease caused by workplace exposure to inhaled agents, it is preventable. A combination of preventive measures and surveillance programs can be implemented to detect airborne exposures to known causes of occupational asthma and to facilitate early detection of allergic sensitization and occupational asthma.

Primary prevention may be achieved by preventing occupational exposure. An effective strategy for reducing or eliminating environmental exposures is based on a number of interventions including improved ventilation, monitoring of aeroallergens, modification of industrial processes to reduce exposures, substitution of known causative agents with other, less toxic ones, and reduction of human exposure by increased use of automation. Atopic individuals and smokers are at increased risk of developing occupational asthma and this should be taken into account in the assignment of tasks to hired workers.

Medical surveillance programs (a form of secondary prevention) are designed to facilitate early detection of occupational asthma. These programs can be justified given that early detection of occupational asthma and prompt removal from exposure improve outcomes, although there is little evidence assessing the efficacy of these programs. Practical methods for medical surveillance include respiratory symptoms questionnaires and screening spirometry. From a surveillance standpoint, tests of nonspecific airway hyperresponsiveness and immunological tests are less useful because of lack of specificity, cost, and the lack of commercially available standardized antigens.

Tertiary preventive strategies focus on modifying disease prevention once it has occurred and are summarized under "Treatment."

Clinical Findings

The diagnosis of occupational asthma should be considered in every adult patient with new-onset asthma. Prompted by an initial suspicion on the part of the clinician, a preliminary evaluation that consists of confirming the diagnosis of asthma and assessing workplace exposures is followed by a confirmatory evaluation in which immunological testing, peak flow monitoring, or specific inhalational challenge testing is performed.

A. History, Symptoms, and Signs

The clinical manifestations of occupational asthma are very similar to those of asthma unrelated to the workplace. Patients may present across a broad spectrum of clinical impairment ranging from mild symptoms to severe and persistent expiratory airflow limitation. Mild cases of occupational asthma may present as episodic shortness of breath, chest tightness, wheezing or cough. In more severe cases, symptoms may increase in intensity and frequency and are associated with dyspnea either on exertion or at rest, or wheezing. Symptoms of rhinoconjunctivitis including rhinorrhea, sneezing, nasal

or ocular itching, and tearing may accompany respiratory symptoms. Systemic symptoms such as fever, myalgia, and arthralgia occasionally occur.

Critical to the evaluation of occupational asthma is a comprehensive employment history. This history should include both current and past job descriptions. Known exposures can be evaluated through inquiry about industrial processes and use of possible sensitizing agents that the patient is able to identify. Material Safety Data Sheets should be obtained from the patient's employer to further establish what agents the patient may have been exposed to in the workplace. Exposure to known culprits such as specific chemicals (eg, isocyanates), animal or vegetable proteins, organic dusts, drugs, metals, and toxic fumes should be evaluated by directed questioning. Because both smoking and atopy are risk factors for occupational asthma, they should be assessed.

The temporal relationship between work and symptoms should be established. Questions about both the onset and worsening of symptoms should be asked, and these should be related not only to at-work periods but also to off-work periods, looking for work-related exacerbation and improvement when away from work on weekends or vacations. In some cases symptoms may develop immediately, or they may not begin until 6 h or more after the beginning of the work shift. In immunological occupational asthma symptoms may not develop until months or years after the onset of workplace exposure. It should be noted that although these historical features are useful in establishing work relatedness, they are rarely diagnostic and should be considered only suggestive of occupational asthma.

The diagnosis of nonimmunological asthma (RADS) is based almost entirely on the clinical history. There is often a history of a single, high-level exposure to an inhaled irritant gas, fume, powder, smoke, or vapor, after which respiratory symptoms begin. This exposure may have occurred in the context of a fire, a chemical spill, or an explosion. Respiratory symptoms should have been absent prior to the exposure, and expiratory airflow limitation and/or airway hyperresponsiveness must also be present. For the diagnosis of RADS to be made, symptoms should persist for at least 3 months after the exposure.

B. Laboratory Findings

Immunological testing has a limited role in the evaluation of occupational asthma because although it is sensitive and specific for immunological sensitization, it is not specific for occupational asthma. Because many cases of occupational asthma are IgE mediated, immunological testing looking for specific IgE to high-molecular-weight and some low-molecular-weight agents may be used to corroborate immunological sensitization. Specific IgE formation is, however, not diagnostic of occupational asthma. Furthermore, the vast majority of causative agents cannot be assayed by commercially available means. Skin prick testing may be useful in cases of latex or lactase sensitization, but many patients with positive skin test responses will not have respiratory symptoms.

C. IMAGING STUDIES

Chest radiographs in occupational asthma are often normal. If expiratory airflow limitation is profound, evidence of thoracic hyperinflation may be present. Chest radiographs may be used to exclude alternative diagnoses.

D. PHYSIOLOGICAL EVALUATION

Spirometric testing is useful in documenting the expiratory airflow limitation seen in asthma. Expiratory airflow limitation is manifested by a reduced forced expiratory volume in 1 s (FEV_1) or forced vital capacity (FVC) or a reduced FEV_1/FVC ratio, but spirometry may be normal and is neither sensitive nor specific for the diagnosis of occupational asthma. If expiratory airflow limitation is present, bronchodilator responsiveness may be confirmed by a 12% and 200 mL improvement in the FEV_1 or FVC following the administration of a short-acting inhaled bronchodilator such as albuterol.

Airway hyperresponsiveness to a nonspecific irritant such as methacholine is manifested by a 20% decrease in FEV_1 at low concentrations of the drug (eg, <8 mg/mL). Nonspecific airways hyperresponsiveness is present in many cases of occupational asthma, but its presence is not specific to asthma alone. Normal nonspecific challenge testing does not exclude occupational asthma, particularly if the patient is currently asymptomatic or has been away from the workplace for a period of time. However, if airway hyperresponsiveness is absent after the patient has worked for 2 weeks under usual conditions, occupational asthma is extremely unlikely.

Once a diagnosis of asthma has been established, peak expiratory flow rate monitoring at and away from work for at least 2 weeks can be a useful step in objectively demonstrating a temporal relation between the workplace and the development or worsening of airflow limitation (Figure 34–1). The optimal frequency of peak flow measurement appears to be four times daily (on awakening, at noon, after work, and at bedtime). It is important that patients note on the diary card which days they are working and that a record of symptoms also be maintained. Unfortunately, patient adherence with serial peak flow monitoring is poor, especially with a measurement frequency of six times per day.

Interpretation of serial peak flow data remains somewhat qualitative, because no uniformly accepted quan-

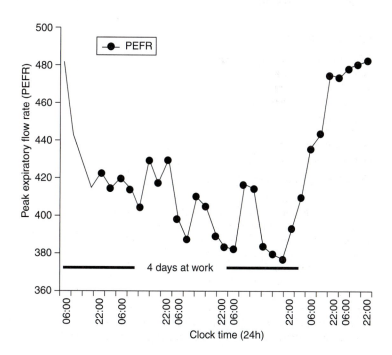

Figure 34–1. Morning (06:00) to night (22:00) peak flow variability in relationship to days at and away from work in a welder with occupational asthma. Note the gradual decline in peak flow over the days when the patient is working, as well as the improvement seen on days away from work. PEFR, peek expiratory flow rate

titative criteria have been established for interpreting peak flow recordings. One group has proposed that deterioration of peak flows during three or four work weeks and improvement in three or four periods away from work are suggestive of occupational asthma, whereas others argue that a 20% variability in peak flow between the at-work and off-work times is suggestive. In addition, FEV_1 may be measured before and after the work shift in an attempt to diagnose changes in airflow over the day. A decrease in FEV_1 of ≥10% is considered objective evidence of work-related bronchoconstriction.

Specific inhalational challenge tests looking for bronchoconstriction in response to a specific inhaled antigen are considered the diagnostic reference standard for occupational asthma. The utility of this test depends on identifying and challenging the patients with the causative agent, which can be difficult, and false-negative results may be obtained if the incorrect antigen is used. Unfortunately, facilities for performing specific inhalational challenge tests are not widely available in the United States.

Differential Diagnosis

The differential diagnosis of occupational asthma includes asthma of nonoccupational etiology and chronic obstructive pulmonary disease (COPD). Other airway diseases such as bronchiectasis, airway sarcoidosis, and bronchiolitis should be excluded. A number of occupational airway diseases other than occupational asthma exist. These include rhinosinusitis due to irritants or allergens, industrial tracheobronchitis due to mineral dusts or sulfur dioxide among others, bronchiolitis from ammonia or chlorine gas, emphysema due to exposures such as coal dust or cadmium pneumonitis, and hypersensitivity pneumonitis due to exposures that can include animal or plant proteins.

Complications

Occupational asthma can range in severity from mild and intermittent to severe and persistent, causing long-term disabling symptoms. It is associated with a high prevalence of unemployment. A diagnosis of occupational asthma is associated with increased all-cause hospitalization rates and decreased quality of life when compared with nonoccupational asthma. Occupational asthma can cause a severe asthma phenotype, putting patients at increased risk of status asthmaticus and death. Continued exposure can lead to worsening of occupational asthma severity, but little is known about the long-term complications of occupational asthma, particularly with regard to chronic airway inflammation, airway fibrosis, airway remodeling, and the risk of developing fixed airway disease.

Treatment

Early diagnosis of occupational asthma and prompt intervention can result in beneficial outcomes for patients, in some cases preventing the development of persistent disease. The treatment of occupational asthma consists of two components: removal from the causative agent and appropriate pharmacotherapy.

Restriction from exposure should be an early goal of therapy, with aggressive efforts directed at either transferring the patient to a job in which the exposure does not occur or retraining the patient to perform a different job altogether. Simply reducing exposure by means of improved ventilation or utilization of a respirator is suboptimal, because patients with occupational asthma will often react to even very low concentrations of the offending agent. Although industrial hygiene measures may reduce symptoms in sensitized patients, these measures are unlikely to reduce the incidence of occupational asthma in at-risk workers. The Americans with Disabilities Act requires that employers provide suitable accommodation once a diagnosis of occupational asthma is made.

Pharmacotherapy for occupational asthma is similar to that for nonoccupational asthma and should follow published guidelines. Current National Heart, Lung and Blood Institute guidelines recommend that short-acting β-agonists be used for reliever therapy, and that inhaled corticosteroids form the foundation of controller therapy in all patients with persistent asthma. These recommendations apply in occupational asthma as well. Inhaled corticosteroids have been shown to be beneficial in occupational asthma following removal from exposure, and they appear to have greater benefits in occupational asthma when administered early in the course of the disease. Even after relocation or retraining at work and the initiation of pharmacotherapy, patients should undergo periodic medical evaluation to ensure that lung function and symptoms are not worsening.

Prognosis

The course of occupational asthma after discontinuing workplace exposure is variable and is highly dependent on restriction from further exposure. Early diagnosis and removal from the offending agent are critical because they increase the likelihood of recovery, whereas continued exposure to a causative antigen is associated with a more severe and progressive course. Some patients will experience an improvement in symptoms within weeks to months after cessation of exposure, although nonspecific airway hyperresponsiveness can persist for years. Complete remission of symptoms is possible, although the majority of patients with immunological asthma will continue to experience symptoms and require pharmacotherapy and follow-up care for a number of years after diagnosis. In many cases, however, patients with occupational asthma can be left with permanent symptoms and chronic expiratory airflow limitation and airway hyperresponsiveness.

A significant proportion of patients with occupational asthma will continue to deteriorate if they continue to work under the same conditions that induced the disease. Longitudinal follow-up studies indicate that measures such as relocation to a different part of the worksite, use of respiratory protective devices, and a change from daily to intermittent exposure do little to alter the progression of disease in these patients.

Occupational asthma can cause disability and prevent patients from working. Evaluation of short- and long-term disability should be performed when asthma is well controlled, and guidelines for evaluating impairment and disability due to asthma have been promulgated by the American Thoracic Society. Patients should be referred to compensation agencies when appropriate.

Beckett WS: Occupational respiratory diseases. N Engl J Med 2000;342:406. [PMID: 10666432]. (Review of differential diagnosis.)

Chan-Yeung M (chair): Assessment of asthma in the workplace. American College of Chest Physicians consensus statement. Chest 1995;108:1084. [PMID: 7555124]. (Guidelines for evaluation and treatment.)

Lombardo LJ et al: Occupational asthma: a review. Environ Health Perspect 2000;108(Suppl 4):697. [PMID: 10931788]. (Comprehensive review of the topic.)

Malo JL et al: Occupational asthma. J Allergy Clin Immunol 2001; 108:317. [PMID: 11544449]. (Review with a focus on pathophysiology and diagnostic algorithms.)

Acute Inhalational Injury

Craig S. Glazer, MD, MSPH

Inhalation is the most common exposure route in reports to national poison control centers and the most common cause of fatalities related to toxic exposures. Acute inhalational injury occurs via two basic mechanisms. Inhaled substances are either absorbed leading to systemic toxicity or they directly injure the pulmonary epithelium at various levels of the respiratory tract. Many exposures (or exposure situations) produce both effects. Systemic toxins include asphyxiants (substances that interfere with oxygen delivery or utilization) and other toxins whose primary effects are on distant organ systems. This chapter will not discuss inhalational toxins whose main effects are on distant organ systems but limited examples are shown in Table 35–1.

The degree of injury after acute inhalational exposure is determined by multiple host and exposure factors. Elderly patients and those with underlying debilitating illness, particularly underlying lung disease that impairs host defense mechanisms, typically fare worse. Important environmental factors include the intensity and duration of exposure as well as the quality of ventilation in the space in which exposure occurs. In general, greater exposure dose (defined as the product of the concentration of exposure and duration of exposure) is associated with greater potential harm.

ASPHYXIANTS

ESSENTIALS OF DIAGNOSIS

- *Patients may be unaware of asphyxiant exposure, as many do not have warning properties.*
- *Consider asphyxiants in patients with a history of working in enclosed spaces prior to symptom onset.*
- *Consider asphyxiant exposure in patients with a history of smoke inhalation.*
- *Consider chemical asphyxiant exposure in patients with unexplained lactic acidosis.*

General Considerations

Asphyxiants are divided into two classes, simple and chemical. Simple asphyxiants act by displacing oxygen from inspired air. Any gas can act as a simple asphyxiant if present in high enough concentration. Typical exposure scenarios include release of compressed gas and work in enclosed spaces. Chemical asphyxiants act by interfering with oxygen delivery or utilization. Examples of both simple and chemical asphyxiants are shown in Table 35–2. The potential number of exposed workers in the United States is unclear, but the National Occupational Exposure Survey estimated that more than 500,000 workers may be exposed annually.

Pathogenesis

Simple asphyxiants act by displacing oxygen from inspired air resulting in a reduced fraction of inspired oxygen and subsequent hypoxemia. Clinically significant effects become apparent when the fraction of inspired oxygen falls below 15–16%. Chemical asphyxiants include carbon monoxide, cyanide and other nitriles, and hydrogen sulfide. Carbon monoxide binds to hemoglobin with a much greater affinity than oxygen, thus reducing the oxygen-carrying capacity of the blood. In addition, carbon monoxide shifts the oxyhemoglobin dissociation curve to the left further limiting oxygen availability. Both cyanide (and the other nitriles) and hydrogen sulfide interfere with the cytochrome oxidase system, thus blocking aerobic metabolism.

Clinical Findings

SYMPTOMS AND SIGNS

Symptoms and signs of asphyxiant exposure are related to hypoxia and occur in four stages. In mild hypoxia, termed the indifferent stage, patients note decreased night vision and physical examination reveals mild tachypnea and tachycardia. As arterial oxygen percent saturation falls into the low 80s patients enter the compensatory stage. They begin to note headaches and tachypnea and tachycardia become more apparent. Pa-

Table 35–1. Systemic toxins absorbed via inhalation.

Agent	Exposure Scenarios	Systemic Effects
Arsine	Chemical industry, smelting, and refining; semiconductor industry; metal pickling and plating	Massive intravascular hemolysis leading to jaundice, hemoglobinuria, and renal failure; also causes pulmonary edema
Solvents	Extensive use in industry and in the home environment (mechanic work)	Central nervous system (CNS) intoxication, similar to alcohol; hepatic damage may occur with heavy exposure to chlorinated solvents
Benzene	Chemical, detergent, pesticide, and solvent manufacture	CNS toxicity, bone marrow suppression; long-term exposure causes hematological malignancy
Nerve gas	Chemical weapons, terrorism	Paralysis, cholinergic crisis (bradycardia, excessive secretions, bronchospasm)
Pesticides	Gardening, farm work	Depends on the agent; organophosphates are similar to nerve gas

tients with underlying coronary artery disease may note angina. Patients with congestive heart failure, respiratory disease, or anemia begin to experience air hunger. When arterial oxygen percent saturation falls into the 70s patients enter the disturbance stage. Symptoms include headache, air hunger, decreased vision, impaired coordination and judgment, numbness in the extremities, mood disturbances, and confusion. Physical examination reveals tachycardia, tachypnea, cyanosis, and abnormal cerebellar findings. The critical stage occurs when arterial oxygen percent saturation falls below 64%. Patients experience a rapid deterioration of coordination and judgment and subsequently lose consciousness within minutes. Seizures may also occur.

Table 35–2. Asphyxiants.

Agent	Exposure Scenarios	Product of Combustion	Other Points
Simple asphyxiants	Similar for all simple asphyxiants: industrial settings with release of compressed gas, confined spaces, or unventilated areas closed for a period of time		
Carbon dioxide	Also a product of carbohydrate fermentation	Yes	
Nitrogen	Ammonia manufacture	No	
Methane	Natural gas	No	
Hydrogen	Metallurgy, vacuum tubes, welding	No	
Chemical asphyxiants			
Carbon monoxide	Raw material in metallurgy and organic synthesis; welding, engine exhaust, use of wood, coal, or propane heaters in enclosed spaces	Yes, product of incomplete combustion of carbon compounds	Patients may have cherry-red lips
Methylene chloride	Paint stripper, varnish remover	No	Releases carbon monoxide
Cyanide	Chemical, plastics, and rubber manufacturing; electroplating, gold extraction, pesticides	Yes, burning cellulose, nylon, wool, polyurethane	Characteristic almond-like odor (can only be smelled by 60% of people)
Hydrogen sulfide	Petroleum and natural gas industry; sewer and septic tank contaminant; animal confinement; raw material for sulfation and sulfuric acid production		Characteristic rotten egg odor; also has irritant properties; high CNS solubility leads to sudden loss of consciousness

B. LABORATORY FINDINGS

Laboratory examination reveals an increased anion gap metabolic acidosis and elevated lactate levels. Arterial blood gases with measured oxygen saturation should be obtained whenever chemical asphyxiant exposure is suspected as pulse oximetry may be falsely elevated due to the presence of abnormal hemoglobin molecules. A lack of correlation between pulse oximetry and measured oxygen saturation should alert the clinician to the possibility of chemical asphyxiant toxicity. Carboxyhemoglobin and methemoglobin levels should be measured if a chemical asphyxiant is suspected. Elevated carboxyhemoglobin levels support a diagnosis of carbon monoxide poisoning and elevated methemoglobin suggests cyanide toxicity. Cyanide levels can also be measured, but results frequently take too long to be clinically useful. Finally, cardiac enzymes should be monitored in patients experiencing angina.

Treatment

Treatment begins with removal from exposure and administration of supplemental oxygen. No other therapy is required for simple asphyxiants. Chemical asphyxiants require additional specific treatment. Carbon monoxide poisoning is managed with 100% oxygen initially. Supplemental oxygen not only increases the amount of oxygen available for binding to hemoglobin but more importantly shortens the half-life of elimination of carbon monoxide through the lungs. Hyperbaric oxygen therapy prevents long-term neurological sequelae from acute carbon monoxide poisoning and should be considered for all symptomatic victims if it is available within 24 h of exposure. Cyanide toxicity is treated with a combination of amyl nitrite, sodium nitrite, and sodium thiosulfate. These are available in a cyanide antidote kit from Lilly Pharmaceuticals (Table 35–3). Alternatively, vitamin B_{12} (5 g intravenously) may be combined with sodium thiosulfate to chelate the cyanide. Hydrogen sulfide toxicity is also managed with sodium nitrite. Hyperbaric oxygen therapy has been used for both hydrogen sulfide and cyanide poisonings, but controlled trials are lacking.

Prognosis

The prognosis is excellent in mild cases. In more severe cases, especially those with loss of consciousness, long-term cognitive and neurological deficits may occur. Hyberbaric oxygen therapy decreases the risk of developing long-term neurological and cognitive deficits associated with severe carbon monoxide poisoning if administered within 24 h.

Forsyth JC et al: Hydroxocobalamin as a cyanide antidote: safety, efficacy, and pharmacokinetics in heavily smoking normal volunteers. J Toxicol Clin Toxicol 1993;31:277. [PMID: 8492341]. (Study describing the use of vitamin B_{12} for the management of acute cyanide toxicity.)

Rorison DG, McPherson SJ: Acute toxic inhalations. Emerg Med Clin North Am 1992;10:409. [PMID: 1559478]. (Thorough review of asphyxiant exposure and management.)

Weaver LK et al: Hyperbaric oxygen for acute carbon monoxide poisoning. New Engl J Med 2002;347:1057. [PMID: 12362006]. (Landmark randomized trial that proves the effectiveness of hyperbaric oxygen for the prevention of long-term neurological sequelae in acute carbon monoxide poisoning.)

Table 35–3. Therapy for cyanide poisoning.

Initial therapy
1. 100% supplemental oxygen administered via facemask.
2. Amyl nitrite pearls—break 0.3-mL ampule onto a piece of gauze, hold in front of patient's nose for 30 s to 1 min. Repeat every 3 min until sodium nitrite administration.

Definitive therapy
1. Sodium nitrite—300 mg intravenously over at least 5 min. For children, the dose is 6–8 mL/m².
2. Sodium thiosulfate—12.5 g intravenously over 10 min. Administer immediately after the sodium nitrite infusion is completed. For children, administer 7 g/m².
3. Observe for 24–48 h. Repeat steps 1 and 2 at one-half the initial dose if signs of poisoning reappear.

IRRITANT-INDUCED LUNG INJURY

ESSENTIALS OF DIAGNOSIS

- *Acute clinical illness ranges from mild irritation of the upper respiratory tract to noncardiogenic pulmonary edema and death.*
- *Accurate exposure history is essential to determine the agent involved and to rule out mixed exposures.*
- *Clinical findings vary depending on the solubility, particle size, and dose of the inhaled substance.*
- *Symptom onset may be delayed up to 24–36 h with some inhalations.*
- *Long-term complications occur in a minority of those exposed.*

General Considerations

Lung irritants are defined as substances that cause cellular injury of the pulmonary parenchyma or epithelium. A large number of irritant substances are used in industry and the household environment (Tables 35–4 and 35–5). There is no national registry of events, so the actual incidence of acute inhalational irritant injury is unknown. The National Occupational Exposure Survey estimated greater than one million workers may be exposed to respiratory irritants annually. However, data from poison control centers suggest that inhalational injuries occur more frequently in the home environment than in the workplace.

Pathogenesis

Clinical manifestations vary depending on the solubility and particle size of the irritant substance. Substances with a high solubility deposit primarily in the nose, upper respiratory tract, and large airways. As a result, highly soluble irritants have better warning properties and exposed individuals tend to leave exposure sooner, thus decreasing the exposure dose. Substances with a low solubility typically bypass the upper respiratory tract and large airways and deposit in small airways and alveoli. The same separation applies to particle size. Particles greater than 10 µm in size deposit in the nose, those between 5 and 10 µm deposit in large airways, whereas particles smaller than 5 µm (respirable particulates) deposit in small airways and alveoli. Importantly, there is overlap in clinical presentations depending on exposure dose. People exposed to high doses of highly soluble substances experience symptoms related to both the upper and lower respiratory tract.

Clinical Findings

A. Symptoms and Signs

Exposure to highly soluble substances or substances with a larger particle size leads to rapid onset of upper respiratory tract symptoms including lacrimation, rhinitis, epistaxis, pharyngitis, and cough. Patients typically note burning of the nose, eyes, mouth, and throat. Skin burns may also occur. Physical examination reveals conjunctivitis, pharyngitis, laryngotracheitis, and expiratory wheezing. Edema may also be seen in the nose, posterior pharynx, and larynx. Patients note hoarseness and difficulty speaking with more severe laryngeal injury and may exhibit stridor on physical examination.

Exposure to irritant substances with low solubility or to respirable particulates causes lower respiratory tract

Table 35–4. High solubility inhalational irritants.

Agent	Exposure Scenario	Product of Combustion	Other Points
Ammonia	Agriculture, mining, plastics, and explosives manufacture; refrigerant, home cleaning products	No	May cause liquefaction necrosis
Hydrogen chloride	Dyes, fertilizers, textiles, rubber, metal ore refining, meat wrappers [heating polyvinyl chloride (PVC) films]	Yes, burning PVC	
Sulfur dioxide	Smelting, paper manufacture, wineries, power plants, kerosene space heaters	Yes, burning of oil and coal	
Hydrogen fluoride	Metal refining and etching, microelectronics and phosphate fertilizer manufacture; rust removal agents	Yes, burning electronics (sulfur hexafluoride is an insulator for electronics)	Can cause clinically important hypocalcemia
Acrolein	Manufacture of plastics, resins, textiles, herbicides, pharmaceuticals	Yes, burning of wood, paper, and cotton	
Methyl bromide	Industrial fumigant	No	Also has prominent CNS effects
Ethylene oxide	Common sterilizing agent in medical centers	No	Poor odor threshold, group 1 carcinogen
Sodium azide	Automotive industry, wreckers, airbag deployment	No	May have cardiovascular effects (hypotension)
Formaldehyde	Production of agricultural, disinfectants, fumigants, and pharmaceutical products; antiseptics	Yes, burning of plywood, particle board, or insulating material	Also a potential immune sensitizer

Table 35–5. Low solubility respiratory irritants.

Agent	Exposure Scenario	Product of Combustion	Other Points
Oxides of nitrogen	Silo filler's disease; manufacture of dyes and fertilizer; welding	Yes, chemical plants and burning of nitrocellulose and mattresses	Reddish-brown gas
Phosgene	Manufacture of dyes, insecticides, plastics, and pharmaceuticals; welding	Yes, burning solvents, paint removers and dry cleaning fluid	Odor of freshly mown hay
Chlorine (moderate solubility so primarily large airway effects)	Manufacture of chemicals, paper production, disinfection, cleaners, swimming pool maintenance	No	Most frequent agent, yellow-green gas
Ozone	Paper manufacture, textiles, welding		
Nickel carbonyl	Nickel processing	No	
Cadmium fume	Welding rods, brazing solder, heating metal coatings; electroplating, battery and semi-conductor manufacture	Yes	Chronic low level exposure can cause emphysema; renal injury also occurs
Mercury fume	Heated metal reclamation, repair of tanks and boilers, manufacture of thermometers and tungsten-molybdenum wire	No	Chronic exposure causes prominent neurological effects

symptoms. Symptom onset is typically delayed for 3–12 h postexposure and delays as long as 48 h may occur. Typical symptoms include cough and dyspnea. Chest tightness and, rarely, hemoptysis may occur. Physical examination reveals wheezes and crackles on lung auscultation. Cyanosis may be seen in severe cases.

The distinction in presentation between low and high solubility compounds is not always perfectly clear. If the exposure dose is high enough overlap occurs and highly soluble agents can cause pulmonary edema. When this occurs symptoms typically follow a proximal to distal gradient with upper airway symptoms greater than those related to lower airways. Likewise, very high exposure to agents of low solubility can cause upper airway symptoms. Once again symptoms follow a gradient, but the gradient is distal to proximal with pulmonary edema greater than upper airway symptoms.

B. LABORATORY AND IMAGING STUDIES

The cornerstone of clinical evaluation for inhalational lung injury is a thorough exposure history. This is essential to determine the causative agent and rule out mixed exposures. Physical examination should focus on the mucous membranes of the eyes, nose, and pharynx as well as the skin. The lungs should be auscultated carefully for stridor, wheezing, and crackles. Chest radiographs may reveal pulmonary edema, atelectasis, or infiltrates. Arterial blood gas analysis may demonstrate hypoxia or an increased $P(A-a)O_2$ gradient. Patients with ocular symptoms require a careful ophthalmological examination with a slit-lamp for corneal burns. Finally, pulmonary function tests should be performed to establish baseline function.

Differential Diagnosis

The differential diagnosis of upper airway symptoms and compromise include thermal injuries and infections, especially epiglottis if severe laryngeal symptoms are present. Anaphylactic reactions could also mimic inhalational exposure, except edema is more prominent. The pathological reaction of the lower respiratory tree to inhalational injury is diffuse alveolar damage (DAD), the same pathology found in acute respiratory distress syndrome (ARDS). The differential for causes of ARDS is broad and is covered in Chapter 15.

Complications

The most feared acute complications are respiratory failure and death. Causes of acute respiratory failure include both severe laryngeal injury and noncardiogenic pulmonary edema. A large variety of chronic pulmonary complications may also occur. These complications are rare, occurring in less than 10% of all exposed victims. This section will describe the range of complications reported following acute inhalational lung injury. Not every agent can cause the whole range of complications. The agents reported to cause each complication will be mentioned where appropriate. A full description of the clinical findings and treatment of each complication is beyond the scope of this chapter.

A. REACTIVE AIRWAYS DYSFUNCTION SYNDROME (RADS)

RADS is the most common sequelae of acute inhalational lung injury. It has been reported with a large variety of irritant exposures. This syndrome features an asthma-like illness with episodic dyspnea, cough, and wheezing that persist for months to years following the acute event. Clinical and physiological abnormalities may be permanent in some patients. Patients demonstrate significant bronchodilator responsiveness on spirometry and/or bronchial hyperresponsiveness on methacholine challenge testing. Treatment consists of avoidance of further irritant exposure and follows the same guidelines as treatment of asthma (see Chapter 6).

B. BRONCHIOLITIS OBLITERANS

Patients present months to years after exposure with symptoms of progressive dyspnea on exertion. Pulmonary function tests typically demonstrate fixed airflow obstruction and chest radiographs show evidence of hyperinflation. Treatment usually consists of oral corticosteroids, but controlled trials are lacking. Some patients, particularly those who develop this syndrome within weeks of exposure, have a more proliferative type of bronchiolitis (as opposed to scarring or constrictive bronchiolitis) and are more likely to respond to steroids. Fortunately, bronchiolitis obliterans is a rare complication. It has been reported most frequently following exposure to oxides of nitrogen or sulfur. There are, however, rare case reports from other exposures including chlorine and phosgene.

C. BRONCHIOLITIS OBLITERANS WITH ORGANIZING PNEUMONIA (BOOP)

BOOP rarely occurs after inhalational injury. It has been reported primarily after exposure to oxides of nitrogen. Patients present within weeks of exposure with dyspnea on exertion, multifocal pulmonary consolidation on chest radiograph, and a restrictive pattern on pulmonary function testing. Treatment is similar to idiopathic BOOP and is discussed in Chapter 14.

D. BRONCHIECTASIS

Bronchiectasis is a rare complication. It has been reported primarily after high-dose ammonia exposure. The clinical findings and treatment are identical to bronchiectasis secondary to other causes (see Chapter 8 for further details).

Treatment

Treatment for acute irritant-induced lung injury is largely supportive and follows the basic approach to resuscitation focusing on airway protection, support of breathing, and maintenance of circulation. Patients with primarily upper respiratory tract symptoms and a history of exposure to only highly soluble agents should be observed for approximately 6 h unless symptoms are severe. Early intubation may be required for severe laryngeal injury. The recommended observation period for people with significant exposure to low solubility agents is longer due to the possibility of delayed-onset noncardiogenic pulmonary edema. These patients should be observed for 24–36 h. A lung protective strategy of ventilation using tidal volumes of 6 mL/kg should be utilized if intubation is required. Supplemental therapy with corticosteroids is recommended for patients with evidence of significant airflow obstruction but has not been studied for patients with noncardiogenic pulmonary edema. Antibiotics should be used only if there is clinical evidence of infection.

Prognosis

The overall prognosis of irritant-induced inhalational lung injury is excellent. Greater than 90% of exposed individuals return to normal health. However, about 5–6% may develop any of a variety of long-term complications.

Acute Respiratory Distress Network: Ventilation with lower tidal volumes as compared with traditional tidal volumes for acute lung injury and the acute respiratory distress syndrome. N Engl J Med 2000;342:1301. [PMID: 10793162]. (Landmark study details the appropriate ventilatory strategy for noncardiogenic pulmonary edema.)

Brooks SM et al: Reactive airways dysfunction syndrome (RADS). Persistent asthma syndrome after high level irritant exposures. Chest 1985;88:376. [PMID: 4028848]. (Landmark paper provides the original case description of RADS.)

Kelleher P et al: Inorganic dust pneumonias: the metal-related parenchymal disorders. Environ Health Perspect 2000;108:685. [PMID: 10931787]. (Thorough review of all the metal-induced lung diseases including noncardiogenic pulmonary edema.)

Leiken JB, Tharratt RS: Part VI. Toxic inhalants. Dis Mon 2000;46:551. [PMID: 11021546]. (Extensive review of acute irritant lung injury.)

Rabinowitz PM, Siegel MD: Acute inhalation injury. Clin Chest Med 2002;23:707. [PMID: 12512160]. (Extensive review of acute irritant lung injury.)

Weiss SM, Lakshminarayan S: Acute inhalation injury. Clin Chest Med 1994;15:103. [PMID: 8200187]. (Extensive review of acute irritant lung injury.)

INHALATIONAL FEVER

ESSENTIALS OF DIAGNOSIS

- *A group of syndromes distinct from inhalation lung injury.*
- *Patients present with a flu-like illness but no clinical evidence of lung injury.*
- *Prognosis is uniformly good and no treatment is required.*

General Considerations

The incidence and prevalence of inhalational fever are unknown. The different syndromes included in this designation are metal fume fever, polymer fume fever, and organic dust toxic syndrome. All share similar clinical findings and prognosis. Metal fume fever is caused by exposure to zinc fume. Copper and magnesium fume may also cause this syndrome. Polymer fume fever occurs after exposure to heated fluoropolymers (Teflon) and organic dust toxic syndrome after exposure to high amounts of endotoxin. A latency period is not required. The presence of lung inflammation in these syndromes has been documented by studies employing bronchoscopy with bronchoalveolar lavage, however clinical findings of lung disease (hypoxia and an abnormal chest radiograph) do not occur. If clinical lung disease is present the clinical syndrome should be characterized as inhalational injury and not inhalational fever.

Clinical Findings

Patients present within hours of exposure complaining of a variety of constitutional symptoms. Fever, chills, arthralgias, myalgias, and fatigue are most common. Dyspnea may also be noted. Physical examination is unremarkable except for fever. Chest radiographs are normal as is oxygen saturation, and laboratory evaluation is unremarkable. All symptoms typically resolve within 24–48 h. In metal fume fever symptom tolerance develops with continued exposure, but symptoms return following breaks in exposure. Patients with metal fume fever thus note symptoms primarily on Monday after returning to work.

Differential Diagnosis

Inhalational fever may be confused with inhalation lung injury, immune-mediated lung diseases such as hypersensitivity pneumonitis, or viral infections. An accurate exposure history is essential for diagnosis.

Treatment and Prognosis

No specific treatment is required. Tylenol may be used for symptomatic therapy. The prognosis is excellent with complete resolution in all affected patients.

Gordon T, Fine JM: Metal fume fever. Occup Med 1993;8:504. [PMID: 8272976]. (Complete review of metal fume fever.)

Shusterman DJ: Polymer fume fever and other fluorocarbon pyrolysis-related syndromes. Occup Med 1993;8:519. [PMID: 8272977]. (Complete review of polymer fume fever and other pulmonary complications of fluorocarbon exposure including acute lung injury.)

Von Essen S et al: Organic dust toxic syndrome: an acute febrile reaction to organic dust exposure distinct from hypersensitivity pneumonitis. J Toxicol Clin Toxicol 1990;28:389. [PMID: 2269997]. (Thorough description of organic dust toxic syndrome.)

SECTION X

Infectious Lung Disease

Bacterial Pneumonia

Kenneth V. Leeper, Jr., MD, & Marc Moss, MD

ESSENTIALS OF DIAGNOSIS

- *Typical symptoms include dyspnea, cough with or without sputum production, fever or hypothermia, chest pain, and chills.*
- *Presence of a parenchymal infiltrate on chest radiograph distinguishes pneumonia from acute bronchitis.*
- *Hospital-acquired pneumonia occurs more than 48 h after admission to the hospital and excludes any infection that is present at the time of admission.*
- *Hospital-acquired pneumonia is especially common in patients who require mechanical ventilation.*

General Considerations

Bacterial pneumonia has been recognized as a common infection for nearly two centuries and remains the sixth leading cause of death in the United States. Community-acquired pneumonia (CAP) is defined as an infection that begins outside of the hospital or is diagnosed within 48 h after admission to the hospital in a patient who has not resided in a long-term facility for 14 days or more before the onset of symptoms. CAP is a major health concern in the United States, accounting for 3.3 to 4 million cases per year. The annual economic impact of CAP includes $20 billion in patient care expenses and lost wages, 64 million days of restricted activity, 39 million days of bed confinement, and 10 million days of work loss. Up to 20% of patients with

CAP require hospitalization, resulting in 600,000 to 1,000,000 hospital admissions per year.

Hospital-acquired pneumonia (HAP) is defined as infection of lung parenchyma occurring more than 48 h after admission to a hospital. When HAP occurs in the subset of patients receiving mechanical ventilation it is termed ventilator-associated pneumonia (VAP). HAP is a common nosocomial infection with a rate of between 5 and 10 cases per 1000 hospital admissions. The incidence in patients who require mechanical ventilation is 6 to 20 times higher. HAP is the leading cause of death from hospital-acquired infections.

Pathogenesis

Bacteria are deposited in terminal bronchioles and alveolar spaces by several mechanisms. These include aspiration of oropharyngeal or gastric contents, inhalation of bacterial laden aerosols, and hematogenous translocation from an infected site to the lung. Aspiration and inhalational mechanisms of entry account for the majority of pulmonary infections. The severity of pneumonia depends on the amount of material aspirated, the quantity of bacteria in the aspirate, the virulence of the organism, and the integrity of host defenses. Community-acquired pathogens such as *Streptococcus pneumoniae, Haemophilus influenzae,* and *Staphylococcus aureus* colonize normal hosts. Colonization by gram-negative bacilli is less common but these organisms are important pathogens in patients with alcoholism, diabetes mellitus, and poor oral hygiene and in the institutionalized elderly. Inhalational entry of organisms is associated with specific pathogens that are able to reach the lower airway. These highly efficient pathogens include *Legionella* species, *Mycoplasma pneumoniae, Chlamydia* species, and *Coxiella burnetii;* they share the ability to resist phagocytosis or to survive intracellularly within phagocytes.

Depending on the virulence of the pathogen and the strength of the patient's host defense system, an intense inflammatory process ensues after propagation of organisms in the lower respiratory tract. Exudation of protein-rich fluid in alveolar spaces is associated with ventilation–perfusion impairment, contributing to increased work of breathing and hypoxia. The inflammatory process is orchestrated by proinflammatory cytokines such as tumor necrosis factor and the interleukin series (IL-1, IL-2, IL-6, and IL-8) and is balanced by antiinflammatory mediators. Cytokines are responsible for the clinical and laboratory manifestations of bacterial pneumonia.

One of three conditions must occur for HAP to develop. The intrinsic host defense must be impaired, sufficient quantities of organisms must reach the lower respiratory tract, or the organism must be sufficiently virulent to induce an inflammatory response. Comorbid illnesses such as diabetes mellitus, alcoholism, malnutrition, chronic obstructive pulmonary disease (COPD), and azotemia impair the immune system and are associated with increased risk of HAP. Two events in patients receiving mechanical ventilation promote development of VAP. These are bacterial colonization of the aerodigestive tract and aspiration of contaminated secretions into more distal airways. Insertion of an endotracheal tube compromises the natural barrier between oropharynx and trachea, facilitates pooling and leakage of contaminated secretions around the endotracheal tube cuff, and eliminates the cough reflex. Endotracheal tubes also impair mucociliary clearance of bacteria from lower airways and become coated with a bacterial biofilm that may subsequently be deposited into the lower respiratory tract. Other factors such as supine position, frequency of ventilator circuit changes, tracheal suctioning, and contaminated respiratory care equipment are additional risk factors for aspiration of colonized secretions. Bacterial colonization of the stomach due to administration of stress ulcer prophylactic medications may also increase the risk of developing HAP; however, this hypothesis is controversial.

A. Microbial Etiology of Community-Acquired Pneumonia

The majority of cases of CAP in the preantibiotic era were caused by S pneumoniae. Recent studies indicate that the etiological agent responsible for CAP cannot be identified in approximately 50% of cases. A specific bacterial pathogen is often difficult to detect due to prior antibiotic therapy that prevents microbiological growth in culture. Therefore the reported prevalence of specific pathogens varies depending on the methods by which the etiological diagnosis is determined and the patient population studied (only ambulatory, mixed ambulatory and hospitalized, or only hospitalized patients).

S pneumoniae still accounts for 30–60% of CAP and is the single most commonly defined pathogen in patients who require hospitalization. Other bacteria that frequently cause CAP include H influenzae, S aureus, and a variety of gram-negative bacilli. Patients with COPD are especially predisposed to infections with H influenzae. Anaerobic bacteria are the predominant flora that colonize the upper respiratory tract and are most likely to be responsible for aspiration pneumonia.

Three agents classically referred to as "atypical" organisms (Legionella species, M pneumoniae, and Chlamydia pneumoniae) are collectively responsible for 10–20% of cases of CAP. M pneumoniae is the most common of the atypical agents and accounts for 9–29% of cases. Although M pneumoniae is generally a pathogen of children and young adults, up to 15% of cases of M pneumoniae occur in individuals older than 40 years. The prevalence of C pneumoniae ranges from 3% to 22%, but has been reported as high as 43% during seasonal outbreaks.

B. Microbial Etiology of Hospital-Acquired Pneumonia

The bacterial etiologies of HAP are different from those that cause CAP. The etiology of HAP depends largely on the spectrum of organisms that colonizes the oropharynx, as microaspiration of upper airway secretions is the most common route of entry into the lower respiratory tract in this infection. The organisms isolated in patients with HAP also vary from institution to institution due to differences in the distribution of organisms colonized in specific hospitals.

HAP is frequently polymicrobial in origin with gram-negative bacilli isolated in 47% of patients, anaerobic bacteria in 35%, and S aureus in 26%. Nosocomial gram-negative pneumonias often occur in patients with serious acute comorbid disease and are associated with high mortality. Pseudomonas, Klebsiella pneumoniae, and Escherichia coli are the most common gram-negative organisms responsible for HAP. Acinetobacter, Citrobacter, Proteus, and Serratia are also important causes of HAP in certain institutions. These organisms are often resistant to multiple antibiotics, making initiation of effective antimicrobial therapy difficult.

Organisms that cause VAP differ depending on the time of onset. VAP that occurs during the first 4 days of mechanical ventilation is associated with recovery of S pneumoniae, H influenzae, Moraxella catarrhalis, oxacillin-sensitive S aureus, or anaerobic bacteria (in patients who aspirated during the periintubation period).

Bacteria associated with VAP that develops 4 or more days after initiation of mechanical ventilation include *Pseudomonas aeruginosa, Acinetobacter* or *Citrobacter*, or methicillin-resistant *S aureus* (MRSA). This difference is linked to use of antimicrobial therapy prior to recognition of late-onset VAP. The paradigm of early- and late-onset VAP loses its significance for those patients who have been on broad-spectrum antibiotics prior to intubation and mechanical ventilation.

Brown PD et al: Community-acquired pneumonia. Lancet 1998;352:1295. [PMID: 9788476]. (Review article with good discussion of the epidemiology of CAP.)

Lynch JP III: Hospital-acquired pneumonia. Risk factors, microbiology and treatment. Chest 2001;119(Suppl):373S. [PMID: 1171773]. (General review article describing clinical characteristics of HAP.)

Mason CM et al: Pulmonary host defenses: implication for therapy. Clin Chest Med 1999;20:475. [PMID: 10516897]. (Review of the inflammatory response of the lung to acute bacterial infection.)

Prevention

Patients at increased risk for developing CAP should be vaccinated with both pneumococcal and influenza vaccines. In addition, because cigarette smoking is a risk factor for CAP, smoking cessation should be promoted.

Pneumococcal vaccine contains 25 μg of capsular polysaccharide from the 23 serotypes that cause 85–90% of invasive pneumococcal infections in adults and children in the United States. The vaccine is cost effective among individuals over the age of 65 years for prevention of bacteremia. In its current form it causes an antibody response and protection rate of at least 85% 5 years after vaccination. However, the level of protection decreases with advancing age, such that individuals in their eighties have only 50% protection 3 years after vaccination.

Currently all immunocompetent individuals age 65 or greater should be immunized with pneumococcal vaccine (Table 36–1). Younger patients should be vaccinated if they have chronic illnesses such as congestive heart failure, COPD, diabetes mellitus, alcoholism, hepatic cirrhosis, cerebrospinal fluid leaks, and anatomic or functional asplenia. Individuals living in special environments or social settings (Native Americans, Alaskans, and individuals in long-term care facilities) should also be vaccinated. The efficacy of pneumococcal vaccine in immunosuppressed patients is less certain. Present recommendations include vaccination of individuals with human immunodeficiency virus (HIV) infection, leukemia, lymphoma, Hodgkin's disease, multiple myeloma, organ transplantation, or chronic use of glu-

Table 36–1. Target groups for influenza vaccination.[1]

Persons of increased risk for complications
Persons 65 years of age or older.
Residents of nursing homes and other long-term care facilities that house persons of any age who have chronic medical conditions.
Adults and children who have required medical follow-up or hospitalization during the preceding year because of chronic metabolic diseases (including diabetes mellitus), renal dysfunction, hemoglobinopathy, or immunosuppression (including immunosuppression caused by medications or infection with the human immunodeficiency virus).
Children and teenagers (aged 6 months to 18 years) who are receiving long-term aspirin therapy and therefore might be at risk for Reyes' syndrome if they contract influenza.
Woman who will be in the second or third trimester of pregnancy during the influenza season.
All persons 50–64 years of age.[2]
Persons who can transmit influenza to those at high risk
Physicians, nurses, and other personnel in both hospital and outpatient-care settings, including emergency response workers.
Employees of nursing homes and long-term care facilities who have contact with residents or patients.
Employees of assisted-living facilities and other residences for persons in groups at high risk.
Persons who provide home care to persons in groups at high risk.
Household members (including children) of persons in groups at high risk.

----

[1]The groups reflect the recommendations of the Advisory Committee on Immunization Practices.
[2]This group has an increased prevalence of persons with high-risk conditions. Persons 50–64 years of age who do not have high-risk conditions also benefit from vaccination through decreased rates of influenza, decreased absenteeism from work, and decreased need for medical visits and medication, including antibiotics.

cocorticoids. Hospital-based immunization for appropriately selected inpatients is highly effective, as more than 60% of all patients with CAP have been admitted to the hospital during the 4 years preceding their pneumonia. Pneumococcal vaccine can be given simultaneously with other vaccines but should be administered at a separate site.

Recommendations concerning the timing and efficacy of revaccination vary as some data suggest the protective effect from vaccination extends beyond 5 years. A single revaccination is appropriate for individuals over the age of 65 who received initial vaccination more than 5 years earlier. Revaccination is also recommended for immunocompromised patients and individuals with functional or anatomic asplenia.

Outbreaks of influenza occur annually, during the winter months. Alterations in bronchopulmonary defense mechanisms from influenza infection promote colonization of the nasopharynx and secondary bacterial pneumonia by certain bacterial organisms. One of the most common bacterial pathogens in this setting is *S pneumoniae*. This scenario occurs frequently in the elderly and in individuals with chronic pulmonary or cardiovascular disorders. Therefore vaccination against influenza is recommended to decrease the risk of CAP.

Influenza vaccine is altered annually to reflect the viral strains that are anticipated in the next season. Vaccination reduces the incidence of laboratory-confirmed infection among healthy individuals less than 65 years old by 70–90% when there is a good match between the actual predominant wild strain and those included in the vaccine.

Individuals at high risk for complications from influenza and those who could transmit the infection to high-risk individuals should be vaccinated. Target groups are listed in Table 36–1. Revaccination is required annually because the viral strains change each year. Patients should be vaccinated between the beginning of September and mid-November.

The majority of strategies to prevent HAP have been directed at critically ill patients receiving mechanical ventilation. These interventions include both nonpharmacological and pharmacological measures.

Strict hand washing between patient contacts is recommended to prevent all nosocomial infections, including HAP. Efforts to reduce the risk of aspiration include keeping mechanically ventilated patients semirecumbent, reducing excessive use of narcotics, and monitoring residual gastric volumes in enterally fed patients. Pooling of secretions above the inflated endotracheal cuff may also be a source of aspiration. One European study demonstrated that continuous subglottic suctioning reduced the risk of VAP.

No pharmacological therapies are prophylactic against development of HAP, but limiting potentially harmful therapies is useful. Specific recommendations include eliminating unnecessary antibiotic therapy to reduce proliferation of antibiotic-resistant organisms and limiting stress ulcer prophylaxis to high-risk critically ill patients such as those who require mechanical ventilation or have a coagulopathy.

Ahmed F et al: Influenza vaccination for healthy young adults. N Engl J Med 2001;345:1543. [PMID: 11794222]. (Review article that discusses the strategy and evidence for influenza vaccination.)

Centers for Disease Control and Prevention: Prevention of pneumococcal disease: recommendations of the Advisory Committee on Immunization Practices (ACIP). MMWR 1997;46(RR-8):1. [PMID: 9132580]. (Review of recommendations for administration of pneumococcal vaccine.)

Kollef MH: The prevention of ventilator-associated pneumonia. N Engl J Med 1999;340:627. [PMID: 10029648]. (Excellent review of preventive strategies associated with reduction in the incidence of VAP.)

Clinical Findings

A. CLINICAL AND RADIOGRAPHIC FINDINGS OF COMMUNITY-ACQUIRED PNEUMONIA

Fever, elevated white blood cell count, and other features of sepsis describe the systemic inflammatory response to pneumonia. Pulmonary symptoms include cough, sputum production, hemoptysis, dyspnea, and pleuritic chest pain. Extrapulmonary symptoms, including headache, diarrhea, myalgia, arthralgia, and gastrointestinal symptoms, occur in 10–30% of patients. Physical findings that correlate with an inflammatory pulmonary parenchymal process include tachypnea, crackles, and signs of consolidation (bronchial breath sounds, dullness to percussion, increased tactile fremitus, and egophony). Arterial blood gases can demonstrate hypoxemia with either hypocapnia or hypercapnia depending on the degree of respiratory muscle fatigue.

Elderly patients may have different clinical presentations and are more likely to present with confusion, weakness, failure to thrive, delirium, abdominal pain, or generalized deterioration of their clinical status. Fever and signs of chest consolidation may be absent. The general lack or nonspecific nature of signs and symptoms of pneumonia in the elderly often leads to delays in diagnosis and initiation of medical therapy.

CAP was historically classified as either typical or atypical. Typical pneumonia presented with acute onset of cough, purulent sputa, dyspnea, high fever, chills, and rigors and was commonly associated with pathogens such as *S pneumoniae* and *H influenzae*. Atypical pneumonia was insidious in onset and was associated with dry cough, low grade fever, and mild dyspnea. It was caused by agents such as *M pneumoniae* and *C pneumoniae*. Choice of initial antibiotics was based on whether pneumonia was typical or atypical. Some atypical agents, however, cause a wide spectrum of illness. Legionnaires' disease, for example, can present with either fulminant or mild symptoms. Subsequent studies have demonstrated that clinical syndromes cannot be used reliably to identify particular pathogens. Therefore, classifying pneumonia as typical or atypical is of limited clinical benefit in choosing empirical antibiotics.

Of patients with CAP 8–10% require intensive care unit (ICU) management for respiratory and/or hemodynamic support. Pneumonia that requires care in an ICU is designated as severe CAP. End organ dysfunction is usually present and patients frequently require mechanical ventilation. The mortality rate of severe CAP ranges between 22% and 50%.

Chest radiographs are critical to the diagnosis of bacterial pneumonia. Radiographic patterns are nonspecific but lobar consolidation is usually associated with acute bacterial pneumonia. Although certain radiographic patterns suggest specific pathogens, microbiological diagnosis cannot be accurately made from radiographic characteristics. Even a normal radiograph does not exclude the diagnosis of pneumonia as high-resolution computed tomography occasionally identifies pulmonary infiltrates in patients with normal chest radiographs but clinical signs of pneumonia.

B. Diagnostic Testing for Community-Acquired Pneumonia

Evaluation of patients with pneumonia includes tests to identify the specific pathogen causing the infection as well as laboratory tests to determine the severity of illness and to monitor for dysfunction in extrapulmonary organs. Identification of the pathogen allows adjustment of the antibiotic regimen to narrow the focus to the specific pathogen. At least one study has documented faster resolution of fever when a specific microbiological diagnosis was determined. Performance of diagnostic testing, however, should not delay initiation of antibiotic therapy. Confirmation of a pathogen requires either strong serological evidence or isolation of the pathogen from respiratory secretions, blood, or a normally sterile body fluid.

Evaluation of patients with CAP who require hospitalization includes complete blood counts, serum electrolytes, blood urea nitrogen, creatinine, liver function studies, and assessment of arterial blood oxygenation. Although most of these tests are nonspecific they help determine the severity of pneumonia (see below) and monitor for dysfunction in nonpulmonary organ systems. An elevated serum lactic dehydrogenase (LDH) level is nonspecific but suggests *Pneumocystis carinii* pneumonia. Assessment of arterial oxygenation by either pulse oximetry or arterial blood gas testing determines whether supplemental oxygen therapy is necessary and identifies patients with respiratory failure.

Blood cultures are positive in only 10% of patients with CAP. *S pneumoniae* accounts for two-thirds of the positive results. Although the value of obtaining blood cultures routinely in patients with CAP has been questioned, blood cultures should be obtained in all patients who require hospitalization. This recommendation will likely become more important as antibiotic resistance increases in common CAP pathogens. The Centers for Disease Control and Prevention recommends serological tests for HIV-1 infection in patients aged 15–54 years with pneumonia who are admitted to a hospital where the proportion of HIV-seropositive patients among those discharged exceeds 1 in 1000.

Sputum gram stains represent lower respiratory tract secretions when more than 25 leukocytes and less than 10 epithelial cells are seen in low-powered microscopic fields. Appropriate antibiotic therapy is chosen greater than 90% of the time when a high-quality gram stain shows a predominant organism. This low-technology, inexpensive, rapid test has been recommended by some organizations for all patients with CAP. Accuracy of sputum gram stains is highly dependent on both proper collection of a deep-cough specimen prior to initiation of antimicrobial therapy as well as prompt delivery to a microbiology laboratory. Sputum may be difficult to obtain from debilitated patients because of a weak cough, obtundation, or dehydration. Inhaled nebulized saline helps induce cough and mobilize secretions in this setting. Nasotracheal suctioning samples the lower respiratory tract directly, but risks oropharyngeal contamination. The clinical history and chest radiograph dictate the use of other stains, such as acid-fast for mycobacteria, modified acid-fast for *Nocardia,* or toluidine blue, silver, and direct fluorescent antibody for *Pneumocystis carinii.*

Serological testing for pathogens such as *Legionella* species, *S pneumoniae,* and *C pneumoniae* is typically performed only when high clinical suspicion exists for infection with one of these organisms. Delays in obtaining results of several days render these tests more valuable to the epidemiologist than the clinician. Serological testing should be performed in the setting of a typical clinical syndrome or in deteriorating patients with no microbiological diagnosis. Serological testing includes sera drawn in both the acute and convalescent phases of the infection. A positive immunoglobulin M (IgM) titer or a 4-fold increase in the immunoglobulin G (IgG) titer is suggestive of recent infection.

Sputum stained for *Legionella* species has 80–90% sensitivity and 100% specificity. Immunofluorescence techniques have a sensitivity of 50–75% whereas DNA probes have a sensitivity of 25–75%. A sensitive urinary assay has been developed for detection of *Legionella* antigen. This test is highly specific (99%), but because urinary antigen persists for up to 1 year after infection, the test does not differentiate past from current infections. The urinary antigen detects only *Legionella* serotype 1; however, this serotype causes 70–90% of *Legionella* pneumonia.

Making a microbiological diagnosis in nonresponsive patients not diagnosed by standard culture techniques requires significant effort, cost, and invasive testing. Tuberculin skin testing may provide a clue to mycobacterial disease. Nasopharyngeal swabs for direct fluorescent antibody testing may yield evidence of viral respiratory antigens. When these procedures fail to yield a microbiological diagnosis, more invasive diagnostic techniques including bronchoscopy with transbronchial biopsy may be indicated. These techniques are primarily utilized in critically ill patients or in patients with nonresolving pneumonia who received initial empirical antibiotic therapy.

C. CLINICAL FINDINGS AND DIAGNOSTIC TESTING IN HOSPITAL-ACQUIRED PNEUMONIA

Clinical findings in patients with HAP are often very subtle. Initial findings may include fever, increased tachypnea, purulent sputum, and leukocytosis. Chest radiographs may demonstrate new infiltrates, although these can be difficult to identify in patients with preexistent diffuse lung disease. Chest radiographs also determine severity by identifying rapidly spreading, multilobar, or cavitary infiltrates. Of blood cultures drawn from febrile patients with HAP, 8–20% isolate the etiological pathogen. Although nonspecific, arterial blood gases or pulse oximetry determines the degree of hypoxemia and guides oxygen therapy. Laboratory evaluation of renal and hepatic function may identify nonpulmonary organ dysfunction.

Diagnostic evaluation for VAP remains controversial. Lower respiratory airways become uniformly colonized within hours of intubation. Therefore the positive predictive value of sputum cultures is relatively low. Additional criteria improve the diagnostic accuracy of sputum culture. For example, if more than 5% of bacteria visualized on gram stain are intracellular, the specificity for VAP is approximately 95%. Presence of more than 10 squamous epithelial cells per low-power field in sputa obtained by endotracheal suction suggests oropharyngeal contamination. These specimens should be rejected for analysis and new samples obtained.

Bronchoscopy can be used to obtain potentially more accurate specimens to differentiate colonization from true pathogens. Three techniques can be performed with bronchoscopy to obtain deep respiratory specimens for stains and cultures. These are bronchoalveolar lavage (BAL) with saline, protected specimen brush (PSB), and transbronchial biopsy. BAL samples large numbers of alveoli (approximately 10^6) and can recover large numbers of organisms. If a threshold of greater than 10^4 colony-forming units (CFU)/mL is used as a positive culture result, sensitivity of lavage is 72–100% and specificity 69–100%. Samples from PSB are placed in transport media that dilutes the number of organisms. A positive cutoff value for quantitative cultures obtained by this technique is 10^3 CFU/mL. This technique has 82% sensitivity and 89% specificity. Transbronchial biopsy of infiltrated lung parenchyma

may reveal alveolar or interstitial pneumonitis, viral inclusion bodies, and invading fungal or mycobacterial organisms.

Proper antibiotic therapy for VAP should not be delayed while waiting for results of these invasive tests. Delays in administration of effective antimicrobial therapy for intubated patients with pneumonia are associated with increased mortality. In addition, it is unclear whether more invasive testing is beneficial in VAP. A morbidity and/or mortality advantage of more invasive tests over standard management based upon clinical criteria and results of endotracheal aspirates has not been consistently demonstrated.

One recent study suggests such a benefit. This study evaluated the efficacy of an invasive strategy utilizing both protected specimen brush and BAL compared to a noninvasive approach. Patients with suspected VAP were randomly assigned to therapy based on results of lower respiratory tract specimens obtained by endotracheal aspiration (noninvasive strategy) or bronchoscopy (invasive strategy). Fourteen day mortality was reduced in patients managed with invasive testing compared to noninvasive testing (16.2% and 25.8%, respectively). Patients in the invasive strategy group also had decreased organ dysfunction and more antibiotic-free days. The major problem associated with the utilization of BAL data is the delay associated with waiting for quantitative culture results. Some recent studies suggest that modification of antibiotic therapy does not impact mortality. This has led to the recommendation that the BAL gram stain, which can be obtained within 3 h of bronchoscopy, should provide an initial guide to appropriate antibiotic selection. Whereas gram stains of expectorated sputum usually do not reflect subsequent culture results in CAP, gram stains of BAL fluid are very predictive of subsequent quantitative cultures.

Fagon JY et al: Invasive and noninvasive strategies for management of suspected ventilator-associated pneumonia: a randomized trial. Ann Intern Med 2000;132:621. [PMID: 10766680]. (Study demonstrating that an invasive strategy for patients with suspected VAP is associated with improved mortality and less antibiotic use.)

Skerrett SJ: Diagnostic testing for community-acquired pneumonia. Clin Chest Med 1999;20:531. [PMID: 10766680]. (Good review of various diagnostic tests that can be used for patients with suspected pneumonia.)

Differential Diagnosis

Rapid onset of fevers, chills, chest pain, and productive sputum is most suggestive of acute bacterial pneumonia. However, other diagnoses should be considered in patients without typical signs and symptoms or those who do not respond to empirical antibiotic therapy. The differential diagnosis in these patients includes pulmonary embolism, sarcoidosis, bronchiolitis obliterans organizing pneumonia (BOOP), hypersensitivity pneumonitis, acute interstitial pneumonitis, Wegener's granulomatosis, and drug-induced pneumonitis. The differential diagnosis of HAP includes congestive heart failure, atelectasis, acute respiratory distress syndrome (ARDS), or pulmonary embolism.

Complications

Patients who remain ill after initiation of appropriate antibiotic therapy may have developed a complication of pneumonia. Common complications include complicated parapneumonic effusions, frank empyema, and ARDS. Initial evaluation of these patients begins with a repeat chest radiograph to monitor for worsening infiltrates or a new effusion. Empyema results most commonly from direct spread of bacteria from lung parenchyma to the pleural space. Patients frequently complain of chest pain, persistent fever, and dyspnea. Diagnostic thoracentesis is indicated if a parapneumonic effusion is greater than 10 mm on lateral decubitus chest radiograph. Thoracentesis can be performed using ultrasound guidance for effusions that are less than 10 mm; however, the indication for thoracentesis in this setting is less clear. Pleural fluid analysis should include gram stain and culture, cell counts and differential, protein, LDH, glucose, and pH. Stains and cultures for mycobacterial and fungal pathogens should be done on selected cases. The need for chest tube drainage is based upon pleural fluid analysis and is discussed in more detail in Chapter 23. Bacteria can also spread by direct extension or hematogenously to sites outside of the lung and pleural space, causing secondary extrapulmonic infections. Potential secondary infections include meningitis, arthritis, endocarditis, pericarditis, and peritonitis.

ARDS presents with progressive dyspnea, hypoxemia, and worsening alveolar infiltrates on chest radiograph. Patients typically deteriorate within 5 days of initial presentation. The majority of patients with ARDS require mechanical ventilation for progressive respiratory failure. ARDS is discussed in detail in Chapter 15. Patients with severe bacterial pneumonia, especially when associated with sepsis, are at risk for developing nonpulmonary organ dysfunction. Renal failure, hepatic failure, disseminated intravascular coagulation, hemodynamic instability, and coma may all occur in this setting; multiorgan system failure occurs when more than one organ is involved.

Treatment

A. THERAPY FOR COMMUNITY-ACQUIRED PNEUMONIA

Prompt initiation of appropriate antibiotic therapy is associated with improved outcomes. The initial choice of antibiotics is empiric and based upon what organisms are anticipated in different clinical settings. Although a number of factors influence which bacteria may be anticipated in different circumstances, a useful approach is based upon severity of the pneumonia as reflected by the need for hospitalization. The most likely organisms in patients whose illness is mild enough to permit treatment as an outpatient are *S pneumoniae*, the atypical organisms *M pneumoniae* and *C pneumonia*, and *H influenzae*. Newer generation macrolides (azithromycin or clarithromycin) or doxycycline (for patients younger than age 40) have good activity against these pathogens and are appropriate empirical therapy in this patient population. Alternative therapy with newer generation fluoroquinolones (levofloxacin, sparfloxacin, grepafloxacin) that have antipneumococcal activity is another option. Although these antibiotics have excellent activity against all the expected organisms, some guidelines recommend reserving them in an effort to prevent emergence of fluoroquinolone-resistant strains.

Choice of antibiotics in patients who require hospitalization is again based upon the severity of illness. The anticipated organisms are different depending on whether the patient has severe CAP (loosely defined as CAP requiring therapy in the ICU) or can be managed on a general medicine ward. The most common bacteria in hospitalized patients with CAP who do not require ICU care are *S pneumoniae*, *H influenzae*, *M pneumoniae*, *C pneumoniae*, enteric gram-negative rods, and occasionally *Legionella* species. Empirical therapy in this setting includes intravenous newer generation fluoroquinolones alone or an antipneumococcal cephalosporin (ceftriaxone or cefotaxime) with or without a macrolide. Addition of the macrolide is driven by concern for *Legionella* and other atypical organisms.

Double antibiotic coverage is recommended for severe CAP. Combinations include an antipneumococcal cephalosporin with either a newer generation fluoroquinolone or a macrolide. Although monotherapy with newer generation fluoroquinolones would appear to be adequate coverage based on the anticipated organisms they have not been adequately studied in severe CAP to allow this recommendation.

Special circumstances may modify these recommendations in hospitalized patients. Of particular concern is CAP in patients with structural lung disease (bronchiectasis or cystic fibrosis) or with risks for aspiration. *P aeruginosa* is a more common pathogen in patients with structural lung disease; antibiotic coverage in this subset of patients must be broadened to include this organism. Patients with suspected aspiration require broadened coverage for anaerobic organisms; recommendations include a newer generation fluoroquinolone with or without a β-lactam/β-lactamase inhibitor, metronidazole, or clindamycin.

Duration of therapy for patients with CAP is dependent on the presence of comorbid illnesses, severity of illness at presentation, presence of bacteremia, and etiological organism. Patients with *S pneumoniae* or other typical pathogens are generally treated for 7–10 days, with atypical pathogens for 10–14 days, and with *Legionella* species for 21 days.

Patients hospitalized for CAP do not require intravenous antibiotics for the entire duration of therapy. Intravenous therapy may be converted to oral administration when (1) the patient has improved clinically, defined as body temperature less than or equal to 101°F, pulse less than or equal to 100 beats/min, systolic blood pressure greater than or equal to 90 mm Hg, respiratory rate less than or equal to 24 breaths/min, and oxygen saturation greater than or equal to 90% and (2) the patient is able to ingest and absorb oral antibiotics. Criteria for hospital discharge include (1) the patient is on oral antibiotics, (2) adequate social support exists to address changes in clinical status, and (3) the patient is able to keep outpatient follow-up visits. Most patients meet these criteria in a median of 3 hospital days.

A major concern in management of CAP is antimicrobial resistance in common CAP pathogens. Although pneumococci have historically been exquisitely susceptible to penicillin, strains with intermediate and high level resistance to penicillin have emerged in the past 15 years. This is a worldwide problem; more than 35% of pneumococcal strains isolated in the United States and Europe exhibit some level of penicillin resistance. Many of these strains are also resistant to cephalosporins, erythromycin, and trimethoprim/sulfamethoxazole. At this time most of the multidrug-resistant strains remain susceptible to the newer fluoroquinolone agents as well as vancomycin and imipenem. However, resistance to these agents has also begun to emerge.

The clinical significance of penicillin resistance is unclear. The definition of resistance is based on the mean inhibitory concentration (MIC) of the antibiotic for the organism. The penicillin MIC of fully susceptible strains *of S pneumoniae* is 0.06 µg/mL or less, intermediate resistant strains have an MIC between 0.1 and 1.0 µg/mL, and highly resistant strains have an MIC of 2.0 µg/mL or greater. Mortality data suggest, however, that the majority of "resistant" strains remain susceptible to higher intravenous doses of β-lactams. Clinical resistance as reflected by increased mortality may occur only in strains with an MIC of 4 µg/mL or greater for penicillin and 8 µg/mL or greater for ceftriaxone.

Local patterns of antimicrobial resistance as well as side effect profiles of newer drugs have significant impact on the selection of antimicrobials. These factors provide powerful arguments for both culture confirmation of the bacterial etiology of pneumonia and pneumococcal vaccination, which is effective against both resistant and susceptible strains.

Erythromycin has long been the drug of choice in *Legionella* infections based on clinical success and a paucity of available alternatives. High-dose erythromycin has drawbacks, however, including venous and gastrointestinal intolerance, reversible ototoxicity, and the large fluid volume required for each dose. The newer macrolide, azithromycin, and newer fluoroquinolones all have excellent *in vitro* activity against *Legionella* species and favorable pharmacokinetic and side effect profiles. Fluoroquinolones and azithromycin also possess excellent intracellular penetration that improves killing of intracellular organisms. For these reasons some guidelines recommend azithromycin, the newer generation fluoroquinolones, and doxycycline over erythromycin for legionellosis.

B. TREATMENT FAILURE

Treatment failures result for a variety of reasons. First, a complication such as empyema or ARDS may have developed. Second, the clinical diagnosis of infection may be wrong. Multiple noninfectious entities, including neoplasms, pulmonary edema, embolism, hemorrhage, connective tissue disease, and drug toxicity, can mimic bacterial pneumonia. Third, there may be problems related to the causative microorganism, antibiotic, or host. For example, the causative organism may be an unusual pathogen such as a fungus, mycobacteria, *Nocardia*, virus, or *P carinii*, or a secondary superinfection may have developed. Treatment failures also occur when a drug-resistant pathogen is present or when systemic antibiotic levels are inadequate due to adverse medication adherence, poor absorption, or drug interactions. Finally, failure to respond may be due to deficits in local or systemic immunity or anatomic abnormalities such as bronchiectasis, emphysema, or obstruction

C. THERAPY FOR HOSPITAL-ACQUIRED PNEUMONIA

Antimicrobial treatment of HAP should cover all relevant pathogens isolated from lower respiratory specimens. Although efforts should be made to obtain an adequate specimen for culture, empirical therapy must be started as early as possible without waiting for microbiological results. If the initial antimicrobial treatment is inadequate, the risk of mortality increases, even when therapy is corrected. Inadequate antimicrobial therapy occurs most frequently when HAP is caused by multidrug-resistant microorganisms.

Combination therapy with either an aminoglycoside or fluoroquinolone and either an antipseudomonal extended-spectrum β-lactam or a carbapenem is indicated if there is concern for multidrug-resistant microorganisms. This recommendation is based on the assumption that at least one of the drugs will be efficacious. However, prospective studies demonstrating the definitive advantage of combination therapy over monotherapy are scarce. The inclusion of vancomycin in empirical treatment is controversial. In one study, vancomycin was necessary for standard empirical therapy to ensure appropriate coverage of the causative pathogens. However, an approach advocated in Europe reserves vancomycin for patients who develop HAP while on antibiotics. This approach is based on the observation that in Europe methicillin-resistant *S aureus* VAP is extremely rare in patients without prior antimicrobial therapy. Treatment of methicillin-sensitive *S aureus* with vancomycin should be avoided because oxacillin is more effective. Therapy that includes drugs active against anaerobic pathogens is indicated if aspiration is likely.

The empirical choice of antibiotics must be adjusted to reflect resistance that may have developed due to previous use of antibiotics. This requires knowledge of the predominant pathogens that occur locally as well as their patterns of antibiotic susceptibility. The distribution of pathogens varies across institutions, implying that uniform empirical therapy may not be effective.

Duration of antimicrobial treatment for VAP has traditionally been 14 days. However, prolonged duration of antibiotic administration may result in both secondary infections that are resistant to antimicrobials and increased risk of antibiotic-related side effects. A recent study evaluated the impact of instituting guidelines for the treatment of VAP. One of the goals of the guidelines was to reduce potentially unnecessary antimicrobial therapy by limiting antibiotics for VAP to 7 days. The guidelines resulted in a reduction of length of antimicrobial treatment from 15 to 8 days with no effect on hospital mortality or length of stay. In addition, second episodes of VAP occurred less often among patients treated with shorter courses of antibiotics (7.7% versus 24.0%, $p = 0.03$). Although the study suggests adequate therapy for VAP may require antibiotics for only 7 days, the presence of multilobar involvement, malnutrition, cavitation, necrotizing gram-negative infections, or persistent signs and symptoms of active infection are associated with delayed resolution. Longer therapy should be used in these situations.

Ibrahim EH: Experience with a clinical guideline for the treatment of ventilator-associated pneumonia. Crit Care Med 2001;29:1109. [PMID: 11395584]. (This original article provides evidence for shorter duration of therapy for VAP.)

Niederman MS: Guidelines for the management of adults with community-acquired pneumonia. Am J Respir Crit Care Med 2001;163:1730. [PMID: 11401897]. (Excellent review of treatment strategies for CAP.)

Official Statement of the American Thoracic Society: Hospital-acquired pneumonia in adults: diagnosis, assessment of severity, initial antimicrobial therapy, and preventative strategies. A consensus statement. Am J Respir Crit Care Med 1996;153:1711. [PMID: 8630626]. (Excellent review of treatment strategies for HAP.)

Prognosis

Several tools help determine the prognosis of patients with bacterial pneumonia. The need for these prognostic scoring tools is motivated by extreme differences in costs of treating patients with CAP on an outpatient basis versus hospitalization. Ninety percent of the estimated cost for care of pneumonia is related to inpatient expenses and the cost of hospitalizing an individual patient exceeds the cost of outpatient care by a factor of 15.

In 1993, the American Thoracic Society identified risk factors that increased the risk of either death or a complicated course for patients with CAP. Inpatient therapy was recommended if one or more of these factors were present (Table 36–2).

Table 36–2. Risk factors for mortality or a complicated course from community-acquired pneumonia.

Historical factors
Age greater than 65 years
Suspicion of aspiration
Congestive heart failure
Chronic obstructive pulmonary disease
Diabetes mellitus
Chronic alcohol abuse
Chronic renal failure
Chronic liver disease of any etiology
Previous splenectomy
Hospitalization during the prior 12 months
Altered mental status
Physical findings
Temperature greater than 38.3°C
Respiratory rate greater than 30 breaths/p min
Systolic blood pressure less than 90 mm Hg
Evidence of extrapulmonary sites of infection
Laboratory abnormalities
White blood cell count <4 or >30 × 10^9
Hematocrit <30%
Pao_2 <60 mm Hg or $Paco_2$ >50 mm Hg on room air
Blood urea nitrogen = 20 mg/dL or creatinine = 1.2 mg/dL
Multilobar or rapidly progressive radiographic infiltrates

Mortality from pneumonia is also related to the causative bacterial pathogen. Mortality is lowest with *M pneumonia* and highest with *P aeruginosa, K pneumoniae, E coli,* and *S aureus.*

Fine and colleagues have developed a two-step prediction rule for patients with CAP that stratifies patients according to estimated mortality. The initial step determines risk based on age, history of coexisting conditions, signs on physical examination, and laboratory abnormalities (Figure 36–1). The patient is risk stratified to Class I if no risk factors are present. Points are assigned based on the presence or absence of additional historical, physical examination, and laboratory findings to classify patients to risk Class II to V. Risk stratification is based on the total points. Class II patients have less than 70 points, Class III patients 71–90

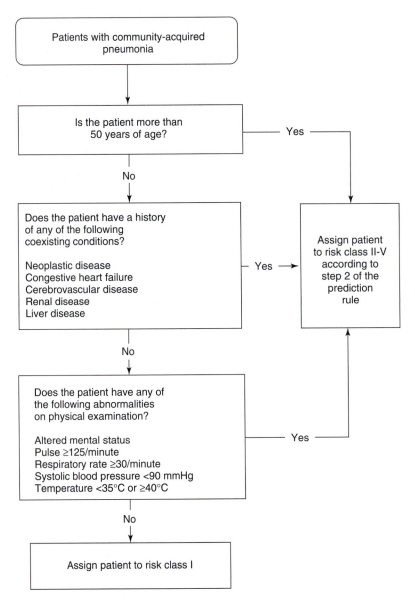

Figure 36–1. Step 1 algorithm of PORT risk stratification for community-acquired pneumonia.

Table 36–3. Port risk stratification for community-acquired pneumonia.

Characteristic	Points Assigned
Demographic factor	
Age	
Men	Age (years)
Women	Age (years) –10
Nursing home resident	+10
Coexisting illnesses	
Neoplastic disease	+30
Liver disease	+20
Congestive heart failure	+10
Cerebrovascular disease	+10
Renal disease	+10
Physical examination findings	
Altered mental status	+20
Respiratory rate ≥30/min	+20
Systolic blood pressure <90 mm Hg	+20
Temperature <35°C or ≥40°C	+15
Pulse ≥125/min	+10
Laboratory and radiographic findings	
Arterial pH <7.35	+30
Blood urea nitrogen ≥30 mg/dL (11 mmol/L)	+20
Sodium <130 mmol/L	+20
Glucose ≥250 mg/dL (14 mmol/L)	+10
Hematocrit <30%	+10
Partial pressure of arterial oxygen <60 mm Hg	+10
Pleural effusion	+10

points, Class IV patients 91–130 points, and Class V patients greater than 130 points (Table 36–3). The estimated 30-day mortality rates by class are 0.1% for Class I, 0.6% for Class II, 0.9% for Class III, 9.3% for Class IV, and 27% for Class V.

This rule results in a reduction in hospitalization rates from 58% to 43% when it is applied as an adjunct to the admission decision process in emergency rooms. Although more patients subsequently fail outpatient management and require readmission (9% versus 0%), no deaths occur as a result of the initial outpatient therapy and measures of recovery between the two groups are comparable.

Dean NC: Use of prognostic scoring and outcome assessment tools in the admission decision for community-acquired pneumonia. Clin Chest Med 1999;20:521. [PMID: 10516901]. (This article reviews different prognostic factors for patients with CAP.)

Fine MJ et al: A prediction rule to identify low-risk patients with community-acquired pneumonia. N Engl J Med 1997; 336:243. [PMID: 8995086]. (This article derives a stratification formula that predicts mortality in patients with CAP.)

Viral & Atypical Pneumonia

Kathryn A. Lee, MD, & Edward D. Chan, MD[1]

Numerous prospective studies examining the etiology for community-acquired pneumonia (CAP) have found that in a significant proportion of cases there is no identifiable cause. This is due, in part, to incomplete or inadequate diagnostic evaluation of all potential pathogens. Although CAP is traditionally divided into typical and atypical pneumonia based on clinical syndromes due to "typical" pathogens (eg, *Streptococcus pneumoniae*) versus "atypical" organisms (eg, *Mycoplasma pneumoniae, Chlamydia pneumoniae,* and *Legionella pneumophila*), it has been repeatedly shown that this dichotomous classification lacks enough predictive value and discriminatory ability to be reliable. As a result, the initial treatment of CAP remains largely empiric. Nevertheless, the term "atypical" is still pervasive in the medical lexicon and useful for discussion. The three major atypical organisms that account for pneumonia and upper respiratory infections are resistant to β-lactam antibiotics: *C pneumoniae* and *L pneumophila* because they are intracellular and *M pneumoniae* because it lacks a cell wall. This chapter discusses these and also discusses some of the important viral causes of CAP, specifically adenovirus, hantavirus, influenza, and varicella pneumonias and Severe Acute Respiratory Syndrome. The key clinical and laboratory features of each of these entities are summarized in Table 37–1. Respiratory viruses such as measles, respiratory syncytial virus, parainfluenza viruses, coxsackievirus, enteroviruses, cytomegalovirus, human metapneumovirus, and herpes simplex viruses are not discussed.

ADENOVIRUS

ESSENTIALS OF DIAGNOSIS

- Polymerase chain reaction (PCR) is the best test to diagnose adenovirus pneumonia. Sensitivity is 90–100% and the specificity is >95%. PCR can be applied to various specimen types including respiratory secretions, urine, stool, blood, and solid tissues.

- Rapid antigen detection (immunoassay) is often part of an antigen panel that includes other respiratory viruses. Sensitivity is low so it should be used in conjunction with cell culture. A nasal wash is the preferred specimen.

- Shell-vial culture (48 h turnaround time) is less sensitive than conventional culture, which may take up to 3 weeks.

- Antibody assays require both acute and convalescent titers. A fourfold rise in immunoglobulin G (IgG) titer over 2–3 weeks is considered positive.

General Considerations

The adenoviruses are nonenveloped double-stranded DNA viruses associated with a wide spectrum of clinical disease in humans. They are most frequently associated with respiratory illness, gastrointestinal disease, and conjunctivitis in young persons. Adenoviruses are highly contagious and have caused large outbreaks in areas in which crowding occurs (especially military recruits and patients in psychiatric care facilities). Nearly 50 serotypes have been identified. Types 3 and 7 are associated with more severe disease and type 4 is associated with outbreaks among military recruits. Adenoviral infections occur year-round but account for a higher proportion of pneumonias in the summer months.

Pathogenesis

The adenoviruses infect epithelial cells of the gastrointestinal, genitourinary, and respiratory tracts. They deliver their genome to the nucleus and can replicate with high efficiency, making them good candidates for delivery and expression of therapeutic genes. Adenoviruses are capable of establishing persistent infection in the host. Reactivation of latent infection may cause disease in immunocompromised hosts.

Prevention

Vaccines for types 4 and 7 have been used successfully in military recruits.

[1]We are grateful to Dr. Adriana Weinberg and Dr. Mary Ann De-Groote for critical review of the manuscript.

Table 37–1. Key features of viral and atypical bacterial pneumonias.

Agent	Key Clinical and Laboratory Features
Adenovirus	Adenovirus is highly contagious and may cause large outbreaks in crowded facilities. It typically causes a self-limited upper respiratory infection although necrotizing bronchitis, bronchiolitis, and pneumonia may occur. Polymerase chain reaction is the best test to diagnose adenovirus pneumonia and can be applied to various specimen types. Cidofovir or Ribavirin has *in vitro* activity against adenoviruses.
Hantavirus	Hantavirus is acquired via direct contact with or inhalation of rodent excreta. Respiratory failure may be due to both noncardiogenic pulmonary edema (from a capillary leak syndrome) and cardiogenic pulmonary edema (from myocardial dysfunction). Hematological tetrad of neutrophilia with left shift, thrombocytopenia, elevated hematocrit, and circulating immunoblasts is characteristic.
Influenza	Influenza typically occurs in the winter months, although sporadic cases of influenza B can occur throughout the year. Primary influenza pneumonia is less common than secondary bacterial pneumonia. The inactivated influenza vaccine is recommended for at-risk individuals. Oral antiviral agents may reduce the duration of illness when begun early in the course of the disease.
Varicella	Respiratory disease due to varicella is most common among adults, pregnant women, and immuno-compromised individuals. It is highly contagious and spreads from person to person via aerosolization. The live attenuated varicella vaccine is effective and is recommended for at-risk individuals who are exposed, except for pregnant women.
SARS-Coronaviris	SARS is a severe respiratory syndrome associated with high infectivity and high mortality. Laboratory findings of lymphopenia and an elevated LDH are common. Treatment with corticosteroids and/or Ribavirin may be beneficial.
Chlamydia pneumoniae	Micrommunofluorescent assay for IgG/IgM or PCR is the preferred method to diagnose acute *C pneumoniae* infection. The spectrum of disease caused by *C pneumoniae* includes pharyngitis, sinusitis, otitis, acute bronchitis, pneumonia, and an "influenza-like" illness. Recovery may be slow and prolonged therapy warranted.
Legionella pneumophila	Antigen detection with the urine antigen assay is sensitive but detects only *L pneumophila* serotype 1. Aspiration of infected potable water is likely the most common mode of acquisition. For severe disease, the fluoroquinolones are recommended as they have the highest bactericidal activity *in vitro*.
Mycoplasma pneumoniae	PCR is highly sensitive and touted to have relatively high specificity for acute infection. Most patients with *M pneumoniae* infection have mild bronchitis or pneumonia, but fulminant pneumonia can occur.

Clinical Findings

In immunocompetent individuals, adenovirus infection usually causes a self-limited upper respiratory tract disease. Conjunctivitis and gastroenteritis are common extrapulmonary manifestations. Adenovirus pneumonia is rare, but may follow more severe lower respiratory disease such as necrotizing bronchitis and bronchiolitis. Patients with adenovirus pneumonia may present with cough and fever for up to 7 days followed by severe dyspnea. Rales and rhonchi are usually heard on lung examination, although wheezing, decreased breath sounds, and signs of consolidation have been noted. Radiographic appearance ranges from patchy lower lobe infiltrates to unilateral lobar consolidation to diffuse interstitial infiltrates. Pleural effusions, diffuse hemorrhagic pneumonia, and diffuse alveolar pneumonia have been reported. Laboratory abnormalities can include leukopenia, mild thrombocytopenia, and elevated transaminases.

In immunocompromised patients, especially bone marrow transplant recipients and patients with acquired immunodeficiency syndrome (AIDS), severe disseminated disease with pneumonitis, hepatitis, gastroenteritis, colitis, encephalitis, cholecystitis, hemorrhagic cystitis, and coagulopathy can occur.

Differential Diagnosis

In immunocompetent hosts, adenovirus pneumonia may be difficult to distinguish from other causes of CAP. In immunocompromised hosts, the clinical and histopathological features can mimic those of cytomegalovirus.

Complications

Acute respiratory distress syndrome (ARDS) and septic shock have occurred in patients infected with adenovirus serotype 35. Central nervous system involvement such as meningitis and viral encephalitis is rare and is most commonly associated with serotype 7. Long-term pulmonary sequelae can include bronchiectasis, chronic restrictive changes, and unilateral hyperlucent lung.

Treatment & Prognosis

Most adenovirus infections are self-limited. Adenovirus pneumonia, however, has been associated with a mortality rate of near 30%, although this is based on few cases. Mortality is higher (up to 50%) in immunocompromised patients who can develop severe disseminated disease. Support of ventilatory function is the major therapeutic priority. Limited data are available on the effect of antiviral agents in humans. Cidofovir has the best *in vitro* activity against adenoviruses. Ribavirin also has *in vitro* activity and has been successful in anecdotal reports of adenovirus pneumonia in adults. Other treatment modalities such as intravenous immunoglobulin have been tried but their benefits have not been proven in clinical trials.

Carrigan DR: Adenovirus infections in immunocompromised patients. Am J Med 1997;102:71. [PMID: 10868146]. (Review of epidemiology and clinical presentation of adenovirus infections in immunocompromised hosts.)

Chien JW, Johnson JL: Viral pneumonias: multifaceted approach to an elusive diagnosis. Postgrad Med 2000;107:67. [PMID: 10649665]. (Basic review of common epidemic respiratory viruses with a focus on diagnostic strategies.)

Gray GC et al: Adult adenovirus infections: loss of orphaned vaccines precipitates military respiratory disease epidemics. Clin Infect Dis 2000;31:663. [PMID: 11017812]. (Discusses the impact of vaccine removal on military recruits. Morbidity has increased significantly since the vaccine was removed in 1995.)

Klinger JR et al: Multiple cases of life-threatening adenovirus pneumonia in a mental health care center. Am J Respir Crit Care Med 1998;157:645. [PMID: 9476884]. (Describes 18 cases of pneumonia during an outbreak of adenovirus infection in a chronic psychiatric care facility. Four developed septic shock. Short review of clinical syndromes and x-ray findings associated with adenovirus pneumonia.)

HANTAVIRUS PULMONARY SYNDROME

 ESSENTIALS OF DIAGNOSIS

- IgM capture enzyme-linked immunosorbent assay (ELISA) has a sensitivity and specificity of close to 100% and is positive early in disease. This test cannot differentiate among the various hantaviruses.
- IgG ELISA is often positive even in the prodromal phase. There is a low prevalence of hantavirus antibodies in the general U.S. population, but this may not be true for other endemic areas.
- Reverse-transcriptase PCR to detect viral DNA will identify virus genotype but is not useful in acute diagnosis because of low sensitivity.
- Culture has a low yield as the virus is very difficult to isolate.
- Immunohistochemistry on formalin-fixed, paraffin-embedded tissue can be used to confirm diagnosis or to make retrospective assessments of suspicious cases.

General Considerations

Hantavirus pulmonary syndrome (HPS) is acquired via direct contact with or inhalation of rodent excreta, especially urine. It was first recognized in 1993, and has occurred only in the Americas to date. Most cases have occurred in the Southwestern region of the United States. Sporadic cases have also been identified in several eastern states and in South American countries. The viruses are found in rodents throughout the Americas. The hantaviruses belong to the family Bunyaviridae. At least 10 hantaviruses causing human disease have been identified. Sin Nombre virus is the most common cause of HPS in North America and is carried by the deer mouse. Infection results in a severe febrile illness associated with cardiopulmonary compromise, hematological manifestations, and a high mortality rate. HPS is largely a rural disease, with most patients acquiring the infection in the home. Patients often note an obvious exposure to rodents or their excreta. Risk factors include rural residence, agricultural activities, opening up and cleaning an uninhabited structure, an excess of small rodents in the home, and possibly hiking and other outdoor activities. In one 1996 epidemic in Patagonia, person-to-person spread was documented with the Andes virus. There is no evidence that this occurs with other hantaviruses.

Pathogenesis

Rodents are chronically infected but have no signs of disease. In humans, the virus infects the pulmonary capillary endothelium after inhalation. The viruses are not very cytopathogenic and host immune response is likely responsible for the disease process. The pathogenesis of myocardial dysfunction is not well understood. Host genetic differences may play a role in severity of disease, or may be protective.

Prevention

To prevent human infection, rodent avoidance and control are important. Care should be taken when handling dead rodents or cleaning rodent nests. Closed structures should be ventilated before entering or cleaning them. No vaccine is currently available.

Clinical Findings

Following an incubation period of about 14–17 days after exposure, the 3- to 5-day prodromal phase consists of abrupt onset of fever, myalgias, malaise, and gastrointestinal symptoms. A cardiopulmonary phase follows, with cough, dyspnea, and hypotension. Gastrointestinal symptoms may worsen as well. After 1–2 days, patients typically develop signs and symptoms of noncardiogenic pulmonary edema, with chest x-ray showing extensive airspace disease and pleural effusions. Rapid decompensation associated with pulmonary capillary leak syndrome, hypoxemia, and myocardial dysfunction is common. Renal involvement may occur, although it is usually not severe. Disseminated intravascular coagulation and frank hemorrhage have been reported. Most deaths occur within 48 h of admission and are related to cardiogenic shock. Several laboratory features can assist in making a clinical diagnosis of HPS. The classic hematological tetrad of thrombocytopenia, a very high white blood cell count with a left shift, hemoconcentration, and circulating immunoblasts is common. Thrombocytopenia occurs early in disease. Other laboratory abnormalities may include a low serum sodium concentration, decreased serum protein concentration, elevated lactate dehydrogenase, a slightly prolonged activated partial thromboplastin time, a mildly increased creatinine, and microscopic hematuria. Bronchoalveolar lavage fluid is remarkable for a lack of inflammatory cells but may show large amounts of proteinaceous fluid. Hemodynamic monitoring will likely reveal a decreased cardiac output, increased systemic vascular resistance, and normal pulmonary capillary wedge pressure suggesting capillary leak.

Differential Diagnosis

The prodrome is typical of many illnesses (such as influenza) but the presence of thrombocytopenia and circulating immunoblasts helps suggest the diagnosis of HPS. HPS differs from ARDS in that there is no peripheral airspace disease in the early stage, and pleural effusions with marked interstitial edema are typically present.

Complications

Whereas Sin Nombre virus infection is dominated by cardiopulmonary and hematological involvement, other hantaviruses may target extrathoracic organs, especially the kidneys.

Treatment & Prognosis

No specific treatment is available for HPS. Many patients will require mechanical ventilation and intensive care support including inotropic agents and pulmonary artery catheter monitoring. Ribavirin benefits patients with hemorrhagic fever with renal syndrome, a disorder caused by other forms of hantaviruses, but is of unknown efficacy in HPS. Experimental therapies such as extracorporeal membrane oxygenator support and nitric oxide have benefited isolated patients. Passive immunotherapy is of theoretical benefit because a poor antibody response is associated with more severe disease. There have been promising anecdotal reports from South America concerning the benefits of using high doses of corticosteroids. HPS is associated with a mortality rate of 30–40%. Survivors tend to do well, but residual pulmonary and cognitive deficits may remain.

Duchin JS et al: The Hantavirus Study Group: Hantavirus pulmonary syndrome: a clinical description of 17 patients with a newly recognized disease. N Engl J Med 1994;330:949. [PMID: 8121458]. (Describes the initial outbreak of HPS in the southwestern United States with detailed clinical information on 17 patients.)

Padula PJ et al: Genetic diversity, distribution, and serological features of hantavirus infection in five countries in South America. J Clin Microbiol 2000;38:3029. [PMID: 10921972]. (Describes the genetic diversity, geographic distribution, and serological features of hantavirus infection in several South American countries.)

Peters CJ, Khan AS: Hantavirus pulmonary syndrome: the new American hemorrhagic fever. Clin Infect Dis 2002;34:1224. [PMID: 11941549]. (The most thorough review of HPS to date. Provides an update of clinical findings associated with HPS since the 1993 epidemic.)

INFLUENZA

ESSENTIALS OF DIAGNOSIS

- *Rapid antigen detection tests are available for influenza A and B, and yield results in 30 min. Sensitivity and specificity are lower than for culture. Nasal washes and swabs, throat swabs, and bronchoalveolar lavage fluid are acceptable specimens.*
- *Shell viral culture is the most sensitive and specific test. Turnaround time is about 48 h.*
- *A fourfold rise in serum antibody titers over 2–3 weeks is diagnostic, but time is a limiting factor.*

General Considerations

Influenza viruses are enveloped, single-stranded RNA viruses of the family Orthomyxoviridae. They are classified as type A, B, or C based on antigenic differences. Influenza A and B are both responsible for epidemics in humans. Epidemics of influenza typically occur during the winter months and are responsible for about 20,000 deaths per year in the United States. Sporadic cases due to influenza B can occur throughout the year. The viruses are spread by close contact and aerosol transmission. Incubation period ranges from 1 to 5 days. Rates of infection are highest among children. Persons over 65 years of age and those with chronic medical conditions are at increased risk for severe disease and death. Pregnancy may also be associated with more severe disease. Primary influenza pneumonia is uncommon and occurs primarily during major influenza A outbreaks.

Pathogenesis

The viruses primarily target the respiratory epithelium including columnar epithelial cells and pneumocytes. Sloughing of epithelial cells, extravasation of fluid, submucosal inflammation, and finally alveolar collapse occur secondary to loss of surfactant.

Clinical Findings

The typical syndrome of influenza starts with rather sudden onset of fever, dry cough, myalgias, headache, and malaise. Nasal congestion and a scratchy throat are common. Gastrointestinal complaints may occur in children, and the elderly may present with lassitude and unexplained fever alone. Disease usually lasts 3–7 days, but cough and fatigue may persist. Primary influenza pneumonia is uncommon, and tends to develop 1–3 days into the illness. Patients complain of severe dyspnea and may note retrosternal chest pain. Sputum production is scant and mild hemoptysis may occur. Physical examination reveals an ill-appearing patient in respiratory distress. Rales, rhonchi, wheezes, and a prolonged expiratory phase may be found on lung exam. Acute respiratory failure is common. Chest x-ray findings vary from local segmental consolidation to diffuse pneumonitis. Laboratory studies may show early lymphopenia and neutrophilia followed by neutropenia later in the course.

Secondary bacterial pneumonia is a more common cause of pneumonia associated with influenza. Factors such as decreased mucociliary clearance, impaired function of phagocytic cells and lymphocytes, and extravasated fluid all contribute to the devlopment of bacterial pneumonia. This tends to occur 5–10 days after the onset of influenza and may follow a brief period of improvement. *Streptococcus pneumoniae*, *Haemophilus influenzae*, and *Staphylococcus aureus* are the pathogens isolated most frequently.

Complications

Exacerbation of chronic disease such as chronic obstructive pulmonary disease (COPD) or congestive heart failure (CHF) contributes to the high mortality observed in the older population. Other potential complications of influenza include myositis (occasionally with myoglobulinemia and renal failure), myocarditis, and pericarditis. Encephalopathy, transverse myelitis, Guillain–Barré syndrome, and Reye's syndrome (especially in association with aspirin use in children) have all been reported. Survivors of severe viral pneumonia may be left with reactive airway disease, pulmonary fibrosis, or respiratory insufficiency of varying degrees.

Prevention

Influenza vaccination with inactivated vaccine is recommended for all adults over age 50, any person 6 months of age or older with certain chronic medical conditions (heart and lung disease, diabetes, immunosuppression), health care workers, persons in close contact with high-risk patients, and anyone who wants to prevent influenza. Universal childhood vaccination is becoming a new recommendation in Japan because it has been shown to produce herd immunity. The vaccine should also be given to women who will be in the second or third trimester of pregnancy during influenza season and is considered safe at any time during pregnancy. It should be administered yearly, preferably during October or November. The vaccine may contain small amounts of egg protein and thimerosal, and should not be given to persons with allergies to these agents. In general, it is 70–90% effective at preventing influenza, although effectiveness varies depending on host factors and degree of similarities between vaccine viruses and those circulating in the community. Among the elderly, it is quite effective in preventing hospitalization, pneumonia, and death from influenza. Development of antibodies can take 2 weeks after vaccination. Immunocompromised patients may produce reduced antibody titers. The antiviral agents listed below can also be used for prevention in unvaccinated persons or those expected to have a poor response to vaccination (such as transplant recipients). They are about 70–90% effective. Chemoprophylaxis is also suggested during institutional outbreaks, regardless of vaccination status of residents. The dosage for each agent in adults is shown in Table 37–2. Efficacy of antiviral agents has not been established in immunocompromised patients.

Treatment

Four influenza antiviral agents are available (Table 37–2). All agents can reduce the duration of uncomplicated illness by about 1 day when started in the first 36–48 h of disease. They have not been shown to prevent complications but most experts advocate treatment of high-risk patients. They have not been studied during pregnancy. Dosages for all but zanamivir must be adjusted for patients with renal insufficiency.

Prognosis

Mortality due to influenza varies from year to year due to antigenic variation and changes in the prevalent types of virus in circulation. Mortality varies from 30 to 150 deaths per 100,000 persons age 65 years and older. Patients with underlying medical illness are at increased risk of complications and death. Primary viral pneumonia due to influenza is associated with a high mortality (about 40%), especially among bone marrow and solid organ transplant patients.

Advisory Committee on Immunization Practices: Prevention and control of influenza. MMWR Morb Mortal Wkly Rep 2001;50(RR-4):1. [PMID: 11334444]. (Provides a thorough review of the demographic characteristics associated with severe influenza infection and its mortality. Summarizes data regarding use of the vaccine and its societal importance. Also addresses chemoprophylaxis and treatment options.)

Table 37–2. Antiviral agents for Influenza.

	Amantadine (Symmetrel)	Rimantadine (Flumadine)	Zanamivir (Relenza)	Oseltamivir (Tamiflu)
Influenza virus inhibited	A	A	A and B	A and B
Mechanism of action	Ion channel M2 blocker, inhibiting viral replication	Same as amantidine	Neuraminidase blocker, preventing release of viral particles	Same as zanamivir
Dosage for treatment	100 mg orally twice a day or 100 mg every day[1] for 24–48 h after symptoms abate	100 mg orally twice a day or 100–200 mg every day[1] for 5–7 days	Same as above	75 mg orally twice a day for 5 days
Dosage for prophylaxis	Same as above	Same as above	10 mg (two inhalations) twice a day for 5 days	75 mg orally daily
Major side effects	Central nervous system (CNS): confusion, tremor, seizures, and coma especially in setting of renal insufficiency; gastrointestinal: loss of appetite, nausea	Same as amantidine, less CNS effects	Bronchospasm (not recommended for patients with underlying airway disease)	Nausea, vomiting
Approximate cost for a 5-day course	$3.50	$8.75	$44.00	$53.00

[1]Preferred dosage for elderly patients.

VARICELLA

ESSENTIALS OF DIAGNOSIS

- *Most patients with varicella zoster virus (VZV) are diagnosed clinically, based on a typical syndrome and characteristic rash.*
- *Antigen detection on skin and bronchoalveolar lavage fluid by direct fluorescent antibody (DFA) is very sensitive and rapid.*
- *A Tzanck smear will allow detection of infected cells in 70% of cases but cannot distinguish VZV from herpes simplex viruses.*
- *Viral culture using shell vial assay or conventional culture has a sensitivity of 30–60% and takes 3–10 days. The specimen must contain cells so a scraping of the base of a lesion is best.*
- *Polymerase chain reaction (PCR) is extremely sensitive and can be used for many specimens such as bronchoalveolar lavage fluid, crust from lesions, and cerebrospinal fluid.*
- *Serological testing using acute and convalescent serum specimens can be used to retrospectively diagnose VZV.*

General Considerations

VZV is a well known member of the herpesvirus family. Primary infection with VZV causes varicella, commonly known as chickenpox. It is highly contagious and spreads from person to person by aerosolization of respiratory tract secretions or by direct contact from skin lesions. The incubation period ranges from 10 to 21 days. Respiratory disease associated with VZV is uncommon. Adults, pregnant and postpartum women, and immunocompromised patients are at increased risk of severe disease due to varicella pneumonia. Smoking may be an additional risk factor. Among adults with varicella, about 5–14% develop lower respiratory tract symptoms, and about 10% of these develop respiratory failure requiring mechanical ventilation. In pregnant women (especially in the third trimester), varicella pneumonia can be particularly severe with mortality rates up to 45%.

Pathogenesis

VZV is spread by airborne transmission from respiratory secretions and from skin lesions. Once the virus comes in contact with the upper respiratory tract mucosa and conjunctiva, it enters mononuclear cells and then disseminates hematogenously to the skin. Following infection, it remains latent in the dorsal root and cranial nerve ganglia. Reactivation of VZV from the ganglia leads to herpes zoster.

Prevention

Varivax, a live attenuated varicella vaccine, is 85% effective at preventing disease and 97% protective against severe varicella disease. It is recommended for all susceptible persons 12 months of age or older, including susceptible household contacts of immunocompromised patients. Vaccinees may develop a rash and there is a small risk of transmitting VZV while the rash is present. Vaccination in adults entails two subcutaneous doses 4–7 weeks apart. Vaccination of immunocompromised patients is under investigation. The vaccine is not recommended for use in pregnant women. Postexposure prophylaxis is recommended for those at high risk for morbidity and mortality from VZV. Intramuscular VZIG, 125 units/10 kg of body weight, up to a maximum of 625 units, can decrease the severity of illness if given within 96 h of exposure. The vaccine is also approved for postexposure prophylaxis. If given within 72 h of exposure, it may modify or prevent disease. Acyclovir, started 7–10 days after the time of exposure, has also been shown to prevent disease.

Clinical Findings

Patients with varicella develop fevers, malaise, and the familiar generalized vesicular rash characterized by "dew drop on rose petal" lesions. Lesions usually begin on the head, followed by the trunk and then extremities. Lesions in different stages of development can usually be seen at the same time. Respiratory symptoms, when they occur, appear 3–5 days into the illness. The pulmonary manifestations tend to correlate with the severity of the rash. Symptoms of VZV pneumonia usually include dyspnea, cough, tachycardia, and fever. Radiographic findings usually reveal patchy diffuse airspace consolidation or a diffuse interstitial infiltrate. Nodular disease, lobar pneumonia, hilar adenopathy, and/or small pleural effusions may also be seen. The infiltrate may be associated with proteinaceous exudates, edema, and hyaline membrane formation, which has been known to progress to ARDS. In immunocompromised patients, the rash may be atypical or absent. Immunocompromised patients with a history of VZV are at increased risk for localized and disseminated zoster, which is related to reactivation of latent virus rather than to a primary infection.

Differential Diagnosis

Smallpox (characterized by multiple lesions in the same stage of development) was often confused with varicella before its eradication. Varicella lesions may also be confused with rash due to impetigo, disseminated herpes simplex virus, and disseminated enteroviral infections.

Complications

The most common complication of varicella is secondary bacterial infection of the skin lesions. Central nervous system complications are rare and include encephalitis, cerebellar ataxia, transverse myelitis, and cerebral vasculitis. Other complications can include hepatitis, nephritis, and myocarditis. After the acute varicella pneumonia, scattered punctate lung calcifications may persist on chest x-ray. Reye's syndrome in association with aspirin use has also been associated with VZV.

Treatment & Prognosis

Acyclovir 10–20 mg/kg every 8 h intravenously for 7–10 days is the treatment of choice for varicella pneumonia. Major side effects include reversible hematological toxicity, renal failure, and seizures or coma. Acyclovir has been used in over 2000 pregnant women with no adverse effects on pregnancy outcome. Foscarnet 40 mg/kg every 8 h should be used in patients who do not respond to acyclovir or who have acyclovir-resistant disease. Cidofovir is also effective. Oral acyclovir, valacyclovir, and famciclovir are available for less complicated VZV infections. Treatment is most effective when started early in the disease, preferably in the first 72 h. Patients should be put in respiratory isolation until the lesions crust. The mortality rate in severe cases of varicella pneumonia is about 10–30% in healthy adults. The mortality rate approaches 50% in pregnant women and immunocompromised patients.

Chien JW, Johnson JL: Viral pneumonias: multifaceted approach to an elusive diagnosis. Postgrad Med 2000;107:67. [PMID: 10649665]. (Reviews major causes of viral pneumonia with a focus on diagnostic strategies.)

Cohen JI et al: Recent advances in varicella-zoster infection. Ann Intern Med 1999;130:922. [PMID: 10375341]. (A thorough review including descriptions of viral pathogenesis and the immune response to VZV. Includes information on treatment of various forms of VZV disease.)

SEVERE ACUTE RESPIRATORY SYNDROME (SARS)

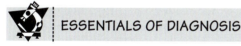

ESSENTIALS OF DIAGNOSIS

- *Severe respiratory symptoms (cough, difficulty breathing) with fever >38°C.*
- *Suspected exposure during the 10 days prior to illness.*
- *Laboratory testing for the probable etiological agent, a coronavirus, is under development.*

General Considerations

SARS is a life-threatening respiratory disease that was first recognized in Guangdong Province, China in late 2002. From there, it quickly spread to many countries. At present (spring 2003) areas of highest risk include the People's Republic of China, Hanoi, Vietnam, Taiwan, Singapore and Canada. The severe nature of the disease and evidence of person-to-person spread in early cases prompted the World Health Organization (WHO) to issue a global alert. Within several weeks, a novel coronavirus (proposed name: Urbani SARS-associated coronavirus) was detected in culture and identified by electron microscopy and molecular studies. This virus was linked to many early cases and is most likely the causative agent. It is presumed that the virus originated in animals, although the actual source is unknown. The virus appears to be highly infectious among humans and certain individuals seem to be "superspreaders" of SARS. Almost all affected patients thus far have a history of contact with another infected patient, but the contact was minor in many cases. SARS affects people of all ages, but may be less severe in children. Transmission is likely by droplets and possibly by fomites. There is currently much to learn about this illness. Because of the severity of the illness, information is quickly being gathered.

Pathogenesis

Autopsy findings on lung tissue have been consistent with early acute respiratory distress syndrome (ARDS) and the organizing phase of alveolar damage without viral inclusions. Other organs are not involved. It appears that much of the illness is due to immunopathological damage rather than viral replication.

Clinical Findings

The incubation period after contact varies from 2 to 16 days (median 6 days). In the first large report of clinical findings, all patients had fever (most >38.4°C). Other common findings included chills, rigors, and myalgias. Cough and headache occurred in over 50% of the patients, and crackles were often heard on lung examination. Sore throat, nausea and vomiting, and diarrhea were present in a minority of patients.

Common laboratory findings include lymphopenia with normal neutrophil counts, thrombocytopenia, elevated lactate dehydrogenase, and creatine kinase levels. Abnormalities on chest radiographs were seen initially in about 80% of cases and progressed over 7–10 days. A typical course was that of unilateral peripheral consolidation on initial chest radiograph, followed by bilateral patchy involvement. Computed tomography (CT) images were helpful in patients with normal chest radiographs and showed peripheral ground-glass opacification similar to that seen with bronchiolitis obliterans with organizing pneumonia (BOOP).

Current case definitions are based on clinical findings and can be found on the listed web sites. A suspect case is defined as a patient with fever >38°C, plus cough or difficulty breathing, plus suspected exposure during the 10 days prior to illness (close contact with a suspect case or travel to an affected area). A probable case is defined as a patient meeting the above criteria plus radiographic or autopsy evidence of pneumonia or respiratory distress syndrome.

At present, no validated specific test is available for diagnosing SARS. Diagnosis is therefore based on clinical and epidemiological factors. Researchers are quickly working toward development of diagnostic tests including both an ELISA and immunofluorescence assay (IFA) for antibody detection. A coronavirus (SARS-CoV) has been isolated in cell culture (Vero cells) from many patients, and can be visualized by electron microscopy. A polymerase chain reaction (PCR) test kit for detection of genetic material of the SARS-associated coronavirus is available from WHO. Care providers should consult the WHO (http://www.who.int/csr/sars/en/), CDC (www.cdc.gov/ncidod/sars), or their local health department for optimal updated testing methods. Upper respiratory specimens are preferred for isolation of the virus, and a nasopharyngeal aspirate is the specimen of choice. The virus can also be recovered from nasopharyngeal and oropharyngeal swabs, lower respiratory secretions, pleural fluid, stool, conjunctival swabs, and biopsy tissue. Acute and convalescent (greater that 21 days after onset of symptoms) serum should also be collected for antibody assays. Because SARS is currently a diagnosis of exclusion, attempts should be made to search for other causes of illness.

Differential Diagnosis

Viral respiratory illnesses such as influenza A and B and respiratory syncytial virus can cause a similar syndrome. Other causes of community-acquired pneumonia and atypical pneumonia should also be considered.

Treatment, Prognosis, & Prevention

The disease is more severe than diseases associated with most respiratory viruses with a mortality rate of >6%.

About 25% of patients will require admission to the intensive care unit and will progress to ARDS and/or require mechanical ventilation. Patients should be treated empirically for common respiratory pathogens (typical and atypical) while awaiting diagnosis. There are no specific treatment recommendations. Ribavirin has been used, but does not appear to be of benefit or to be active *in vitro*. Corticosteroids may be useful, given that the immune system may be responsible for much of the disease syndrome. To prevent spread, hospitalized patients should be isolated. Contact and airborne (N-95 respirator) precautions should be exercised and eye protection is recommended. Patients treated at home should also limit contact with others. Please consult the CDC or WHO for up-to-date recommendations on treatment, quarantine, and travel.

Lee N et al: A major outbreak of severe acute respiratory syndrome in Hong Kong. N Engl J Med 2003;348:1986. [PMID: 12682352]. (A description of 138 suspected cases of SARS associated with a hospital outbreak in Hong Kong. Clinical findings including symptoms, laboratory values, and radiographic changes are discussed. Factors associated with ICU admission and poor prognosis are identified.)

Web Sites

CDC. Web site of the Centers for Disease Control with updated information on SARS. www.cdc.gov/ncidod/sars

WHO. Web site of the World Health Organization with frequently updated information on this rapidly evolving clinical illness. http://www.who.int/csr/sars/en/

CHLAMYDIA PNEUMONIAE

 ESSENTIALS OF DIAGNOSIS

- *PCR is as least as sensitive as culture and is the preferred method of detection in most laboratories. PCR methods have not been standardized or approved by the Food and Drug Administration (FDA).*

- *The microimmunofluorescent (MIF) IgG or IgM blood test (utilizing the TW 183 antigen) is the serological testing method of choice for diagnosis of acute C pneumoniae infection. It is quite species specific but requires an experienced reader. MIF is ~90% sensitive. Acute and convalescent titers are generally required, although a single IgM ≥1:16 or IgG ≥1:512 is suggestive.*

- *C pneumoniae isolation requires special transport medium and growth in cell culture. Further-*

more, isolation of the organism from the upper respiratory tract may reflect only colonization.

General Considerations

Infection with *C pneumoniae* is common but many cases are asymptomatic. In preschool-aged children, the presence of antibodies to *C pneumoniae* is rare. In adults, up to 80% are seropositive. Data from cultures, however, indicate the prevalence in young children is similar to that of adults. *C pneumoniae* is transmitted predominantly from human-to-human via the respiratory route. As with *M pneumoniae*, outbreaks of *C pneumoniae* have occurred in enclosed populations such as military recruits and members of the same household. It can occur at any age although the incidence peaks among teens and young adults. It is considered the third or fourth most common identifiable cause of CAP, and may account for 5–15% of all cases of CAP.

Pathogenesis

C pneumoniae is an obligate intracellular organism that grows in macrophages, smooth muscle cells, and endothelial cells. It can inhibit ciliary action, accounting for its ability to cause a persistent cough. The development of specific anti-*C pneumoniae* IgE may account for the ability of this organism to induce asthma, although the association of *C pneumoniae* with asthma is controversial.

Clinical Findings

No signs or symptoms are specific for *C pneumoniae* infection. In fact, it is estimated that ~80% of infections are asymptomatic or mildly symptomatic. Clinical manifestations include upper respiratory tract symptoms, pharyngitis, otitis, sinusitis, acute bronchitis, an "influenza-like illness," and pneumonia. The presentation of pneumonia may range from a subacute and mild pneumonia to an abrupt-onset and severe bronchopneumonia resulting in respiratory failure. Fever, cough, headache, and mental status changes are common signs and symptoms. A biphasic illness may occur: upper respiratory tract symptoms, especially pharyngitis with hoarseness, may precede the onset of cough and pneumonia by several days or weeks. Sputum production is minimal and rarely purulent. Associated sinusitis or otitis may accompany the pneumonia. There are no characteristic radiographic findings for *C pneumoniae* pneumonia. A unilateral subsegmental or segmental infiltrate is the most common abnormality. An associated

pleural effusion occurs in 20–25% of the cases. Laboratory findings are nonspecific. The peripheral white blood cell count may be quite high but is usually <15,000 cells/mm^3. A chronic cough and wheeze may linger leading to the suggestion that *C pneumoniae* may precipitate or exacerbate asthma.

Complications

Persistent nasopharyngeal infection following an acute infection may occur for several years. The significance of this is not known. A number of chronic diseases are linked to *C pneumoniae* with variable strengths of evidence: chronic bronchitis, asthma, myocarditis, atherosclerotic disease, reactive arthritis, and erythema nodosum-type vasculitis.

Treatment & Prognosis

Recovery may be slow (lasting weeks to months) even with proper antibiotic treatment. Prolonged therapy (up to 3 weeks) with erythromycin (500 mg orally four times daily), doxycycline (100 mg orally twice daily), or azithromycin (standard 5-day course) is recommended. The fluoroquinolones also show promise. If symptoms fail to respond after a treatment course, a second antibiotic may be tried.

Dowell SF et al: Standardizing *Chlamydia pneumoniae* assays: recommendations from the Centers for Disease Control and Prevention (USA) and the Laboratory Centre for Disease Control (Canada). Clin Infect Dis 2001;33:492. [PMID: 11462186]. (A comprehensive review by a large panel of experts on recommendations for diagnosing *C pneumoniae* infections.)

Hammerschlag MR: *Chlamydia pneumoniae* and the lung. Eur Respir J 2000;16:1001. [PMID: 12090910]. (A thorough review on the epidemiology, clinical spectrum of diseases, diagnosis, and treatment of *C pneumoniae* infection.)

LEGIONELLA PNEUMOPHILA

 ESSENTIALS OF DIAGNOSIS

- *Culture is a widely used test for diagnosing Legionella infection. It picks up all Legionella species. Its sensitivity is poor and the required selective medium is not always available. Saline and lidocaine used in bronchoalveolar lavage may inhibit Legionella growth. Culture has a very high positive predictive value of an active infection.*

- Detection of L pneumophila *in respiratory specimens by DFA is rapid and has high specificity but lacks sensitivity.*
- *Serological testing by indirect immunofluorescent antibody requires acute and convalescent titers over several weeks. A presumptive diagnosis of Legionnaires' disease may be made in the proper clinical setting with a single titer of 1:256.*
- *Antigen detection with the urine antigen assay is sensitive but detects only* L *pneumophila serotype 1. This serotype accounts for ~90% of infections caused by* L pneumophila. *Antigenuria may be prolonged after infection.*

General Considerations

Legionellosis refers to infection by *Legionella* species. It is comprised of two clinical syndromes: (1) Legionnaires' disease, a pneumonia with or without extrapulmonary manifestations caused by *L pneumophila*, and (2) Pontiac Fever, an acute, self-limiting illness caused by other *Legionella* species but mainly by *L micdadei*. Infections due to *Legionella* species are caused mainly by *L pneumophila*, of which there are 14 known serotypes. In general, the overall incidence of CAP due to *L pneumophila* is low but *Legionella* species account for up to 16% of cases of CAP in hospitalized patients. The incidence may be higher among patients in intensive care units. *Legionella* species are widespread in man-made aquatic environments, including potable water systems. Aspiration after colonization of the oropharynx with infected potable water is likely the most common mode of acquisition. Outbreaks of Legionnaires' disease have also been linked to inhaled aerosols from showers, whirlpools, evaporative condensors, respiratory care devices, and grocery store misting machines. *L pneumophila* is also a well-known cause of nosocomial pneumonia. Human-to-human transmission does not occur.

Pathogenesis

In water sources, environmental protozoa are vital for survival of *Legionella* species. The organism also produces an endotoxin that is weakly biologically active, hemolysins, proteases, and acid phosphatase.

Clinical Findings

The clinical features of *L pneumophila* pneumonia are generally nonspecific and can vary from mild manifes-

tations to fulminant disease. The following clinical and laboratory features, although nonspecific, should raise one's suspicion for Legionnaires' disease: temperature >39°C (102.2°F), watery diarrhea, abdominal symptoms such as nausea and vomiting, encephalopathy, hyponatremia, hypophosphatemia, rhabdomyolysis, abnormal liver function tests, elevated serum lactate dehydrogenase, and hematuria. A relative bradycardia may also occur with *Legionella* infection. Neurological abnormalities include headache, confusion, and more localized deficits. Unilateral lower lobe consolidation is the most common radiographic finding in legionellosis. Initially, *Legionella* infection may present as a pulmonary nodule. Progression to multilobar involvement may be seen and may be due to inadequate coverage for the organism. Cavitation, large effusions, or empyema are rarely seen. Severe pneumonia resulting in nonfatal or fatal respiratory failure is more likely to occur in the elderly, the immunosuppressed, and those with chronic illnesses such as emphysema, heart failure, chronic renal failure, and diabetes mellitus.

Complications

Legionella infection, although most commonly affecting the lungs, may also involve the heart (pericarditis, native or prosthetic valve endocarditis), gastrointestinal tract (colitis, peritonitis, pancreatitis), lymph nodes, and urinary tract (pyelonephritis, rhabdomyolysis-induced nephropathy).

Treatment & Prognosis

L pneumophila is uniformly resistant to the β-lactam antibiotics. The macrolide antibiotics including erythromycin, clarithromycin, and azithromycin, and the newer "respiratory" fluoroquinolones such as levofloxacin, moxifloxacin, and gatifloxacin, are generally considered to be the drugs of choice against *L pneumophila*. For severe disease, the fluoroquinolones are recommended as they have the highest bactericidal activity *in vitro*. Rifampin may also be added to a failing regimen but should not be used as a single agent. Pneumonia due to *L pneumophila* is generally more severe and is associated with a higher mortality than that due to *C pneumoniae* or *M pneumoniae*.

Hindiyeh M, Carroll KC: Laboratory diagnosis of atypical pneumonia. Sem Respir Infect 2000;15:101. [PMID: 10983928]. (Review on the laboratory diagnosis of *M pneumoniae*, *Chlamydia* species, *Legionella* species, *Bordetella* species, and *Coxiella burnetti*.)

Waterer GW, Baselski VS, Wunderink RG: *Legionella* and community-acquired pneumonia: a review of current diagnostic tests from a clinician's viewpoint. Am J Med 2001;110:41.

[PMID: 11152864]. (A very comprehensive section on the laboratory diagnosis of *L pneumophila* infection.)

MYCOPLASMA PNEUMONIAE

 ESSENTIALS OF DIAGNOSIS

- *Serological methods include ELISA, indirect fluorescent antibody assay, and particle agglutination to detect IgM and IgG. Acute and convalescent titers are required although a single titer of ≥1:64 is suggestive of an acute infection.*

- *PCR is highly sensitive and touted to also have high specificity for acute infection. Carriage of M pneumoniae in the population may lower its positive predictive value.*

- *Culture of M pneumoniae in respiratory specimens requires special medium and prolonged incubation. Specificity for active infection is not known. It is infrequently useful in the clinical setting.*

- *Cold agglutinin test has a relatively poor specificity because viral infections, lymphoma, and collagen vascular disease may also give a positive test. A cold agglutinin titer >1:128 is suggestive of an acute mycoplasmal infection but it is not diagnostic. A bedside cold agglutinin test may be performed with a blue top tube. Smooth coating of the tube by red blood cells occurs with body heat, but in an ice bath, there is macroscopic agglutination of the erythrocytes on the side of the tube. Such a finding is indicative of a titer of ~≥1:64.*

General Considerations

Mycoplasma species are the smallest free-living organisms known. Overall, *M pneumoniae* is considered to be the second or third most common cause of CAP, accounting for ~15% of all CAPs. In large prospective CAP studies performed in the 1990s, *M pneumoniae* accounted for up to 29% of pneumonia in hospitalized patients. Epidemics of *M pneumoniae* respiratory infection are typically seen among people living in closed conditions such as college dormitories, military barracks, and prisons. Most patients with *M pneumoniae* infection have mild bronchitis or pneumonia but severe CAP can occur. Fulminant cases resulting in respiratory failure and death have been reported. Risk factors for

severe disease include sickle cell anemia, sickle-related hemoglobinopathies, and hypogammaglobulinemia. Disease typically affects individuals 5–15 years old, with a second peak at 25–35 years (although it may be seen in all age groups including the elderly). There is an increased incidence in the fall and winter. Transmission is from person to person via respiratory droplets produced by coughing. A history of upper and/or lower respiratory illness can usually be elicited in a family member within the the past few weeks.

Pathogenesis

The pathogenic mechansisms of *M pneumoniae* include attachment to respiratory epithelium by cytadhesins, production of hydrogen peroxide and superoxide by the organism, and the elicitation of autoantibodies such as cold isohemagglutinins (IgM) directed against an altered I antigen on the surface of erythrocytes of infected patients. A 190-kDa adhesin protein known as P1 mediates the attachment of the organism to specific glycolipids and sialated glycoproteins present on the bronchial epithelium. Mycoplasmas activate T cells and B cells in a polyclonal fashion, stimulate macrophages, and can induce the expression of several cytokines and growth factors including granulocyte-macrophage colony-stimulating factor (GM-CSF) and interferon-α. It has been suggested that the humoral arm of the immune system, especially IgG and IgA, is important in host defense against *M pneumoniae*, and that an exuberant cell-mediated response may be responsible for some of the severe cases seen.

Clinical Findings

The original report of an "atypical pneumonia," characterized by lack of sputum production, leukocytosis, or dense lobar consolidation, likely described infection due to *M pneumoniae*. Most infections due to *M pneumoniae* are mild and involve only the upper respiratory tract. In a small proportion of individuals, the infection progresses to a tracheobronchitis or pneumonia. The typical clinical presentation includes subacute onset of fever, headache, malaise, myalgias, sore throat, and cough (which is usually dry but may be productive of mucoid or blood-streaked sputum). Pharyngeal erythema, crackles, and wheezes may be found. Bullous myringitis is rarely seen in naturally occurring infections. In addition to tracheobronchitis and pneumonia, the spectrum of respiratory diseases due to *M pneumoniae* is diverse and includes cellular bronchiolitis, bronchiolitis obliterans with or without organizing pneumonia, bronchiectasis, pneumatoceles, Swyer–James syndrome, pleural effusion, pulmonary embolism, chronic interstitial fibrosis, and lung abscess. Although the pneumonia is generally considered to be benign and self-limited, fulminant disease leading to respiratory failure and death may occur. Severe hypoxemia may accompany mycoplasma-associated inflammatory bronchiolitis, even when the chest radiograph is relatively unimpressive. Radiographically, unilateral patchy alveolar infiltrates are most commonly seen, although an array of radiographic findings may accompany the respiratory disorders outlined above.

Complications

Extrapulmonary complications of mycoplasma infection include pharyngitis, sinusitis, myocarditis, pancreatitis, hepatitis, polyarthralgias, polyarthritis, hemolytic anemia, meningoencephalitis, morbilliform skin rashes, and erythema multiforme major.

Treatment & Prognosis

Treatment of symptomatic *M pneumoniae* infections can shorten the illness. Because they lack a cell wall, these Mollicutes are uniformly resistant to β-lactam antibiotics. Effective agents against *M pneumoniae* include the macrolides (erythromycin, clarithromycin, and azithromycin), fluoroquinolones, and tetracyclines. The treatment period should be 7–14 days. With azithromycin, the standard 5-day treatment is used.

Chan ED, Welsh CH: Fulminant *Mycoplasma pneumoniae* pneumonia: a review of the English literature. West J Med 1995;162:133. [PMID: 7725685]. (A literature review of *M pneumoniae* pneumonia that resulted in respiratory failure and/or death.)

Chan ED et al: *Mycoplasma pneumoniae*-associated bronchiolitis causing severe restrictive lung disease in adults: report of three cases and literature review Chest 1999;115:1188. [PMID: 10208228]. (Three case reports of inflammatory bronchiolitis associated with acute *M pneumoniae* infection resulting in severe gas-exchange abnormalities.)

Fungal Pneumonias

38

Laurie A. Proia, MD

The human respiratory tract serves as the principal route of entrance for most major fungal pathogens. These fungi are classified as endemic mycoses, fungal opportunists, and emerging pathogens (Table 38–1). Fungal pneumonia poses a unique problem for clinicians in that diagnosis is often made late in the course of a patient's illness. It is common for fungal etiologies to be considered only after a patient has failed to respond to treatment for bacterial pneumonia. The ability of clinicians to recognize and effectively treat invasive fungal infections impacts on the morbidity and mortality associated with these diseases. Enhanced knowledge of the epidemiology, clinical pattern, diagnostic methodologies, and therapy of fungal pneumonia may enable clinicians to more effectively identify and manage these types of infections.

HISTOPLASMOSIS

ESSENTIALS OF DIAGNOSIS

- *Endemic to Ohio and Mississippi River valley regions; the causative fungus is found in soil contaminated by bird or bat droppings.*
- *Acute infection is usually asymptomatic or flu-like; chronic cavitary pneumonia occurs in smokers with emphysema; it is a disseminated disease, especially in human immunodeficiency virus (HIV)-infected individuals.*
- *Diagnosis is by bronchoalveolar lavage (BAL) or tissue biopsy, by blood and bone marrow cultures for disseminated infection, and by urine Histoplasma antigen for severe pulmonary or disseminated disease.*

General Considerations

Histoplasmosis, a disease caused by the dimorphic fungus *Histoplasma capsulatum*, is the most common mycosis occurring in the United States. *H capsulatum* is found predominantly in the mid- and south-central United States, especially in the Ohio and Mississippi River valley regions. Histoplasmosis also occurs in other areas of the world, including Africa, Central and South America, and the Caribbean.

Pathogenesis

Because *H capsulatum* grows well in soil enriched with bird and bat guano, exposure may occur in or around caves (spelunking), barns, bird roosts, and chicken coops. *H capsulatum* spores are aerosolized, especially with soil excavation, and inhaled. Once inhaled, spores are deposited into pulmonary alveoli where they revert to yeast forms. This genetically controlled switch from mold form at ambient temperature to yeast form at body temperature is called thermal dimorphism and is a property of *H capsulatum* and other endemic fungi. The presence of *H capsulatum* in the lung causes an influx of inflammatory cells (primarily lymphocytes and macrophages) that attempt to control and contain infection. Macrophages phagocytose and in turn disseminate *H capsulatum* throughout the reticuloendothelial system of the body during primary infection. T cell immunity develops in immunocompetent hosts approximately 2 weeks after infection. Individuals who fail to mount a protective T cell response, such as those with HIV infection or hematological malignancy, develop progressive and severe pneumonia or disseminated infection.

Clinical Findings

A. Symptoms and Signs

Symptomatic disease occurs in only 1% of infected individuals. Pulmonary disease is the most common manifestation of *H capsulatum* infection.

1. Primary pulmonary histoplasmosis—Primary pulmonary histoplasmosis produces few or no symptoms. Symptoms of primary infection develop after a 1- to 3-week incubation period and include fever, chills, myalgias, dry cough, dyspnea, and pleurisy. Inhalation of a large inoculum of organisms may predispose individuals to severe pneumonia or the acute respiratory distress syndrome (ARDS). Some patients with primary infection develop immune-mediated rheumatological syndromes, such as arthritis, pericarditis, and erythema nodosum, which are self-limited.

Table 38–1. Common and emerging pathogens associated with fungal pneumonia.

Pathogenic dimorphic fungi
  Histoplasma capsulatum
  Blastomyces dermatitidis
  Coccidioides immitis
  Paracoccidioides brasiliensis
  Penicillium marneffei
  Sporothrix schenckii
Opportunistic yeasts and molds
  Aspergillus spp.
  Cryptococcus neoformans
  Candida spp.
  Pneumocystis carinii
Emerging fungal opportunists
  Fusarium
  Zygomycetes (Mucor, Rhizopus)
  Trichosporon
  Pseudallescheria
  Scedosporium

---

2. Chronic cavitary histoplasmosis—A sequelae of primary infection, chronic cavitary histoplasmosis is often mistaken for pulmonary tuberculosis. Individuals who develop chronic cavitary histoplasmosis are generally middle-aged men (>50 years old) with a history of tobacco use and centrilobular emphysema. Typical symptoms include fatigue, fever, night sweats, weight loss, dyspnea, productive cough, and hemoptysis. Multilobar involvement can occur due to bronchogenic spread. Progressive pulmonary dysfunction results without treatment.

3. Progressive disseminated histoplasmosis—Progressive disseminated histoplasmosis may develop secondary to postprimary spread of infection or reactivation of latent disease. Progressive disseminated histoplasmosis is usually associated with impaired cell-mediated immunity, such as in patients with advanced HIV infection or hematological forms of cancer. Patients receiving cytotoxic chemotherapy, corticosteroids, or immunosuppression for solid organ or bone marrow transplantation are also at risk. Clinical manifestations are typically extrapulmonary. Symptoms and signs include fever, cough, dyspnea, diarrhea, weight loss, and mucosal ulcerations. Yeast are concentrated in the reticuloendothelial organs causing diffuse lymphadenopathy, hepatosplenomegaly, and pancytopenia. Cutaneous dissemination manifests as a maculopapular rash. Infiltration of the adrenal glands may cause adrenal insufficiency or adrenal crisis.

4. Granulomatous mediastinitis and fibrosis—These occur when primary infection is associated with robust local inflammation resulting in mediastinal and hilar lymphadenitis. Lymph nodes during this stage may necrose, coalesce, and attach to adjacent structures such as the mainstem bronchi, pulmonary arteries, pericardium, esophagus, and trachea. The fibrosis that occurs with healing can result in airway obstruction, fistula formation, postobstructive pneumonia, traction bronchiectasis, esophageal or tracheal dysfunction, superior vena cava syndrome, or cor pulmonale.

B. LABORATORY FINDINGS AND DIAGNOSIS

Definitive diagnosis of histoplasmosis is made by direct examination and culture of tissue specimens. Expectorated sputum may be positive in up to 60% of patients with chronic cavitary pneumonia. However, sputum cultures are rarely positive in acute primary histoplasmosis, progressive disseminated histoplasmosis, or mediastinal disease. Histopathological examination and culture of BAL fluid or transbronchial biopsy tissue may be diagnostic in patients with radiographic abnormalities. Cultures of blood, bone marrow, or skin lesions may yield *H capsulatum* in cases of progressive disseminated infection. Histopathological examination of specimens reveals small intracellular and extracellular yeast forms as well as caseating or noncaseating granulomas. Serological tests that measure anti-*Histoplasma* antibody by immunodiffusion or complement fixation aid in diagnosis of acute histoplasmosis or chronic pneumonia, but are less useful in cases of disseminated infection owing to the underlying immunosuppression present in these patients.

An assay is available for testing BAL fluid, serum, or urine for the presence of *Histoplasma* polysaccharide antigen. Antigen is present in urine in 90% of patients with disseminated histoplasmosis and 75% of patients with acute infection. The sensitivity of this test falls to 10–25% in cases of localized subacute or chronic pneumonia. The sensitivity and specificity of the urine assay are greater than for serum. False positives may occur with blastomycosis, paracoccidioidomycosis, and infections caused by *Penicillium marneffei*. *Histoplasma* antigen should fall in response to appropriate therapy and a rise may herald disease relapse.

C. IMAGING STUDIES

Interstitial pneumonitis, patchy alveolar infiltrates, and mediastinal adenopathy may be seen with acute infection, even in immunocompetent hosts. Parenchymal radiographic abnormalities either resolve completely or become solitary pulmonary nodules as primary infection wanes. Pulmonary nodules or adjacent lymph nodes may necrose and calcify. Some infiltrates heal to larger nodules, termed histoplasmomas, which are sometimes mistaken for neoplasm. Cavitary histoplasmosis affects predominantly the lung apices. Upper lobe cavities and changes due to chronic obstructive pulmonary disease (COPD) may coexist but adenopathy is rare. Chest radiographs are normal in 30% of patients with disseminated disease. The remainder demonstrate diffuse reticulonodular or miliary disease. More subtle pulmonary abnormalities that may be missed on chest radiograph are often detected by computed tomography (CT). CT is generally indicated in cases of chronic pneumonia or mediastinal fibrosis to determine the extent of disease.

Differential Diagnosis

The differential diagnosis of chronic pulmonary histoplasmosis includes other endemic mycoses, such as blastomycosis, tuberculosis, and other atypical mycobacteria, sarcoidosis, and neoplasm.

Treatment

The decision to treat histoplasmosis is based on the severity of infection and the immune status of the host. Treatment of acute histoplasmosis in immunocompetent hosts is generally not indicated as infection is usually self-limited. However, treatment may be useful for patients with persistent fever lasting more than 3 weeks, symptoms lasting more than 1 month, diffuse radiographic abnormalities, or hypoxemia. Oral itraconazole (200–400 mg/day) may be given for 6–12 weeks in mild to moderate localized pulmonary disease. Intravenous itraconazole is also available for treating moderate pulmonary disease. Fluconazole should be used only in patients intolerant of itraconazole, but higher doses are required (400–800 mg/day). For severe pneumonia or disseminated histoplasmosis, initial treatment with amphotericin B deoxycholate (0.7–1.0 mg/kg/day) is preferred. Patients may be switched to oral itraconazole after clinical improvement to complete 12–18 months of treatment. Patients with ongoing immunosuppression or HIV infection require chronic maintenance therapy with oral itraconazole (200 mg/day). Lipid formulations of amphotericin B (3 mg/kg/day) may be used in patients intolerant of conventional amphotericin B. Additional clinical data are needed regarding the extended spectrum azoles, voriconazole and posaconazole. The *in vitro* activity of the echinocandin class of antifungals (eg, caspofungin) is modest, limiting their use as monotherapy.

Goldman M et al: Fungal pneumonias. The endemic mycoses. Clin Chest Med 1999;20:507. [PMID: 10516900]. (Excellent and thorough review of the endemic fungal pneumonias.)

Wheat LJ: Laboratory diagnosis of histoplasmosis: update 2000. Semin Respir Infect 2001;16:131. [PMID: 11521245]. (Review of laboratory tests for histoplasmosis.)

Wheat J et al: Practice guidelines for the management of patients with histoplasmosis. Infectious Diseases Society of America.

Clin Infect Dis 2000;30:688. [PMID: 10770731]. (A must read for anyone who treats histoplasmosis.)

BLASTOMYCOSIS

 ## ESSENTIALS OF DIAGNOSIS

- *Endemic to midwestern and southern United States along the Ohio and Mississippi Rivers (similar to histoplasmosis).*
- *Soil association; infection occurs in those who work outdoors or with outdoor recreational activities.*
- *May cause asymptomatic infection or acute or chronic pneumonia; dissemination is to skin, bone/joints, or genitourinary tract.*
- *Characteristic broad-based budding yeast are seen in tissue.*

General Considerations

Blastomycosis is a disease caused by the dimorphic fungus *Blastomyces dermatitidis*. Similar to *H capsulatum*, this fungus is associated with the rich soil found along the Ohio and Mississippi Rivers. *B dermatitidis* is endemic to the midwestern, southeastern, and south central United States. *B dermatitidis* may also be found along the St. Lawrence River valley of New York and in the Canadian provinces bordering the Great Lakes. Infection has also been reported in Africa and South America. Blastomycosis is a disease of young and middle-aged men and women who work outdoors or who engage in recreational activities along riverbanks or in wooded areas, such as hunting, camping, or fishing. Dogs have a unique vulnerability to infection and can serve as harbingers for human illness.

Pathogenesis

Infection occurs when *B dermatitidis* spores are released from soil, inhaled, and deposited into pulmonary alveoli. The spores revert to yeast form and cause an influx of inflammatory cells, particularly macrophages that phagocytose the organisms. Yeast that escape killing may disseminate lymphohematogenously throughout the body. As immunity develops the inflammatory response becomes primarily polymorphonuclear. Both microabscesses and granulomas may be seen on histopathological examination of infected tissue. This pyogranulomatous reaction is unique to blastomycosis.

Immunocompromised individuals who fail to develop protective immunity, such as those with advanced HIV infection, may develop severe pneumonia or disseminated infection.

Clinical Findings

A. SYMPTOMS AND SIGNS

Symptomatic blastomycosis develops in less than 50% of those infected. Infection remains localized to the lungs in the majority (60–75%) of infected individuals. Extrapulmonary infection, most commonly of the skin, bones/joints, genitourinary tract, and central nervous system (CNS), occurs in 25–40% of those infected.

1. Acute pulmonary blastomycosis—Acute pulmonary blastomycosis is the most common presentation of patients with symptomatic infection. An influenza-like illness with fever, chills, myalgias, arthralgias, pleurisy, and dry cough develops 4–6 weeks (range 2 weeks to 3 months) after exposure. Some patients develop erythema nodosum with acute disease. A minority of patients presents with fulminant, multilobar pneumonia that can progress rapidly to respiratory failure and ARDS. Spontaneous resolution of acute pneumonia may occur.

2. Chronic pulmonary blastomycosis—Chronic pulmonary blastomycosis may develop after acute infection. Patients often have symptoms lasting 2–6 months and complain of fever, night sweats, anorexia, weight loss, productive cough, chest pain, and occasionally hemoptysis.

3. Extrapulmonary blastomycosis—Extrapulmonary blastomycosis occurs following postprimary spread of infection in 25–40% of infected individuals. Approximately 50% of patients with extrapulmonary blastomycosis have concomitant chest radiograph abnormalities. Cutaneous, osteoarticular, or genitourinary involvement is most common with disseminated blastomycosis. Other sites of dissemination include the liver, spleen, gastrointestinal tract, thyroid, and adrenal glands. Meningoencephalitis or brain abscesses are rare complications, occurring more commonly in immunocompromised hosts.

B. LABORATORY FINDINGS AND DIAGNOSIS

Diagnosis of blastomycosis is made by identification of the organisms in sputum, BAL fluid, or tissue and confirmed by culture. The characteristic broad-based budding yeast forms with double refractile cell walls are readily recognized in clinical specimen. Fresh sputum specimen or BAL fluid can be directly examined by wet mount or after preparation with 10% potassium hydroxide (KOH). Special fungal staining of biopsy tissue enhances identification of *B dermatitidis*. On histopathological examination, noncaseating granulomas and a polymorphonuclear infiltrate may also be observed. Serological assays, such as skin testing and serum antibody measurements, have low sensitivity and specificity and are not clinically useful.

C. IMAGING STUDIES

Chest radiographs in acute pulmonary blastomycosis reveal patchy alveolar infiltrates or lobar consolidation. Pleural effusions and mediastinal or hilar adenopathy are rare. Infiltrates of chronic pulmonary blastomycosis occasionally cavitate, but less frequently than in histoplasmosis or tuberculosis. These dense radiographic lesions are often mistaken for a neoplastic process.

Treatment

Because the majority of cases of acute blastomycosis are self-limited, immunocompetent patients with mild pulmonary disease, normal oxygen saturation, and no evidence of dissemination may be monitored and treatment withheld. However, some experts recommend treatment of all cases of acute infection to reduce the likelihood of progressive disease, dissemination, or late relapse. All immunocompromised patients and patients with progressive pneumonia or extrapulmonary infection require treatment. Mild to moderate pneumonia or extrapulmonary, nonmeningeal, infection can be treated with oral itraconazole (200–400 mg/day) for 6–12 months. Amphotericin B deoxycholate is the treatment of choice for severe pulmonary or disseminated infection, including CNS disease. The lipid formulations of amphotericin B may be used in those patients intolerant of conventional amphotericin B. As for histoplasmosis, fluconazole has less activity compared to itraconazole, but may be used at higher doses (400–800 mg/day) in patients unable to take itraconazole. The newer azoles, voriconazole and posaconazole, appear to have good activity but more clinical data are needed. The echinocandins (eg, caspofungin) have only modest *in vitro* activity, which limits their use as monotherapy.

Bradsher RW: Histoplasmosis and blastomycosis. Clin Infect Dis 1996;22:S102. [PMID: 8722836]. (Good review of the epidemiology and clinical features of these infections.)

Chapman SW et al: Practice guidelines for the management of patients with blastomycosis. Infectious Diseases Society of America. Clin Infect Dis 2000;30:679. [PMID: 10770729]. (A must read for anyone who treats blastomycosis.)

Pappas PG et al: Blastomycosis in patients with the acquired immunodeficiency syndrome. Ann Intern Med 1992;116:847. [PMID: 1567099]. (A classic article.)

COCCIDIOIDOMYCOSIS

 ESSENTIALS OF DIAGNOSIS

- *Found in the desert soil of the southwest, especially southern California, New Mexico, Arizona, and northern Mexico.*
- *Cause of "San Joaquin Valley Fever"; the primary infection is often self-limited; it may cause acute or chronic pneumonia; disseminated infection occurs in immunocompromised hosts.*
- *Definitive diagnosis is made by the presence of spherule in or positive culture from involved tissue. Presumptive diagnosis is based on serological testing.*

General Considerations

Coccidioidomycosis is a disease caused by the dimorphic fungus, *Coccidioides immitis*. *C immitis* is endemic to the southwestern United States, primarily the San Joaquin Valley in southern California, southern Arizona, and New Mexico, and west Texas. Coccidioidomycosis occurs outside of the United States in northern Mexico and Central and South America. Coccidioidomycosis may occur in nonendemic regions when individuals are diagnosed with primary infection or reactivation disease upon return from travel to endemic areas. Exposure to *C immitis* in nonendemic regions occurs when spores are carried to distant locations on fomites, fresh fruits and vegetables, or automobiles. In the past 20 years, coccidioidomycosis has become an important cause of opportunistic infection in immunocompromised individuals, particularly those with HIV infection.

Pathogenesis

C immitis thrives in the soil of the Southwest, particularly the San Joaquin Valley and lower Sonoran Desert. Increased infection rates have been documented after rainy seasons, dust storms, and earthquakes, which cause spores to be aerosolized and blown for many miles. Archaeologists and construction workers are at increased risk for infection. Inhaled spores deposit in pulmonary alveoli where they enlarge and develop into large spherules containing endospores. Spherules rupture and release these endospores, beginning the cycle again. Pneumonitis develops at the site of infection with the initial inflammatory response comprised of macrophages, neutrophils, and lymphocytes. Spherules, however, are relatively resistant to phagocytosis and oxidative killing. Resolution of primary infection correlates with the development of T cell immunity. Individuals with impaired cell-mediated immunity may develop progressive primary infection or reactivation of latent disease.

Clinical Findings

A. SYMPTOMS AND SIGNS

Although *C immitis* produces approximately 100,000 new infections per year, 60% of infected individuals are asymptomatic or have subclinical disease.

1. Acute pulmonary coccidioidomycosis—Acute pulmonary coccidioidomycosis may cause influenza-like symptoms and subacute pneumonitis 1–3 weeks after exposure. Fever, fatigue, headache, arthralgias, dry cough, dyspnea, and pleuritic chest pain are common symptoms, sometimes referred to as "San Joaquin Valley Fever." Immune-mediated erythema nodosum, erythema multiforme, and arthritis, called "desert rheumatism," occur in 20% of patients. This must be differentiated from true septic arthritis caused by *C immitis*. Acute coccidioidomycosis resolves spontaneously in the vast majority of those exposed. Progression of acute infection to severe pneumonia and respiratory failure develops in some patients; this is more likely to occur in immunocompromised patients or after inhalation of high titers of organisms.

2. Persistent pulmonary coccidioidal nodules and cavities—Of infected individuals 5–10% have sequelae of acute infection, most commonly evolution of pneumonia to a solitary pulmonary nodule or thin-walled cavity. Pulmonary nodules are often found incidentally, with the patient and clinician unaware of prior *C immitis* infection, and cancer may be suspected. *C immitis* cavities are often asymptomatic and up to 50% resolve spontaneously within 2 years. Enlarging cavities may produce symptoms such as cough, chest pain, and hemoptysis. Mycetomas ("fungus balls") comprised of *Aspergillus* or *C immitis* can form within cavities and cause intermittent, but rarely life-threatening, hemoptysis. Pyopneumothorax, a rare complication, results from cavity rupture into the pleural space producing dyspnea and chest pain.

3. Chronic progressive pulmonary coccidioidomycosis—Patients with diabetes mellitus are more prone to develop chronic pneumonia, although there is often an absence of apparent underlying risk factors. Symptoms are subacute and include fever, productive cough, weight loss, pleuritic chest pain, and hemoptysis.

Symptoms and signs are often attributed incorrectly to tuberculosis or cancer.

4. Disseminated coccidioidomycosis—Disseminated coccidioidomycosis occurs in <1% of infected immunocompetent individuals. Persons of African or Filipino descent, men, pregnant women, and individuals with HIV infection, diabetes mellitus, or receiving steroids are at greater risk for disseminated infection. The most common sites of dissemination are skin, bones/joints, lungs, and CNS. Approximately 30% of patients with disseminated infection have single organ spread to the CNS. Coccidioides meningitis, although rare, is rapidly fatal without treatment.

B. Laboratory Findings and Diagnosis

Diagnosis of *C immitis* infection is usually based on histopathological examination and culture of purulent clinical specimen. Sputum, BAL fluid, synovial fluid, or skin biopsy is more likely to yield growth of the organism. Blood, cerebrospinal fluid (CSF), and pleural or peritoneal fluids are less likely to be culture positive. In the presence of cavitary lung disease, fresh sputum specimens collected on two to three consecutive days show a high yield. In the absence of sputa, BAL, transbronchial biopsy, percutaneous lung biopsy, or open lung biopsy may obtain culture specimen. Pleural biopsy is usually required to diagnose pleural disease. It is imperative to notify laboratory personnel when coccidioidomycosis is suspected so that precautions may be instituted when handling patient specimens. *C immitis* reverts back to the highly infectious mold form when cultured, thus care must be taken to prevent aerosolization and accidental exposures in the laboratory.

On histopathological examination of tissue, the presence of the typical giant spherule of *C immitis* containing multiple endospores is diagnostic of infection. Serological testing for coccidioidomycosis, in contrast to blastomycosis or histoplasmosis, may be helpful. Serum immunoglobulin M (IgM) antibodies are detected in up to 75% of individuals in the first 4 weeks of symptomatic primary infection. Serum immunoglobulin G (IgG) antibodies become evident after 2 weeks of infection. The IgG response persists for 6–8 months and should fall with therapy. IgG antibodies remain positive in chronic pulmonary coccidioidomycosis and rising titers predict worsening disease, such as dissemination or relapse.

C. Imaging Studies

Primary *C immitis* infection is characterized by lower respiratory tract infection. Chest radiographs in acute pulmonary coccidioidomycosis demonstrate a single parenchymal infiltrate in 60–70% of individuals. Patchy alveolar infiltrates or multilobar involvement also occur. Pleural effusions or hilar adenopathy occur in up to 20% of those infected. Adenopathy can persist for many months and be mistaken for lymphoma or bronchogenic cancer. Pulmonary infiltrates in the majority of acute infections evolve into peripherally located, thin-walled, solitary cavities or nodules. Sometimes cavities persist and exhibit air-fluid levels intermittently. A pleural air-fluid level may be seen when enlarging or subpleural cavities rupture into the pleural space. Cavity rupture may also lead to formation of a bronchopleural fistula. Chronic progressive pulmonary coccidioidomycosis may present with lobar consolidation, pleural effusion, or an upper lobe cavitary infiltrate, mimicking tuberculosis. Reticulonodular infiltrates or a miliary pattern may be seen with disseminated infection, often in patients with severe underlying immunosuppression.

Treatment

Most immunocompetent patients with primary pulmonary coccidioidomycosis require no therapy other than close clinical and radiographic follow-up to ensure resolution of infection. Patients with progressive or severe primary infection, persistence of symptoms for more than 6–8 weeks, or multilobar involvement warrant treatment. All cases of disseminated coccidioidomycosis should be treated. Individuals with underlying chronic diseases (diabetes mellitus, asthma, COPD), immune impairment (eg, HIV infection, hematological cancer, organ transplant, or pregnancy) should be treated. Consideration should be given to treating other groups at increased risk for dissemination, such as infants and nonwhite individuals. Laboratory personnel with accidental exposure to a large inoculum of spores should be treated. High antibody titers (>1:16 or >1:32) predict dissemination and are considered an indication for therapy.

Asymptomatic coccidioidal nodules do not require treatment in immunocompetent hosts. Asymptomatic cavities should be monitored as many resolve in the absence of treatment. When cavities become symptomatic, causing persistent local pain or hemoptysis, surgical intervention may be required. Antifungal therapy alone does not heal cavities or ameliorate symptoms produced by them. Surgical resection is also necessary when a cavity is enlarging and rupture into the pleural space is imminent. Pyopneumothorax from cavity rupture may require lobectomy and decortication in addition to systemic antifungal therapy.

Galgiani JN: Coccidioidomycosis: a regional disease of national importance. Rethinking approaches for control. Ann Intern Med 1999;130:293. [PMID: 10068388]. (Dr. Galgiani is the Cocci-guru; this article reviews the epidemiology and groups at risk for coccidioidomycosis.)

Galgiani JN et al: Practice guidelines for the treatment of coccidioidomycosis. Infectious Diseases Society of America. Clin Infect Dis 2000;30:658. [PMID: 10770727]. (A must read for anyone who treats coccidioidomycosis.)

Stevens DA: Coccidioidomycosis. N Engl J Med 1995;332:1077. [PMID: 7898527]. (A classic article for anyone's journal collection.)

PARACOCCIDIOIDOMYCOSIS

 ESSENTIALS OF DIAGNOSIS

- *Also referred to as "South American blastomycosis," it is an important cause of systemic fungal infection in Latin America.*
- *Primary site of infection is the respiratory tract; it can disseminate to skin, mucous membranes, lymph nodes, and adrenal glands.*
- *Diagnosis is based on culture of involved tissue or presence of characteristically shaped budding yeast on histopathology.*

General Considerations

Paracoccidioidomycosis is a disease caused by the dimorphic fungus, *Paracoccidioides brasiliensis*. The epidemiology of *P brasiliensis* is not completely understood. Paracoccidioidomycosis is restricted geographically to Central and South America from Mexico to Argentina. Chile and some Caribbean islands are excluded. The environmental source of *P brasiliensis* is unknown. Soil isolation of the fungus has been rare. Infection occurs almost exclusively in young and middle-aged men. Malnutrition and alcoholism are predisposing risk factors. Infection has been reported outside of endemic regions, suggesting a long latency period, perhaps decades, between acquiring the infection and developing overt disease. There is no evidence of person-to-person transmission.

Pathogenesis

P brasiliensis infection is likely acquired through inhalation from an environmental source. Most infections are probably asymptomatic or subclinical in immunocompetent hosts, although symptomatic disease does occur with both primary and reactivated infection. Lympho-hematogenous dissemination is likely to occur during primary infection, with fungi becoming dormant in the reticuloendothelial system and other organs of the body. Immunocompromised individuals, including those with advanced HIV infection, are more likely to develop severe forms of primary and disseminated disease, or reactivation of latent infection.

Clinical Findings

A. SYMPTOMS AND SIGNS

The most common sites of infection with *P brasiliensis* are the lungs, skin, mucous membranes, lymph nodes, and adrenal glands.

1. Pulmonary paracoccidioidomycosis—Pulmonary paracoccidioidomycosis may manifest as acute or subacute pneumonia resulting from either primary or reactivated infection. Typical symptoms include fever, productive cough, dyspnea, chest pain, hemoptysis, and weight loss.

2. Disseminated paracoccidioidomycosis—Disseminated paracoccidioidomycosis presents most commonly with ulcerated lesions of the lips, mouth, tongue, and palate. Ulcerations and edema of the nasopharynx or larynx may cause vocal cord damage. Granulomatous lesions of the skin, usually the face, may be ulcerated, wart-like, crusted, or necrotic. Massive lymphadenopathy, with formation of draining sinuses, is common. Dissemination to adrenal glands may cause adrenal insufficiency. Chronic pneumonia may be seen with disseminated forms of the disease. Other sites of involvement include liver, spleen, gastrointestinal tract, bones, and CNS.

B. LABORATORY FINDINGS AND DIAGNOSIS

P brasiliensis may be detected in clinical specimens by histopathological examination and culture. Single or multiple expectorated sputum specimens may reveal the fungus after digestion with KOH. The characteristic yeast form is the spherical parent cell with multiple daughter cells budding from it, similar to a "pilot wheel on a ship." Serological testing by gel immunodiffusion may be useful for diagnosing paracoccidioidomycosis. This test has both high sensitivity and specificity for detecting serum antibodies to *P brasiliensis*. Complement fixation (CF) allows measurement of antibody titers and may provide better assessment of therapeutic response. False-positive CF results may be seen with histoplasmosis.

C. IMAGING STUDIES

Lung infection with *P brasiliensis* may reveal nodular infiltrates or focal consolidation on chest radiograph. Lesions are often bilateral and affect predominantly the central and lower lung fields. Cavitation or hilar adenopathy may also develop. As pneumonia progresses from a subacute to chronic form, pulmonary fibrosis leads to chronic respiratory insufficiency. Cor pulmonale may arise as a result of restrictive lung disease.

Treatment

Paracoccidioidomycosis responds to treatment with amphotericin B, the azole antifungals, or sulfa-based antibiotics. Oral trimethoprim-sulfamethoxazole should be given at high doses for 6–9 months, followed by maintenance doses for 3–5 years to prevent disease relapse. Alternatively, oral itraconazole (100–200 mg/day) may be administered for 6 or more months depending on response to therapy. Amphotericin B is reserved for severe forms of disease or when there is no response to other antibiotics. Oral maintenance therapy should follow treatment with amphotericin B.

Lortholary O et al: Endemic mycoses: a treatment update. J Antimicrob Chemother 1999;43:321. [PMID: 10223586]. (Paracoccidioidomycosis is briefly covered here.)

PENICILLIOSIS

 ESSENTIALS OF DIAGNOSIS

- *Acquired immunodeficiency syndrome (AIDS)-defining illness in Southeast Asia.*
- *Causes pneumonia, skin lesions, lymphadenopathy, and bone marrow suppression; mimics tuberculosis (TB) or histoplasmosis.*
- *Diagnosed by culture of blood or involved tissue.*

General Considerations

Penicilliosis, a disease caused by the dimorphic fungus *Penicillium marneffei*, is endemic to Thailand, Hong Kong and Southern China, Malaysia, and Vietnam. The majority of those infected are men who are immunocompromised. In endemic regions of Southeast Asia, penicilliosis is considered an AIDS-defining illness and is the third most common opportunistic infection following tuberculosis and cryptococcosis. Infection in the United States may be diagnosed in Southeast Asian immigrants, individuals from nonendemic countries who travel to Southeast Asia, Vietnam War veterans, or other military personnel. Bamboo rats are carriers of *P marneffei* but not an apparent source of transmission to humans. A common environmental source, such as soil, may serve to infect both rats and humans.

Pathogenesis

P marneffei is highly infectious and, although not definitively established, is likely inhaled, ingested, or directly inoculated into skin. The lungs, skin, and reticuloendothelial system are affected in disseminated penicilliosis. Tissue reaction in involved organs may be granulomatous, suppurative, or necrotizing. Immunocompetent individuals are more likely to develop granulomatous or suppurative forms of the disease. Cell-mediated immunity is important in controlling infection.

Clinical Findings

A. SYMPTOMS AND SIGNS

Penicilliosis may cause localized or disseminated disease that develops weeks to years after infection. Reactivation of latent disease is common. Typical symptoms include fever, weight loss, dry cough, pleuritic chest pain, and diarrhea. Physical examination may reveal generalized lymphadenopathy and hepatosplenomegaly. Skin lesions, prominent on the face, trunk, and arms, may be papular, pustular, or nodular. Genital ulcers, pericarditis, meningitis, and osteomyelitis have also been reported.

B. LABORATORY FINDINGS AND DIAGNOSIS

Anemia is a common laboratory abnormality. Blood cultures may yield growth of *P marneffei*. In the absence of positive blood cultures, sputum, skin lesions, bone marrow, or lymph node tissue should be examined histologically and cultured. Small, oval-shaped, intracellular and extracellular yeast-like organisms are seen with special fungal staining. Differentiation from *H capsulatum* is necessary.

C. IMAGING STUDIES

Pneumonia is a common manifestation of *P marneffei* infection and may result from localized infection or disseminated disease. Infection may involve any portion of the lung. Chest radiograph findings include lobar infiltrates, nodular densities, abscess, or cavitation.

Treatment

Untreated penicilliosis is associated with a 90–100% mortality rate. Treatment with intravenous amphotericin B followed by oral itraconazole is very effective for severe disease. Oral itraconazole alone may be used in cases of mild disease. Itraconazole has been shown to be superior to fluconazole in clinical studies. The extended spectrum azoles, voriconazole and posaconazole, have been shown to have good *in vitro* activity, but *in vivo* data are lacking. Chronic suppressive therapy with oral itraconazole (200 mg/day) is recommended to prevent relapse in HIV-seropositive patients.

Duong TA: Infection due to *Penicillium marneffei*, an emerging pathogen: review of 155 reported cases. Clin Infect Dis 1996;23:125. [PMID: 8816141]. (A landmark article.)

Supparatpinyo K et al: A controlled trial of itraconazole to prevent relapse of *Penicillium marneffei* infection in patients infected with human immunodeficiency virus. N Engl J Med 1998;339:1739. [PMID: 9845708]. (Itraconazole prevents relapse in HIV seropositive patients treated for penicilliosis.)

SPOROTRICHOSIS

 ## ESSENTIALS OF DIAGNOSIS

- *Pulmonary sporotrichosis is rare.*
- *Sporotrichosis may cause chronic pneumonia in elderly men with obstructive lung disease or pneumonia with disseminated infection in immunocompromised individuals.*
- *Diagnosis is based on culture of involved tissue; histopathology demonstrates typical cigar-shaped yeast forms.*

General Considerations

Sporotrichosis is a disease caused by the dimorphic fungus *Sporothrix schenckii*. Infection manifests commonly as lymphocutaneous or osteoarticular infection following direct traumatic inoculation, but pneumonia is rare. *S schenckii* is associated with soil, decaying vegetation, sphagnum moss, and hay. Individuals with outdoor vocations or hobbies are most commonly affected.

Clinical Findings

Pulmonary infection likely develops with aerosolization and inhalation of *S schenckii* spores from soil. Middle-aged, alcoholic men with obstructive lung disease are at risk for developing chronic pneumonia. Fever, night sweats, fatigue, weight loss, productive cough, chest pain, and hemoptysis are common symptoms. Apical cavitary lesions on chest radiograph may resemble tuberculosis. If untreated, chronic pulmonary sporotrichosis leads to progressive symptoms and respiratory insufficiency.

Disseminated sporotrichosis usually presents with widespread cutaneous disease in immunocompromised hosts, but visceral dissemination to lungs, bones, joints, and CNS can occur. Alcoholism, diabetes mellitus, and advanced HIV infection are risk factors for dissemination.

Isolation of organisms from infected sites is necessary to diagnose sporotrichosis. Sputum cultures may be positive in chronic cavitary pneumonia. Histopathological examination of tissue specimens reveals typical cigar-shaped yeast forms.

Treatment

Amphotericin B or itraconazole are both effective for pulmonary sporotrichosis. However, surgical resection of cavitary lesions may be required to improve cure rates. Disseminated sporotrichosis in immunocompromised hosts is usually treated with intravenous amphotericin B followed by oral itraconazole after clinical improvement. Chronic, perhaps lifelong, suppression may be necessary for individuals with advanced HIV infection.

Kauffman CA: Sporotrichosis. Clin Infec Dis 1999;29:231. [PMID: 10476718]. (Overall, a very thorough review and interesting read.)

Kauffman CA et al: Practice guidelines for the management of patients with sporotrichosis. For the Mycosis Study Group. Infectious Diseases Society of America. Clin Infect Dis 2000;30:684. [PMID: 10770730]. (Guidelines with recommendations for treatment of various forms of sporotrichosis.)

ASPERGILLOSIS

 ## ESSENTIALS OF DIAGNOSIS

- *There are three forms of disease: allergic, saprophytic, and invasive; the lungs are a major site for infection.*
- *Invasive aspergillosis is associated with high morbidity and mortality in immunocompromised hosts.*
- *Establishing a definitive diagnosis of invasive disease may be difficult and often comes late in the course of illness.*

General Considerations

Aspergillus is a ubiquitous mold that usually causes disease in immunocompromised hosts. Most infections are caused by *Aspergillus fumigatus*, but species such as *A flavus* and *A niger* are also occasionally pathogenic. Pulmonary manifestations include allergic, saprophytic, and invasive forms.

Pathogenesis

Allergic forms of aspergillosis result from an immunological reaction directed against *Aspergillus* antigens that are inhaled into the upper and lower respiratory tract. No direct tissue invasion occurs. The allergic response in allergic bronchopulmonary aspergillosis is IgE mediated. *Aspergillus* takes a saprophytic form when it colonizes a preexisting lung cavity or the airways of children with cystic fibrosis and bronchiectasis. A mass of hyphae, an aspergilloma, forms within the cavity. Invasive aspergillosis, the most severe form of disease, occurs predominantly in immunocompromised patients. Invasive infection generally complicates neutropenia or defective neutrophil function, as seen in patients with hematological cancer or bone marrow transplantation. However, other conditions also pose a risk for infection including solid organ transplantation, chronic steroid use, systemic lupus erythematosus, and HIV infection.

Clinical Findings

A. SYMPTOMS AND SIGNS

1. Allergic bronchopulmonary aspergillosis (ABPA)—*Aspergillus* does not cause invasive disease, but rather the presence of *Aspergillus*, usually *A fumigatus*, in the airways stimulates an allergic response. Bronchospasm or asthma-like symptoms result from IgE-mediated type 1 hypersensitivity reactions. ABPA may worsen the bronchospasm of preexisting asthma or complicate cystic fibrosis. Low grade fever, dyspnea, wheezing, and cough are common symptoms. Affected patients frequently expectorate brown mucous plugs.

2. Aspergilloma—The saprophytic form of aspergillosis is referred to as an aspergilloma when *Aspergillus* colonizes a preexisting lung cavity, such as from old tuberculosis, histoplasmosis, healed lung abscess, or sarcoidosis. *Aspergillus* spores, after being inhaled into a lung cavity, replicate and mix with fibrin, mucous, and cellular debris forming a fungus ball. Children and adolescents with cystic fibrosis may develop *Aspergillus* colonization of bronchiectatic airways. Aspergillomas are often asymptomatic and detected incidentally on chest radiographs. Aspergillomas produce symptoms when local replication leads to erosion into adjacent bronchial arteries. Semiinvasive or invasive aspergillomas have

also been described. Symptoms in these conditions result from direct invasion into surrounding lung parenchyma or from the inflammatory process extending into adjacent lung tissue and pleura. The most common symptom associated with an aspergilloma is hemoptysis, which may be mild or progressively fatal. Life-threatening hemoptysis occurs in 20–30% of patients. Other less severe symptoms include chest pain and cough.

3. Invasive pulmonary aspergillosis—Invasive pulmonary aspergillosis has an extremely high mortality rate. Individuals with prolonged (more than 10–12 days) and significant [absolute neutrophil count (ANC) <500 cells/mm^3, especially ANC <100 cells/mm^3] neutropenia from hematological cancer or bone marrow transplantation are at greatest risk, but other immunodeficiency disorders also predispose to infection. Invasive aspergillosis may cause infection in any organ after hematogenous dissemination from the lungs. However, 60% of patients have disease localized only to the lungs. Symptoms are frequently insidious in onset, occurring over days to months. Fever, dry cough, dyspnea, and pleuritic chest pain are common. Other than fever, tachypnea, and sometimes hypoxia, the physical examination is usually normal. The angioinvasiveness of *Aspergillus* may cause mild hemoptysis or fatal pulmonary hemorrhage. *Aspergillus* may also cause necrotizing tracheobronchitis, rhinosinusitis, or CNS infection in high-risk patients. Symptoms of tracheobronchitis include fever, chest pain, productive cough, and often hemoptysis.

B. LABORATORY FINDINGS AND DIAGNOSIS

Patients with asthma and characteristic fleeting pulmonary infiltrates or central bronchiectasis on chest radiographs may have ABPA. Other criteria for diagnosing ABPA include peripheral eosinophilia, increased serum IgE levels, and immediate wheal and flare skin reactivity to *Aspergillus* antigens. *A fumigatus* or other *Aspergillus* species are frequently cultured from sputum.

Finding a fungus ball within a cavity on chest radiograph or CT is often sufficient to diagnose aspergilloma, although other molds and sometimes bacteria may colonize cavities. Although rarely necessary, positively identifying *Aspergillus* within a lung cavity may be made by sputum culture or examination of tissue obtained by biopsy or surgical resection.

Definitive diagnosis of invasive aspergillosis requires histopathology that demonstrates characteristic acute-angle branching, septated hyphae, and culture confirmation. Blood cultures are seldom positive. Sputum cultures lack sensitivity, but have high specificity in neutropenic patients. Sputum cultures in immunocompetent hosts are not specific and often represent benign airway colonization. BAL fluid has high specificity in immunocompromised patients, but sensitivity varies depending on the underlying disease and the extent of radiographic abnormalities. BAL fluid yields a diagnosis in 30–70% of patients with invasive aspergillosis and underlying neutropenia. Transbronchial biopsy may be falsely negative due to sampling error and bronchial brushings add little to the sensitivity of BAL. Occasionally percutaneous or open lung biopsy is required for diagnosis. The safety of these procedures is often limited, however, by potential bleeding related to the thrombocytopenia that frequently accompanies hematological cancers. A presumptive diagnosis of invasive aspergillosis is frequently made based on clinical suspicion and radiographic findings, especially high-resolution CT.

Infection is often diagnosed late because symptoms are insidious in onset and standardized, noninvasive diagnostic tests are not available. These factors contribute directly to the high mortality rate observed with this infection. Promising developments have been made recently in serodiagnosis and polymerase chain reaction (PCR)-based methodologies. Galactomannan, a component of the cell wall of *Aspergillus*, can be detected by enzyme-linked immunosorbent assay (ELISA) in the serum of patients at earlier stages of infection. Some studies have shown good sensitivity and specificity (>90%) of this test for early diagnosis of invasive aspergillosis in high-risk populations. PCR-based assays that measure *Aspergillus* DNA are also under intense investigation. These non-culture-based tests, although currently investigational in the United States, may allow earlier initiation of therapy and improve outcomes.

C. Imaging Studies

Bilateral, usually upper lobe, interstitial infiltrates are often seen on chest radiograph or CT in ABPA. These infiltrates may be fleeting or wax and wane, depending on the severity of symptoms. Chronic inflammation leads to central bronchiectasis and pulmonary fibrosis. A pulmonary aspergilloma appears as a round density within a cavity, usually apical, on chest radiograph or chest CT. A clue to the presence of an aspergilloma is a crescent sign created by air between the superior aspect of the aspergilloma and the wall of the cavity. Pleural thickening may occur adjacent to peripheral lesions.

Chest radiographs are abnormal in 90% of patients with invasive pulmonary aspergillosis, but are often nondiagnostic due to other infections or conditions that produce similar findings. Chest CT abnormalities precede those seen on plain radiographs. High-resolution CT offers an advantage over routine chest CT for earlier presumptive diagnosis of invasive aspergillosis. Radiographic findings include diffuse interstitial infiltrates, wedge-shaped or lobar consolidation, nodular densities, and pleural effusion. The earliest finding may be a small pleural-based nodule with a halo sign, seen as an area of low attenuation surrounding the nodular lesion. Late findings include cavitation of consolidated or nodular lesions and an "air crescent" sign, representing infarcted and contracted lung tissue.

Treatment

The primary treatment of ABPA consists of oral corticosteroids to decrease bronchospasm and tissue inflammation. Antifungal therapy may also play a role in treating ABPA by eradicating *Aspergillus* from the airways. In one randomized, placebo-controlled trial, oral itraconazole was effective in the treatment of ABPA and was useful as a corticosteroid-sparing agent. ABPA patients treated with itraconazole had improved exercise tolerance and pulmonary function, and a reduction in serum IgE levels and steroid dose.

Asymptomatic aspergilloma generally requires no therapeutic intervention. However, semiinvasive or invasive aspergillomas benefit from antifungal therapy. Inhaled, intracavitary, and systemic antifungal therapies have been tried, but data obtained from randomized, controlled trials are lacking. Hemoptysis may be ameliorated by bronchial artery embolization. Although bleeding often recurs after 1–2 years, it is the treatment of choice in patients deemed poor surgical candidates due to severe underlying diffuse lung disease. Definitive treatment for symptomatic aspergillomas is surgical resection, particularly when life-threatening hemoptysis develops. Surgery, however, is associated with significant morbidity and mortality in patients with severe chronic lung disease.

Mortality of untreated invasive aspergillosis in immunocompromised hosts is nearly 100%; treatment is associated with a complete or partial response in only 30%. Therefore, it is imperative to begin systemic antifungal therapy in this population if invasive aspergillosis is suspected. Investigation to establish the diagnosis of invasive aspergillosis should continue even after empiric antifungal therapy has been started.

Intravenous therapy is preferred with amphotericin B being the standard first-line agent. Lipid-based formulations of amphotericin B should be given to patients with underlying renal insufficiency or intolerance to conventional amphotericin B. Lipid-based agents are at least equivalent in efficacy to conventional amphotericin B. To date, no prospective, randomized, controlled study has proven superiority of the lipid preparations. It has also not been established that higher doses (>5 mg/kg/day) of lipid-based amphotericin B are more effective than lower doses in humans. Limited studies suggest that itraconazole, available in both the intravenous and oral route, may be a suitable alternative to amphotericin B. Most clinicians initiate treatment with amphotericin B, followed by oral itraconazole for prolonged treatment once a patient's condition has improved.

The echinocandins (eg, caspofungin) and extended spectrum azoles (eg, voriconazole and posaconazole) may play a larger role in the treatment of invasive aspergillosis in the future. These agents may replace amphotericin B as preferred first-line therapy for invasive aspergillosis because of better efficacy and tolerance. Results from comparative trials are only preliminary. Another promising area of research involves combining antifungal agents with different mechanisms of action to improve outcome (eg, amphotericin B plus an echinocandin or an azole plus an echinocandin). Surgical resection of isolated pulmonary lesions has been successful in some cases, but operative risks are significant. Adjuvant therapies, such as colony-stimulating factors (CSF) (granulocyte-CSF or granulocyte–macrophage-CSF), interferon-γ, or related-donor white blood cell transfusions, enhance fungal cell killing but are not recommended for routine use at this time.

Patterson T et al: Invasive aspergillosis: disease spectrum, treatment practices, and outcomes. 13 Aspergillus Study Group. Medicine 2000;79:250. [PMID: 10941354]. (Questionnaire-based survey; good clinical statistics on *Aspergillus* infections.)

Stevens DA et al: A randomized trial of itraconazole in allergic bronchopulmonary aspergillosis. N Engl J Med 2000; 342:756. [PMID: 10717010]. (Randomized trial suggesting patients with ABPA treated with itraconazole require less corticosteroid.)

Stevens DA et al: Practice guidelines for diseases caused by *Aspergillus*. Infectious Diseases Society of America. Clin Infect Dis 2000;30:696. [PMID: 10770732]. (A must read for anyone who treats *Aspergillus* infections; good review of diagnostic modalities.)

CRYPTOCOCCOSIS

 ESSENTIALS OF DIAGNOSIS

- *Associated with pigeon droppings.*
- *Inhalation into lungs where it may cause asymptomatic or subclinical infection or pneumonia.*
- *Spontaneous healing is common in immunocompetent hosts; dissemination (especially to the meninges) occurs frequently in immunocompromised hosts.*
- *Diagnosis is based on culture of sputa, BAL fluid, lung, CSF, or skin tissue or presence of large encapsulated yeast forms on histopathology.*
- *Presumptive diagnosis is based on positive serum or CSF cryptococcal antigen assay.*

General Considerations

Cryptococcosis refers to a disease caused by the fungus *Cryptococcus neoformans*. *C neoformans* is abundant in dried pigeon droppings found in soil, bird roosting sites, old towers, barns, and stables. It has been isolated from the excrement of chickens, parrots, sparrows, starlings, and canaries, but does not cause avian infection. It has been cultured from the beaks and feet of pigeons suggesting that birds act as mechanical carriers. There is no defined geographic focus for *C neoformans*; cryptococcosis occurs throughout the United States and the world. Person-to-person spread of infection does not occur.

Pathogenesis

Dried yeast cells of *C neoformans* are inhaled and deposited into pulmonary alveoli. Yeast cells rehydrate in the lung and acquire the thick polysaccharide capsule that helps *C neoformans* resist phagocytic killing. Cell-mediated immunity is important in limiting infection to the respiratory tract. Immunocompetent hosts may clear infection spontaneously. However, individuals with impaired immune defenses are prone to developing cryptococcal pneumonia and/or disseminated infection. The meninges are the most common site of extrapulmonary dissemination, followed by blood, skin, bone, and genitourinary tract.

Clinical Findings

A. SYMPTOMS AND SIGNS

The presentation of cryptococcal lung infection is highly variable, ranging from asymptomatic illness to severe pneumonia progressing to the acute respiratory distress syndrome. *C neoformans* may act as a saprophyte, colonizing airways of patients with COPD and producing mild respiratory symptoms. Cryptococcal pneumonia may develop in normal hosts, but severe infection occurs more commonly in immunocompromised patients. More than 90% of individuals have an underlying debilitating condition or immunodeficiency and 40% of these have concurrent extrapulmonary infection. Absolute CD4+ T cell counts are usually <50 cells/mm^3 in HIV-seropositive patients who develop cryptococcosis.

Symptoms associated with pulmonary cryptococcosis may take weeks to months to develop and include fever, malaise, weight loss, dyspnea, chest pain, and cough. Hemoptysis is rare. Headache associated with respiratory symptoms suggests concomitant cryptococcal meningitis.

B. LABORATORY FINDINGS AND DIAGNOSIS

No specific laboratory findings suggest cryptococcal disease and patients often deny exposure to pigeon droppings or bird habitats. Diagnosis of cryptococcal pneumonia is made by histopathological examination and culture of sputum, BAL fluid, or lung tissue. Blood, cerebrospinal fluid (CSF), or skin lesions aid in diagnosing disseminated infection. A large, encapsulated yeast form of *C neoformans* is typically found on histopathological examination.

The non-culture-based latex agglutination test is highly sensitive and specific for cryptococcal infection. This test quantitates the amount of cryptococcal capsular polysaccharide antigen present in blood or CSF. The assay has >90% sensitivity in serum from patients with moderate to severe pneumonia or disseminated infection. False-negative results can occur if the test is performed early in infection, when fungal burden is very low, or in cases of isolated pulmonary disease. False-negative results may also occur when the fungal burden is large. Further dilution of the specimen is required in this situation, especially when clinical suspicion for cryptococcosis is high.

C. IMAGING STUDIES

Radiographic findings in pulmonary cryptococcosis are nonspecific and varied. Chest radiographs may demonstrate alveolar or interstitial infiltrates, lobar consolidation, abscess, nodular lesions, a miliary pattern, hilar adenopathy, or pleural effusions. Some patients have more than one type of lesion on radiograph. Spontaneous resolution of radiographic abnormalities prior to the initiation of antifungal therapy has been described.

Treatment

All patients with pulmonary and extrapulmonary cryptococcosis must undergo lumbar puncture to exclude concomitant CNS infection. Asymptomatic immunocompetent patients with only pulmonary disease may be monitored clinically. Alternatively, treatment with fluconazole (200–400 mg/day for 3–6 months) may be given. Duration of therapy should be extended to 6–12 months for mild to moderate cryptococcal pneumonia. Itraconazole or amphotericin B may be substituted in patients intolerant of fluconazole.

Amphotericin B is first-line therapy for patients with severe pneumonia or underlying immunodeficiency. Oral fluconazole or itraconazole may be used after clinical improvement for long-term treatment.

Lipid formulations of amphotericin B appear equivalent in efficacy to conventional amphotericin B and may be substituted as needed. The echinocandins (eg, caspofungin) have little or no activity *in vitro* against *Cryptococcus*, which limits their use in monotherapy. Extended spectrum azoles (eg, voriconazole and posaconazole) are active against *Cryptococcus*, but comparative clinical studies have not been done.

Saag MS et al: Practice guidelines for the management of cryptococcal disease. Infectious Diseases Society of America. Clin Infect Dis 2000;30:710. [PMID: 10770733]. (Article contains easy to read tables that list treatment regimens based by type of cryptococcal infection and host immune status.)

PULMONARY CANDIDIASIS

Candida pneumonia is rare and is usually diagnosed in patients with hematological cancers and severe immunosuppression. Primary pneumonia may occur following aspiration of *Candida*-laden oropharyngeal secretions but is uncommon. Secondary *Candida* pneumonia usually develops as a result of hematogenous dissemination to the lungs during an episode of candidemia.

Patients on antibiotics, corticosteroids, or mechanical ventilation frequently develop overgrowth of *Candida* in the oropharynx. Cultures of sputa or respiratory specimens contaminated by oral secretions exhibit growth of *Candida*, reflecting benign airway colonization and not true infection. Thus, diagnosis of *Candida* pneumonia cannot be made based on microbiological data alone. When feasible, lung biopsy showing tissue invasion by *Candida* aids in the diagnosis of *Candida* pneumonia.

No treatment guidelines exist specifically for the management of *Candida* pneumonia. Therapy for *Candida* pneumonia should follow treatment guidelines for disseminated candidiasis. Amphotericin B or fluconazole is generally effective, but consideration must be given to the particular *Candida* species causing infection, prior azole exposure, severity of infection, and underlying medical conditions. The echinocandins (eg, caspofungin) and extended spectrum azoles (eg, voriconazole and posaconazole) look promising as therapeutic options, particularly for the treatment of azole-resistant *Candida* species. Clinical studies are ongoing.

Rello J et al: The role of Candida species isolated from bronchoscopic samples in non-neutropenic patients. Chest 1998; 114:146. [PMID: 9674461]. (Concludes that *Candida* is often a respiratory contaminant, not a pathogen.)

Rex JH et al: Practice guidelines for the treatment of candidiasis. Infectious Diseases Society of America. Clin Infect Dis 2000;30:662. [PMID: 10770728]. (Very thorough review that covers much more than just therapy for *Candida* infections.)

PNEUMOCYSTOSIS

Please refer to Chapter 40, "Pulmonary Complications of HIV Disease," for a discussion of *Pneumocystis carinii* pneumonia.

EMERGING OPPORTUNISTIC PATHOGENS

Uncommon fungal pathogens that were once considered to be rare causes of human infection have increased in incidence over the past decade. These pathogens include the *Zygomycetes* (eg, *Mucor* and *Rhizopus*), *Fusarium, Trichosporon, Pseudallescheria,* and *Scedosporium.* The morbidity and mortality associated with these infections are extremely high, particularly in immunocompromised hosts. Unfortunately, this population is at greatest risk for developing overwhelming infection. Pneumonia occurs with disseminated infection. No uniform guidelines exist for optimal management of these infections and susceptibility to any particular antifungal agent is variable.

Perfect JR, Schell WA: The new fungal opportunists are coming. Clin Infect Dis 1996;22:S112. [PMID: 8722837]. (Good overview of the rare, and not so rare anymore, fungal organisms that are on the rise.)

Mycobacterial Diseases of the Lungs 39

Michael D. Iseman, MD

THE MYCOBACTERIA

Mycobacteria are slender, rod-like bacilli. They belong to the order of Actinomycetales, microbes of the soil. The mycobacteria have complex cell walls rich in lipids and waxes. These cell walls are related to several distinctive features including their staining properties and growth rates.

Although classified as gram-positive, the mycobacteria usually do not take up gram stain and thus appear as "ghost" or gram-neutral forms. Classically the mycobacteria have been stained with the red dye, carbol fuchsin, enhanced by heating or alkalinity. So stained, the mycobacteria are resistant to decolorizing with the potent agent acid-alcohol. This has given rise to the designation "acid-fast bacilli," or AFB. Modern laboratories may use the fluorochrome technique employing a dye, auramine-o, which fluoresces yellow when excited by ultraviolet light.

Most species of mycobacteria are characterized by very slow growth on culture media, replicating usually in the range of 18–24 h. Thus, laboratory isolation of mycobacteria usually requires 5–15 days in liquid media and 15–30 days on solid media.

The most common human pathogens are *Mycobacterium tuberculosis* and *M leprae* (Hansen's bacillus, which causes the cutaneous-neural disease leprosy). However, there is an array of related microbes found widely in the soil and water that cause lung and extrapulmonary disease in humans. These latter organisms have been referred to variably as atypical TB, mycobacteria other than TB (MOTT), nontuberculous mycobacteria (NTM) or environmental mycobacteria (EM). In this chapter, "environmental mycobacteria" will be used.

MYCOBACTERIUM TUBERCULOSIS (TB)

ESSENTIALS OF DIAGNOSIS

- *Tuberculosis organisms are spread from human to human but are not exquisitely communicable.*
- *Only 10% of people with normal immune function develop active disease following a primary infection.*
- *Primary tuberculosis is most often a nondescript infiltrate with ipsilateral reactive hilar or mediastinal nodes.*
- *Reactivation tuberculosis is characterized by respiratory symptoms with upper lobe fibronodular infiltrates with or without cavitation.*
- *Tuberculosis is usually limited to the lungs, with lymph nodes and pleura the only common sites of extrapulmonary spread.*
- *Identification of acid-fast organisms by staining or culture is diagnostic of disease.*

Among the mycobacteria there is a group of closely related microbes that is referred to as the "tuberculosis complex." The group includes *M tuberculosis, M bovis, M canetti, M africanum,* and *M microti.* Although the microbes are highly comparable by DNA analysis, they are generally distinguishable in terms of natural reservoirs, human pathogenicity, and transmission patterns. Thus, I believe it is appropriate clinically to preserve the term "tuberculosis" or TB for diseases caused by *M tuberculosis.* Disease caused by other mycobacteria should, I believe, be referred to as "mycobacteriosis" due to "*M x.*"

General Considerations

TB is arguably the most "successful" parasite of humans. The World Health Organization (WHO) estimates that roughly one-third of the world's population or 2 billion persons are infected with *M tuberculosis.* However, the patterns of infection are extremely heterogeneous, ranging from 40–50% of the populations in India, the Philippines, Indonesia, and sub-Saharan Africa to only 5–10% in the United States and some countries in western Europe.

Disease rates generally follow this pattern as well. WHO calculates there were roughly 9 million new cases in 2000. India yielded 1.9 million and China 1.4 million of these cases whereas the United States experienced approximately 16,000. Case rates for TB are referred to as the annual number of new active disease cases per 100,000 population. Rates for selected countries are given in Table 39–1. The high prevalence of infection and disease outside the United States is cen-

Table 39–1. TB morbidity by country, 2000.[1]

Country	Estimated Case Numbers (Million)	Case Rates/100,000
India	1.85	184
China	1.36	102
Indonesia	0.59	280
Nigeria	0.35	305
Philippines	0.25	330
Pakistan	0.25	175
Russian Federation	0.20	130
Vietnam	0.15	66
Thailand	0.09	142

[1]The data are estimated by WHO for these selected countries for the year 2000. By contrast, in 2001 the United States reported 15,900 cases for a case rate of 5.6/100,000 population.

tral to understanding the role of TB in the foreign born in the United States today (see below).

Within the United States TB case rates are also heterogeneous in terms of race, geography, age, and country of origin. Data for 2000 are displayed in Table 39–2. Disparities in case rates by race or ethnicity may be substantially explained by socioeconomic factors including access to or utilization of health care; however,

there may also be genetic differences in innate resistance to this disease.

TB is spread almost exclusively by airborne, human-to-human spread. There are no natural reservoirs for *M tuberculosis* other than humans. Persons most likely to spread TB are those with respiratory tract diseases associated with sputum that is positive on microscopy for AFB; however, a modest proportion of new cases appears to be due to transmission from patients with pulmonary disease that is smear-negative but culture-positive. Patients with cavitary lung disease are of particular concern because cavitation is generally associated with high numbers of bacilli in the respiratory secretions.

TB, in comparison to some other airborne infections, is not usually highly communicable. Transmission typically involves exposure to the source case in an indoor, confined environment for days or weeks. This limited transmissibility is directly related to the portal of entry. TB cannot invade across the respiratory mucous membranes but must be transported through the complex, ramifying bronchial tree to the alveolae. To make this journey, the exhaled particles containing bacilli must undergo dehydration to form tiny particles termed "droplet nuclei." Available evidence suggests these particles are 1 μm or smaller and thus have so little inertial mass that they float with the air rather than impacting on the mucous membrane (where they

Table 39–2. TB cases in the United States, 2000, by race and age.[1]

	Group				
	White	Black	Hispanic	Asian/P.I.	Native American
Case numbers	3674	5162	3805	3451	236
% Total	22	32	23	21	1
Case rates (per 100,000)	1.8	15.1	11.5	32.1	11.3
Cases by age (group)(#/rate per 100,000)					
<5 years	71/0.6	173/6.5	220/6.1	65/7.5	18/10.5
5–14 years	35/0.1	156/2.6	158/2.5	60/3.6	9/2.3
15–24 years	131/0.5	480/8.5	635/11.0	357/23.0	14/3.8
24–44 years	840/1.4	1962/18.5	1445/13.8	1261/34.7	64/10.2
45–64 years	1186/2.4	1593/24.9	852/17.1	940/42.7	75/19.9
65+ years	1411/4.7	795/27.5	495/24.9	768/93.0	56/36.0

[1]"Persons of color" now contribute 78% of the annual TB morbidity. The case rates in these groups are far higher than the white population: blacks 8-fold, Hispanics 6-fold, Asian/Pacific Islanders (P.I.) 18-fold, and Native Americans 6-fold greater. Note that in all groups, rates in ages 5–14 are very low, the so-called "favored age" effect. Case rates in the elderly are increased presumably due to greater risks of exposure to TB in their youth; the relative risk with aging is greatest among the whites.

would be carried out by mucociliary clearance before they could invade or replicate). So, although the usual untreated patient with cavitary lung disease may have up to 10,000,000 bacilli/mL of sputum, the number of infectious particles is far lower. It should be noted that there are variations in transmission patterns (the proportion of contacts infected) among cases that cannot be explained simply by the bacillary burden in the sputum or radiographic extent of disease. Among the potentially relevant variables included are strain virulence and characteristics of the cough or respiratory secretions.

Rarely, TB may be transmitted by aerosols generated from other sources including debridement of soft-tissue wounds, autopsy procedures, or direct inoculation in laboratory or postmortem accidents.

Pathogenesis

Following deposition of the bacillus in the distal airspaces of the lung beyond the distribution of the ciliated epithelium, the microbe *must* be taken up by an alveolar macrophage for invasion to occur. Alveolar macrophages, depending upon genetic factors, provide a variably cordial environment for intracellular replication of the bacilli. For immunologically significant infection to occur, the bacilli must undergo intracellular replication, induce destruction of the engulfing macrophages, and proliferate. This sequence initiates a complex cascade involving mycobacterial antigen presentation by dendritic cells and the attraction and activation of monocyte-derived macrophages, γ/δ T cells, and CD4 and CD8 lymphocytes. Important protective cytokines mediating this process include tumor necrosis factor-α, interferon-γ, and interleukins 1 and 12 (IL-1 and IL-12).

Assuming that a single bacillus induces the primary infection and that the initial host response is incapable of halting bacillary replication, within weeks or months there would be millions of bacilli within the body. The bacilli are presumed to spread in sequence from the primary lung site to the hilar-mediastinal lymph nodes, then via the thoracic lymphatic duct to the subclavian vein, back to the right ventricle, out via the pulmonary artery through the pulmonary circulation, back to the left heart, and ultimately via the systemic circulation through the various organs and tissues of the body.

In most normal hosts, an effective immune response evolves within 3–8 weeks, which results in involution of the lesions at the sites within the lung and throughout the body. This immune response is generally associated with the appearance of a delayed-type hypersensitivity reaction to cell wall proteins of the bacilli. This is responsible for the positive tuberculin skin test, which usually appears 4–12 weeks after infection. However,

this immune response generally is not sufficient to "sterilize" the tissues. Latent foci may persist in the lungs or other organs capable of producing "reactivation"-type disease—either pulmonary or extrapulmonary—months, years, or decades later. Surveys suggest that the majority of TB cases seen in the United States are due to such recrudescence of remote infections.

In some cases the initial host response is not able to cause involution of the infection. In these cases, the patient is said to experience "progressive primary disease." Situations in which this is most likely to occur include infancy or immunosuppressed states including acquired immunodeficiency syndrome (AIDS) (see below). In a considerable proportion of these cases, the disease is disseminated or multifocal.

Clinical Presentation & Diagnosis

TB may present as a pulmonary, extrapulmonary, or disseminated illness, depending primarily on the host's immune response.

A. PULMONARY TB

There are three fairly distinctive pulmonary presentations of TB—"primary," "reactivation," and "miliary" (pleural TB is discussed under extrapulmonary TB).

1. Primary—"Primary" TB is generally recognized in newly infected infants and children, although it may be seen as well in occasional adults and persons with AIDS (see below). The hallmarks of primary-type TB are a parenchymal focus (where the infecting bacillus is presumed to have lodged) and prominent ipsilateral reactive hilar or mediastinal lymphadenopathy. Occasionally a small to moderate pleural effusion may accompany primary TB. The parenchymal focus is generally a nondescript, noncavitary infiltrate. These cases are typically found during contact investigations and are usually associated with the development of a newly positive tuberculin skin test (TST).

2. Reactivation—"Reactivation" or "adult type" TB most commonly consists of upper lobe, fibronodular infiltration with variably present consolidation and/or cavitation. The most common sites are the posterior-apical segments of the right or left upper lobes followed by the superior segments of the lower lobes. Isolated involvement of the anterior segments is exceedingly rare. However, in roughly one-third of human immunodeficiency virus (HIV)-negative adults there is an "atypical" pulmonary presentation with prominent lower lobe disease and sparing of the upper zones (the proportion of "atypical" findings is considerably higher in persons with AIDS, see below). The classic upper lobe disease is believed to be due to hematogenous seeding during the primary infection. Reactivation TB involves the reappearance of symptomatic, radiographically progressive disease following a postprimary hiatus of clinical quiescence. It has been estimated that only 10% of normal hosts will develop active disease following their primary infection. Roughly half of those cases will appear in the first 2–3 years after the infection; the remainder appear sporadically over the remainder of life. Factors increasing the likelihood of active disease include extremes of age or immunocompromised states, the most potent of these being AIDS (see below).

3. Miliary—"Miliary" or disseminated infection in the lungs occurs when there is hematogenous seeding. In the classic picture there are fine, well-demarcated nodules, uniform in size and mindful of millet seeds, initially manifest in the lower lung zones. Early in the course of the illness, they may not be visible on a plain radiograph but are discernible on computed tomographic scanning. Disseminated TB is seen most often in persons in the extremes of age or immune compromised conditions. However, it does occur occasionally in persons who are otherwise "normal hosts." As the miliary process evolves from its early stages, the nodules enlarge, become fluffy, and may even result in diffuse airspace filling that resembles acute respiratory distress syndrome (ARDS). (See *Extrapulmonary TB* below) for more details on miliary disease.

B. Extrapulmonary TB (XPTB)

XPTB embraces all disease outside the tracheobronchial tree and lung parenchyma including laryngeal and pleural disease.

XPTB generally evolves in sites that were infected during the bacillemia of the primary infection. However, certain forms of disease involve other pathways (see below). XPTB, particularly pleurisy, may occur simultaneously with the primary infection, or, more often, as a form of reactivation disease.

In most cases one site or organ is involved. Synchronous pulmonary and XPTB are seen in a distinct minority of cases, less than 10% of the time, except in those with AIDS (see below).

The epidemiological patterns (age, sex, race) differ modestly between various forms of XPTB and pulmonary disease. Particular profiles will be noted by form of XPTB below. XPTB in relationship to HIV infection is discussed in a separate section.

Historically, XPTB comprised about one in six cases observed in the United States during the period 1965–1985. As AIDS began to influence the profile of tuberculosis, XPTB increased in relative incidence until it now comprises nearly one-quarter of the annual morbidity.

Among those without HIV infection the commonest forms of XPTB are pleural and lymph node; others, in terms of descending frequency, include genitouri-nary, bone and joint (including spinal), gastrointestinal, and, less commonly, miliary, pericardial, and meningeal disease.

C. Pleural TB

Pleural TB occurring in association with primary infection presumably evolves secondary to inflammation of the pleural surface abutting the primary pulmonary parenchymal lesion. This has been described as a delayed-type hypersensitivity (DTH) phenomenon rather than true infection. Yet the presence of tubercle bacilli in some of the pleural effusions obscures this distinction. Tuberculous pleurisy occurring in elderly persons generally represents reactivation disease with clear-cut infection of the pleural space.

Clinically, pleural TB usually presents with varying patterns of cough, chest pain (classically "pleuritic" or nonspecific), fever, and dyspnea. Malaise, sweats, and weight loss are associated with longer standing, more extensive disease. Occasionally, asymptomatic pleural TB may be detected on radiography done for other purposes.

Laboratory studies typical of pleural TB include a unilateral effusion of small to moderate extent; sometimes a parenchymal lesion may be seen as well. Leukocytosis or thrombocytosis is uncommon. The TST is falsely negative in a significant proportion of cases. For patients with cough it is appropriate to obtain sputum for smear and culture.

The primary thrust of diagnosis lies with analysis of the pleural fluid and biopsy of the parietal pleura. Thoracentesis typically yields a lymphocytic exudate; rarely a neutrophil dominant pattern is seen. AFB are rarely seen on microscopic examination of the fluid; culture of the fluid is positive in roughly one-half of the proven cases. If the clinical picture and/or pleural fluid analysis are consistent with TB, a biopsy should be done promptly. Generally a closed technique such as a Cope needle is indicated; if the first biopsy is nondiagnostic, a second procedure will increase the diagnostic yield.

D. Lymph Node TB

Lymph node TB most commonly involves the supraclavicular, posterior, or anterior cervical chains, primarily because these nodes drain the thorax. By contrast, lymphadenitis due to environmental mycobacteria predictably involves the preauricular, submandibular, or sublingual nodes, systems that drain the oropharynx. Occasional cases of TB lymphadenitis involve other sites such as axillary or inguinal chains. By contrast, persons with AIDS develop a unique syndrome with disseminated lymphadenitis.

Notable epidemiological features of tuberculous lymphadenitis include the relative predilection for females, particularly those from the Orient and Indian subcontinent.

Distinguishing childhood lymphadenitis due to TB from environmental mycobacteria may be problematic. Too often, cultures have not been done because the objective of the biopsy has been to "rule out cancer." Even if culture is performed, positive results (for TB or EM) are seen in less than 50% of cases. Histopathology is generally similar or indistinguishable. Further, a considerable portion of children with proven EM infection have significant reactions—in the range of 8–15 mm induration—to purified protein derivative of tuberculin (PPD-T). Helpful discriminating features include the nodes involved (see above), race or immigrant status, socioeconomic factors that influence the likelihood of TB exposure, and age. The overwhelming majority of EM lymphadenitis occurs in children, presumably associated with primary exposure to these organisms; hence, mycobacterial lymphadenitis in an adult, even a teenager, is far more likely due to TB.

E. GENITOURINARY TB

Genitourinary TB includes renal, ureteral, bladder, uterine-fallopian, prostatic, and epididymal disease. It is slightly more common in women than men and tends to involve older populations. Generally patients present with "local" symptoms related to irritation or dysfunction of the affected organ(s); constitutional symptoms such as fever, chills, sweats, malaise, or weight loss appear late in the course.

Diagnosis relies on microbiological confirmation, often by culture of urine. Caution must be taken that the patient has not received antibiotics prior to submitting the urinary specimen; due to renal concentration, even penicillin can inhibit the growth of tubercle bacilli in urine.

F. BONE AND JOINT TB

Bone and joint TB most commonly involves weight-bearing structures such as hips, knees, and vertebrae. However, TB can involve virtually any bone including the flat bones of the skull or pelvis. Pathogenesis usually involves reactivation of a focus at a growth plate, a true osteomyelitis. Commonly the infection spreads to a nearby joint resulting in arthritis. In the spine, analogous conditions would be spondylitis and diskitis.

The site of vertebral TB varies rather predictably according to age. In adolescents and young adults mid-to-high thoracic vertebrae are involved. Because the size of the cord more closely approximates the dimension of the spinal canal, there is a more critical risk of cord compression in these higher lesions. By contrast, in middle-aged or older persons, low thoracic or lumbosacral vertebrae are more likely to be involved.

Clinically there usually are minimal constitutional symptoms, even with fairly advanced infection; this has given rise to the description, "cold abscesses." Local pain or a "lump" usually brings the patient to medical attention.

Radiological studies commonly show bony destruction and a surrounding collection in the joint and soft tissue. Diagnosis usually involves needle aspiration and/or biopsy.

Unique aspects of the management of bone–joint/spinal TB include the questions of surgical drainage or stabilization procedures. Debridement is not required to "cure" the infection, but surgery may be important in conserving the function and anatomical integrity of the involved skeleton.

G. MILIARY TB

Miliary TB refers to disseminated infection simultaneously involving several to many organs. "Miliary" refers to the appearance on the chest x-ray; but it should be stressed that in some patients, pulmonary radiographic findings lag behind involvement of other organs. Organs most typically involved include lung, liver, spleen, bone marrow, kidneys, and meninges. Persons at particular risk for disseminated TB include those with AIDS and the immunosuppressed, the young and the elderly, and African-Americans. Clinically the disease may advance slowly or rapidly depending upon the host's immune capacity. Unusual manifestations of miliary TB include bone marrow failure, disseminated intravascular coagulation, noncardiogenic pulmonary edema, or even abrupt cardiovascular collapse mindful of gram-negative sepsis. Diagnosis is usually established by biopsy and microscopic staining for AFB in involved organs; blood cultures are useful only in persons with AIDS. Therapy should be initiated empirically in suspected cases; awaiting culture results entails considerable jeopardy.

H. PERICARDIAL TB

Pericardial TB is believed often to result from invasion via pretracheal lymph nodes that become adherent to the abutting pericardium. Persons at particular risk include those with AIDS and African-Americans. Clinically those with pericarditis typically complain of cough, which may be triggered by pericardial irritation. Dyspnea or exercise limitation may reflect either an effusion or fibrotic constriction. Chest radiography commonly shows diffuse enlargement of the cardiac silhouette; occasionally this may be accompanied by a left pleural effusion. The electrocardiogram usually shows low voltage and ST-segment depression, not the elevations typical of acute pericarditis. Echocardiography is a primary diagnostic tool, indicating the presence of fluid and/or thickening. When pericardial involvement is suspected, either a closed or open biopsy and aspiration is indicated. If there is evidence of pericardial thickening, an open procedure affords the opportunity to perform a simultaneous pericardiectomy. Corticosteroids are useful to acutely decompress hemodynamically significant effusions but do not obviate the need for ongoing surveillance for fibrotic constriction.

I. MENINGEAL TB

Meningeal TB is an uncommon but potentially lethal form of XPTB. It may occur as an isolated phenomenon or as a component of disseminated TB. Classically there is arachnoiditis around the base of the brain. Rarely it is accompanied by a mass lesion in the brain, a "tuberculoma." Early recognition is essential to decrease the risk of irreversible neurological sequelae or death. Typically, meningeal TB presents initially with headache, feverishness, irritability, and stiff neck or back; this is Stage I. As the disease progresses to Stage II, confusion or subtle neurological deficits appear, reflecting cranial nerve entrapment and/or vascular compromise. It is not rare for such patients to be referred for psychiatric evaluation for altered or unusual behavior. Untreated, there is progression to altered consciousness and/or seizures, Stage III. Diagnosis generally is made by lumbar puncture and cerebrospinal fluid (CSF) analysis; caution must be exercised, however, in case of increased intracranial pressure. If the CSF profile is typical for TB, empirically initiating chemotherapy is indicated. Corticosteroids are of clear benefit for those in Stages II or III, and may be appropriate for those in Stage I as well.

The antimicrobial therapy of meningeal TB must take into account differential passage of the various drugs across the blood–brain barrier. In the presence of severe inflammation all agents pass; but as the inflammation subsides, only isoniazid and pyrazinamide achieve consistently high levels in the CSF. Aminoglycosides and ethambutol cross poorly through uninflamed meninges; rifampin passage is intermediate.

J. OTHER FORMS

Other forms of XPTB are diverse and pleomorphic, requiring broad clinical awareness.

Complications

By depleting the numbers and compromising the function of CD4 lymphocytes, HIV infection increases both the risk and severity of TB. Early in the course of HIV infection patients present with typical forms of TB including upper lung zone cavitary disease. But, as immunity wanes, there is a progressive trend toward uncharacteristic pulmonary disease (lower zone infiltrates, prominent hilar adenopathy and large pleural effusions). Also, with low CD4 counts multifocal or disseminated disease emerges.

Treatment of TB in persons with AIDS is complicated primarily by drug–drug interactions related to the rifamycins. Rifampin is an extremely potent inducer of hepatic cytochrome P-450 pathways, accelerating the elimination of many antiretroviral agents as well as various other drugs. Rifabutin, which has less of an effect upon the cytochrome system, may be substituted. The current guidelines continue to support 6-month regimens for TB in persons with AIDS; however, extended treatment is advised for those whose sputum cultures remain positive at or after 2 months of therapy (see below).

Treatment

Multidrug regimens are indicated for all cases of active disease to prevent acquired drug resistance, improve cure rates, and accelerate response to therapy. Replicating tubercle bacilli undergo random, spontaneous mutations that spawn organisms resistant variously to all drugs. These are unlinked chromosomal alterations and they confer resistance to single drugs or classes. These mutations occur at a low frequency, typically in the range of 1 per 1,000,000 to 10,000,000 replications. Because they are unlinked, mutants resistant to "drug A" are killed by "drug B." The risk for acquired resistance is greatest when large numbers of bacilli are proliferating rapidly; examples of this include untreated cavitary lesions or persons with AIDS and extensive TB.

The central drugs in modern regimens include the rifamycins (rifampin, rifabutin, and rifapentine), isoniazid, and pyrazinamide. Regimens including these agents given for 6 months yield cure rates of 95% or more. Ethambutol or streptomycin is given to decrease the likelihood of failure or relapse in populations among whom there is a significant risk of initial resistance to one or more of the standard drugs. See Table 39–3 for a list of usual medications.

The central issue in contemporary TB control is noncompliance. The failure to consistently administer drugs drives treatment failures, acquired drug resistance, and relapse rates. To combat nonadherence, the United States Centers for Disease Control and Prevention (CDC), ATS, and WHO all embraced directly observed therapy (DOT) in the 1990s. The philosophy of DOT relates to the unique situation of TB: the public expects protection against casual, airborne transmission of a potentially lethal infection. To fulfill this mandate, the public health agencies become responsible for seeing that patients either take their drugs reliably or be quarantined. In compelling treatment, government thereby assumes responsibility for provision of all treatment and diagnostic services.

To make DOT feasible, intermittent regimens have been employed. Multiple studies document that regi-

Table 39–3. Standard antituberculosis medications for adults.

Drug	Daily	Usual Adult Dose Three Times (or Twice) a Week	Toxicity	Special Considerations	Comments
Isoniazid (INH)	300 mg orally	600 (900) mg	Hepatitis, neuritis, mood/cognition, Lupus reaction	Pregnancy: safe Liver disease: caution Renal impairment: decrease dose if severe	Monitor liver function tests monthly in most patients; clinically significant interactions with phenytoin and anti-fungal agents (azols)
Rifampin (RIF)[1]	600 mg orally; 450 mg in persons < 50 kg body weight	600 (600) mg	Hepatitis, thrombopenia, nephritis, flu syndrome	Pregnancy: acceptable Liver disease: caution Renal impairment: safe	Key: multiple, profound drug interactions possible (see later); turns urine and fluids red
Rifapentine (RPT)	Not recommended	Not recommended (600 mg orally once weekly)	Similar to RIF	Similar to RIF	The primary role for RPT is in *once-weekly* therapy for patients with non-cavitary TB; not indicated for persons with AIDS
Rifabutin (RBU)	150–300 mg orally	300 (300) mg	Similar to RIF; modestly more neutropenia and thrombopenia than RIF	Similar to RIF	The primary role for RBU is in persons with AIDS to lessen drug–drug interactions.
Pyrazinamide (PZA)	25–30 mg/kg orally	30–35 mg/kg (same)	Hepatitis, arthralgias and arthritis secondary to hyperuricemia, gastrointestinal (GI) distress, rash	Pregnancy: unknown (avoid) Liver disease: caution Renal impairment: caution	Urate levels always rise; do not treat or stop PZA unless unmanageable gout develops
Ethambutol (EMB)	15 mg/kg orally	35 (50) mg/kg	Optic neuritis; GI distress; rare peripheral neuritis	Pregnancy: safe Liver disease: safe Renal impairment: decrease dose/frequency	Monitor visual acuity and color vision regularly
Streptomycin (SM)	12–15 mg/kg intramuscularly	15 mg/kg (same)	Vestibular and auditory, cation depletion	Pregnancy: high risk (avoid) Liver disease: safe Renal impairment: decrease dose/frequency	Reduce dose and/or frequency in case of renal impairment

[1]Rifampin drug interactions have been reported with antiretroviral agents including protease inhibitors and nonnucleoside reverse transcriptase inhibitors, oral contraceptives, anticoagulants, methadone, corticosteroids, estrogen replacement, calcium channel blockers, β-blockers, cyclosporine, antifungal agents (azols), phenytoin, theophylline, sulfonylureas, haloperidol, and others (see *Physicians' Desk Reference*).

mens given 2 or 3 days per week are comparable in efficacy to daily therapy. Thus, patients need be seen only 62–78 times over a 6-month period to ensure administration of all drugs. To make DOT programs effective, cordial and convenient programs have been established that include a variety of "incentives" and "enablers." The use of DOT in the United States has risen from 4% to over 75% of eligible patients between 1990 and 2001. Due in significant measure to such programs, TB cases in the United States have fallen from 26,678 in 1992 to 15,900 in 2001; case rates declined from 10.5 to 5.6 per 100,000 in this period putting America among the countries with the lowest incidence of TB in the world. It is inferred that DOT impacts case rates by halting transmission in the community.

Typical DOT regimens are represented in Table 39–4. Although recommended, DOT is not mandated for all patients. However, physicians who elect to treat TB patients by self-administration of drugs must bear the onus for noncompliance and any adverse conse-

quences including ongoing transmission of infection and/or acquired drug resistance.

Drug resistance arises due to "inadequate" therapy. Modern regimens are so constructed that if taken predictably, failure and resistance are extremely rare. "Inadequate" regimens can entail irregular administration, too few drugs, suboptimal doses, or malabsorption. The prevalence of drug-resistant strains gradually rose in the United States through the 1980s reaching peak levels in the early 1990s when roughly 14% of strains showed resistance to one or more drugs and nearly 3.5% were resistant to the major agents, rifampin (RIF) and isoniazid (INH). Strains resistant to both INH and RIF were designated as "MDR-TB" (multidrug resistant).

Drug resistance that evolves in a patient undergoing treatment is called "acquired" resistance. If that strain is transmitted to another person who subsequently develops active TB with preformed resistance, it is called "initial" resistance. At present, the overall prevalence of INH-resistant TB in the U.S.-born population is about

Table 39–4. Contemporary antituberculosis regimens.[1]

Regimen	Medications	Total Duration/ Number of Doses	Comments
Denver	INH, RIF, PZA, and EMB or SM daily for 2 weeks; then twice weekly for 6 weeks. Follow with INH and RIF twice weekly for 18 weeks. *Note:* All intermittent regimens must be given as DOT.	6 months/62 doses	EMB has replaced SM in most cases. Stop PZA and EMB at 8 weeks if strain is susceptible; continue through 6 months; if there is initial INH resistance may continue all medications through 6 months; 24 weeks of twice weekly therapy facilitates directly observed therapy.
Hong Kong	INH, RIF, PZA, and SM or EMB three times a week for 6 months (may stop PZA, SM, or EMB after 2 months). *Note:* All intermittent regimens must be given as DOT.	6 months/78 doses	All intermittent. If strain is susceptible, may stop PZA and SM or EMB after 2 months. If there is INH resistance, may continue all medications through 6 months.
CDC Trial 22	INH, RIF, PZA, and EMB for 2 months; may be given daily, per the Denver regimen or intermittently per the Hong Kong regimen; then INH and rifapentine once a week for 4 months (not for persons with AIDS or cavitary lung disease).	6 months/42–74 doses	Rifapentine is a potent and long-acting rifamycin. In trials comparing once weekly INH and rifapentine with twice weekly INH and RIF, the rifapentine regimen performed slightly less well. But for those who had become culture negative at 2 months, the results were comparable. Currently advocated in the United States only for patients without cavities on chest x-ray.
ATS/CDC	INH and RIF daily for 6 months; PZA and SM or EMB daily for initial 2 months.	6 months/180 doses	The standard self-administered regimen. Add SM or EMB in areas/patients at risk for initial drug resistance. Stop PZA, EMB, or SM after 2 months if strain susceptible; continue or modify regimen if resistance is present.

[1]Currently, the ATS and CDC advocate initial four-drug therapy for cases in communities with a background prevalence of initial drug resistance of 4% or greater. If susceptibility has been demonstrated or if resistance is deemed very unlikely, initial three-drug regimens may be used. INH, isoniazid; RIF, rifampin; PZA, pyrazinamide; SM, streptomycin; EMB, ethambutol.

5% and the prevalence of MDR-TB is less than 1%. Persons at greatest risk are immigrants with a prior history of TB therapy; their risk of MDR-TB in 2000 was almost 8%.

Currently in the United States all new isolates of *M tuberculosis* should be tested for *in vitro* resistance. Modern laboratory techniques usually allow reporting of drug susceptibility within 3–4 weeks of receiving a specimen that is positive by microscopy. Starting treatment with a four-drug regimen is usually sufficient protection while awaiting susceptibility results. However, for patients who are at high risk historically (prior therapy) or epidemiologically, and who have very extensive or serious forms of TB such as miliary or meningeal disease, an empirically extended initial regimen might be appropriate. Adding a second- or third-generation fluoroquinolone (levofloxacin, moxifloxacin, or gatifloxacin), cycloserine, or amikacin to INH, RIF, and pyrazinamide (PZA) would generally be appropriate. This decision should be made in conjunction with expert consultation whenever possible.

The ongoing management of patients with MDR-TB is complicated. Preventing nosocomial transmission, coping with drug side effects and toxicity, and considerations of surgical intervention all mandate that such cases promptly be referred to specialized centers.

Prevention

In the 1960s public health experts in the United States chose to rely upon a strategy of preventive chemotherapy (to stop progression from latent infection to active disease) rather than vaccination to protect the American public. This was based on two central tenets: (1) Most cases of TB in the United States occurred due to reactivation of prior infection and thus would not be prevented by vaccination, which was directed to those without prior infection, eg, those who were not reactive to tuberculin. (2) There was uncertainty about the protection afforded by the available vaccine, the bacillus of Calmette–Guérin or (BCG). Note that it was impossible to do both because vaccination with BCG would induce tuberculin reactivity and nullify the ability of the TST to identify those with prior infection by TB.

A. Treatment of Latent TB Infection (TLTI)

TLTI is the new designation for preventive therapy. New guidelines from the CDC/ATS were published in 2000. However, some have found them difficult to interpret and one of the recommended regimens has been badly compromised by unexpected toxicity and mortality.

The basic strategy of TLTI is to identify persons who are both infected with TB *and* likely to progress to active disease and then to encourage medical therapy to eliminate the viable bacilli in those individuals. Historically, INH has been the only agent with rigorously proven efficacy, and the 2000 guidelines still advocate INH for 9 months as the primary regimen. However, other therapeutic options were described (see Table 39–5). One of the options, an RIF–PZA regimen, to be given for 2 or 3 months, unfortunately resulted in 20 cases of serious hepatitis and 5 deaths among no more than 10,000 recipients. Based on this initial experience, additional cautions included careful clinical and biochemical monitoring. However, the risks do not seem to justify its utilization.

Individuals for whom TLTI might be advised can be classified into two groups: (1) Those identified during contact investigations around a new case of communicable TB who are presumed to be newly infected; they

Table 39–5. Regimen options for treatment of adults with latent TB infection.[1]

Regimen	Comments
A. INH, 300 mg daily for 6 months	Acceptable option for all indications except HIV-infected persons and those with inactive fibronodular scars in upper zones; these groups should receive 9 months of INH.
B. INH, 300 mg daily for 9 months	The preferred option for all groups in the 2000 ATS/CDC guidelines; but the modest improvement in outcome versus 6 months of INH may not be worth the struggle for reluctant subjects.
C. INH, 900 mg twice weekly for 6 or 9 months [directly observed preventive therapy (DOPT)]	High dose, twice weekly INH is recommended in correctional facilities or in a household in which a parent or other patient is receiving DOT; DOPT.
D. RIF, 600 mg daily for 4 months	For contacts to INH-resistant TB, those intolerant of INH, or those for whom shorter therapy is important. Its use in persons with HIV/AIDS is discouraged due to risk of acquired resistance to RIF.

[1]The 2000 ATS/CDC guidelines also advocated a 2- or 3-month regimen of RIF/PZA. However, due to a considerable risk of serious, even lethal hepatitis, this regimen does not seem to be an acceptable alternative.

are at particular risk during the ensuing 2 or 3 years. Those at greatest risk are persons who are at the extremes of age or otherwise are immunologically compromised. (2) Persons who are screened or otherwise identified as being at particular risk; the high-risk groups are noted in Table 39–6.

The TST is the only tool to identify latent TB infection. Following new infection, TST reactivity typically

Table 39–6. Candidates for treatment of latent TB infection.[1]

Certain patients among the infected population are at greater risk than others and should be considered for TLTI. *In the United States, persons with any of these risk factors should be considered regardless of age:*

1. Persons with HIV infection (TST ≥ 5 mm) and persons with risk factors for HIV infection whose HIV infection status is unknown but is suspected to be positive.
2. Close contacts of persons with newly diagnosed infectious tuberculosis (TST ≥ 5 mm). In addition, tuberculin-negative children and adolescents who have been in close contact with infectious persons within the past 3 months are candidates for preventive therapy until a repeat tuberculin skin test is done 3 months after exposure.
3. Recent TST converters, as indicated by a ≥ 10 mm increase of induration within a 2-year period.
4. Persons with abnormal chest radiographs that show fibrotic lesions likely to represent old healed tuberculosis (TST ≥ 5 mm).
5. Intravenous drug users known to be HIV seronegative (TST ≥ 10 mm).
6. Persons with medical conditions that have been reported to increase the risk of tuberculosis (TST ≥ 10 mm). This includes type I diabetes mellitus, immunosuppressive therapy such as prolonged steroids or tumor necrosis factor-α inhibitors, end-stage renal disease, organ transplantation, and solid organ or hematolymphatic neoplasms.

In addition, in the absence of any of the above risk factors, persons younger than 35 years of age in the following high-incidence groups are appropriate candidates for preventive therapy if their reaction to a TST is ≥ 10 mm.

1. Foreign-born persons from high-prevalence countries.
2. Medically underserved low-income populations, including high-risk racial or ethnic minority populations, especially blacks, Hispanics, and Native Americans.
3. Residents of facilities for long-term care (eg, correctional institutions, nursing homes, and mental institutions).

---

[1]The 2000 ATS/CDC guidelines also advocated a 2- or 3-month regimen of RIF/PZA. However, due to a considerable risk of serious, even lethal hepatitis, this regimen may not be an acceptable alternative.

develops in around 5–8 weeks. Among patients with active TB the range of induration measured following the TST is 15 ± 5 mm. However, the TST is neither *sensitive* (roughly 25% of those with known TB have negative TSTs) nor *specific* (a considerable number of persons infected with environmental or nontuberculous mycobacteria react with 10–15 mm of induration to the TST). Thus, clinicians must make clinical judgments about the significance of reactions or nonreactions to the TST in identifying candidates for TLTI. Preventive chemotherapy might be offered to some subjects who do not react to the TST but are at high risk: eg, an HIV-infected adult who has spent his entire life in Haiti where TB is endemic or an infant in a household in which an active case has apparently infected many other contacts.

B. Preventing Nosocomial Transmission

This has become an important element of modern TB control. "Genetic fingerprinting" (molecular epidemiology) studies showed in retrospect that roughly 80% of the MDR-TB cases seen in New York City in the early 1990s were transmitted in hospitals, not in the community. Because patients with MDR-TB do not enjoy the prompt response to therapy that those with susceptible strains do, they represent a special challenge to infection control. To combat nosocomial transmission, Occupational Safety and Health Administration (OSHA) guidelines were published calling for administrative policies, engineering controls, and personal respiratory protection. Essentially, the program consists of early recognition of those suspected of TB, removing them from the mainstreams of the institution, placing them in negative-pressure isolation rooms that undergo six or more air changes per hour, promptly obtaining and promptly reporting sputum smears, and using personal respiratory protection devices (respirators) when sharing the air with these patients. Basically, the OSHA recommendations indicate that if a clinician thinks the possibility of pulmonary TB is sufficient to order sputum tests, the patient should be isolated. However, many institutions do not have adequate numbers of isolation rooms to accommodate this practice and clinical prioritization is used to determine which patients are to be isolated.

The issue of prior BCG vaccination, TST reactivity, and recommending TLTI merits mention. Many of the immigrants who come to the United States have previously received BCG. Thus, they either decline TSTs or, when a TST is done and demonstrates reactivity, they decline preventive chemotherapy. However, U.S. authorities maintain that most adults who received BCG in their childhood do not react to the TST unless they have had intervening infection with *M tuberculosis*. Hence, given the high risk of TB among immigrants despite prior BCG, the ATS/CDC guidelines advocate TLTI for TST-positive persons from countries with endemic TB.

Ultraviolet germicidal irradiation (UVGI) or high-efficiency particulate air (HEPA) filtration has also been advocated to lessen transmission. UVGI has demonstrated efficacy in killing airborne mycobacteria and is relatively easy, safe, and economical to deploy.

C. VACCINATION

BCG has been given to more persons (between 3 and 5 billion) than any other vaccine. Many of the countries in which the TB epidemic continues out of control report BCG coverage of 97% or more of their newborns and children making claims of the vaccine's efficacy dubious. That BCG significantly lessens the risk of certain forms of TB in infants and young children (miliary, meningeal, or spinal) is *not* contested. However, it does not—even when given repeatedly through childhood and adolescence—consistently diminish adult pulmonary disease. Thus, it has failed to curtail the ongoing TB epidemic. Currently, considerable research is being directed toward identification of a more effective vaccine.

American Thoracic Society: Treatment of tuberculosis and tuberculosis infection in adults and children. Am J Respir Crit Care Med 1994;149:1359. [PMID: 8173779]. (Most recent guidelines for treatment of adults, children, and infants. Excellent overview of contemporary issues. New guidelines in 2000 superseded the 1994 recommendations on preventive therapy. Revised guidelines for treatment are now available: Am J Respir Crit Care Med 2003;167:603 [PMID 12588714].)

American Thoracic Society, Centers for Disease Control and Prevention: Targeted tuberculin testing and treatment of latent tuberculosis infection. Am J Respir Crit Care Med 2000;161(Suppl):S221. [PMID: 10764341]. (These guidelines indicate that tuberculin skin testing should be done only for those individuals who, if reactive, should be offered treatment for latent infection. They identify high-risk individuals or groups and describe various regimens with evidence-based support.)

Centers for Disease Control and Prevention: *Reported Tuberculosis in the United States, 2000.* US Department of Health and Human Services, CDC, August 2001. (A review of TB case numbers, age, race, and country of origin by state and city. Also, data regarding drug resistance are provided.)

Centers for Disease Control and Prevention: Update: fatal and severe liver injuries associated with rifampin and pyrazinamide for latent tuberculosis infection, and revisions in the American Thoracic Society/CDC recommendations—United States, 2001. MMWR Morb Mortal Wkly Rep 2001;50:733. [PMID: 11787580]. (This initial report documented 20 cases of severe hepatitis and 5 deaths associated with the RIF/PZA TLI regimen; more cases have subsequently been noted. The update called for more limited use of the regimen and stricter monitoring.)

Iseman MD: *A Clinician's Guide to Tuberculosis.* Lippincott, Williams & Wilkins, 1999. (A textbook that focuses upon
diagnosis, treatment, and prevention of tuberculosis. This monograph provides expanded discussion of the various topics addressed in this chapter.)

ENVIRONMENTAL MYCOBACTERIA (EM)

ESSENTIALS OF DIAGNOSIS

- *Nontuberculous mycobacterial organisms (environmental TB) are increasingly recognized due to improved laboratory culture techniques and frequent CT scanning identifying bronchiectasis.*
- *Several organisms cause disease, with* Mycobacterium avium *complex and* M. kansasii *most common.*
- *Symptoms and signs may mimic classic tuberculosis, however, different clinical presentations such as chronic lobar bronchiectasis or disseminated disease for HIV-infected patients are common.*

The EM are an array of organisms that cause sporadic disease in humans (see Table 39–7). The usual habitats for these microbes are soil and water; it is presumed that infections are acquired from environmental sources, not by human-to-human transfer. Low numbers of cases were described in Europe and North America throughout the first 75 years of the twentieth century. Then, in the last decades of the century, case numbers appeared to rise considerably in the United States, western Europe, and Japan.

Explanations for this putative surge in cases range from "laboratory artifact" to changes in water processing and hygienic practices. Two possible laboratory elements that may have influenced the frequency with which EM lung disease has been recognized include the widespread use of agar culture media (which is superior to Lowenstein–Jensen egg medium in recovering EM) and the introduction of CT lung scanning (which led to recognition of bronchiectasis, which in turn led to obtaining more cultures for mycobacteria). Changes in potable water treatment may also have increased the prevalence of EM in the human ecosystem. In the latter twentieth century the temperatures in institutional and home water heaters were reduced from ~165°F and 140°F, respectively, to 120°F to 125°F. This was done to both reduce energy expenditures and lessen the risk of scalding accidents. However, the lowered temperatures favor survival of EM in these water systems. There was also a distinct shift in personal hygiene from tub

Table 39–7. The Runyon classification of environmental mycobacteria.

Group	Characteristics	Typical Pathogens
I. Photochromogens	When grown in dark, colonies are cream colored; on exposure to light, changes to yellow-orange; slow growing	M kansasii M marinum
II. Scotochromogens	Colonies pigmented even in dark; slow growing	M scrofulaceum M gordonae M szulgai
III. Nonchromogens	Always cream or buff colored	M avium M intracellulare M xenopi M malmoense
IV. Rapid growers	Visible colonies appear on solid medium in 3–7 days (Note: may grow slowly on initial recovery from sputum or tissue)	M abscessus M chelonae M fortuitum

bathing to showering, particularly in closed stalls. These factors theoretically could result in increases in airborne/aerosol exposures to the EM.

This model could not explain shifts in the patterns of EM disease in the United States and Japan from males with underlying chronic obstructive pulmonary disease (COPD) to females without clear risk factors. Recent series in the United States have emphasized the apparent vulnerability of slender women, overwhelmingly white, to EM lung disease. Phenotypic features in these women include subtle scoliosis, occasional straight back syndrome, narrow anterior–posterior chest diameter (sometimes with sternal depression or pectus excavatum), and mitral valve prolapse. Possible specific host factors conveying vulnerability to the EM have been identified including mild variants of cystic fibrosis, anomalies of the α_1-antitrypsin system, and relative deficiencies of estrogen (which appears to enhance cellular immunity against mycobacteria, at least in a murine model).

Mycobacteria avium Complex (MAC)

The M avium complex includes M avium and M avium intracellulare (MIC) as well as some strains that appear intermediate between M scrofulaceum and MAC. These organisms are slow growing, nonpigmented, and classified as Runyon Group III.

Pulmonary disease associated with MAC ranges from upper-lobe fibronodular, cavitary disease that is quite mindful of classic TB (seen mostly in males with COPD or inorganic dust exposure) to a more subtle disorder characterized by bronchiectasis, most prominently in the right-middle lobe and/or lingula (seen primarily in slender women).

Diagnosis in the former group is usually straightforward: these patients usually complain of cough, sputum, hemoptysis, feverishness, chills, sweats, and weight loss. Their sputa are usually positive on smear (and culture). Commonly, the initial diagnosis is TB and they are begun on TB therapy until the laboratory reports identification of MAC.

By contrast, those patients with bronchiectasis commonly have a protracted history of cough, congestion, recurrent "pneumonia," malaise, and lassitude. Plain chest x-rays commonly are read as nonspecific abnormalities. Diagnostic criteria were described by an expert ATS panel in 1997. Although academically appropriate, these criteria were probably too restrictive and were also confusing to apply. A simpler model generally suffices to establish the diagnosis. For women with typical symptoms, the above-described body habitus, scattered areas of bronchiectasis, nodules on CT scans, and the presence of MAC [or rapidly growing mycobacteria (RGM)] on sputum or bronchial aspiration/lavage culture, the diagnosis may be reasonably established. Nonetheless, it is prudent to recall that MAC or the other EM *may* be present in a saprophytic or commensal status in some minority of these cases.

The natural course and requirement for treatment of bronchiectatic MAC disease have not been fully clarified. Certainly, for some patients the disease may progress to disabling and potentially lethal ends. However, it seems likely that series reported from referral centers are biased toward those with more aggressive disease. It *may* be appropriate to observe some patients who report minimal respiratory or constitutional symptoms; but it is incumbent upon the clinician to follow such patients at regular intervals to detect progression at an early point.

For those with the cavitary, destructive variety of MAC the decision to treat is simple; medications used for MAC and other slow-growing EM are represented in Table 39–8. Generally, an aggressive regimen employing three oral agents and an injectable drug is appropriate (see Table 39–9). The 1997 ATS recommendations encourage empirical selection of medications. The ATS and National Committee for Clinical Laboratory Standards (NCCLS) recommendations endorse *in vitro* susceptibility testing only for clarithromycin (or

Table 39–8. Medications commonly used in the treatment of slow-growing environmental mycobacterial disease.

Medication and Dosage	Side Effects/Toxicity	Comments
Clarithromycin (CLA): 500–750 mg daily; 500 mg twice a day; 750 mg three times a week	Metallic bitter taste; anorexia; griping abdominal distress; loose stools; tinnitus and high-frequency hearing loss are rare	May be given three times a week; cytochrome P-450 inhibitor; drug interactions
Azithromycin (AZI): 250–500 mg daily/ 500 mg three times a week	Fewer but similar GI effects than CLA; tinnitus and high-frequency hearing loss are rare	Long half-life favors intermittent use; but is moderately less active than CLA; minimal effects on cytochrome P-450 system
Ethambutol (EMB): 25 mg/kg daily for 2 months, then 15 mg/kg daily; 25–30 mg/kg three times a week	Optic neuritis with potential for vision impairment or blindness; rash; rare peripheral neuropathy; GI distress; mild hyperuricemia	Has predictable additive effect with CLA or AZI; may be synergistic with rifamycins; must monitor vision; reduce dose with renal insufficiency
Rifampin (RIF): 600 mg daily if ≥50 kg body weight, 450 mg if ≤50 kg; 600 mg three times a week	Hepatitis, thrombopenia, mild GI upset, rash	Additive or synergistic with ethambutol versus many MAC strains; potent cytochrome P-450 inducer; major effect, lowering CLA bioavailability
Rifabutin (RBU): 150–300 mg daily; 300 mg three times a week	Hepatitis; neutropenia and thrombopenia more frequently than RIF	Additive/synergistic effects comparable to RIF; less effect on cytochrome P-450 (may be advantageous with CLA) (*Note:* CLA slows catabolism of RBU; use lower dose of RBU with CLA
Ciprofloxacin (CIP): 500–750 mg twice a day; 750 mg daily; 750 three times a week	Tremors, insomnia, bad dreams; GI upset; rare hepatitis; very rare, Achilles rupture	CIP and LQN usually active versus *M kansasii;* variable versus MAC and RGMs; CIP, an inhibitor of cytochrome P-450
Levofloxacin (LQN): 500–750 daily; 750 mg three times a week	Less CNS stimulation than CIP; GI upset; very rare, Achilles rupture	Higher maximum concentration and longer half-life than CIP, but slightly higher MICs versus MAC than CIP
Amikacin (AK): 12–15 mg/kg intravenously daily; 15–22 mg/kg intravenously three times a week	High-frequency hearing loss; tinnitus; less vestibular toxicity than streptomycin; renal impairment (may be amplified by nonsteroidal antiinflammatory drugs)	AK probably preferred agents versus MAC, *M kansasii,* or other slow-growing EM; may be given intramuscularly, but this may be problematic in slender subjects without much soft tissue

azithromycin) as these are the only agents for which there is unequivocal evidence linking *in vitro* susceptibility and clinical efficacy. However, earlier experience from the National Jewish Center showed a clear association between administration of medications to which there was *in vitro* susceptibility and clinical response in a large series of patients with pulmonary MAC. Although it appears appropriate to initiate therapy for previously untreated pulmonary MAC with an empirical regimen, performing *in vitro* testing to guide therapy for patients who have failed prior treatment or are intolerant of standard agents is indicated.

For patients with bronchiectatic disease, bronchial hygiene measures are important to optimize lung function. Inhaled β-agonists may both bronchodilate and accelerate mucociliary clearance. Mechanical devices such as the Flutter, PEP, or Acapella valve are useful in

mobilizing and clearing tenacious secretions. Clinicians should also be aware of the propensity of patients with bronchiectasis to become superinfected with gram-negative bacilli such as *Pseudomonas aeruginosa, Alcaligenes xylosoxidans,* or *Stenotrophomonas maltophilia.* Episodic clinical deterioration may be related to these gram-negative organisms, and an intensive course of antibiotics, usually given intravenously, can be quite beneficial.

Resectional surgery appears indicated for patients with severely damaged lobes or even lungs. This is an issue particularly when there is chronic disease in dependent zones where drainage is problematic. Particularly troublesome are combined bronchiectasis and atelectasis in the lingula and/or right middle lobe. Although intensive antimycobacterial therapy and bronchial hygiene can affect improvement, these damaged structures act as reservoirs for recurring infections throughout the pa-

Table 39–9. Regimens for the treatment of slow-growing environmental mycobacterial lung disease.[1]

Regimen		Comments
MAC or other slow-growing EM except *M kansasii*		
CLA 500 or 750 mg RIF 600 mg EMB 15 mg/kg	Daily	May substitute rifabutin 150 mg daily for RIF to lessen CLA elimination; use AK for more extensive or refractory disease
± Ak 15 mg/kg	Three times a week	
CLA 750 mg RIF 600 mg EMB 25 mg/kg ± AK 15 mg/kg	Three times a week	Experience from Tyler, Texas indicates three times a week therapy to be comparable to daily therapy for MAC disease; also, it is less expensive and has fewer side effects
The above regimens, substituting AZI 250 mg daily or 500 mg three times a week for CLA		AZI is better tolerated but slightly less active than CLA
M kansasii		
RIF 600 mg daily EMB 15 mg/kg daily	9 months	Extrapolating from British Thoracic Society study, should see high cure rates with this regimen; use higher dose of CLA if tolerable
CLA 500–750 mg daily	2 months	
RIF 600 mg daily EMB 15 mg/kg daily	9 months	
CLA 500–750 mg daily AK 15 mg/kg three times a week	2 months	Use AK with more extensive disease
RIF 600 mg daily EMB 15 mg/kg Isoniazid 300 mg daily	15–18 months	The 1997 ATS recommendations advocated this regimen; use AK or SM for more extensive disease; probably a less attractive option than regimens IIA or IIB
± AK or streptomycin 15 mg/kg three times a week	2 months	

[1]The usual duration of treatment for slow-growing EM other than *M kansasii* is 18–24 months. But for patients who find the treatment very difficult to tolerate, shorter treatment with the expectation of suppression, not cure, is acceptable.

tient's life. Because chronic infection and scarring tend to obliterate normal anatomic features, resectional procedures should be done only by experienced surgeons.

Lymphadenitis or disseminated infections due to MAC in persons with AIDS or other immunosuppressed states will not be addressed in this chapter.

Mycobacterium kansasii

M kansasii (*Mk*) is the second most common EM pathogen in the United States. Disease due to *Mk* is largely centered in the south-central region. These organisms involve both those with obvious predispositions (COPD or inorganic dust pneumoconioses) and young otherwise healthy persons. In general, *Mk* is rarely involved with the bronchiectatic disease involv-

ing the right middle lobe and lingula that is typical of MAC and the RGMs. More typically, *Mk* causes upper lobe, fibronodular cavitary disease similar to TB. Thin-walled cavities are seen more frequently with *Mk* than TB or other EM.

The therapy of *Mk* is more straightforward and predictable than for any other EM. Wild strains of *Mk* (untreated) typically show resistance only to PZA (*all* EM are resistant to PZA) and low-level resistance to INH. Historically the ATS has advocated an 18-month regimen of INH, RIF, and EMB with an initial 2-month course of streptomycin for pulmonary *Mk* disease. However, based on a 90% "cure rate" with 9 months of RIF and EMB in a British Thoracic Society trial, a 9-month regimen employing these two agents and a macrolide appears more suitable (see Table 39–9).

Therapy of *Mk* is compromised if there is acquired resistance to or intolerance of the rifamycins. In such cases, a tailored retreatment regimen based on *in vitro* susceptibility and consideration of resectional surgery is warranted.

Rapid-Growing Mycobacteria (RGM): *M chelonae* & *M abscessus*

RGM are biologically rather distinctive among the EM. *In vitro* these microbes grow more quickly (usually 3–10 days) on mycobacterial media and may grow on some standard media. They are resistant to most of the oral agents to which TB and the other EMs are susceptible. Also, the immune responses to RGM may be dimorphic with mixed granulomatous and pyogenic features.

The current impression is that pulmonary disease due to RGM is increasing, both absolutely and proportionately to the aggregate EM morbidity.

Pulmonary disease related to RGM most typically resembles the bronchiectatic forms described above under MAC. In fact, a considerable share of EM patients present with one pathogen, usually MAC, then subsequently manifest disease from the RGM. Classic TB-like cavitary disease is relatively rare. The same predispositions discussed for MAC apply to patients with RGM lung disease. One particular factor should be emphasized in relation to RGM—esophageal dysfunction and aspiration. Although aspiration pneumonitis may act as a general predisposition to subsequent EM disease, RGM are particularly linked to achalasia. It has been assumed, but not proven, that the dilated esophagus becomes colonized with RGM, which are then aspirated into the lungs.

Treatment of RGM lung diseases is extremely challenging due to limited agents with activity and an extremely high risk of relapse following cessation of antibiotics. Agents that are most likely to have clinical utility include cefoxitin, imipenem or meropenem, clarithromycin, linezolid, amikacin, tobramycin, and gentamicin. *M abscessus* typically is inhibited by cefoxitin and amikacin with fewer strains susceptible to imipenem and clarithromycin. By contrast, most strains of *M chelonae* are resistant to cefoxitin but susceptible to clarithromycin and amikacin. No randomized trials have been conducted for treatment of RGM. However, it is my firm clinical impression that *in vitro* susceptibility testing (from a qualified laboratory) is critical in selecting therapy.

In view of the nearly universal tendency for recurrence and the finite tolerance for the medications employed (especially ototoxicity from the aminoglycosides), it may be preferable to consider RGM chemotherapy as analogous to the management of *Pseudomonas aeruginosa* in CF: episodic treatment (for weeks or months) when symptomatic or physiological deterioration occurs rather than intensive treatment to cure.

Because of the propensity for relapses, resectional surgery is an obvious consideration. However, such surgery is quite complex and poses more risks for operative complications than for MDR-TB or other EM lung disease.

Other EM

A wide variety of EM have been associated with pulmonary (or extrapulmonary) disease. *M xenopi* and *M malmoense* are relatively common in Europe and appear sporadically in the United States. Clusters of *M simiae* have been noted in the southwestern United States. *M gordonae* is infamous as an environmental contaminant of laboratories; in particular, when renovations are being done in institutions that agitate the plumbing, these "tap water scotochromogens" may be recovered frequently from contaminated reagents and equipment.

American Thoracic Society: Diagnosis and treatment of disease caused by nontuberculous mycobacteria. Am J Respir Crit Care Med 1997;156:S1. [PMID: 9279284]. (An expert panel convened by the ATS developed recommendations for diagnostic criteria and treatment programs for EM disease.)

DeGroote MA et al: Retrospective analysis of aspiration risk and genetic predisposition in bronchiectasis patients with and without non-tuberculous mycobacteria infection. Am J Respir Crit Care Med 2001;163:A763. (A survey of a large cohort of patients with EM lung diseases documenting high rates of esophageal dysfunction, cystic fibrosis variants, and α_1-antitrypsin anomalies.)

Falkinham JO: Epidemiology of infection by nontuberculous mycobacteria. Clin Microbiol Rev 1996;9:177. [PMID: 8964035]. (A comprehensive review of the distribution of EM in the environment.)

Iseman MD, DeGroote M: Environmental mycobacterial (EM) infections. In: *Infectious Diseases,* ed 3 (Gorbach SL, Bartlett JG, Blacklow NR, editors). Lippincott, Williams & Wilkins, in press. 2003 (This chapter provides a comprehensive overview of pulmonary and extrapulmonary disease due to EM.)

Lieberman J: Augmentation therapy reduces frequency of lung infections in antitrypsin deficiency. A new hypothesis with supporting data. Chest 2000;118:1480. [PMID: 11083705]. (An unusual survey that suggests that repletion of α_1-antitrypsin reduces the frequency of bronchial infections in patients with A1-AT emphysema.)

Pulmonary Complications of HIV Disease

40

John Segreti, MD

General Considerations

The lungs are major target organs in patients infected with the human immunodeficiency virus (HIV) and in patients with acquired immunodeficiency syndrome (AIDS). In the United States and Europe use of highly active antiretroviral therapy (HAART) and prophylaxis for *Pneumocystis carinii* pneumonia (PCP), cytomegalovirus, and *Mycobacterium avium* complex (MAC) have changed the incidence and spectrum of diseases affecting the lungs. There has been a decline in the incidence of opportunistic infection, progression to AIDS, and mortality from the disease. The epidemiology of HIV infection has also changed in the United States. In new cases of AIDS patients are increasingly likely to have acquired HIV from intravenous drug use or heterosexual contact.

Pathogenesis/Epidemiology of HIV/AIDS

Infection with HIV produces multiple defects in the immune system resulting in dysfunction of humoral, cell-mediated, and phagocytic immunity. Thus patients with HIV/AIDS are at greater risk for infection with a variety of bacterial, mycobacterial, and fungal organisms. They are also predisposed to a variety of noninfectious diseases of the lungs such as Kaposi's sarcoma and non-Hodgkin's lymphoma. Because of the widespread use of HAART in the United States since 1996, the number of persons diagnosed with AIDS has declined substantially. At the same time, the number of people living with AIDS has steadily climbed. This has and will continue to place a greater burden on the health care system. The incidence of AIDS increased rapidly in the 1980s and peaked in the 1990s. The peak in new diagnoses was in 1993 with over 80,000 new cases. In 1996, a sharp decline in new cases was observed for the first time and since 1998 the incidence has leveled off at about 40,000 new cases per year. Mortality from AIDS has also declined over the past 5 years to about 40%. The number of new cases has declined most dramatically in men who have sex with men and to a lesser degree in intravenous drug users. During this time, however, the number of new cases attributable to heterosexual contact has increased.

As of December 2000 there were about 350,000 people with AIDS living in the United States. The proportion of African-American patients, heterosexual females, residents of the South, and persons acquiring AIDS via heterosexual contact has increased. AIDS also is disproportionately affecting subgroups that have poor access to health care and preventive care. Because almost one-quarter of persons with AIDS are not aware of their diagnosis and an additional third are aware of it but are not receiving care, it is expected that there will continue to be patients with PCP, tuberculosis, and other mycobacterial infections despite availability of HAART.

Almost 65% of persons with AIDS in the pre-HAART era had evidence of pulmonary disease. PCP was the most common cause, followed by other fungi, bacteria, *Mycobacterium tuberculosis,* and MAC. Viral pneumonia due to cytomegalovirus (CMV) was distinctly uncommon despite evidence of almost 100% prior infection. With the advent of HAART and subsequent immune system reconstitution, there are now fewer cases of opportunistic infection and some patients have been able to discontinue primary and secondary PCP prophylaxis. The incidence of Kaposi's sarcoma of the lung also may be decreasing. At the same time, however, bacterial pneumonia (especially from *Streptococcus pneumoniae*) and non-Hodgkin's lymphoma have become more common.

Clinical Presentation of Pulmonary Diseases in Persons with HIV/AIDS

Patients with HIV frequently present with respiratory complaints. The patient's risk factors, degree of immunosuppression, and chest radiographic appearance provide important initial clues and help guide the formulation of the initial diagnostic strategy. The clinical presentation of lung disease associated with HIV infection is nonspecific and similar to that of patients without HIV. Signs and symptoms may include fever, cough, shortness of breath, dyspnea on exertion, hemoptysis, weight loss, and night sweats. The more chronic the symptoms are, however, the less likely is the diagnosis of bacterial pneumonia. Subacute or chronic presentations should raise suspicion for PCP, tuberculosis and atypical mycobacterial infections, fungal pneumonia, Kaposi's sarcoma, and non-Hodgkin's lymphoma.

The degree of immunosuppression may also provide a clue in establishing the etiology of lung disease. PCP, MAC, and Kaposi's sarcoma are uncommon in patients with CD_4^+ T lymphocyte counts greater than 200. However, a CD_4^+ T lymphocyte count over 200 does not discount tuberculosis, fungal pneumonia, or non-Hodgkin's lymphoma. The radiographic patterns on presentation, although nonspecific, may also provide useful clues to the etiology of the underlying pulmonary disease (Table 40–1). A diffuse reticulonodular infiltrate is suggestive of PCP, disseminated tuberculosis, disseminated fungal disease, and Kaposi's sarcoma. Focal airspace consolidation occurs with bacterial pneumonia, Kaposi's sarcoma, cryptococcosis, legionellosis, and *Mycoplasma pneumoniae* infection. Hilar and mediastinal adenopathy suggest tuberculosis, MAC, Kaposi's sarcoma, and non-Hodgkin's lymphoma. Presence of a pleural effusion may be indicative of Kaposi's sarcoma, tuberculosis, empyema, and non-Hodgkin's lymphoma. The absence of radiographic findings, however, does not rule out pulmonary disease. In the patient with respiratory complaints, PCP and tuberculosis must be considered even when the radiograph is normal.

Table 40–1. Radiographic appearance of pulmonary diseases in HIV.

Diffuse interstitial infiltrates
  Pneumocystis carinii pneumonia
  Tuberculosis
  Fungal pneumonias
  Viral pneumonia
Nodules or masses
  Tuberculosis
  Kaposi's sarcoma
  Pulmonary lymphoma
  Cryptococcosis
  Aspergillosis
  Mycobacterium avium complex
Cavities
  Bacterial pneumonia
  Tuberculosis
  Aspergillosis
Focal consolidation
  Bacterial pneumonia
  Tuberculosis
Normal chest radiograph
  Pneumocystis carinii pneumonia
  Tuberculosis

Diagnosis and reporting of HIV and AIDS in states with HIV/AIDS surveillance—United States, 1994–2000. MMWR 2002;51:595. [PMID: 12139203]. (Discussion of trends in newly diagnosed cases of HIV infection following introduction of HAART.)

Lee LM et al: Survival after AIDS diagnosis in adolescents and adults during the treatment era, United States, 1984–1997. JAMA 2001;285:1308. [PMID: 11255385]. (The authors found that AIDS-related mortality fell, resulting in more patients living with AIDS.)

Murphy EL et al: Highly active antiretroviral therapy decreases mortality and morbidity in patients with advanced HIV disease. Ann Intern Med 2001;135:17. [PMID: 11434728]. (HAART-related reduction in mortality and opportunistic infections occurs even in patients with advanced disease.)

BACTERIAL PNEUMONIA

 ESSENTIALS OF DIAGNOSIS

- *Acute onset of fever, cough, sputum production, dyspnea, and chest pain.*
- *Chest radiograph demonstrates lobar or segmental infiltrate.*
- *Sputum gram stain/culture and blood culture aid diagnosis.*
- *Empiric therapy for common pathogens.*

General Considerations

Bacterial pneumonia is more common in HIV seropositive persons than in seronegative control subjects. The rate of bacterial pneumonia increases with a decline in CD_4^+ T lymphocyte counts. Injection drug users have a greater risk of pneumonia than men who have sex with men. As in non-HIV patients, cigarette smoking is associated with a higher risk of pneumonia. HIV patients who develop pneumonia have a four-fold higher mortality than persons who did not develop pneumonia. Trimethoprim/sulfamethoxazole (TMP/SMX) prophylaxis decreases the risk of pneumonia. The most common cause of bacterial pneumonia is *S pneumoniae* followed by *Haemophilus influenzae*.

Pathogenesis

The pathogenesis of bacterial pneumonia in HIV patients is identical to that in non-HIV patients. Patients with HIV have a higher incidence of bacterial pneumonia secondary to their abnormal humoral immunity.

Prevention

There is no effective way to reduce exposure to *S pneumoniae* and *H influenzae*. HIV seropositive adults and adolescents with CD_4^+ T lymphocyte counts of ≥ 200 cells/µL should receive a single dose of 23-valent polysaccharide pneumococcal vaccine if they have not received the vaccine in the previous 5 years (Table 40–2). Multiple observational studies have found that this vaccine is safe and beneficial in this group. Immunization should also be considered in patients with a CD_4^+ T lymphocyte count of <200/ µL. However, data supporting vaccination in this group are lacking. Revaccination should be considered for patients who were initially immunized when their CD_4^+ T lymphocyte count was less than 200 and whose cell count has increased to over 200 cells/µL in response to HAART. Vaccination is becoming more important as the rate of antibiotic resistance increases among pneumococci. The duration of protective effect of primary pneumococcal immunization is unknown. Periodic revaccination should be considered every 5 years. However, there is no clinical evidence that this is of benefit.

The incidence of *H influenzae* type B infection among adults is low. Therefore routine vaccination with *H influenzae* B vaccine is not recommended. TMP/SMX prophylaxis for PCP also decreases the incidence of bacterial respiratory infections. This should be considered when selecting an agent for PCP prophylaxis. Azithromycin and clarithromycin prophylaxis for MAC also appears to decrease the risk of bacterial respiratory tract infections.

Because bacterial infections are more common after viral infections such as influenza, many experts recommend that HIV seropositive patients receive annual influenza vaccination. In the pre-HAART era there was disagreement on the benefit of annual immunization because some studies indicated there was a poor antibody response to vaccination, especially in patients with low CD_4^+ T lymphocyte counts. More recent studies in patients on HAART document good antibody responses in a greater proportion of patients. Vaccination induces antigenic stimulation raising viral loads. However, this elevation is transient and viral loads quickly decline to baseline levels. Given that influenza vaccine is safe and inexpensive, it is cost effective in all HIV-positive patients and should be given annually. Oseltamivir, rimantidine, or amantidine given during outbreaks of influenza offers alternative approaches to prophylaxis.

Clinical Manifestations

The presentation of bacterial pneumonia in patients with HIV is different than that of PCP. It is similar to that of non-HIV patients with bacterial pneumonia. There is more acute onset of fever, chills, and cough. Duration of symptoms is usually less than 1 week and physical examination may reveal evidence of consolidation. Laboratory findings may include leukocytosis with a left shift and hypoxemia. Blood cultures should be obtained, as bacteremia is more common than in non-HIV patients. Chest radiographs usually demonstrate segmental or lobar infiltrates, however, diffuse infil-

Table 40–2. Prophylaxis to prevent first episode of opportunistic disease among adults infected with HIV.

Pathogen	Indication	First Choice	Alternative
Pneumocystis carinii	CD_4^+ T lymphocyte count <200/µL or oropharyngeal candidiasis	TMP/SMX 1 double-strength orally daily or 1 single-strength orally daily	Dapsone 50 mg orally twice a day or 100 mg orally daily; aerosolized pentamidine 300 mg monthly
Mycobacterium tuberculosis	Tuberculin skin test (TST) reaction $\geq$ 5 mm or prior positive TST result without previous treatment or contact with person with active infection	Isoniazid 300 mg orally plus pyridoxine 50 mg orally daily for 9 months	Rifampin 600 mg orally daily for 4 months or rifabutin 300 mg orally for 4 months
Streptococcus pneumoniae	CD_4^+ T lymphocyte count $\geq$ 200 µL	23-valent polysaccharide vaccine, 0.5 mL intramuscularly	
Influenza virus	All patients	Inactivated trivalent influenza virus vaccine 0.5 mL intramuscularly annually	Oseltamivir, 75 mg orally daily; rimantidine, 100 mg orally twice a day or amantidine 100 mg orally twice a day

trates occur in up to 40% of cases. Diagnosis of bacterial pneumonia is made clinically and management is the same as in non-HIV patients. Management is covered in detail in Chapter 36.

Complications/Prognosis

Bacteremia is more common in patients with HIV than in those who are HIV seronegative. Long-term declines in pulmonary function including permanent decreases in forced expiratory volume (FEV_1), forced vital capacity (FVC), FEV_1/FVC, and the diffusing capacity of carbon monoxide are also more common following bacterial pneumonia in HIV seropositive patients. Otherwise complications are similar to those seen in patients without HIV.

Hirschtick RE et al: Bacterial pneumonia in persons with the human immunodeficiency virus. Pulmonary Complications of HIV Infection Study Group. N Engl J Med 1995; 333:845. [PMID: 7651475]. (The authors conclude bacterial pneumonia is more common in HIV seropositive persons and identify risk factors for infection.)

Salvato PD, Thompson CE: Clinical, virologic, and immunologic features of influenza vaccination in HIV infection. AIDS Reader 1999;9:624. (A review of clinical issues regarding influenza vaccination in HIV seropositive persons.)

Wolff AJ, O'Donnell AE: Pulmonary complications of HIV infection in an era of highly active antiretroviral therapy. Chest 2001;120:1888. [PMID: 11742918]. (Retrospective review identifying changes in pulmonary complications following institution of HAART. Bacterial pneumonia was more common with HAART.)

PNEUMOCYSTIS CARINII PNEUMONIA (PCP)

 ESSENTIALS OF DIAGNOSIS

- *Subacute onset of fever, dyspnea on exertion, shortness of breath, and nonproductive cough.*
- *Hypoxemia on arterial blood gas.*
- *Diffuse interstitial infiltrate on chest radiograph.*
- *CD_4^+ T lymphocyte count <200/μL.*
- *Stains demonstrate Pneumocystis carinii in a clinical specimen (sputum, bronchoalveolar lavage, or lung biopsy).*

General Considerations

P carinii is currently classified as a fungus. In the pre-AIDS era it was seen primarily in patients with acute lymphocytic leukemia or in those receiving high-dose corticosteroids and presented with acute onset of fever and respiratory failure. The incidence of PCP was less than 100 cases/year. The incidence increased dramatically with the onset of the AIDS epidemic over 20 years ago. PCP is one of the most common pulmonary infections in patients with AIDS. The number of cases peaked in 1990 at about 20,000 cases/year, but has subsequently declined due initially to PCP chemoprophylaxis and later from the effects of HAART. Nonetheless, PCP remains a common opportunistic infection in persons with AIDS, especially if their HIV infection is not recognized or if they are unresponsive or nonadherent with HAART.

Pathogenesis

PCP has been diagnosed in patients throughout the world. The mode of transmission in humans is unknown but is presumed to be via the respiratory route. Reservoirs for human infection are unknown, but may include environmental sources or other humans. Serological studies indicate that healthy humans have a high rate of prior infection. In cross-sectional and longitudinal studies two-thirds of normal children were found to have antibody titers to *P carinii* of 1:16 or greater by age 4. Therefore it is likely that subclinical infection is highly prevalent at an early age. This observation suggests that PCP in persons with AIDS represents reactivation of latent infection. However, newer studies utilizing molecular typing of isolates indicate that recurrent infection may be due to reinfection with a new strain rather than reactivation of the previously acquired strain. In a recent study 54% of patients with PCP were infected with strains characterized by mutations that imparted sulfa resistance, suggesting their infection was recently acquired from someone receiving PCP prophylaxis.

Prevention

Prevention of PCP is an extremely successful public health strategy that is associated with a significant decline in morbidity and mortality from this infection. Strategies include preventing exposure, preventing disease, and preventing recurrence (Table 40–2). Although some authorities recommend that HIV-infected persons at risk for PCP not share a hospital room with a patient with PCP, data are insufficient to support this as standard practice.

The primary approach to prevention of PCP is chemoprophylaxis. All HIV-infected patients, regardless of history of previous PCP, should receive chemoprophylaxis against PCP if they have a CD_4^+ T lymphocyte count of <200 cells/μL. TMP/SMX is the recommended prophylactic agent. One double-strength tablet daily is the preferred regimen, although one single-strength tablet daily is also effective and might be better tolerated than the double-strength tablet regimen. One double-strength tablet three times weekly is also effective. Treatment with TMP/SMX may be continued in patients who have an adverse reaction to it that is not life-threatening. If TMP/SMX is discontinued, reinstituting therapy should be strongly considered after the adverse event resolves. If TMP/SMX cannot be tolerated, alternative prophylactic regimens include dapsone, dapsone plus pyrimethamine plus folinic acid, aerosolized pentamidine, and atovoquone. Atovoquone appears as effective as dapsone or aerosolized pentamidine.

Primary and secondary PCP prophylaxis may be discontinued in patients who have responded to HAART with an increase in CD_4^+ T lymphocyte counts to >200 cells/μL for 3 or more months. Discontinuing prophylaxis in these patients is recommended because prophylaxis provides limited disease prevention in this population and discontinuation decreases pill burden, potential for drug toxicity, drug interactions, selection of resistant pathogens, and cost.

Clinical Manifestations

The presentation of PCP in persons with AIDS is different compared to that in the pre-AIDS era. In non-AIDS patients the typical presentation is acute onset of fever and respiratory failure that develops concomitant with tapering of the corticosteroid dose. Symptoms of fever, shortness of breath, dyspnea on exertion, chest pain, and nonproductive cough are usually mild and slowly progressive in persons with AIDS. Chest radiographs characteristically show bilateral interstitial infiltrates that progress to an alveolar pattern. The chest radiograph is normal, however, in up to 10% of cases. High-resolution computed tomography of the chest in these cases usually shows ground-glass attenuation. Arterial blood gases should be obtained if PCP is suspected as hypoxemia may be severe and life-threatening. The degree of hypoxemia also appears to identify patients who benefit from corticosteroid therapy. The serum lactate dehydrogenase (LDH) is extremely high in some patients and may be a clue for PCP. However, other pulmonary diseases also cause elevated serum LDH. Some experts recommend gallium-67 scanning of the lungs to look for pulmonary inflammation if the chest radiograph is normal. Unfortunately, pulmonary uptake of gallium is not specific for PCP and the test may take several days to perform.

Although some experts believe that PCP can be accurately diagnosed based on a typical clinical presentation and compatible chest radiograph, tuberculosis, fungal infection, lymphoma, or Kaposi's sarcoma occasionally have identical presentations. Although a typical presentation should trigger empiric institution of PCP therapy, efforts should be made to establish a specific diagnosis. Clinical improvement while on empiric therapy does not establish a diagnosis. This is especially true if corticosteroids have been used, as the antiinflammatory effect of these drugs may mask symptom progression.

The gold standard for diagnosis of PCP is demonstration of the organisms in sputum, bronchoalveolar lavage (BAL), or tissue biopsy. Organisms were identified in the pre-AIDS era primarily by using stains, such as Gomori methenamine silver, specific for the cyst form of the organism. More experienced pathologists used Giemsa stains to identify the trophozoite form of *P carinii*. Diagnosis usually required lung biopsy as most patients were unable to produce sputum. The introduction of fiberoptic bronchoscopy in the early 1970s facilitated specimen acquisition by transbronchial biopsy (TBBx) and BAL. These specimens have sensitivities comparable to those of open lung biopsy. There were reports in the mid-1980s that sputum induction using nebulized saline could provide specimens with a sensitivity of 60–90%. However, many centers were unable to achieve these results. Introduction of monoclonal antibodies that react with *P carinii* and are sensitive and specific has led to the development of fluorescent antibody tests that allow detection of the organism within hours. Patients with AIDS typically have a large burden of PCP in their lungs, which increases the sensitivity of BAL. A negative BAL is usually adequate to rule out PCP in most patients. Patients who have failed primary or secondary prophylaxis, however, have a smaller burden of organisms and an increased frequency of false-negative results. Further diagnostic tests such as TBBx or open biopsy may be required in these patients.

Differential Diagnosis

Infection by other organisms such as *M tuberculosis, Histoplasma capsulatum, and Penicillium* and noninfectious diseases such as non-Hodgkin's lymphoma and Kaposi's sarcoma occasionally mimic the clinical presentation of PCP.

Complications

The primary complication of PCP infection is respiratory failure requiring mechanical ventilation and leading to death. There is a greater risk of subsequent infection in persons who survive the initial infection. Survivors of PCP can also develop lung cysts that cause spontaneous pneumothorax. Finally, infection with PCP and to some extent bacterial pneumonias may be associated with expiratory airflow obstruction that persists after resolution of the acute infection as well as long-term decline in pulmonary function including permanent decreases in FEV_1, FVC, FEV_1/FVC, and the diffusing capacity of carbon monoxide.

Treatment

TMP/SMX is the mainstay of treatment of PCP. It should be initiated in any person in whom PCP is suspected. The usual intravenous dose is 15 mg trimethoprim and 75 mg sulfamethoxazole per kg/day in three or four divided doses. If therapy is started with an oral preparation the usual dose is 20 mg trimethoprim and 100 mg sulfamethoxazole per kg/day in three or four divided doses. The typical duration of therapy for persons with AIDS is 2–3 weeks. Recent studies indicate that up to 50% of cases of PCP without previous exposure to TMP/SMX are due to organisms that harbor mutations that confer resistance to trimethoprim. Patients with prior exposure to TMP/SMX had such organisms 70–90% of the time. Although the clinical significance of this mutation is probably minimal it is not known if additional mutations will result in degrees of resistance that lead to therapeutic failures. Adverse reactions to TMP/SMX are very common in patients with AIDS and include fever, rash, bone marrow suppression, hepatitis, gastrointestinal symptoms, and metabolic acidosis. Therapy with TMP/SMX may be continued if adverse events are not life-threatening, however, up to 50% of treated patients require a change in therapy.

Pentamidine is the other first-line treatment of PCP. It is available in intravenous, intramuscular, and aerosolized forms, however, only intravenous formulations should be used for treatment of PCP. Aerosolized pentamidine is inferior to both the intravenous formulation and TMP/SMX and should be used only for PCP prophylaxis. Intramuscular pentamidine causes sterile abscesses at the site of injection; its routine use is not recommended. The usual dose of intravenous pentamidine is 3 mg/kg/day in a single dose infused over 60 min. Therapy is usually continued for 2–3 weeks. Adverse events are very common with intravenous pentamidine and include renal dysfunction, hypoglycemia, bone marrow suppression, and pancreatitis.

Adjunctive corticosteroids are effective in preventing respiratory failure and subsequent mechanical ventilation in persons with moderately severe to severe PCP. The threshold for initiating corticosteroids is a room air arterial oxygen tension/pressure (PaO_2) of less than 70 mm Hg or an alveolar–arterial oxygen tension gradient [$P(A–a)O_2$ of greater than 30 mm Hg while breathing room air. The usual dose of corticosteroids is 40 mg of prednisone twice daily for 5 days, followed by 40 mg daily for 5 days, followed by 20 mg daily for the duration of antipneumocystis therapy.

Seventy-five percent of patients respond to either TMP/SMX or pentamidine as initial therapy. However, a change in therapy is often required due to drug toxicity or failure to improve within 4 days. Usually the substitution of pentamidine for TMP/SMX or vice versa is effective. However, 5–20% of patients fail to improve despite this switch in therapy. The optimal salvage therapy for patients unresponsive to conventional therapy is unclear. Alternative therapies include atovaquone, clindamycin–primaquine, trimethoprim–dapsone, and trimetrexate.

Atovaquone is less effective than TMP/SMX for primary treatment of PCP, but also has fewer treatment-limiting adverse events. It is a reasonable alternative for patients with mild to moderately severe PCP who cannot tolerate TMP/SMX. It is also available for oral use. The usual dose is 750 mg orally twice a day. Trimetrexate is an analogue of methotrexate. It is better tolerated than TMP/SMX but has lower response rates for primary treatment of PCP and is effective in only 30% of TMP/SMX and pentamidine treatment failures. It is available only in intravenous forms. The usual dose is 45 mg/m^2 along with folinic acid at a dose of 20 mg/m^2. The combination of clindamycin and primaquine is the most successful salvage therapy for patients failing conventional treatment. This combination was successful in about 90% of patients initially failing TMP/SMX or pentamidine. It is unclear why clindamycin–primaquine is more effective as salvage therapy than other drugs. It does not appear to be related to differences in severity of illness, duration of failed treatment, or underlying disease. The most serious adverse events associated with clindamycin–primaquine include neutropenia, anemia, thrombocytopenia, and methemoglobinemia. The usual dose of chloroquine is 30 mg base and clindamycin 600 mg intravenously every 6 h or 300–450 mg orally every 6 h.

Prognosis

Patients who respond to initial therapy have a good prognosis. Patients who fail initial therapy do very poorly with salvage therapy. Reduction in pulmonary function and recurrent pneumothorax occur in some long-term survivors.

Kaplan JE et al: Guidelines for preventing opportunistic infections among HIV-infected persons—2002. Recommendations of the U.S. Public Health Service and the Infectious Diseases Society of America. MMWR 2002;51(RR-8):1. [PMID: 12081007]. (The most recent edition of evidence-based guidelines for the prevention of opportunistic infections.)

Kovacs JA et al: New insights into transmission, diagnosis and drug treatment of *Pneumocystis carinii* pneumonia. JAMA 2001;

286:2450. [PMID: 11712941]. (Case report and discussion of modes of transmission, diagnosis, and treatment of PCP.)

Smego RA et al: A meta-analysis of salvage therapy for *Pneumocystis carinii* pneumonia. Arch Intern Med 2001;161:1529. [PMID: 11427101]. (Meta-analysis of 27 studies. Authors conclude clindamycin plus primaquine is the most effective agent for patients failing conventional antipneumocystis agents.)

PULMONARY TUBERCULOSIS

 ESSENTIALS OF DIAGNOSIS

- *Gradual onset of fever, cough, and sputum production associated with night sweats and weight loss.*
- *Abnormal chest radiograph that may show scarring, fibrosis, infiltrates, or cavitary lesions.*
- *Positive acid-fast bacillus (AFB) smear of sputum.*
- *Nucleic acid amplification methods.*
- *Culture of M tuberculosis.*

General Considerations

Tuberculosis remains one of the most common and deadliest infections in the world. It is estimated that the annual incidence of tuberculosis is over 8 million with 3 million deaths. About 15 million people in the United States are infected with tuberculosis, although over the past few years the incidence has progressively declined. In the mid-1980s an increase in new cases of tuberculosis occurred with the emergence of multidrug-resistant strains. Much of this resurgence was attributed to the HIV epidemic. *M tuberculosis* is a highly virulent organism that is spread from person to person via airborne droplet nuclei. The prevalence of active tuberculosis among HIV-infected patients is as high as 3.8%. The prevalence in the general American population is only about 0.01%. The incidence of new cases of tuberculosis is higher in the eastern United States, in patients with CD_4^+ T lymphocyte counts <200 cells/mm^3, and in patients who have a positive reaction (≥5 mm of induration in patients with HIV) to purified protein derivative (PPD). This is especially true if the PPD has become positive in the past 12 months.

Pathogenesis

The pathogenesis of pulmonary tuberculosis is discussed in Chapter 39. HIV-infected persons are at greater risk of infection with tuberculosis when exposed to someone with active pulmonary disease. This increased risk is primarily due to depression in cellular immunity that is the hallmark of HIV infection. HIV-infected persons rapidly develop disease after becoming infected with *M tuberculosis*, especially if the CD_4^+ T lymphocyte count is low. It is estimated that after infection with *M tuberculosis* 50% of patients will develop disease. Persons with previously untreated tuberculous infection who acquire HIV develop active tuberculosis at a rate of about 5–10% per year.

Prevention

Tuberculosis can be prevented in HIV-infected persons by avoiding exposure and by preventing active disease through targeted tuberculin testing and subsequent treatment of latent infection (Table 40–2). HIV-infected persons should avoid activities that increase the risk of exposure to tuberculosis. This may include avoidance of volunteer work in health care facilities, correctional institutions, or homeless shelters.

A more efficacious approach involves targeted screening and treatment of latent infection. Patients should receive a tuberculin skin test (TST) by administration of a 5-TU PPD as soon as HIV infection is recognized. Routine evaluation for anergy is not recommended. All HIV-infected persons with a positive TST (≥5 mm of induration) should undergo chest radiography and clinical evaluation for active disease. HIV-infected patients with a positive TST but no evidence of active tuberculosis or history of previous treatment should be treated for latent tuberculosis. Options include isoniazid, 300 mg daily with pyridoxine 50 mg orally daily for 9 months. An alternative treatment is isoniazid 900 mg with pyrazinamide 100 mg orally twice weekly for 9 months. Two months of therapy with rifampin and pyrazinamide is as effective as the 9-month regimens, however, recent reports of fatal liver injury has cooled the excitement about this regimen. HIV-infected persons who are close contacts of persons with active pulmonary tuberculosis should also be treated for latent infection regardless of TST results, age, or prior courses of treatment.

Clinical Manifestations

The presentation of tuberculosis in persons with AIDS is similar to that in persons without AIDS. Occasionally the diagnosis is confounded by the tendency of persons with AIDS to develop fever, night sweats, and weight loss due to their underlying disease. Therefore pulmonary tuberculosis must be kept in the differential diagnosis of all patients with these symptoms. Extrapulmonary involvement also seems to be much more common in persons with AIDS; the incidence of extrapulmonary disease increases with declining immuno-competence. Pulmonary tuberculosis is almost always associated with radiographic abnormalities. However, up to 10% of persons with AIDS with pulmonary tuberculosis have normal chest radiographs. Persons with AIDS are also more likely to have atypical radiographic findings. Cavitation is less common whereas lower lung or diffuse infiltrates and lymphadenopathy are more common.

Laboratory diagnosis of tuberculosis in persons with AIDS is identical to that in the general population. The only caveat is that persons with AIDS are more likely to be colonized and infected with MAC and therefore growth of mycobacteria from a clinical sample does not confirm tuberculosis. Definitive diagnosis requires identification of the mycobacterial species.

Differential Diagnosis

The clinical presentation of tuberculosis is nonspecific in persons with AIDS. The differential diagnosis includes atypical mycobacteria, fungi, Kaposi's sarcoma, and lymphoma.

Complications

Complications of tuberculosis are more common in persons with AIDS than in persons not infected with HIV. HIV infected persons are more likely to develop extrapulmonary disease. HIV-infected persons on HAART are also more likely to experience adverse drug events and to develop paradoxical worsening of tuberculosis following immune reconstitution. The latter includes transient exacerbations with recurrent fever, enlarging or worsening pulmonary infiltrates, and/or the appearance of new radiographic lesions. Paradoxical worsening is more likely to occur in patients treated for tuberculosis who are then placed on HAART. Up to 35% of such patients may experience paradoxical worsening, typically within the first few weeks or months of therapy. These patients are usually not toxic and subjectively feel well despite fever and worsening radiographic appearance. It is important to recognize that exacerbation does not necessarily represent infection with drug-resistant bacteria, noncompliance, drug fever, or an alternative diagnosis, especially if these events appear temporally associated with initiation of HAART and evaluation for alternative diagnosis is negative.

Treatment

Treatment of tuberculosis in persons with AIDS who are not receiving antiretroviral therapy is identical to that of patients who are not infected with HIV. However, concomitant use of HAART complicates the treatment of tuberculosis because of overlapping drug toxicities and significant drug–drug interactions (Table 40–3).

Skin rashes, nausea, vomiting, and hepatitis occasionally occur with use of pyrazinamide, rifampin, rifabutin, and isoniazid. Nevirapine, delavirdine, efavirenz, and abacavir are all associated with skin rashes whereas zidovudine, ritonavir, amprenavir, and indinavir have been associated with nausea and vomiting. Nevirapine and protease inhibitors may cause hepatitis. Therefore some experts recommend delaying initiation of HAART for 1–2 months until there has been time to detect and manage toxicities to antituberculous chemotherapy.

The major pharmacokinetic issue complicating treatment of tuberculosis in HIV-infected patients is drug–drug interactions, especially those between rifamycins and antiretroviral drugs. Rifamycins, nonnucleoside reverse transcriptase inhibitors (NNRTIs), and protease inhibitors are all affected by and affect the cytochrome P-450 system, especially CYP3A. The rifamycins are inducers of CYP3A and decrease serum concentrations of drugs metabolized by this enzyme system. Rifampin is the most potent inducer and rifabutin is the least. Protease inhibitors and NNRTIs undergo a significant amount of metabolism by CYP3A. Therefore concomitant use of these drugs with rifamycins leads to very low serum concentrations of protease inhibitors and NNRTIs. Rifampin reduces serum levels of protease inhibitors, with the exception of ritonavir, by 75–95%. Such dramatic declines are likely to result in decreased antiviral activity and increase the chance of selecting drug-resistant viral mutants. Delavirdine concentrations decline by 90% when given with either rifampin or rifabutin. Protease inhibitors also inhibit the metabolism of rifabutin resulting in drug concentrations that are two to four times higher. This may cause rifabutin toxicity and require a reduction in dose. Overall, rifabutin offers greater flexibility in the choice of antiretroviral drugs and is generally preferred to rifampin. The dose of rifabutin should be decreased to 150 mg/day when it is given with protease inhibitors other than saquinavir to avoid toxicity and it should not be used with delavirdine. Although it is possible to treat tuberculosis with a regimen that does not include rifamycins, the routine use of such a regimen is not recommended. The only trial that assessed the efficacy of a rifamycin-free regimen demonstrated that these regimens were inferior to rifampin-based regimens. There were higher relapse rates with regimens that limited rifampin to the first 2 months of therapy. Non-rifamycin-containing regimens should be reserved only for patients with severe side effects.

The decision to treat an HIV-infected patient who has tuberculosis with antiretroviral agents depends on

Table 40–3. Effects of antituberculosis medications on antiretroviral medications.

Affected Drug	Interacting Drug	Mechanism Effect	Recommendation
Amprenavir, delavirdine, indinavir, lopinavir–ritonavir, nelfinavir, saquinavir	Rifampin	Induction of metabolism; marked reduction in concentration of protease inhibitor	Avoid concomitant use
Efavirenz, nevirapine	Rifampin	Induction of metabolism; decreased nevirapine levels	Consider efavirenz 800 mg orally daily
Delavirdine	Rifabutin	Induction of metabolism; 50–60% decrease in delavirdine levels	Avoid concomitant use
Indinavir, nelfinavir, amprenavir	Rifabutin	Induction of metabolism; 50% decrease in protease inhibitor levels	Increase indinavir dose to 1000 mg orally every 8 h; decrease rifabutin to 150 mg orally daily
Ritonavir, ritonavir–lopinavir, ritonavir–saquinavir	Rifabutin	Induction of metabolism of ritonavir	Consider rifabutin 150 mg orally every other day or 3 times weekly
Efavirenz	Rifabutin	Decreased rifabutin levels	Increased rifabutin to 450–600 mg daily or 600 mg twice weekly
Saquinavir	Rifabutin	Decreased saquinavir levels	Increase saquinavir to 1600 mg orally PO every 8 h

the stage of HIV infection. For patients with early HIV disease (CD$_4^+$ T lymphocyte counts >300) it may be prudent to treat tuberculosis with a rifampin-based regimen for 6–9 months and forgo HAART while closely monitoring CD$_4^+$ T lymphocytes counts. Patients with more advanced HIV disease who are already on effective HAART should receive rifabutin-containing regimens. Discontinuation of all antiretrovirals for the first 2 months of antituberculous therapy should be considered in patients failing HAART. HIV-infected patients with tuberculosis should be comanaged with someone experienced in the treatment of HIV and tuberculosis.

Prognosis

Although untreated tuberculosis has a very high mortality rate, the prognosis is comparable to that in non-HIV patients when adequate treatment is employed.

American Thoracic Society: Diagnostic standards and classification of tuberculosis in adults and children. Am J Respir Crit Care Med 2000;61:1376. [PMID: 10764337]. (Official statement of the American Thoracic Society and Centers for Disease Control regarding the diagnosis and classification of tuberculosis.)

Burman WJ, Jones BE: Treatment of HIV-related tuberculosis in the era of effective antiretroviral therapy. Am J Respir Crit Care Med 2001;64:7. [PMID: 11435232]. (Review of issues involved in the management of tuberculosis in persons receiving HAART.)

Kaplan JE et al: Guidelines for preventing opportunistic infections among HIV-infected persons—2002. Recommendations of the U.S. Public Health Service and the Infectious Diseases Society of America. MMWR 2002;51(RR-8):1. [PMID: 12081007]. (The most recent edition of evidence-based guidelines for the prevention of opportunistic infections.)

NONINFECTIOUS LUNG DISEASES

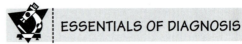 ESSENTIALS OF DIAGNOSIS

- *Negative cultures.*
- *Subacute onset of symptoms.*
- *Usually requires histopathological confirmation.*

General Considerations

Persons with AIDS are more susceptible to a variety of noninfectious diseases including Kaposi's sarcoma and non-Hodgkin's lymphoma. One retrospective study found that pulmonary involvement with non-Hodgkin's lymphoma was higher in the era of HAART.

Pathogenesis

The pathogenesis of Kaposi's sarcoma and non-Hodgkin's lymphoma is unknown. Although Kaposi's sarcoma appears to be linked to prior infection with human herpes virus type 8 (HHV8), the mechanism by which the virus contributes to development of Kaposi's sarcoma is unknown. It is postulated that duration of HIV infection and degree of immunosuppression are primary risk factors for development of Kaposi's sarcoma and non-Hodgkin's lymphoma. HAART would be expected to improve immunosuppression and reduce the risk of these conditions. Therefore it is likely that factors other than CD_4^+ T lymphocyte counts are important. It has been suggested that long-term B cell stimulation contributes to the development of HIV-related non-Hodgkin's lymphoma. It is possible that such B cell stimulation is unaffected or perhaps enhanced by HAART. Alternatively, HAART itself may trigger development of non-Hodgkin's lymphoma.

Prevention

There is currently no method to prevent Kaposi's sarcoma or non-Hodgkin's lymphoma.

Clinical Manifestations

HIV-infected patients who develop pulmonary involvement with non-Hodgkin's lymphoma usually present with nonspecific respiratory complaints in addition to systemic symptoms such as fever, weight loss, and night sweats. The disease is often widely disseminated at presentation with frequent involvement of extranodal sites including the central nervous system, bowel, and liver. Diagnosis of pulmonary non-Hodgkin's lymphoma usually requires biopsy of a suspicious lesion by TBBx or open lung biopsy.

Pulmonary Kaposi's sarcoma is often associated with dyspnea, nonproductive cough, fever, and hemoptysis. Chest radiographs may show diffuse parenchymal lesions, nodules, hilar adenopathy, or a pleural effusion. The presence of pleural effusions is not pathognomonic for Kaposi's sarcoma, occurring more frequently with bacterial pneumonia or tuberculosis. However, the presence of a bloody effusion on thoracentesis is very suggestive of Kaposi's sarcoma. Although Kaposi's sarcoma is typically a multicentric neoplasm with skin, gastrointestinal, and lymph node involvement, many patients with pulmonary Kaposi's sarcoma do not have the characteristic cutaneous violaceous macules, papules, or nodules or clinical evidence of disease in other organs. Endobronchial involvement is frequent with pulmonary Kaposi's sarcoma; lesions appear as red plaques most commonly occurring at the bronchial bifurcations. Bronchial washings, brushings, and transbronchial biopsies are of limited utility in establishing the diagnosis due to the small size of the specimen obtained, but are of value in excluding other conditions in the differential diagnosis.

Complications

Complications of untreated pulmonary non-Hodgkin's lymphoma and Kaposi's sarcoma include respiratory failure and death. In addition, treatment of non-Hodgkin's lymphoma and Kaposi's sarcoma with chemotherapy is frequently complicated by immunosuppression and may result in neutropenia, gram-negative bacillary infection, and invasive aspergillosis. Additional complications of pulmonary Kaposi's sarcoma include upper airway obstruction, massive pleural effusions, and pulmonary edema.

Treatment

Treatment of pulmonary Kaposi's sarcoma and non-Hodgkin's lymphoma usually consists of combination chemotherapy administered under the direction of an oncologist.

Prognosis

The prognoses of pulmonary non-Hodgkin's lymphoma and Kaposi's sarcoma are very poor with 2-year survival rates less than 50%.

Afessa B et al: Pulmonary complications of HIV infection: autopsy findings. Chest 1998;113:1225. [PMID: 9596298]. (Retrospective review of complications of HIV infection identified at autopsy.)

Wolff AJ, O'Donnell AE: Pulmonary complications of HIV infection in an era of highly active antiretroviral therapy. Chest 2001;120:1888. [PMID: 11742918]. (Retrospective review identifying changes in pulmonary complications following institution of HAART. Non-Hodgkin's lymphoma was more common with HAART.)

SECTION XI

Neoplastic Lung Diseases

Bronchogenic Carcinoma & Solitary Pulmonary Nodules

41

Robert L. Keith, MD, FCCP

LUNG CANCER

 ### ESSENTIALS OF DIAGNOSIS

- *Worsening or chronic cough, shortness of breath, weight loss, fatigue. More common in patients with chronic obstructive pulmonary disease (COPD).*
- *Dyspnea, hemoptysis, anorexia, many patients are asymptomatic (with abnormalities detected on thoracic imaging).*
- *Chest x-ray or chest computed tomography (CT): nodule, enlarging mass, persistent/nonresolving infiltrate, atelectasis, mediastinal or hilar adenopathy, pleural effusion; patients may present with manifestations of metastatic disease.*
- *Histological confirmation of lung cancer on biopsy specimens (sputum cytology, bronchial biopsies, pleural fluid, lymph node sampling, needle aspirations).*

General Considerations

Lung cancer is the leading cause of cancer death in men and women in both the United States and the world. More Americans die each year of lung cancer than of colon, breast, and prostate cancer combined. The overall 5-year survival of lung cancer is 15% or less and has only shown minimal improvement over the past 30 years. The vast majority (85–90%) of cases of lung cancer are attributable to smoking, and intensive research efforts have identified hundreds of carcinogens contained in both mainstream smoke (smoke directly inhaled by the smoker) and sidestream smoke (smoke released from burning tobacco between puffs plus smoke exhaled by the smoker). Although risk for lung cancer decreases significantly after smoking cessation, overall disease risk reduction takes years and an individual's risk never returns to that of a never smoker (never smoker is defined as fewer than 100 cigarettes in an individual's lifetime). Historically, 20 pack-years of tobacco exposure or more has been considered to contain the highest risk populations. Due to the large number of former smokers, new cases of lung cancer in the United States are diagnosed more commonly in former smokers than current smokers.

Other environmental factors can contribute to the development of lung cancer. Table 41–1 contains a list of proven and suspected agents that have been implicated in the development of lung cancer in current, former, and never smokers. Of particular note, many of these exposures, when coupled with smoking, lead to exponential increases in the risk of developing lung cancer. For example, smokers with asbestos exposure have a 50–100 times increased risk of developing lung cancer.

There are also disease states that are associated with an increased risk of lung cancer. First, patients who develop COPD [defined as chronic bronchitis or emphysema with pulmonary function testing showing at least mild airflow limitation, forced expiratory volume in is (FEV_1) <70% predicted and/or FEV_1/forced vital capacity (FVC) <0.70] secondary to smoking have been shown to have higher rates of lung cancer. Ongoing

Table 41–1. Environmental risk factors for developing lung cancer.

Proven
  Passive/environmental tobacco smoke
  Radon gas
  Asbestos
  Metals (chromium, arsenic, iron oxide)
  Industrial (bischloromethyl ether)
  Polycyclic aromatic hydrocarbons
Suspected
  Air pollution
  Vinyl chloride
  Silica
  History of tuberculosis

---

large epidemiological studies have shown that hazard ratios for the development of lung cancer are the highest in the lowest quartile of percentage predicted FEV_1. There is also a genetic predisposition to lung cancer as evidenced by increased lung cancer mortality rates in nonsmoking relatives of lung cancer cases when compared with nonsmoking relatives of matched controls. In addition, females have a higher rate of developing lung cancer when compared to males and controlled for amount of tobacco exposure. The genetic contribution, along with common genetic susceptibilities to developing COPD and lung cancer, is currently an area of intensive research and may in the future allow better identification of "genetically" high-risk groups. In addition to COPD, sarcoidosis and pulmonary fibrosis/interstitial lung disease (ILD) are also associated with increased risk. Lastly, the highest risk groups are those with a history of a previous lung cancer or a head and neck cancer.

Pathogenesis

Cancer develops in a multistep fashion in which cells become malignant by multiple genetic alterations affecting cellular growth, differentiation, and survival. This can include the mutation of tumor suppressor genes (for example p53), the activation of oncogenes (for example, *myc, jun*, and *fos*), and the transformation of apoptotic genes. The overwhelming majority of cases of lung cancer are due to cigarette smoking. It is estimated that of cases of lung cancer, 90% in men and 80% in women are smoking related. Smoke contains hundreds of known carcinogens, including free radical oxidants and nonradical oxidants, which can damage DNA, proteins, and lipids. The chronic inflammation accompanying repeated smoke exposure also leads to genetic alterations in bronchial cells and contributes to development of lung cancer.

Lung cancer is classified into two main categories, non-small cell (NSCLC) and small cell (SCLC). Within these two major categories are four basic histological types that account for over 90% of the cases. NSCLC has three main types: squamous cell carcinoma (25–35% of cases) arising from the bronchial epithelium and typically more central in location; adenocarcinoma (25–35% of cases) arising from mucous glands and typically more peripheral in location; and large cell carcinoma (10% of cases), a heterogeneous group of poorly differentiated tumors that does not have features of adenocarcinoma, squamous cell, or SCLC. A distinct subtype of adenocarcinoma is bronchoalveolar cell carcinoma (2% of cases), which arises from distal airway epithelial cells and typically presents as an unresolving infiltrate or as multiple nodules. Small cell carcinoma (20–25% of cases) is of bronchial origin and typically begins as a central lesion that can often narrow or obstruct bronchi. Hilar and mediastinal adenopathy as well as evidence of metastatic disease are often present on initial presentation. For staging and treatment purposes, NSCLC and SCLC are viewed very differently.

Growth factors and growth factor receptors are also involved in the pathogenesis and progression of both SCLC and NSCLC. Many of these factors or receptors are preferentially produced by the tumor cells and they induce cell-specific growth. Classic SCLC has a neuroendocrine origin accounting for many of the paraneoplastic syndromes, which can be seen at presentation or during disease progression. Paraneoplastic syndromes are also seen in patients with NSCLC due to accumulated genetic alterations in tumor cells.

Clinical Findings

The majority of lung cancers are symptomatic at the time of diagnosis, and clinical presentation is largely dependent on the tumor type, tumor location, and tumor stage (local or distant spread), and whether paraneoplastic syndromes are present. The clinical presentation often contains clues as to tumor type (NSCLC or SCLC).

A. SYMPTOMS AND SIGNS

In its earliest stages, lung cancer is asymptomatic. Primary lung cancers can reach a large size without causing any symptoms, although careful history and physical examinations reveal that only about 5% of lung cancer presentations are truly asymptomatic. Many of these are solitary pulmonary nodules, a topic discussed at length later in this chapter. Cough, anorexia, weakness, and weight loss are the most common presenting symptoms in patients with undiagnosed lung cancer. Other common presenting symptoms include new cough or a change in a chronic cough (60+%), hemoptysis

(10–25%), and pain, either local at a thoracic site or secondary to metastatic disease (25–35%). Presentation also depends on tumor location, for example, endobronchial obstruction can lead to postobstructive pneumonia, atelectasis, and pleural effusions. Enlarging tumor size and/or lymph node involvement can lead to hoarseness (secondary to recurrent laryngeal nerve injury), superior vena cava syndrome (ie, supraclavicular venous engorgement, much more common in SCLC), Horner's syndrome (ptosis, anhidrosis, and miosis from inferior cervical ganglion and sympathetic chain involvement), and dysphagia (secondary to esophageal obstruction from bulky mediastinal adenopathy). The Pancoast syndrome is shoulder and upper chest wall pain caused by a tumor in the apex of the lung. A tumor in this location can also be accompanied by Horner's syndrome, brachial plexopathy, and reflex sympathetic dystrophy. Bronchoalveolar cell tumors may induce copious amounts of "salty" sputum (a condition termed bronchorrhea).

Symptoms of metastatic disease are also relatively common presentations. Lung cancer commonly spreads to the adrenal glands, liver, brain, and bone. Central nervous system (CNS) spread may lead to headache, nausea, altered mental status, and possibly seizures. SCLC typically metastasizes at a much earlier time point than NSCLC.

Paraneoplastic syndromes are remote effects of the primary tumor leading to organ dysfunction. Up to 20% of lung cancer patients develop paraneoplastic syndromes, but these syndromes may not necessarily indicate metastatic disease. The more common paraneoplastic syndromes are listed in Table 41–2.

B. LABORATORY FINDINGS

The diagnosis of lung cancer is completely dependent on a tissue sample containing malignant cells. There are a variety of ways to obtain diagnostic tissue, including sputum cytology (best for central airway lesions); bronchoscopy with endobronchial or transbronchial biopsies; thoracentesis with cytological examination of the cellular component; and fine needle aspiration of intrathoracic masses, lymph nodes, or metastatic foci. The sensitivity of bronchoscopy in making the diagnosis is variable and depends on the size and location of the lesion. Transbronchial needle aspiration, video-assisted thoracoscopic surgery (VATS), mediastinoscopy, and thoracotomy may also be needed to adequately diagnose and stage patients. Other laboratory abnormalities may be present due to the paraneoplastic syndromes (listed in Table 41–2).

C. IMAGING STUDIES

Virtually all patients with lung cancer have abnormal chest x-rays or chest CT scans. Patients may present

Table 41–2. Lung cancer paraneoplastic syndromes.

Cachexia (anorexia, weight loss, weakness)
Fever
Hypertension
Endocrinological
  Hypercalcemia
  Hyponatremia
  Cushing's syndrome
  Gynecomastia
  Acromegaly
  Hypoglycemia
Neurological
  Lambert–Eaton myasthenic syndrome
  Peripheral neuropathy
  Cerebellar degeneration
  Limbic encephalitis
  Encephalomyelitis
Musculoskeletal
  Clubbing
  Hypertrophic pulmonary osteoarthropathy
  Dermatomyositis
  Polymyositis
Hematological
  Anemia
  Autoimmune hemolytic anemia
  Leukocytosis/thrombocytosis
  Vasculitis
  Noninfectious thrombotic endocarditis
  Idiopathic thrombocytopenic purpura

with a solitary pulmonary nodule, and this particular clinical scenario is discussed at length later in the chapter.

D. SPECIAL TESTS

1. Staging—Correctly staging patients with lung cancer is crucial in determining the proper therapeutic approach. One of the most important parts of staging is a thorough history and physical examination. These components directly determine blood work and further imaging. All patients need electrolyte testing, liver function tests [including alkaline phosphatase and lactate dehydrogenase (LDH)], and a chest x-ray. Elevated alkaline phosphatase suggests bone metastases. In the past, patients routinely had head CTs and radionuclide bone scans as part of the diagnostic workup, but large studies have shown that these tests should be ordered only if the patient's signs and symptoms indicate they are necessary. For example, CNS symptoms or an abnormal neurological examination necessitate a brain CT with contrast.

NSCLC and SCLC are staged differently. Due to the high incidence of micrometastases early in the disease state, SCLC is divided into two stages: limited disease (25–30%), in which the tumor is limited to ipsilateral hemithorax (including contralateral mediastinal nodes), and extensive disease (70–75%), in which the tumor extends beyond the hemithorax (including pleural effusions). SCLC is typically treated with chemotherapy and radiation therapy. NSCLC is staged using the TNM staging system (T is tumor size, N is nodal involvement, and M is presence or absence of metastases). Table 41–3 contains the TNM descriptors and staging for lung cancer.

Table 41–3. TNM descriptors and staging for lung cancer.

TNM descriptors

T (primary tumor)

Tis—carcinoma *in situ*

T1—tumor <3 cm (not in mainstem bronchus)

T2—tumor >3 cm or present in mainstem bronchus but not within 2 cm of carina, invasion of visceral pleura, associated atelectasis or pneumonitis extending to hilar region

T3—tumor of any size that invades the chest wall, diaphragm, mediastinal pleura, parietal pericardium; tumor <2 cm from carina, associated atelectasis or pneumonitis of entire lung

T4—tumor of any size with invasion of mediastinum, heart, great vessels, trachea, esophagus, vertebral body, or carina; malignant pleural or pericardial effusion; satellite tumor nodules in ipsilateral tumor lobe

N (nodal status)

N0—no nodal involvement

N1—metastases to ipsilateral peribronchial or ipsilateral hilar region (including direct extension)

N2—metastases to ipsilateral mediastinal and/or sub-carinal lymph nodes

N3—metastases to supraclavicular or contralateral mediastinal, hilar, or scalene nodes

M (distant metastases)

M0—no distant metastasis

M1—distant metastasis

Staging

Stage	TNM Descriptor
0	Tis (carcinoma *in situ*)
IA	T1N0M0
IB	T2N0M0
IIA	T1N1M0
IIB	T2N1M0 or T3N0M0
IIIA	T3N1M0 or T1–3N2M0 (N2 disease)
IIIB	Any TN3M0 or T4, any NM0
IV	Any T, any N, M1

In general, patients with NSCLC at an earlier stage with disease amenable to surgery have the best chances to be cured. Patients being considered for surgery must be thoroughly evaluated to determine if they have resectable disease. The decision for surgical resection is largely based on tumor invasion and lymph node status, along with underlying medical comorbidities. CT imaging and, to a larger extent, positron emission tomography (PET) scanning are important staging modalities. Chest CT scanning is performed with contiguous sections through the liver and adrenal glands to aid in staging. Lymph nodes larger than 1 cm in diameter suggest tumor involvement and should be surgically sampled at the time of resection, or in procedures to help determine the stage (ie, mediastinoscopy, transbronchial needle aspiration, or VATS). CT scanning does have limitations, for instance, determination of chest wall invasion has a sensitivity of 38–87% and a specificity of 40–90% and determination of mediastinal invasion is difficult. Patients should not be denied surgery based on unproven CT findings. In fact, many patients have their stage altered based on surgical pathology. A comprehensive discussion of staging can be found in Mountain (1997).

One new addition to many staging algorithms is 2-[^{18}F]fluoro-2-deoxyglucose (FDG)-PET scanning. PET scans exploit differences between normal and neoplastic tissue. Transformed cells exhibit increased glucose metabolism resulting in increased accumulation of FDG. Sensitivity and specificity of PET for detecting mediastinal metastases is superior to CT scans. PET is also used to evaluate patients with multiple nodules, although it does have limitations in the resolution of nodules <1 cm. As clinical experience with PET scanning continues, it likely will attain a more prominent role in staging algorithms.

2. Pulmonary function testing—This is thoroughly discussed in Chapter 4. Many patients with NSCLC have concomitant chronic lung disease that increases the risk of thoracic surgery. All patients considered for surgery need complete pulmonary function testing. A predicted postresection FEV_1 >800 mL (or >40% predicted FEV_1) is indicative of decreased postoperative complications. A quantitative lung perfusion scan (Q scan) can be used to improve the estimate of the patient's postoperative FEV_1. Patients with an estimated postoperative FEV_1 <800 mL, but who otherwise have a favorable performance status, may be evaluated with cardiopulmonary testing (discussed in Chapter 4).

E. Screening

The remarkable improvements in survival achieved in other common cancers such as breast and colon cancer have not been realized in lung cancer. This is due to many factors, most importantly the inability to create reliable screening methods. Smoking cessation is crucial to decreasing rates of lung cancer, but even with this intervention there is still a large at-risk population. Because of the heavy burden of disease and the large number of current and former smokers, considerable research has focused on the best way to screen asymptomatic persons at highest risk. Early detection or screening for lung cancer has been a highly controversial topic for many years. In the mid-1970s, several large trials were organized to determine the efficacy of sputum cytology and chest radiography either in combination or separately for early detection of lung cancer. The design and results of these trials have been extensively reviewed, criticized, and debated. In all of the trials, screening resulted in detection of earlier stage disease with better lung cancer-specific survival, but no reduction in lung cancer-specific mortality. Therefore, at present, screening for lung cancer is not recommended by any of the major advisory groups. These recommendations may change as knowledge regarding the epidemiology and biology of premalignant airway lesions advances. For instance, studies have shown that those with 30 pack-years of tobacco exposure or greater who develop at least mild airflow limitation and have cellular atypia on sputum cytology represent the highest risk cohort. Although many of the early screening studies did not concentrate on these high-risk patients, studies currently in progress are doing so.

Advances in imaging technology are also being applied to lung cancer screening. Recently, there has been considerable interest in using low-dose, helical CT (spiral CT) as a lung cancer screening modality. CT is a more sensitive test than chest x-ray and can be used to accurately identify pulmonary nodules. Large-scale trials funded by the National Cancer Institute and the American College of Radiology are underway, and these trials will attempt to address directly many of the issues raised by earlier studies, including the question of whether screening will result in a decreased mortality rate. Improved understanding of the distinct morphological and genetic changes that occur in the airways will allow the highest risk patients and those who may benefit from screening and chemoprevention to be targeted. The indentification of this population may ultimately be based on a variety of factors (tobacco exposure, pulmonary function testing, and sputum cytology).

Treatment

The 5-year survival for lung cancer has shown relatively little improvement in the past 50 years, predominantly due to the late stage presentation in the majority of patients. The treatment regimens discussed below are those currently in use, but they are subject to change based on large, multicenter trials that are currently in progress. Predictors of survival are tumor type, stage, and patient's performance status.

A. SMALL CELL LUNG CANCER

SCLC is classically treated with cisplatin and etoposide, with responsive rates directly related to disease stage. Two-year survival is around 20% in limited disease and 5% in extensive disease. Remissions tend to be relatively short, with a median duration of 7–9 months. Once SCLC recurs, survival is 3–4 months. Radiation therapy, which is used to treat symptomatic metastases, such as those in bone and the CNS, improves survival in patients with limited stage disease. Patients with SCLC are not treated surgically, although in rare instances patients who have solitary pulmonary nodules resected turn out to have SCLC. These patients tend to have an improved survival compared to patients with limited disease SCLC.

B. NON-SMALL CELL LUNG CANCER

Surgical resection provides the best opportunity for cure. Many features will preclude resection, including extrathoracic metastases; malignant pleural effusions; tumors involving the contralateral mediastinal nodes; and tumors that invade the heart, great vessels, pericardium, esophagus, or trachea, or are within 2 cm of the main carina. For those proceeding to surgery, the type of surgery does affect the outcome. For example, trials comparing lobectomy to "limited resection" found a higher incidence of local recurrence in the limited resection group, along with a trend toward decreased mortality at 5 years in the lobectomy cohort (44% versus 27% survival, $p = 0.09$).

Neoadjuvant therapy, the administration of chemotherapy or radiation prior to surgery, is gaining favor as an initial therapy for NSCLC. Studies suggest there is an improved survival rate in patients with earlier stage (I and II) disease who receive chemotherapy prior to surgery. In general, nonadjuvant therapy is being studied in earlier stage disease (in combination with surgery) and may be one important avenue to improve the survival rates.

Adjuvant chemotherapy, the administration of chemotherapy after radiation or surgery, is commonly used in treating NSCLC. In patients with stage IIIA disease and node-positive stage II disease, adjuvant chemotherapy probably improves survival, but mostly in those with a good performance status. Patients with advanced stage disease (IIIA and IIIB), which comprises the majority of patients diagnosed with lung cancer, who are not surgical candidates do have an improved survival when treated with chemotherapy and radiation. Patients with advanced disease (stages IIIB and

IV) have an increased survival at 1 year with such treatments, provided they exhibit a good performance status on presentation. Overall, multiple trials have shown that patients with stage IIIB and stage IV disease who are treated with chemotherapy and/or radiation have better symptom control and performance compared to patients receiving only palliative care. Newer chemotherapeutic agents are continually being evaluated, which may result in some improvements in survival. It is imperative that patients placed on newer regimens do so as part of an organized, multicenter protocol that acts to best evaluate efficacy.

Prognosis

The cumulative 5-year survival rate for lung cancer is 14% based largely in part on the large percentage of patients who present with late stage (IIIA or greater) disease. Survival best correlates with surgical–pathological stage of disease, and can vary from 74% 5-year survival for stage IA NSCLC to roughly 5% 5-year survival for stage IIIB NSCLC. Most large studies have failed to find a significant difference in prognosis for the variety of NSCLC types when adjusted for stage and performance status.

Henschke CI et al: Early Lung Cancer Action Project: overall design and findings from baseline screening. Lancet 1999;354:86. [PMID: 10538481]. (One of the first studies reporting the use of spiral CT in early detection of lung cancer. Discusses the difficulties in designing lung cancer screening trials and potential uses for helical CT.)

Jemal A et al: Cancer statistics, 2002. CA Cancer J Clin 2002; 52;23. [PMID: 11814064]. (Annual publication reporting the cancer frequency, incidence, mortality, and survival rates for U.S. residents.)

Mountain CF: Revisions in the International System for Staging Lung Cancer. Chest 1997;111:1710. [PMID: 9187198]. (Original manuscript describing the current TNM system for staging lung cancer. Database represents all clinical, surgical–pathological, and follow-up information for 5319 patients treated for primary lung cancer.)

Patz EF Jr., Goodman PC, Bepler G: Screening for lung cancer. N Engl J Med 2000;343:1627. [PMID: 11096172]. (A comprehensive review of past screening trials and future directions in early lung cancer detection.)

Pretreatment Evaluation of Non-Small Cell Lung Cancer. Official Consensus Statement of the American Thoracic Society. Am J Crit Care Med 1997;156:320. [PMID: 9230769]. (A comprehensive review of the literature on screening, clinical evaluation, staging, and management of lung cancer. Includes discussions of the role of bronchoscopy, mediastinoscopy, and preoperative evaluation.)

Rom WN et al: Molecular and genetic aspects of lung cancer. Am J Respir Crit Care Med 2000;161:1355. [PMID: 10764334]. (A thorough review of the molecular biology of lung cancer with a concentration on more recent advances and future directions.)

SOLITARY PULMONARY NODULE

ESSENTIALS OF DIAGNOSIS

- A solitary mass, typically <3 cm in size, outlined by a normal lung and not associated with atelectasis or adenopathy.
- The majority of patients are asymptomatic with the nodule representing an unexpected finding detected on chest x-ray.
- Radiological imaging is used to determine which nodules are malignant and should be resected and which are benign. Differential diagnosis includes benign causes (infectious, benign neoplasms) and malignant etiologies (primary bronchogenic carcinoma, carcinoid tumors, metastatic disease).

General Considerations

Solitary pulmonary nodules (SPNs) are <3 cm in size, are surrounded by normal lung, and are not associated with atelectasis or adenopathy. Historically these were referred to as "coin lesions." Lesions >3 cm are referred to as pulmonary masses, and have a much greater chance of being malignant. SPNs are relatively common, with approximately 1 out of 500 chest x-rays revealing a nodule. Most of the patients are without symptoms and the nodule is detected on a film obtained for some other clinical indication. The goals of further evaluation are to determine which nodules should be resected (ie, which patients will benefit from resection) and to limit invasive procedures for benign disease.

Pathogenesis & Differential Diagnosis

The potential benign and malignant etiologies of solitary pulmonary nodules are listed in Table 41–4. Roughly 10–20% of bronchogenic carcinomas present as SPNs or pulmonary masses (this number may increase in light of new screening trials involving spiral CT scans). Clues can be obtained from the history and physical examination, along with previous and current imaging studies.

Clinical Findings

A. SYMPTOMS AND SIGNS

Many patients are truly symptomatic when the SPN is discovered if a careful history and physical examination

Table 41–4. Causes of solitary pulmonary nodules.

Benign
    Infectious granulomas: tuberculosis, coccidioidomycosis, histoplasmosis, blastomycosis
    Viral infections: measles, cytomegalovirus
    Pneumocystis carinii
    Round pneumonia
    Lung abscess
    Hamartoma
    Chondroma
    Pulmonary infarct
    Arteriovenous fistula or malformations
    Pulmonary amyloidosis
    Sarcoidosis
    Pseudotumors (collections of fluid in the lung fissures)
Malignant
    Bronchogenic carcinoma
    Bronchial carcinoid tumors
    Other primary lung tumors: carcinosarcoma, lymphoma, hemangioendothelioma
    Metastatic tumors: most commonly colorectal, breast, renal cell, testicular, malignant melanoma, sarcoma

are performed. Additional clinical and radiographic data can assist in assessing the likelihood of cancer. Key historical findings include age, smoking history, environmental exposures, potential infectious exposures, residence or travel to areas with endemic pulmonary mycoses, history of cancer (particularly lung or head and neck), and any coexisting lung disease. For example, in patients younger than 35 years of age and without a history of smoking or previous cancer, the probability of primary bronchogenic carcinoma is < 1%. This likelihood increases with age and tobacco exposure. Occupational exposure to asbestos, silica, radon, or uranium, particularly in smokers, increases the risk of lung cancer.

Other pertinent historical information includes residence or travel in areas of endemic mycoses. In the United States, histoplasmosis and coccidioidomycosis are major concerns. Coccidioidomycosis is caused by a soil organism endemic to the desert southwest, southern California, and northern Mexico. Case series from Arizona have determined that 60% of SPNs were due to coccidioidomycosis exposure. Histoplasmosis is caused by a fungus that lives in soil fertilized by bird or bat droppings and is commonly found in the central and south-central United States. A history of previous cancer is very important, as these may metastasize to the lungs. Cancers that commonly metastasize to the lung are listed in Table 41–4. In 60% of patients with a prior history of cancer, pulmonary nodules represent metastasis from an extrathoracic primary cancer. These patients should expeditiously undergo further imaging. A tissue diagnosis is mandatory to differentiate metastatic disease, a second primary cancer, and a benign etiology.

Physical examination can also provide clues to the etiology of an SPN. Lymphadenopathy, particularly supraclavicular or scalene nodes, suggests cancer, and generalized lymphadenopathy raises concern for lymphoma or an infectious process. A fixed or localized wheeze suggests an endobronchial location and may indicate a tumor (particularly in current and former smokers with COPD). Clubbing and joint tenderness (hypertrophic pulmonary osteoarthropathy) may be associated with bronchogenic carcinoma. Unexplained hypoxemia may signify pulmonary atrioventricular malformations, and one such disease [hereditary hemorrhagic telangiectasia (HHT); Osler–Weber–Rendu syndrome] is characterized by telangiectasia or angiomata on the face, nasopharyngeal mucous membranes, skin, lips, and nail beds.

B. Laboratory Findings

There are no specific laboratory findings in patients with solitary pulmonary nodules other than those listed in the section on lung cancer. Rarely patients with bronchogenic carcinoma will present with manifestations of a paraneoplastic syndrome.

C. Imaging Studies

The most critical step in evaluating pulmonary nodules is reviewing old chest x-rays to determine nodule stability. The presence and pattern of calcification within a nodule can indicate whether it is benign. Characteristic benign patterns have been described and include lamination or a "bull's eye" pattern characteristic of granulomas, a chondroid or "popcorn" pattern occurring in hamartomas, or a dense, central core of calcification. The likelihood of a diagnosis of cancer rises significantly if the SPNs lack calcification. Most lesions that lack calcification are termed indeterminate until a tissue diagnosis is obtained. Malignant lesions can contain calcium, but it is usually eccentrically located and does not conform to the patterns listed above.

Comparison with older radiographic studies allows doubling time, an important marker of cancer, to be estimated. Benign nodules typically have rapid (<20 days) or long (>450 days) doubling times, whereas malignant nodules typically double in 30–450 days. Shape, size, and cavitation on the chest x-ray are other important features that suggest cancer, although none of these factors is pathognomonic. A spiculated appearance, along with irregular or poorly defined borders, suggests cancer. Smooth borders can suggest a benign lesion, but often this will require biopsy confirmation. Size is a very important factor, particularly for larger lesions. Lesions 5 cm or more in diameter have a 95% chance of being malignant. Small size should not be equated with a lesion being benign, as many studies report a 15% chance of nodules less than 1 cm in size being malignant. In fact, CT scan and biopsy data show that 1% of nodules 2–5 mm, 24% of nodules 6–10 mm, 35% of nodules 11–20 mm, and 80% of nodules 20–45 mm are malignant. Location and the presence of cavitation have not proven helpful in differentiating benign from malignant etiologies.

Computed tomography (CT) is the accepted way to further evaluate SPNs. CT is better than chest radiography in detecting calcification patterns and nodule density. Nodules must remain stable is size over at least 2 years to be considered benign. Malignant lesions typically have eccentric calcification patterns on CT, whereas the presence of fat density within a nodule is pathognomonic of hamartomas. Cavitary lesions with thick walls (>16 mm) are much more common in cancers. One CT technique that can better define nodules is a nodule enhancement study (the differential enhancement following the injection of intravenous contrast). After injection of contrast, malignant nodules exhibit greater enhancement due to qualitative and quantitative differences in blood supply. This also allows vascular lesions to be identified. In a prospective study of SPNs without calcification or fat on CT scan, malignant nodules were accurately identified if they enhanced by at least 15 Houndsfield units within the first 2 min of contrast injection. Large changes in contrast enhancement are indicative of arteriovenous fistulas or other vascular lesions. Nodule enhancement studies require a special CT protocol and should be discussed with the radiology department prior to ordering.

Other imaging modalities are gaining favor in the evaluation of SPNs. PET scanning can be used to characterize and stage lesions. PET exploits the biochemical differences between normal and neoplastic tissue and can evaluate lesions that are indeterminate in nature. Transformed cells exhibit increased glucose metabolism resulting in accumulation of FDG. The intensity of accumulation in the nodule is then compared with the background activity. Increases in activity suggest cancer. For SPNs, PET has reported sensitivies of 85–95% and specificities of 75–85%. PET scans do have limitations, including lack of resolution below 1 cm, high cost, and limited availability (PET scanners are not universally available at this time in the United States). Overall, PET has also been proven to be cost effective in the staging of patients with NSCLC because

it reduces the number of surgical procedures in patients with unresectable disease. Magnetic resonance imaging is of little benefit in diagnosis, but can aid in determining chest wall or mediastinal invasion, such as in the evaluation of superior sulcus (pancoast) tumors.

D. MULTIPLE PULMONARY NODULES

The evaluation of a patient with an SPN at times reveals multiple nodules. The more common etiologies of multiple nodules are contained in Table 41–5. The time course of the nodules' appearance and the calcification patterns are important as they may represent independent disease processes. The most common cause is metastatic disease, which occurs more often than all of the other causes combined. Benign tumors of the lung, infectious nodules, and noninfectious granulomas comprise the other causes. CT scans are the most commonly employed imaging modality, and transthoracic needle aspiration (TTNA) under CT or ultrasound guidance is often the safest and simplest method to obtain tissue for diagnosis. Nondiagnostic TTNA should be followed by thoracoscopic open lung biopsy. Rapid diagnosis is essential in immunocompromised individuals to allow for appropriate treatment of opportunistic infections.

Treatment

Based on the clinical and radiographic data, the clinician must decide which nodules should be biopsied and determine the best method to obtain a tissue diagnosis. Each clinical situation is unique, and the following discussion will focus on guidelines. A variety of biopsy techniques, including bronchoscopy, TTNA, and surgi-

Table 41–5. Causes of multiple pulmonary nodules.

Benign
  Infectious: granulomas, septic emboli, parasites
  Noninfectious granulomas: Wegener's granulomatosis, sarcoidosis, rheumatoid arthritis
  Pulmonary arteriovenous malformations
  Silicosis
  Vasculitis
  Broncholithiasis
Malignant
  Metastatic cancer
  Lymphoma
  Metastatic bronchogenic carcinoma
  Kaposi's sarcoma
  Synchronous primary bronchogenic carcinomas

---

cal resection, can determine whether an SPN in high-risk patients is benign or malignant. The efficacy of bronchoscopy depends on nodule size and location. If a nodule is <2 cm in size, the sensitivity of biopsies and brushings taken during bronchoscopy is 10%. With malignant nodules 2–3 cm in diameter, the sensitivity rises to 50%. If CT imaging shows a bronchus entering the nodule, then bronchoscopy has a higher diagnostic yield. TTNA is usually carried out under ultrasound, fluoroscopic, or CT guidance. TTNA is diagnostic in 80–95% of cancers, although the false-negative rate has been reported to be as high as 29%. The indications for TTNA are controversial, but include establishing if SPNs in patients with a history of a nonpulmonary tumor are the same tumor type, establishing a diagnosis in high-risk surgical patients, and aiding in tissue diagnosis in presumed benign lesions. Tumor dissemination along the needle track is extremely rare.

VATS and exploratory thoracotomy for resection of SPNs are the most definitive diagnostic procedures. CT scans, besides evaluating the nodule, may also reveal hilar or mediastinal lymphadenopathy (a finding that is present in about 20% of SPN patients). If the CT scan fails to detect lymphadenopathy, thoracotomy can occur without mediastinoscopy. Surgical mortality for malignant nodules may be as high as 4%, and can rise to 9% in patients over the age of 70. For benign lesions, the mortality is 0.3%, mainly because these patients are less likely to have a history of heavy tobacco abuse with concomitant COPD and coronary artery disease. For patients with an intermediate probability of cancer,

VATS is likely the best treatment. During these procedures, if cancer is revealed on the frozen sections the surgical procedure can be extended to a lobectomy with lymph node sampling for staging. In some patients lobectomy can be accomplished via VATS. VATS will likely decrease morbidity secondary to nodule resection and has been used successfully in patients with severely compromised pulmonary function.

Coleman RE: PET in lung cancer staging. Q J Nucl Med 2001;45:231. [PMID: 11788815]. (Complete discussion of PET in the diagnosis, staging, and restaging of patients with non-small cell lung cancer. PET is accurate in staging the mediastinum, adrenals, and skeletal system, but is not as accurate for brain metastases.)

Gould MK et al: Accuracy of positron emission tomography for diagnosis of pulmonary nodules and mass lesions. A meta-analysis. JAMA 2001;285:914. [PMID: 11180735]. (A systematic review of the published literature on PET scans that concludes PET has a high sensitivity for cancer but is limited in the ability to detect nodules <1 cm.)

Ost D et al: Evaluation and management of the solitary pulmonary nodule. Am J Respir Crit Care Med 2000;162:782. [PMID: 10988081]. (Comprehensive review of causes and management of pulmonary nodules.)

Swensen SJ et al: Lung nodule enhancement at CT: multicenter study. Radiology 2000;214:73. [PMID: 10644104]. [Large multicenter study evaluating nodule enhancement illustrating that absence of significant nodule enhancement (<15 Houndsfield units) is strongly predictive of a lesion being benign. Malignant lesions enhanced significantly more than benign or granulomatous lesions.]

Pleural Malignancies & Benign Neoplasms of the Lung

42

Howard West, MD, & Karen Kelly, MD

MALIGNANT PLEURAL MESOTHELIOMA

 ESSENTIALS OF DIAGNOSIS

- Associated with asbestos exposure.
- Nonexertional chest pain and dyspnea are presenting symptoms.
- Pleural effusion is common.
- Pleural thickening and/or nodules are present on chest computed tomography (CT).
- Thoracoscopy or thoracotomy is often required for definitive diagnosis.

General Considerations

Malignant pleural mesothelioma (MPM) is a rare tumor with only 2000–3000 new cases each year in the United States. MPM is strongly associated with asbestos exposure, which can be documented in up to 80% of cases. Thus, workers with heavy industrial exposure to asbestos, such as pipe fitters, naval yard workers, plumbers, welders, and asbestos factory workers, have a remarkably higher risk of developing MPM than the general population. Asbestos fibers are found more frequently and in larger concentrations in the lung parenchyma of patients with MPM than in the general population. Animal studies also corroborate a role of asbestos in the pathogenesis of MPM.

Recent interest has focused on a potential role of simian virus 40 (SV40) in the etiology of this malignancy. Several lines of preclinical research support this hypothesis such as the presence of SV40 sequences in MPM tumors. It has been suggested that SV40 may interact with asbestos fibers to induce MPM. This issue is controversial, but provides a basis for investigational approaches to management of MPM such as vaccine therapy against the SV40 tumor antigen.

MPM is generally a disease of advanced age. The median age is approximately 60, consistent with prolonged latency between asbestos exposure and clinical manifestation of disease, which is typically two to five decades. The male:female ratio is 4–5:1.

There are three main pathological subtypes: epithelial, sarcomatoid, and mixed histology. The sarcomatoid variant is relatively uncommon and has the worst prognosis. The epithelial subtype is associated with better survival.

As described below, management of MPM has largely been characterized by pessimism, but recent developments have provided an increasing number of treatment options.

Clinical Findings

A. Symptoms and Signs

Nonexertional, nonpleuritic chest pain and/or dyspnea are the presenting symptoms in 90% of patients. These symptoms typically wax and wane but do not resolve. Over time MPM encases the lung and progressively invades the chest wall, leading to worsening dyspnea and constant pain. Other symptoms include cough, weight loss, and fever. Spontaneous pneumothorax is occasionally the presenting symptom of the disease.

Physical examination typically demonstrates decreased breath sounds and associated dullness to percussion in areas of marked pleural thickening and/or pleural effusion. A chest wall mass may be evident late in the course of the disease.

B. Laboratory Findings

There are no specific laboratory findings that are diagnostic for MPM, but mild thrombocytosis and anemia are common.

C. Imaging Studies

Chest radiographs reveal a pleural effusion with pleural thickening and/or nodules, predominantly in more basilar lung regions. In more advanced disease, encasement of the lung leads to evidence of consolidation and mediastinal shift secondary to volume loss. Chest CT is optimal for defining the extent of disease by identifying the location and degree of pleural plaques and thickening, areas of fluid accumulation, and to some degree chest wall invasion. Magnetic resonance imaging (MRI) may be superior to CT in characterizing the degree of tumor spread into bone, fissures, and diaphragm, but is not routinely incorporated into clinical practice. In addition to these anatomic imaging studies, functional imaging with fluorodeoxyglucose (FDG) positron emission tomography (PET) is being increasingly employed. MPM typically demonstrates abnormally increased radiotracer uptake. One study of 28 patients with suspected mesothelioma (confirmed later in 22) revealed that increased radiotracer uptake by tumor was associated with shorter survival. Patients with tumor standard uptake values (SUV) greater than the median had a cumulative survival estimate of 0.17 at 12 months compared to 0.86 for the group with tumor SUV lower than the median. Smaller studies also suggest that the accuracy of PET for assessing disease extent is superior to chest CT. The ultimate utility of PET scanning for initial staging of MPM and assessment of response to therapy is being addressed in ongoing trials.

D. Pleural Fluid and Pathological Examination

Thoracentesis is often performed at the time of initial presentation. Pleural fluid is typically serous and exudative, occasionally with frank blood. Cytological studies of the fluid reveal suspicious but nondiagnostic cells because it is difficult to distinguish between normal reactive mesothelial and malignant cells; therefore cytology provides a definitive diagnosis of mesothelioma in only 35–50% of cases.

Closed pleural biopsy may be employed to provide tissue for definitive diagnosis, but pathological diagnosis is more frequently made from tissue obtained by thoracoscopy.

Despite expert pathological evaluation, a precise diagnosis of MPM can be very challenging. MPM is easily mistaken histologically for adenocarcinoma, necessitating detailed immunohistochemical studies to confirm the diagnosis. Unlike adenocarcinoma, MPM stains positive for calretinin and negative for carcinoembryonic antigen (CEA) and Leu-M1 (Table 42–1). Electron microscopy may also be helpful in distinguishing MPM from carcinomas, although this technique is infrequently used.

E. Pulmonary Function Tests and Electrocardiography

Pulmonary function tests typically document restrictive lung physiology due to encasement of a lung. Electrocardiographic abnormalities are observed in the majority of cases. These are generally arrythmias such as sinus tachycardia; atrial fibrillation or flutter, premature atrial

Table 42–1. Stains for differentiation of MPM and adenocarcinoma.

Marker	MPM	Adenocarcinoma
CEA	–	+
Leu-Mi	–	+
Mucicarmine	–	+
Calretinin	+	–
Hyaluronic acid	++	±
Keratin proteins	++ (diffuse cytoplasmic)	+ (peripheral cytoplasmic)
Vimentin	+	–

or ventricular contractions, conduction abnormalities, or nonspecific changes occur less frequently.

Benard F et al: Prognostic value of FDG PET imaging in malignant pleural mesothelioma. J Nucl Med 1999;40:1241. [PMID: 10450672]. (Descriptive study of mesothelioma correlating activity on FDG-PET with prognosis.)

Differential Diagnosis

Several conditions have a radiological or pathological appearance similar to MPM. Benign, reactive, and inflammatory processes may induce mesothelial hyperplasia that results in pleural thickening with or without an effusion. Benign hyperplasia, however, does not exhibit tissue invasion, cytological atypia, or hyperchromatism. Benign pleural mesothelioma (solitary fibrous tumor of the pleura) arising from the visceral pleura presents with the same clinical symptoms and has a radiographic appearance similar to MPM. However, unlike MPM, pleural effusions are not common with benign mesothelioma and there is no association with asbestos exposure. Benign mesothelioma is usually well defined, localized, and sometimes pedunculated. It is rarely diagnosed correctly preoperatively; resection establishes the diagnosis and provides a cure in most cases.

A difficult challenge occurs when patients present with a malignant pleural effusion but without specific features, such as pleural nodules or thickening, that suggest MPM. The differential diagnosis in this setting consists primarily of adenocarcinoma and MPM. Adenocarcinoma may metastasize from many different sites prompting an exhaustive search for a primary lesion. Detailed immunohistochemical stains and electron microscopy are invaluable in differentiating between the two malignancies (Table 42–1).

The sarcomatoid variant of MPM may be difficult to distinguish from fibrosarcoma, malignant fibrous histiocytoma, hemangiopericytoma, and malignant schwannoma. Carcinosarcomas and synovial sarcomas are more likely to present as a discrete mass within lung parenchyma as opposed to a lesion surrounding the lung.

Staging

Although multiple different staging systems for MPM exist, the American Joint Committee on Cancer system has become most accepted (Table 42–2).

Prognosis

The growth pattern of MPM is characterized by local rather than distant spread. Typically originating in one hemithorax, the disease tends to encase the lung and spread contiguously rather than metastasize to distant sites. At the time of diagnosis most cases are advanced to the point that curative resection is precluded, making symptom palliation the primary goal of therapy. The median survival is 6–8 months from diagnosis in the absence of treatment. Results with treatment are variable, but median survival of a year or more has been reported using aggressive surgical therapy, multimodality treatment, and/or palliative systemic therapy.

Death most commonly occurs due to local complications such as respiratory and/or cardiac compromise, sometimes with direct myocardial invasion. Although distant/noncontiguous metastases may eventually develop, they rarely cause mortality.

Treatment

Treatment options and median survival for patients with MPM are summarized in Table 42–3.

Table 42–2. AJCC staging system for malignant mesothelioma.

Stage 1: Disease confined within the capsule of the parietal pleura: ipsilateral pleura, lung, pericardium, and diaphragm

Stage 2: All of stage 1 with positive intrathoracic (N1 or N2) lymph nodes

Stage 3: Local extension of disease into the following: chest wall or mediastinum; heart or through the diaphragm, peritoneum; with or without extrathoracic or contralateral (N3) lymph node involvement

Stage 4: Distant metastatic disease

Table 42–3. Median survival for MPM by treatment strategy.

Therapy	Median Survival (Months)
Best supportive care	6–8
Pleurodesis	7–9
Extrapleural pneumonectomy	13–17[1]
Pleurectomy/decortication	13
Single-agent chemotherapy	6–9
Combination chemotherapy	6–17
Multimodality: EPP with chemotherapy ± radiation	13–34[2]

[1] Patients with disease localized to the chest without invasion or mediastinal involvement (Stage I).
[2] Early stage patients only (Stage I and II).

A. SURGERY

Surgical resection may be attempted in patients who present with disease that is limited to a single hemithorax without evidence of invasion or mediastinal involvement and who have acceptable cardiopulmonary function. Although apparent cures have been achieved in individual cases with surgery, single-modality extrapleural pneumonectomy (EPP) has not prolonged median survival. Operative mortality is generally less than 10% and in the largest series is less than 5%. Aggressive surgery is feasible only for patients with a Karnofsky performance status of greater than 70, cardiac ejection fraction greater than 45%, and predicted postoperative forced expiratory volume (FEV$_1$) of greater than 1 L.

A less extensive debulking surgery such as decortication/pleurectomy may also be undertaken. This approach is feasible for patients who cannot tolerate the physiologic demand of EPP; mortality rates range from 1.5 to 5%. It is only palliative, as complete resection of tumor is not possible.

Dyspnea and discomfort secondary to a pleural effusion may be quite severe in patients with MPM. These symptoms can frequently be controlled with pleurodesis to eliminate the effusion. The preferred approach is by video-assisted thoracoscopic surgery (VATS) with infusion of tetracycline, doxycycline, bleomycin, or talc. Eighty to 100% of effusions can be controlled in this manner. There are no differences in success rates among the agents commonly used.

B. RADIATION

The role of radiation therapy in MPM is limited to palliation of local pain and control of tumor spread at incision sites and needle tracks. External beam radiation to a large treatment volume may lead to significant side effects such as esophagitis and diminished pulmonary function. For this reason it is not a feasible single-modality therapy for MPM, as curative radiation therapy would require irradiation of an entire hemithorax. Radiation therapy is not associated with proven survival benefit for patients with MPM.

C. CHEMOTHERAPY

Systemic therapy with conventional chemotherapy has been the cornerstone of treatment for the majority of patients in whom aggressive surgical management is not an option. Multiple single-agent or combination regimens, frequently incorporating platinums, antimetabolites, and anthracyclines, have been reported to have modest activity against MPM in phase I and II trials. Clinical trials have been limited by the rarity of MPM and difficulty in assessing tumor response. In general, response rates of less than 20% are reported. This has led to some of the nihilism surrounding the management of MPM.

The most widely used regimen has been combination therapy with cisplatin and gemcitabine. This regimen produced an objective response rate of 48%, a median response duration of 25 weeks, and a median survival of 41 weeks in a trial of 21 patients with advanced MPM. It also has the advantage of being widely used in the management of advanced non-small cell lung cancer, making this regimen an appealing option for cases in which adenocarcinoma of the lung and MPM cannot be reliably distinguished by pathological examination.

Preliminary results from a recently completed large multicenter randomized trial of chemotherapy for advanced MPM may have established a new standard of care for the management of unresectable patients. Four hundred patients were randomized to receive either cisplatin alone or a combination of cisplatin and the multitargeted antifolate pemetrexed (ALIMTA). The two-drug combination was associated with significant improvement in median survival from 10 to 13 months along with significant improvement in tumor response rates, pain control, dyspnea, and lung function compared with single-agent cisplatin. Pemetrexed is awaiting Food and Drug Administration (FDA) approval.

D. MULTIMODALITY TREATMENT

Several single-institution case series describe bimodality or trimodality treatment strategies that incorporate various combinations of chemotherapy, surgery, and radiation. Numerous sequences have been reported and remain the focus of single-institution approaches.

Adjuvant radiation or chemoradiation is generally administered 4-6 weeks after surgical resection. Radia-

tion after EPP does not have a risk of pulmonary toxicity and can potentially reduce the risk of local recurrence, particularly if there are positive surgical margins. In a series of 176 patients treated by Sugarbaker and colleagues with EPP followed by chemoradiation, the 2- and 5-year survivals were 38% and 15%, respectively. Rusch and associates treated 88 patients with EPP followed by adjuvant radiation therapy alone and reported a median survival of 34 months for early stage (I/II) patients. Although local control was achieved, patients developed distant metastases suggesting that future studies should include chemotherapy.

Intrapleural chemotherapy has also been employed in single-institution studies, but is rarely used due to difficulty in assessing its efficacy.

Among the most promising sequences has been the use of induction chemotherapy followed by extrapleural pneumonectomy and adjuvant radiation therapy. This approach has the advantage of potentially making surgery feasible if induction chemotherapy is associated with tumor shrinkage; postoperative radiation therapy can also provide additional local therapy against residual MPM tissue. Patients treated in such series have demonstrated encouraging survival results compared to historical controls. A planned multiinstitutional trial for resectable MPM will entail administration of cisplatin and pemetrexed as induction chemotherapy, followed by surgery and then adjuvant radiation.

E. CLINICAL TRIALS

There are several avenues of ongoing clinical research in the management of MPM. A trial in the United Kingdom with a targeted accrual of 840 patients will investigate survival benefit for chemotherapy compared to symptomatic management alone; careful assessment of cancer symptoms with treatment will also be performed. Other research explores the optimal integration of two or three treatment modalities. Brachytherapy, intrapleural photodynamic therapy, gene therapy, cytokine administration, novel cytotoxic chemotherapeutic agents, antiangiogenic agents, and or other systemic targeted molecular approaches have also been proposed. Ongoing phase II trials of agents that inhibit the structure or function of the epidermal growth factor receptor, which is overexpressed in the majority of MPM tumors, are currently the focus of considerable attention. With the exception of palliative chemotherapy, much of the research on MPM is performed at a small number of specialized treatment centers. This is especially true of multimodality approaches to the disease. Patients interested in clinical trials or who are candidates for aggressive therapy should be referred to a center with a research interest in MPM to maximize management options.

Byrne MJ et al: Cisplatin and gemcitabine treatment for malignant mesothelioma: a phase II study. J Clin Oncol 1999;17:25. [PMID: 10458214]. (Phase II study documenting effect of combined cisplatin and gemcitabine therapy in mesothelioma.)

Kindler HL: Malignant pleural mesothelioma. Curr Treat Options Oncol 2000;1:313. [PMID: 12057157]. (General review of therapy of mesothelioma, with emphasis on chemotherapy.)

Rusch VW et al: A phase II trial of surgical resection and adjuvant high-dose hemithoracic radiation for malignant pleural mesothelioma. J Thorac Cardiovasc Surg 2001;122:788. [PMID: 11581615]. (Phase II study of bimodal therapy with surgery followed by radiation for mesothelioma.)

Sugarbaker SJ, Norberto JJ: Multimodality management of malignant pleural mesothelioma. Chest 1998;113:61S. [PMID: 9438692]. (Discussion of survival rates for mesothelioma treated with surgery followed by combination chemoradiotherapy.)

Vogelzang NJ et al: Phase III single-blinded study of pemetrexed + cisplatin vs. cisplatin alone in chemonaive patients with malignant pleural mesothelioma. Proc Am Soc Clin Oncol 2002;21:A#5.

Zellos LS, Sugarbaker SJ: Multimodality treatment of diffuse malignant pleural mesothelioma. Semin Oncol 2002;29:41. [PMID: 11836668]. (General discussion of rationale for and preliminary results of multimodality therapy of mesothelioma.)

BENIGN NEOPLASMS OF THE LUNG

 ESSENTIALS OF DIAGNOSIS

- *Rare, slow growing tumors.*
- *Discovered as an incidental nodule on chest radiograph.*
- *Hamartoma is the most frequent benign neoplasm.*
- *Hamartomas have characteristic radiographic findings including popcorn calcification or fat deposits.*

General Considerations

Benign pulmonary neoplasms (BPNs) are rare tumors that are occasionally diagnosed during evaluation of solitary pulmonary nodules. Most solitary nodules are benign granulomas. Less than 15% are BPNs. Table 42–4 lists the types of benign tumors that have been identified. The most common benign tumor is hamartoma, which accounts for 6–8% of resected pulmonary nodules. The other BPNs listed in the table are so uncommon that they will not be discussed in further detail.

Table 42–4. Benign pulmonary neoplasms.

Hamartoma
Inflammatory pseudotumor
Schwannoma
Clear cell tumor
Sclerosing hemangioma
Meningioma
Granular cell tumor
Leiomyoma
Myoepithelioma
Amyloidoma
Fibroma
Chondroma
Lipoma
Neurofibroma
Neurilemona
Chemodectomas

It is controversial whether hamartomas represent true benign neoplasms or tumor-like developmental abnormalities. Regardless, hamartomas are believed to arise as an outgrowth from normal mesenchymal and epithelial lung elements. They contain a mixture of cartilage, mature adipocytes, smooth muscle, bone, and respiratory epithelium. A cytogenetic analysis of 30 pulmonary hamartomas identified chromosomal abnormalities in 6p21 or 12q14 –15 in 60% of cases. Molecular analyses on these same samples revealed rearrangements of the HMG1-C gene (high mobility group protein gene family) in 70% of the tumors suggesting that HMG1-C plays a major role in pathogenesis. This evidence of a clonal process supports a neoplastic etiology. Investigation continues into the possible mechanism by which HMG1-C leads to hamartoma formation.

A review of 215 cases revealed a male:female ratio of 2:1. Average age at diagnosis was 62 years and most were white. Eighty-two percent of patients smoked an average of 44 pack-years.

Kazmierczak B et al: HMGI-C rearrangements as the molecular basis for the majority of pulmonary chondroid hamartomas: a survey of 30 tumors. Oncogene 1996;12:515. [PMID: 8637707]. (Cytogenetic analysis documenting chromosome abnormalities in 30 pulmonary hamartomas.)

Clinical Findings

A. SYMPTOMS AND SIGNS

Patients with pulmonary hamartomas or other BPNs are frequently asymptomatic due to the peripheral location of the lesion and their small size (mean 1.5 cm, range 0.2–6 cm). Most BPNs are found incidentally on chest radiographs obtained for other reasons. Hamartomas are evenly distributed throughout all lung fields. The median age for the development of hamartoma is in the sixth decade, which parallels the age group for lung cancer. Obtaining pertinent information about predisposing risk factors for cancer such as smoking history, previous history of cancer or emphysema, and a family history of cancer is essential in determining how aggressive of an evaluation is required. Physical examination is unrevealing. A rare, central intrabronchial hamartoma has been described that can produce respiratory symptoms.

B. Imaging Studies

Continued advances in radiology have led to increased confidence in distinguishing benign and malignant lesions. This is especially true for hamartomas. Hamartomas appear as moderately smooth or lobulated small lesions with popcorn calcification on chest radiograph. Unfortunately only 25–30% of hamartomas fulfill these criteria, necessitating further evaluation with chest CT. In one retrospective study of 47 patients with hamartomas (histologically proven in 31 patients and presumed in 16), high-resolution CT correctly identified 18 lesions with fat only (38%), 10 lesions with fat and calcium (21%), and 2 lesions with calcium only (4%). Seventeen lesions (36%) did not display fat or calcium. These 17 patients underwent a biopsy for definitive diagnosis while 16 of 28 patients with assessable fat content were observed. All remaining patients underwent biopsy or surgical resection.

Recently PET was approved for evaluation of solitary pulmonary nodules. FDG–PET is extremely accurate in distinguishing benign from malignant lesions. In a meta-analysis of 40 studies, the sensitivity was 97% with a specificity of 78%, however, accuracy decreased slightly for lesions less than 1.5 cm. Lesions less than 1 cm are not evaluable by current PET scanners. Although PET cannot distinguish between hamartoma and other types of BPN, the benign nature of the lesion is what is most important in avoiding unnecessary biopsies or resections.

Another important feature supporting a diagnosis of BPN is a slow growth rate. In 16 patients presumed to have hamartoma without a definitive diagnosis, radiographic follow-up revealed no detectable growth for 2 years in 12 patients and only a 1.0 mm increase in size in the remaining four. This emphasizes the importance of obtaining old radiographs. Minimal or no growth of a lesion on chest radiograph over a 2-year period suggests a benign process and no additional studies other than continued radiographic observation are warranted.

C. Diagnostic Tests

If a nodule is categorized as indeterminant after radiographic testing, three options are available to the patient: (1) serial radiographs to assess growth, (2) biopsy by bronchoscopy, CT guidance, or surgery, or (3) surgical removal of the lesion without prior biopsy. All options should be discussed with the patient and placed into context with the patient's overall clinical picture. If a patient chooses observation, radiographs should be repeated at 3–6 month intervals for a period of at least 2 years. Several semiinvasive approaches are available for patients electing biopsy: endobronchial or transbronchial biopsy (TBBx), transbronchial needle aspiration (TBNA), transthoracic needle aspiration (TTNA), or a combination of techniques. Biopsies for benign disease are problematic due to the wide variability in etiology and technically challenging when sampling fibrosis, sclerotic granulomas, or inhomogeneous lesions. This leads to lower diagnostic yield compared to biopsies of malignant disease. Advances in biopsy techniques have made these procedures easier and safer with higher diagnostic yield. The choice of biopsy procedure is dependent upon the size and location of the lesion. In a retrospective review of 928 consecutive cases undergoing biopsy for solitary pulmonary nodules, 714 of 750 patients (95%) with malignancy but only 106 of 178 patients (60%) with benign disease had diagnostic biopsy samples. Of the patients in this series 2% had hamartomas. A benign diagnosis was made in 41% of patients undergoing TBBx, 17% having TBNA, and 47% electing to have TTNA. Approximately half of the patients had more than one procedure. The low accuracy of TBNA was thought to be due to the use of small gauge needles. More adequate samples are being obtained with larger-bore cutting needles. The complication rates from the large series described above were low. Severe hemoptysis occurred in 1% and moderate hemoptysis in 2.7% of patients undergoing TBBx or TBNA. Moderate pneumothorax developed in 9% of patients following TTNA, but only 3% required tube thoracostomy. In another review of 1412 patients with pulmonary nodules, TTNA resulted in a diagnosis of hamartoma in 15 patients (1%). Four of these were subsequently confirmed at surgery and 11 were indirectly confirmed by radiographic follow-up, further supporting the value of TTNA for presumed hamartoma.

Video-assisted thoracoscopic surgery (VATS) or thoracotomy with biopsy may be indicated for patients in whom less invasive biopsies are nondiagnostic or not technically feasible. Minimally invasive surgery by VATS is preferred for patients with high suspicion of benign disease. The surgery can be converted to an open thoracotomy if frozen section pathology reveals malignancy. Although removal of the entire lesion can be accomplished by either surgical approach, thoracotomy for benign lesions should be avoided whenever possible.

Gasparini S et al: Integration of transbronchial and percutaneous approach in the diagnosis of peripheral pulmonary nodules or masses. Experience with 1,027 consecutive cases. Chest 1995;108:131. [PMID: 7606947]. (Study suggesting TBBx and TTNA are complementary in the evaluation of lung nodules and masses.)

Gjevre JA, Myers JL, Prakash UBS: Pulmonary hamartomas. Mayo Clin Proc 1996;71:14. [PMID: 8538225]. (Retrospective review of clinical and pathological features of 104 biopsy-proven hamartomas.)

Gould MK et al: Accuracy of positron emission tomography for diagnosis of pulmonary nodules and mass lesions: a meta-analysis. JAMA 2001;285:914. [PMID: 11180735]. (Sensitivity and specificity of FDG–PET in distinguishing benign and malignant pulmonary nodules.)

Reichenberger F et al: The value of transbronchial needle aspiration in the diagnosis of peripheral pulmonary lesions. Chest 1999;116:704. [PMID: 10492275]. (Retrospective study of the safety and efficacy of TBNA in the evaluation of peripheral lung nodules.)

Seemann MD et al: Differentiation of malignant from benign solitary pulmonary lesions using chest radiography, spiral CT and HRCT. Lung Cancer 2000;29:105. [PMID: 10963841]. (Prospective study evaluating the ability of chest radiography, spiral CT, and HRCT to distinguish benign from malignant nodules.)

Thomas JW, Staerkel GA, Whitman GJ: Pulmonary hamartoma. AJR 1999;172:1643. [PMID: 10350308]. (Case report and review of typical radiographic features of pulmonary hamartomas.)

Wiatrowska BA et al: Fine needle aspiration biopsy of pulmonary hamartomas. Radiologic, cytologic and immunocytochemical study of 15 cases. Acta Cytol 1995;39:1167. [PMID: 7483993]. (Prospective series documenting radiological and cytological features obtained by TTNA of surgically resected hamartomas.)

Treatment

Treatment is not indicated for asymptomatic, small peripheral hamartoma or BPN diagnosed by imaging studies or semiinvasive biopsy. However, these lesions must be followed radiographically for at least 2 years to establish a growth rate and to confirm their benign nature. Additional therapy is also not required for patients who undergo surgical resection of lesions that are subsequently found to be benign neoplasms. Surgery in these cases is both diagnostic and curative. Hamartomas are well encapsulated and can be easily removed by enucleation from surrounding lung tissue or with a limited wedge or segmental resection. Surgical resection is necessary for patients with respiratory compromise from a BPN. In one series of 212 patients, no recurrent hamartomas were observed in the 128 patients who had adequate follow-up.

Index

Page numbers followed by an *t* and *f* indicate table and figures, respectively.